Ophthalmology

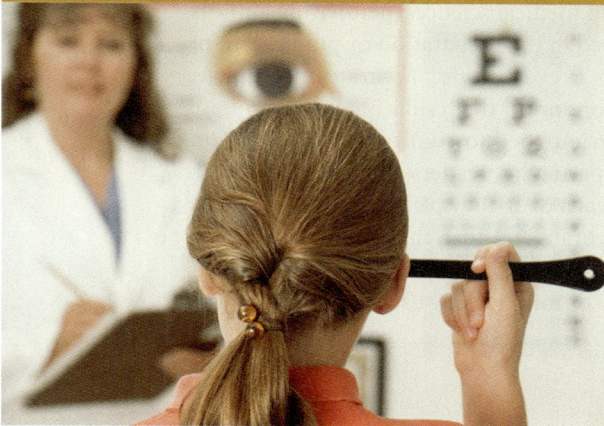

PEDIATRIC PRACTICE

Ophthalmology

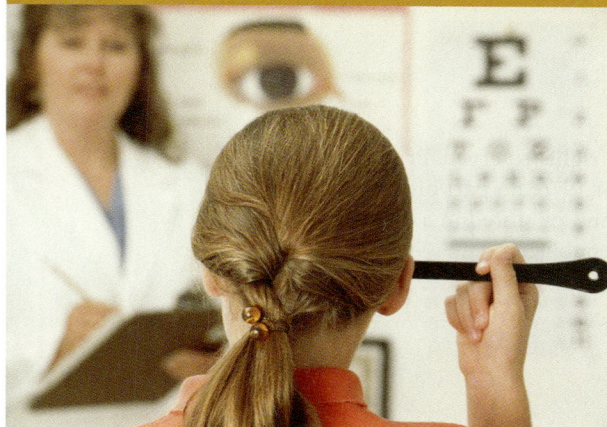

EDITOR

Gregg T. Lueder, MD, FAAO, FAAP
Professor of Ophthalmology and
  Visual Sciences, and Professor of Pediatrics
St. Louis Children's Hospital
Washington University School of Medicine
St. Louis, Missouri

McGraw Hill **Medical**

New York Chicago San Francisco Lisbon London Madrid Mexico City
Milan New Delhi San Juan Seoul Singapore Sydney Toronto

Pediatric Practice: Ophthalmology

Copyright © 2011 by The **McGraw-Hill Companies**, Inc. All rights reserved. Printed in China. Except as permitted under the United States Copyright Act of 1976, no part of this publication may be reproduced or distributed in any form or by any means, or stored in a data base or retrieval system, without the prior written permission of the publisher.

1 2 3 4 5 6 7 8 9 10   CTP/CTP   14 13 12 11 10

ISBN 978-0-07-163380-2
MHID 0-07-163380-4

This book was set in Minon by Thomson Digital.
The editors were Alyssa Fried and Christie Naglieri.
The Production supervisor was Sherri Souffrance.
Project management was provided by Aakriti Kathuria, Thomson Digital.
The cover designer was David Dell'Accio.
China Translation & Printing Services, Ltd. was printer and binder.

This book was printed on acid-free paper.

Library of Congress Cataloging-in-Publication Data

Pediatric practice. Ophthalmology / editor, Gregg T. Lueder. – 1st ed.
    p. ; cm.
  Other title: Ophthalmology
  Includes bibliographical references and index.
  ISBN-13: 978-0-07-163380-2 (hardcover : alk. paper)
  ISBN-10: 0-07-163380-4 (hardcover : alk. paper)
  ISBN-13: 978-0-07-163965-1 (ebook (pdf)
1. Pediatric ophthalmology. I. Lueder, Gregg T. II.
Title: Ophthalmology.
  [DNLM: 1. Eye Diseases. 2. Child. 3. Infant. WW 600 P37185 2011]
  RE48.2.C5P445 2011
  618.92'0977—dc22
                2010016523

McGraw-Hill books are available at special quantity discounts to use as premiums and sales promotions, or for use in corporate training programs. To contact a representative please e-mail us at bulksales@mcgraw-hill.com.

To my wife, Cindy, our four daughters, and my patients. I get up in the morning and look forward to going to work. At the end of the day I look forward to going home. You can't ask for more than that.

Contents

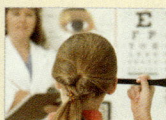

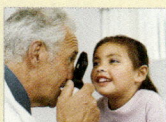

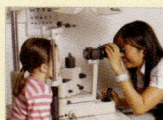

Acknowledgments

I want to thank Alyssa Fried, Christie Naglieri, and the people at McGraw-Hill for asking me to write this book, and for the flexibility to let me design it the way I wanted.

I have been blessed to work in an outstanding environment at St. Louis Children's Hospital for the past 17 years. I thank my partners and the superb staff in the Children's Eye Center. The greatest things in life are accomplished through teamwork, and these people allow us to provide excellent care to our patients. Special thanks go to Judy Stockstad for her tireless administrative work, Dave Garibaldi for his photographic skills, and Aakriti Kathuria for her production assistance.

I have been fortunate to have outstanding teachers during my career. I hope that this book carries this gift forward.

I thank my parents for their constant support during many years of education, and for providing a wonderful role model for a balanced life and loving marriage.

Most importantly, I thank my wife, Cindy, and our daughters. They have been fully supportive of this endeavor, despite my greater-than-usual under-estimation of the time that it would require.

Introduction

I love practicing pediatric ophthalmology, but I admit that we ophthalmologists often do not do a very good job of teaching others about our specialty. The reasons (excuses?) for this are twofold. First, there is an increasing time crunch during medical education, with students expected to master an ever-expanding body of knowledge. Unfortunately something has to give, and often that means students get little, if any, exposure to ophthalmology. Second, ophthalmology is a very specialized area. Learning to use even basic ophthalmic examination equipment, such as the direct ophthalmoscope, takes time and practice. Mastering more specialized equipment, such as the slit lamp and indirect ophthalmoscope, usually requires several months. In addition, the language, abbreviations, and notations that ophthalmologists use are arcane, such that an ophthalmology note often looks like it's written in hieroglyphics.

I have had the good fortune to do residencies and become board-certified in both pediatrics and ophthalmology, so I have firsthand experience with both sides of this knowledge gap. This book sprang from a desire to narrow that gap. The basic idea was based on this question: if I were practicing pediatrics and could have only one pediatric ophthalmology book on my shelf, what would it be? Most currently available pediatric ophthalmology books are either relatively short guides that cover the basics, or detailed texts designed for pediatric ophthalmologists. This book attempts to strike a balance between these two.

The book is divided into three parts:

- The first section (Evaluation of the Eye: Chapters 1 and 2) deals with the evaluation of pediatric ophthalmology patients. The first chapter describes the examination. It is divided into a section on the eye examination for pediatricians and a section on the techniques and instruments used by pediatric ophthalmologists. The second chapter describes ancillary tests used for evaluation of pediatric eye disorders.
- The next section (Symptoms: Chapters 3 to 23) provides a straightforward, focused, how-to approach based on specific clinical problems. This is the part of the book that can be taken off the shelf and used quickly when evaluating a patient in the office.
- The third section (Diseases: Chapters 24 to 34) is written in the style of a traditional medical textbook, based on diseases affecting different parts of the eye. It provides more detailed information than the second section, but not the voluminous amount found in textbooks written specifically for pediatric ophthalmologists.

The recommended evaluation and management of problems described in this book is based on a combination of personal experience and, when available, evidence-based medicine. Many medical problems can be addressed effectively in more than one way, and there are other acceptable approaches to many of these conditions. If possible, I recommend that you establish a relationship with a pediatric ophthalmologist, someone you can contact when you have questions or need a patient seen quickly. Together you can develop a plan for caring for your patients who have eye problems.

Finally, life is a work in progress. If you have any suggestions or recommendations for making this book better, please let me know.

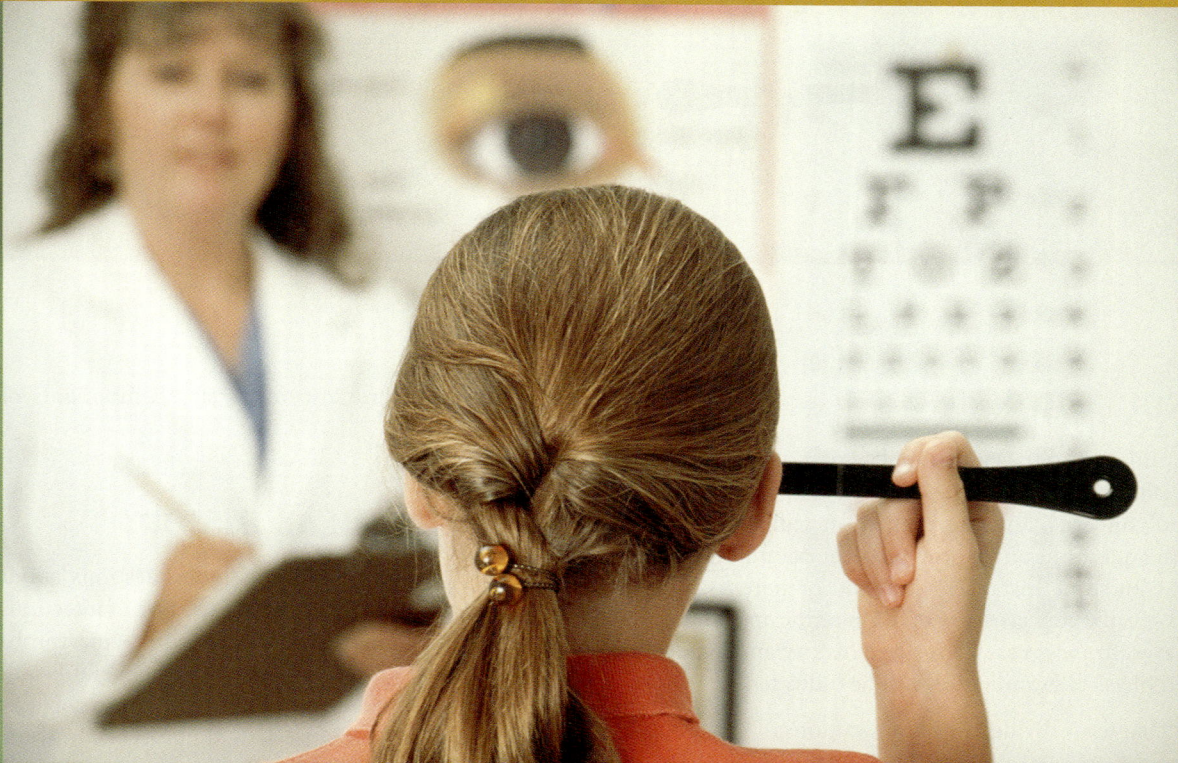

Evaluation of the Eye

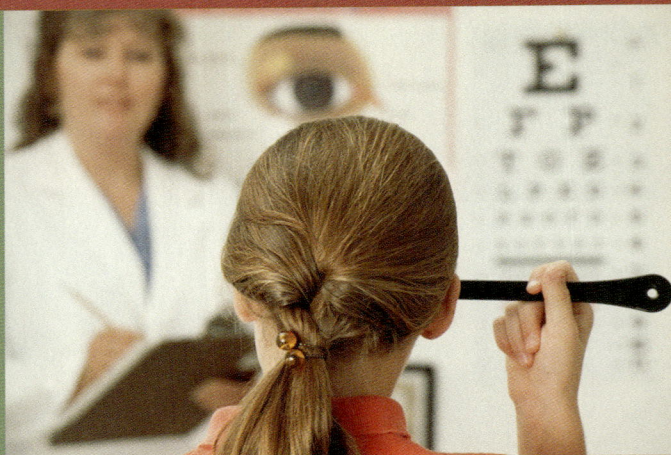

CHAPTER 1

The Eye Examination

INTRODUCTION

An examination of the eyes should be part of every well-child visit. In most cases the children and parents will have no concerns, and the evaluation will consist of screening questions and a brief physical examination of the eyes. In some instances, the child or parents may express specific concerns about vision or the appearance of the eyes. In these cases, a focused history and a more detailed physical examination will be indicated.

This chapter is divided into four sections:

- The first section describes the important aspects of the medical history for children with ocular problems.
- The second section describes a quick screening examination for eye problems that can be performed during well-child evaluations in the pediatric office.
- The third section describes additional examination techniques that pediatricians can use for evaluation of children with specific ocular problems.
- The fourth section describes the examination techniques and tools used by pediatric ophthalmologists.

HISTORY

As with any well-child examination, basic questions about the child's general medical history should be asked. This is part of the routine evaluation of new patients, and the information will already be known for established patients. General questions about vision and the eyes should be included in well-child visits, whereas additional questions may be indicated if specific problems are identified. A family history and review of systems are also important components of the evaluation.

GENERAL MEDICAL HISTORY

The pediatric history should include questions about the pregnancy and birth. Prenatal exposure to infectious diseases or teratogens may cause specific ocular problems. The parent's reports of the child's general health and development should be obtained. Vision problems may occur in many pediatric systemic diseases. In some diseases, specific ocular abnormalities are present. In many systemic disorders associated with developmental delay, however, the ocular problems are nonspecific. Delayed visual tracking and strabismus are common features of global developmental delay from many causes (Table 1–1). The appropriate evaluation is influenced by this information. For instance, it will take longer for an infant born at 28 weeks gestation to begin tracking consistently than it will for a full-term infant. Therefore, additional investigations might not be indi-

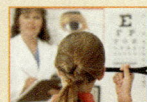

Table 1–1.

Systemic Disorders Associated With Delayed Vision and Strabismus

- Marked prematurity
- Trisomy-21
- Serious systemic illnesses in infancy
- Many metabolic disorders
- Infantile spasms
- Perinatal asphyxia

cated unless a tracking problem in a pre-term infant persists beyond the first few months of life.

OCULAR HISTORY

During General Well-child Screening

General questions about vision should be part of every well-child evaluation. This may be as simple asking the parents whether they have any specific concerns about their child's vision and whether they feel their child sees well. Additional questions could address whether the eyes track normally and whether there are any concerns about the appearance of the eyes or periocular structures. If specific problems are identified by the parents or noted during examination, more specific questions will be indicated.

If Specific Eye Problems Are Noted

The appropriate history for ocular problems follows the same principles as those for any other medical problem. These include questions about timing, duration, exacerbating factors, and previous treatments:

- When was the problem first noted?
- How frequently does it occur?
- Is it getting worse?
- Does anything seem to make it better or worse?
- Have you tried any treatments?

The specific questions themselves will depend on the nature of the ocular problem being evaluated. These are addressed in more detail in the sections of the book that deal with the evaluation and initial management of specific ocular problems.

Review of Systems

In addition to specific eye-related questions, the review of systems in children with ocular complaints should include questions about the child's neurological status (e.g., whether the patient has had any headaches, nausea, vomiting, change in behavior, clumsiness, etc.) Additional review of systems may be indicated in certain situations. For instance, a child with new onset of iritis should be questioned about symptoms of arthritis (due to the association of iritis with juvenile idiopathic arthritis). These specific questions are addressed in their respective chapters in the book.

Family History

Many ocular problems have genetic components, and the family history is useful in their assessment. In addition to specific medical information, the number of siblings a patient has is important when asking questions about the patient's eye problem. If a child has older siblings, the parents will have a better understanding of the development of normal visual behavior than if the patient is the only child.

- With any family history, the larger the number of siblings and first-degree relatives the more informative the family history will be, particularly with regard to inherited diseases. For example, if an autosomal recessive disorder is being considered, the risk to each child is 1 in 4. Therefore, the absence of disease in several siblings would be informative, whereas it would be much less helpful if there were only one sibling (unless that sibling was affected with the same disorder). Similarly, questions about male relatives on the maternal side may assist in evaluating potential X-linked disorders.

Many systemic and ocular disorders are inherited in a mendelian fashion (autosomal dominant, autosomal recessive, and X-linked). Specific questions about these should be asked, based on the diagnoses being considered. Other ocular problems, particularly strabismus, are multifactorial. They have a genetic component, but are not linked to specific genetic mutations. This information may be particularly useful in assessing a child with the new onset of strabismus. If the child has several relatives with strabismus, there will be less concern that a central nervous system tumor or other underlying problem is causing the problem.

ROUTINE SCREENING EXAMINATION IN THE PEDIATRICIAN'S OFFICE

A routine eye screening examination should include an assessment of vision, eye movements, structural abnormalities, and the red reflex. The methods to assess these are based on age.

ROUTINE SCREENING IN AN INFANT OR TODDLER

Vision

Because infants and young children are not able to comprehend or comply with visual acuity testing, the assessment of vision is primarily based on the child's behavioral responses. The initial assessment is made by simply noting whether the infant responds to the examiner's face. A toy or interesting object is then held in front of the child and the examiner monitors the infant's behavior (Figure 1–1).

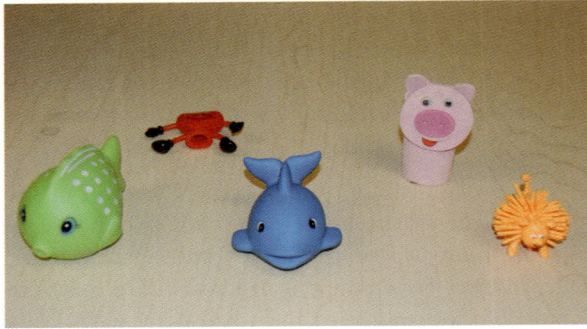

FIGURE 1–1 ■ A variety of different small toys can be used to get a child's attention.

A normal visual response requires the following: the child's eye must be able to see the object. The eye then sends visual information to the occipital cortex, where it is processed. This information is then sent to other areas of the brain that stimulate a behavioral response. If a toy is held in front of a child and the child reaches for it, this indicates that the child must have seen the ball. The test is performed with both eyes open, then with each eye individually (by occluding the opposite eye with a hand or some other object).

A normal behavioral visual response indicates that the child does not have a profound visual problem, but there are several caveats:

■ It does not rule out a moderate problem. This is because most young children adapt to and function well with visual problems, such that their behavior may make it appear that the vision is better than it is.
■ It is important that the toy not make a noise and that the examiner be quiet while performing this test. Children may be attracted to noise, and this could be erroneously interpreted as a visual response.

■ When testing the eyes individually, the visual responses should be similar. Some children reflexively object to having their eyes covered. It is important to determine whether this is due to decreased vision, or simply an aversion to something coming near them. If the child always responds negatively with one eye covered, but tracks well with the other, then the vision is probably decreased in the eye that the child does not track with (Figure 1–2A–C). However, if the child reacts equally negatively to either eye being covered, then little information can be gleaned from the test (Figure 1–3).

Eye Movements

During the same portion of the examination, the eye movements should be assessed. The toy is moved from side to side and up and down and the child's tracking is monitored. The eyes should move symmetrically horizontally and vertically and there should be no limitation of movement. The presence of nystagmus can also be noted at this time.

Strabismus

There are 2 main methods for assessing strabismus. The first (the corneal light reflex test) is a quick screening tool. The second (cover testing) is used when there is concern that the patient might have strabismus.

The corneal light reflex

This is a quick and effective screening test. The light from a penlight or other handheld light is held in front of the child. Most children will find this interesting and look toward the light. In normal patients, the reflex from the light will fall on the same spot in each cornea. If the patient is esotropic, the reflex on the in-turned eye will be displaced temporally. In exotropia, it will be displaced

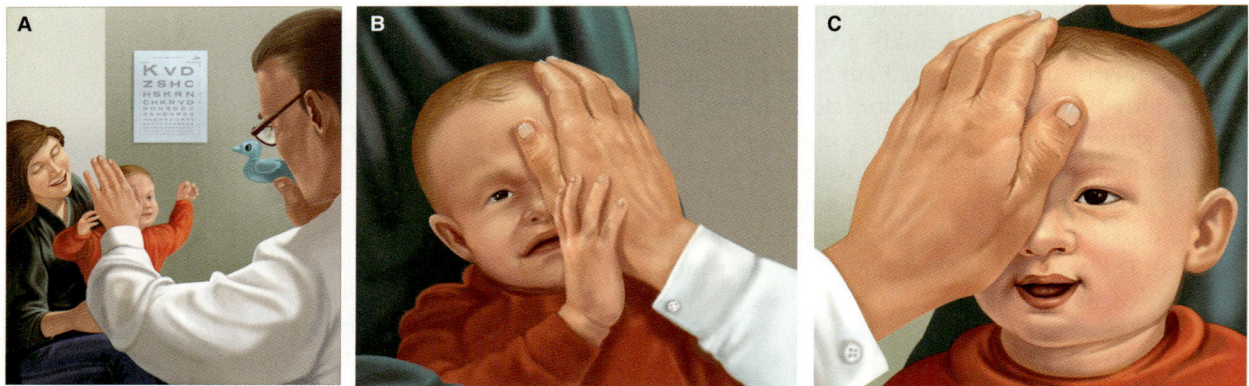

FIGURE 1–2 ■ Behavioral evidence of decreased vision in right eye. (A) A small toy is used to get the child's attention, and the examiner covers the right eye to monitor fixation of the left eye. The child fixates on the toy without objecting. (B) When the left eye is covered, the child objects and tries to move the examiner's hand. (C) When the right eye is covered, the child does not object and tracks the object.

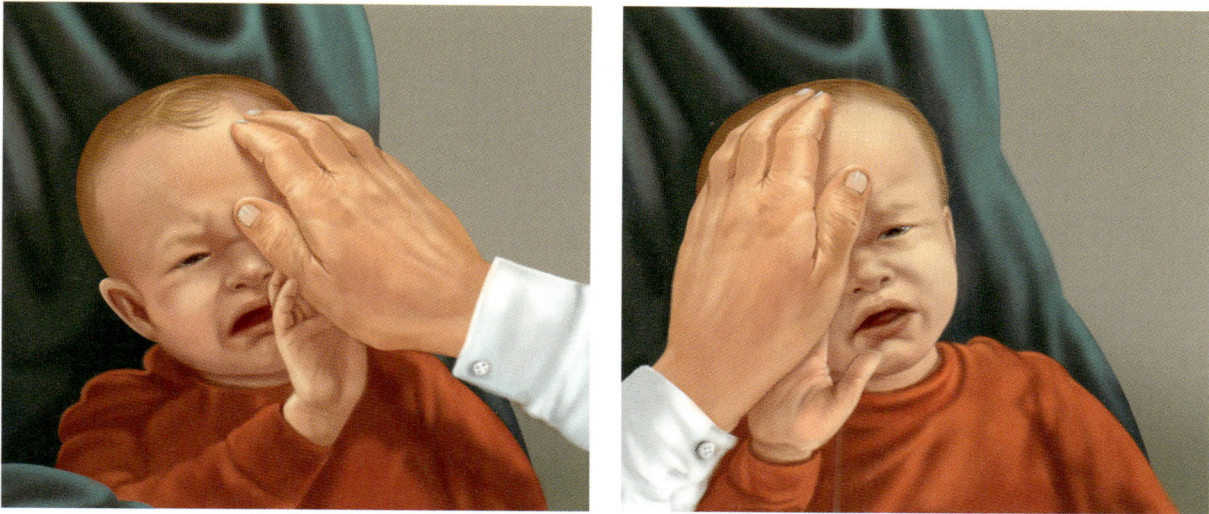

FIGURE 1–3 ■ Some children object to having either eye covered, simply because they do not like having the examiner's hand near their face. If this is the case, this test cannot accurately determine whether there is a difference in vision between the eyes.

medially (Figure 1–4). This test is particularly useful in assessing pseudostrabismus, in which the patient appears esotropic due to epicanthal folds, but the light reflex test shows that the eyes are straight. The light reflex can be used to estimate the degree of strabismus, based on how far the reflex is deviated from a central position.

In certain conditions, the eyes may be optically straight, but the corneal reflexes are not symmetric. A frequent type of this form of pseudostrabismus is called positive angle kappa, in which the light reflex makes it appear that the patient has exotropia. This most commonly occurs in patients who have retinopathy of prematurity that causes the fovea (responsible for central vision) to be dragged temporally. The eye, therefore, must be in an outward position to align the fovea with the visual axis (Figure 1–5). These patients do not demonstrate a shift when checked with the alternate cover test (described in the following sections) (Figure 1–6A–C).

The cover test

This test is not always necessary during routine screening, but should be attempted if there is a concern about strabismus. In patients with normal vision, both eyes look at an object at the same time. Therefore, if one eye is occluded, the opposite eye should not move. In patients with strabismus one eye is deviated. In children the vision from this eye is usually ignored, and the patient is not aware that the eye is not being used. If the straight eye is covered, the other eye will make a movement to line up the visual target. If a patient is exotropic, the eye will make an inward movement. If an eye is esotropic, it will make an outward movement (Figure 1–7).

There are 2 caveats to this test:

■ Similar to what may occur when covering an eye to assess vision, some young children will object to having anything held in front of their eyes. Some of these children may settle down and allow testing with time, particularly if the toy used for a target is changed frequently to maintain the child's interest. In others, repeated attempts are unsuccessful, in which case the test cannot be performed.
■ Many normal people have a *phoria.* This is a tendency for the eyes to drift if binocular vision is interrupted.

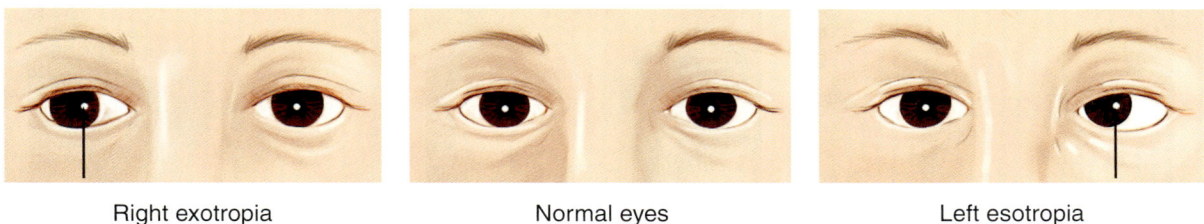

Right exotropia   Normal eyes   Left esotropia

FIGURE 1–4 ■ The corneal light reflex test, used to screen for strabismus. When the eyes are straight (middle figure), the corneal light reflex is centered on both corneas. If the patient is exotropic, the light reflex is displaced medially; if the eye is esotropic, the light reflex is displaced temporally (arrows).

Examiner's view

Normal central location of corneal light reflex

Corneal light reflex displaced nasally

Light ray hits center of fovea

Normal location of fovea

Displaced fovea

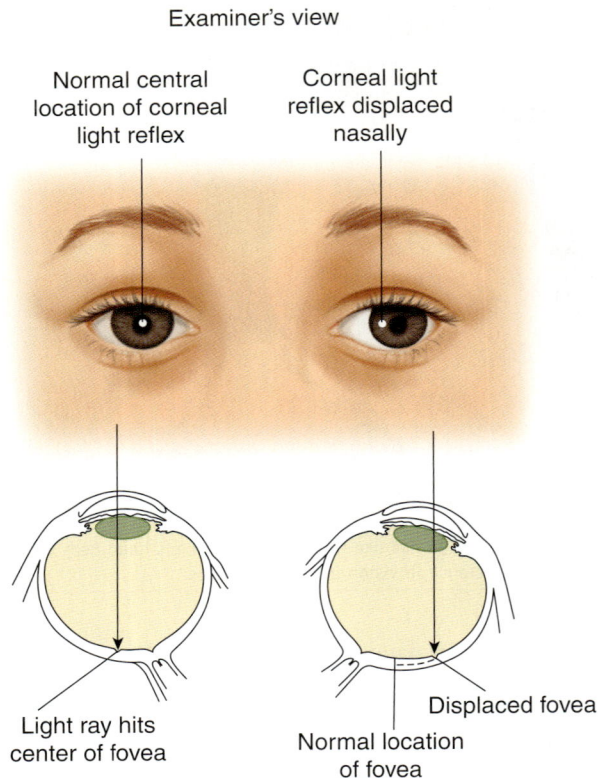

FIGURE 1–5 ■ Positive angle kappa, a form of pseudostrabismus that often results from an abnormal location of the fovea. In the left eye the fovea is displaced temporally. The eye therefore turns outward in order for light to focus on the displaced fovea, creating the appearance of exotropia.

In these patients, the eye moves slightly after it is covered. When it is uncovered, it makes a movement to return to normal. A phoria is present if there is no movement of an eye when the opposite eye is initially covered, but the eye begins to drift if the cover is left in place. Therefore, in a screening examination the examiner should look for movement of the uncovered eye when the opposite eye is initially occluded, rather than looking at the occluded eye after the occluder is removed. This is discussed further in the section on the ophthalmologist's examination later in this chapter.

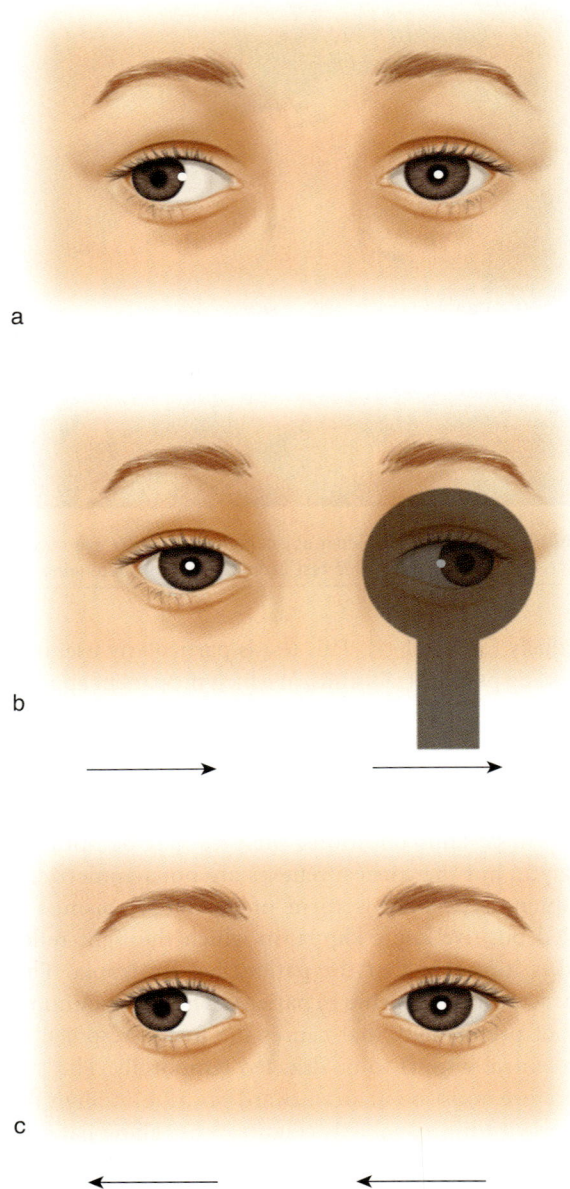

a

b

c

FIGURE 1–7 ■ The cover test for strabismus. Top: The patient has a right exotropia. Middle: When the left eye is covered, the right eye moves inward to fixate, which causes the left eye to move outward behind the cover. Bottom: When the cover is removed, the patient reverts to fixating with the left eye, causing both eyes to move to the right.

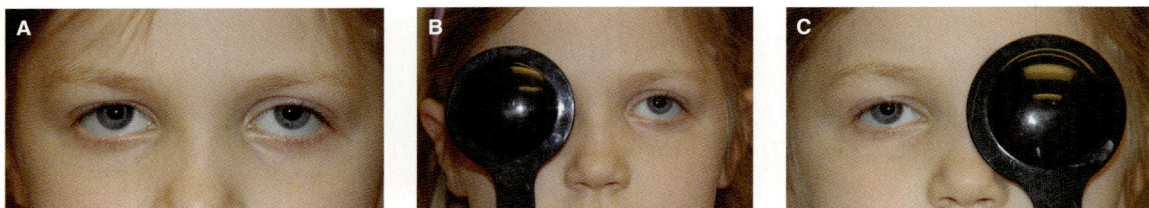

A   B   C

FIGURE 1–6 ■ Pseudoexotropia due to positive angle kappa. (A) The left eye appears exotropic because the corneal light reflex is decentered nasally and more sclera is visible nasally in the left eye compared to the right. However, neither the eyes nor the corneal reflexes shift when either the (B) right eye or the (C) left eye is covered, indicating that the patient has pseudostrabismus.

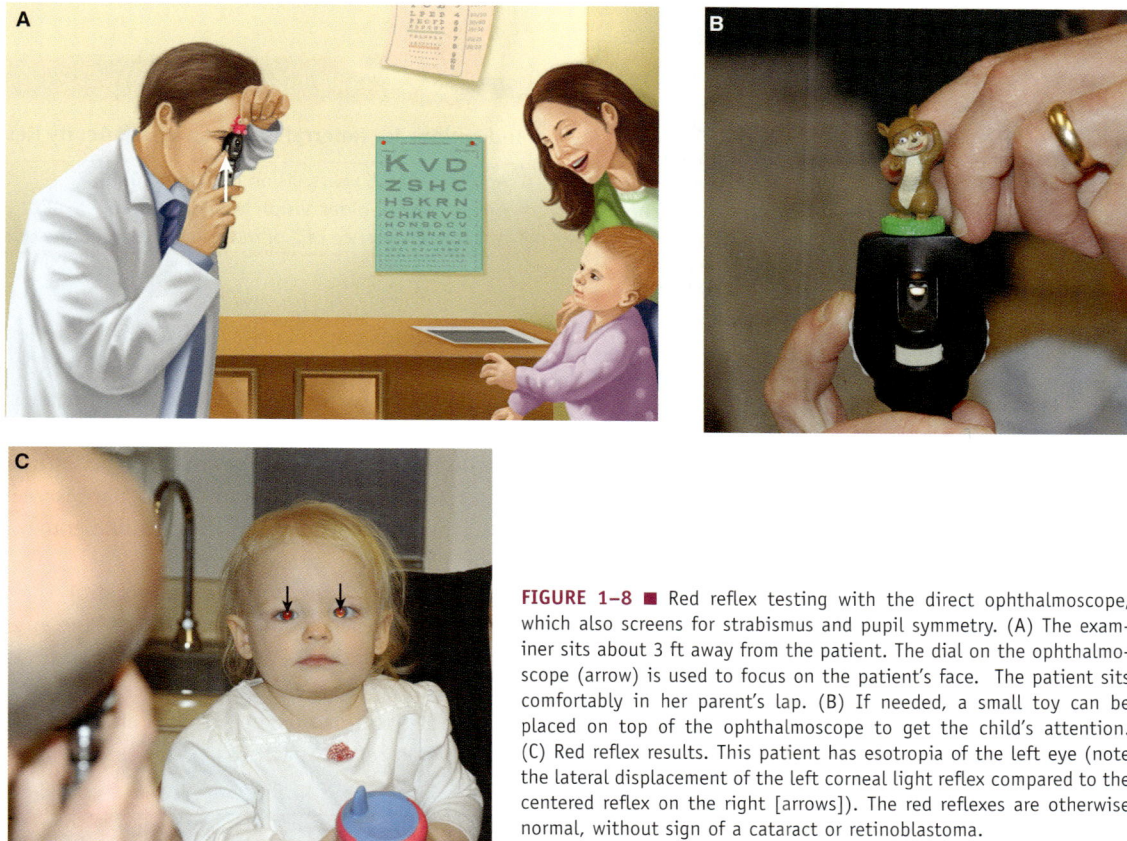

FIGURE 1–8 ■ Red reflex testing with the direct ophthalmoscope, which also screens for strabismus and pupil symmetry. (A) The examiner sits about 3 ft away from the patient. The dial on the ophthalmoscope (arrow) is used to focus on the patient's face. The patient sits comfortably in her parent's lap. (B) If needed, a small toy can be placed on top of the ophthalmoscope to get the child's attention. (C) Red reflex results. This patient has esotropia of the left eye (note the lateral displacement of the left corneal light reflex compared to the centered reflex on the right [arrows]). The red reflexes are otherwise normal, without sign of a cataract or retinoblastoma.

The Red Reflex

Cataracts and retinoblastoma are rare in childhood, but it is very important that they be diagnosed as early as possible. They most commonly present as abnormalities of the red reflex. This can be easily assessed using a direct ophthalmoscope from 2 to 3 ft away from the patient in a darkened room. The infant will usually be interested in the light and look directly toward it. The focusing dial on the ophthalmoscope should be adjusted so the child's face is in focus. As the child looks at the light, the red reflex from both eyes should be symmetric (Figure 1–8A–C). If one eye appears white, this suggests the child may have a cataract or intraocular tumor.

An advantage of this technique is that the symmetry of the corneal light reflex can be assessed at the same time, which provides a quick screen for strabismus, and the pupils can be evaluated for symmetry.

External examination

For practical purposes, most parents will bring to your attention any concerns regarding visible abnormalities of the eyeball, eyelids, or orbit. Nevertheless, a brief inspection should be part of routine screening.

ROUTINE SCREENING IN AN OLDER CHILD

Visual Acuity

By ages 4 to 5 years, most children will be able to cooperate with visual acuity testing (American Academy of Pediatrics Committee on Practice and Ambulatory Medicine and Section on Ophthalmology. *Pediatrics.* 2003;111:902–907). This is most commonly done using a wall chart at a standard distance. Charts are available for young children that have drawings of figures, rather than letters. Most school-aged children can cooperate for standard testing with Snellen letters.

Vision is measured by a ratio comparing what the patient sees at a standard distance compared to what a normal patient can see. Normal vision is 20/20, meaning the patient can read an object from 20 ft away that normal individuals can also read. The ratio is greater than 1 if patients see better than normal (e.g., 20/15 vision means the patient can identify a letter from 20 ft away that normal individuals can only see from 15 ft). The ratio is less than 1 if the vision is worse than normal (e.g., a patient with 20/40 vision must be 20 ft away from a letter to identify it, compared to normal individuals, who can see the letter from 40 ft away). In countries that use the metric system normal vision is often notated as 6/6 (using 6 m instead of 20 ft as the standard testing distance).

Before age 5, vision of 20/40 or better is considered normal. After age 5, vision should be 20/30 or better. A difference between the two eyes of one line is normal. A difference of 2 lines or greater, even if both eyes are in the normal range (e.g., one eye 20/20 and the other 20/30), is abnormal (Table 1–3). Children who fail the screenings should be referred to an optometrist or ophthalmologist for further evaluation.

Other

A quick screening for eye movements, strabismus, and examination of the red reflex should be performed using the same techniques described above.

Instrument-based Vision Screening Tests

A number of different machines have been developed to facilitate vision screening by pediatricians and lay personnel. There are two basic types:

■ *Photoscreening* machines are based on evaluation of the red reflex (the same reflex that can be seen in photographs). The test can screen for 3 potentially ambly-

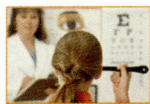

Table 1–2.

Quick Vision Screen in Infants (The 30-Second Eye Examination)

■ Check red reflex with direct ophthalmoscope
  □ At the same time, check light reflex on cornea to screen for strabismus
  □ At the same time, check pupils for symmetry
■ Assess vision by infant's fixation behavior
  □ At the same time, check eye movements
■ Assess for any obvious abnormalities of eye, eyelid, and orbit

Table 1–3.

Indications for Referral Based on Visual Acuity Results

■ Age less than 5 years: vision less than 20/40
■ Age 5 years or older: vision less than 20/30
■ Any age: Difference of 2 or more lines between the two eyes

ogenic conditions: (1) opacities of the red reflex could indicate a cataract, tumor, or other lesion, (2) asymmetry of the cornea light reflex could indicate strabismus, and (3) abnormalities of the light reflected through the pupil can be analyzed to estimate the refractive error. The advantage of photoscreeners is that the two eyes are examined simultaneously and all 3 of these factors are assessed.

■ *Autorefractors* assess vision by estimating the refractive error of each eye independently, using analysis of the light reflection. They are generally less expensive and easier to use than photoscreeners, but they do not screen for strabismus and are less effective at screening for red reflex opacities.

ADDITIONAL OCULAR EXAMINATION TECHNIQUES FOR PEDIATRICIANS

Additional tests beyond those used for routine screening discussed may be indicated, based on concerns raised by the parents or by identification of possible problems during the examination.

TESTS OF BINOCULAR VISION

If the two eyes work together, patients normally will have depth perception (the ability to perceive where objects are in space). This can be measured in the office by using polarized glasses and stereoscopic targets. These tests are similar to those used when viewing a 3-D movie. Some tests have pictures in which a portion of the object appears to stick up from the page when viewed through the glasses (Figure 1–9A and B). Random dot stereograms have no discernible objects when viewed without polarized glasses, but figures are visible when the glasses are used (Figure 1–10A and B).

PUPILS

The pupils in normal individuals should be equal in size and both should react to light symmetrically. Specific evaluation of the pupils may be indicated if

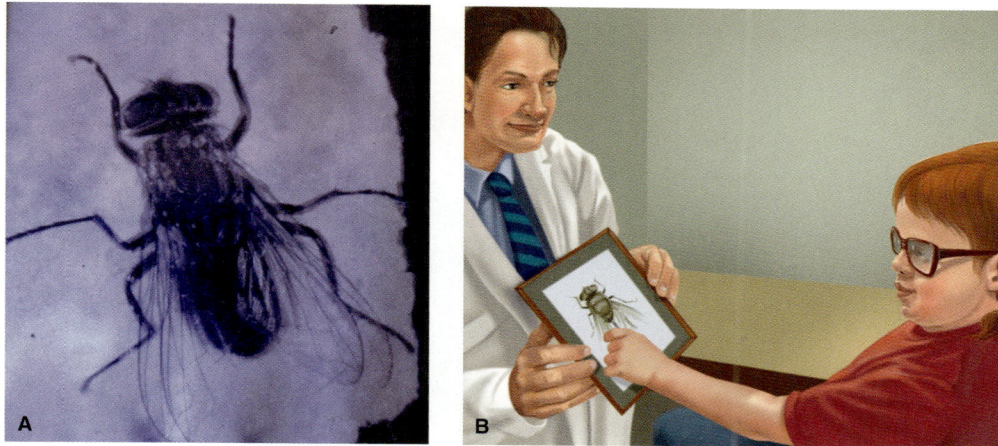

FIGURE 1–9 ■ Stereoacuity (depth perception). (A) The test uses a picture of a fly whose wings appear to stick out from the page when viewed through polarized glasses. (B) The child attempts to "grab the wings," indicating that depth perception is present.

unequal pupil size is noted, or as part of a neurological examination. The pupils are best assessed in a dark room. The examiner asks the patient to fixate on an object on the other side of the room. As a penlight is shined into the eyes, the pupil should constrict briskly.

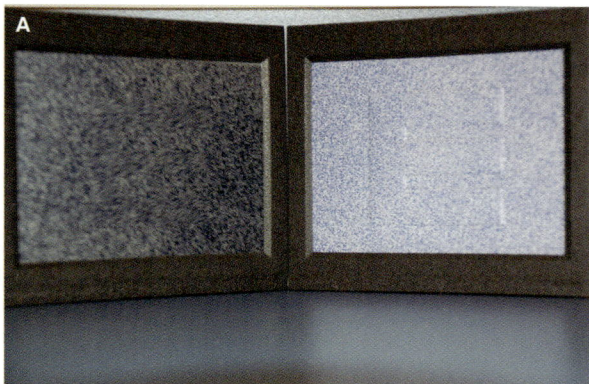

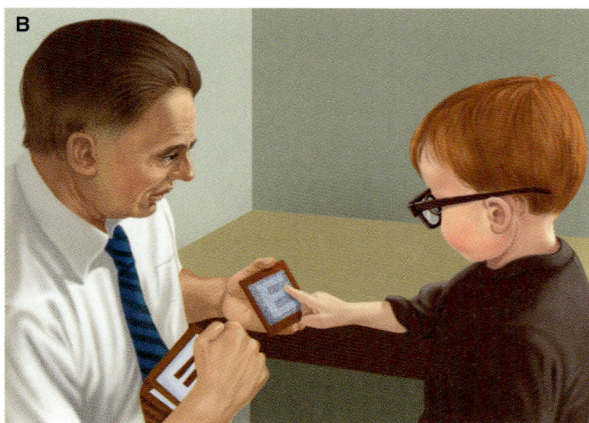

FIGURE 1–10 ■ Random dot stereoacuity testing. (A) Without polarized glasses, no pattern is visible (left). With glasses, the letter E appears elevated above the test plate (right). (B) The child traces the letter E with his finger, indicating that depth perception is present.

The light beam should be directed in the same orientation in both eyes. The 2 pupils should react equally to the bright light.

Testing the pupils in infants and toddlers may be difficult, and is prone to erroneous results. Young children will not consistently fixate on distant objects, and therefore the light may be directed unequally into the two eyes, which can affect the pupil response. More importantly, the normal pupil constricts when a person focuses on a near object (the *accommodative pupil response*). Because the attention in young infants frequently shifts between distance and near, the normal constriction of the pupil due to accommodative response may be mistaken for a reaction to light.

A more detailed assessment of the pupils, the relative afferent pupillary test, is discussed in the in the section on the ophthalmologist's examination.

VISUAL FIELDS

Assessment of the peripheral vision is important in the evaluation of patients with suspected optic nerve or central visual pathway disorders. The type of visual field defect may provide specific localizing information.

Assessing Visual Fields in Infants and Toddlers

As with visual acuity, assessment of the visual fields in young children is based on behavioral responses to light stimuli. This is performed using the *evoked saccade test*. The examiner sits in front of the child in a dimly lit room. While the child is looking at the examiner's face, a light is held in the child's peripheral field of vision. Because the light stimulus is interesting, most young

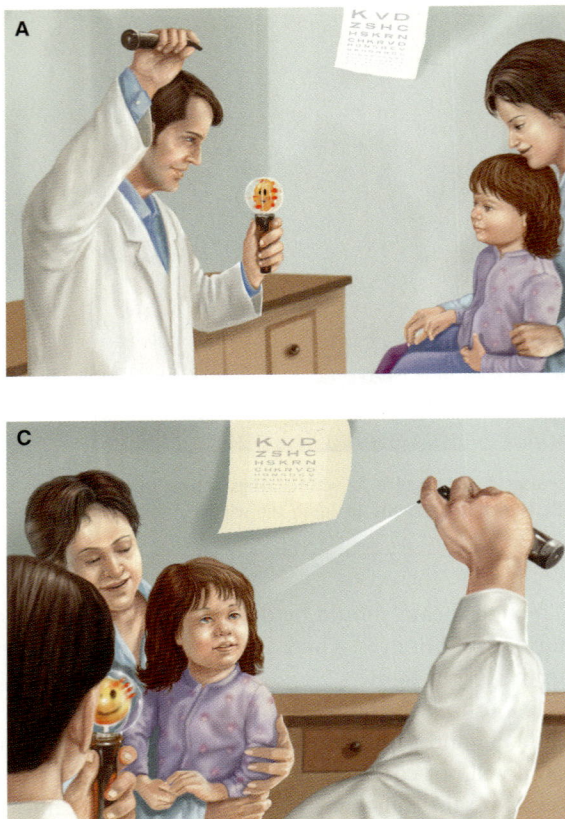

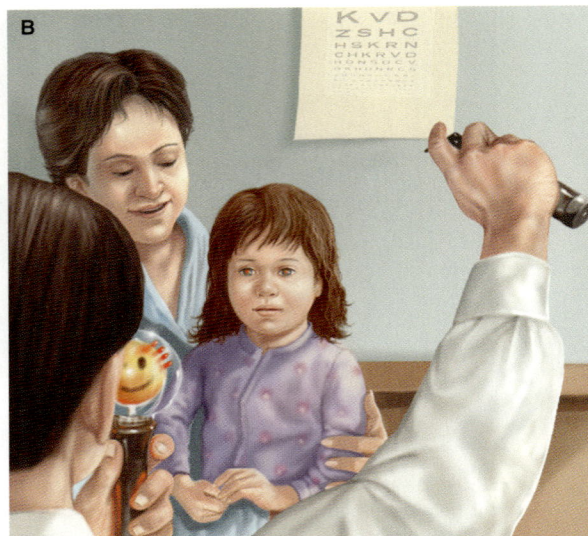

FIGURE 1–11 ■ Evoked saccade for testing peripheral vision in infants and young children. The test is best done in a dimly lit room. (A) The child fixates on a centrally located target. With the child's attention on the central target, a bright light is turned on in the peripheral field. (B) View from the examiner's perspective before the peripheral light is turned on. (C) After the peripheral light is turned on, the child immediately looks toward this light, indicating that the peripheral field is intact. The test is repeated in different peripheral fields. To test each eye independently, a patch should be placed on the eye not being tested.

children will move their eyes to look toward it. This indicates that the peripheral field is intact (Figure 1–11A–C). The light is then turned off and moved sequentially to each side horizontally and vertically. The caveats to this test are as follows:

- The test is good for screening, but cannot rule out a moderate visual field defect. If there is some residual function in the peripheral field, the child may still notice the light and turn toward it.
- It is important to turn off the peripheral light and keep the child's attention toward the examiner's face while moving the light. The light should be turned on once it is in position in the peripheral field and the child is looking straight ahead. If the child watches the light as it is moved, he or she may keep looking in its direction, anticipating that it will be turned on. If the child does this, visual fields cannot be assessed accurately.
- The visual fields between the two eyes overlap substantially, so that if one eye is normal and the other has a visual field defect, the child will appear to respond normally if the test is performed with both eyes open. To assess each eye separately, an adhesive patch should be placed over the nontested eye. Covering the eye with a hand or other object does not work well because the peripheral light may be visible around the object blocking the eye.

Assessing Visual Fields in Older Children

In children who are old enough to understand and cooperate, visual fields are performed using the *confrontation test*. The child covers one eye and looks at the examiner's face. While the child looks straight, the examiner holds up fingers in the peripheral visual field briefly (1 second) and asks the child how many fingers were held up (Figure 1–12). It is not uncommon for

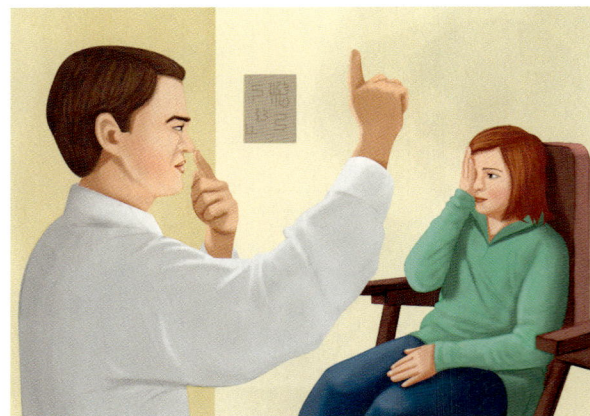

FIGURE 1–12 ■ Confrontation visual field testing in older children. The child is asked to look at the examiner's nose. The examiner's hand is held up in the peripheral field and fingers are flashed briefly. The child then reports how many fingers were seen.

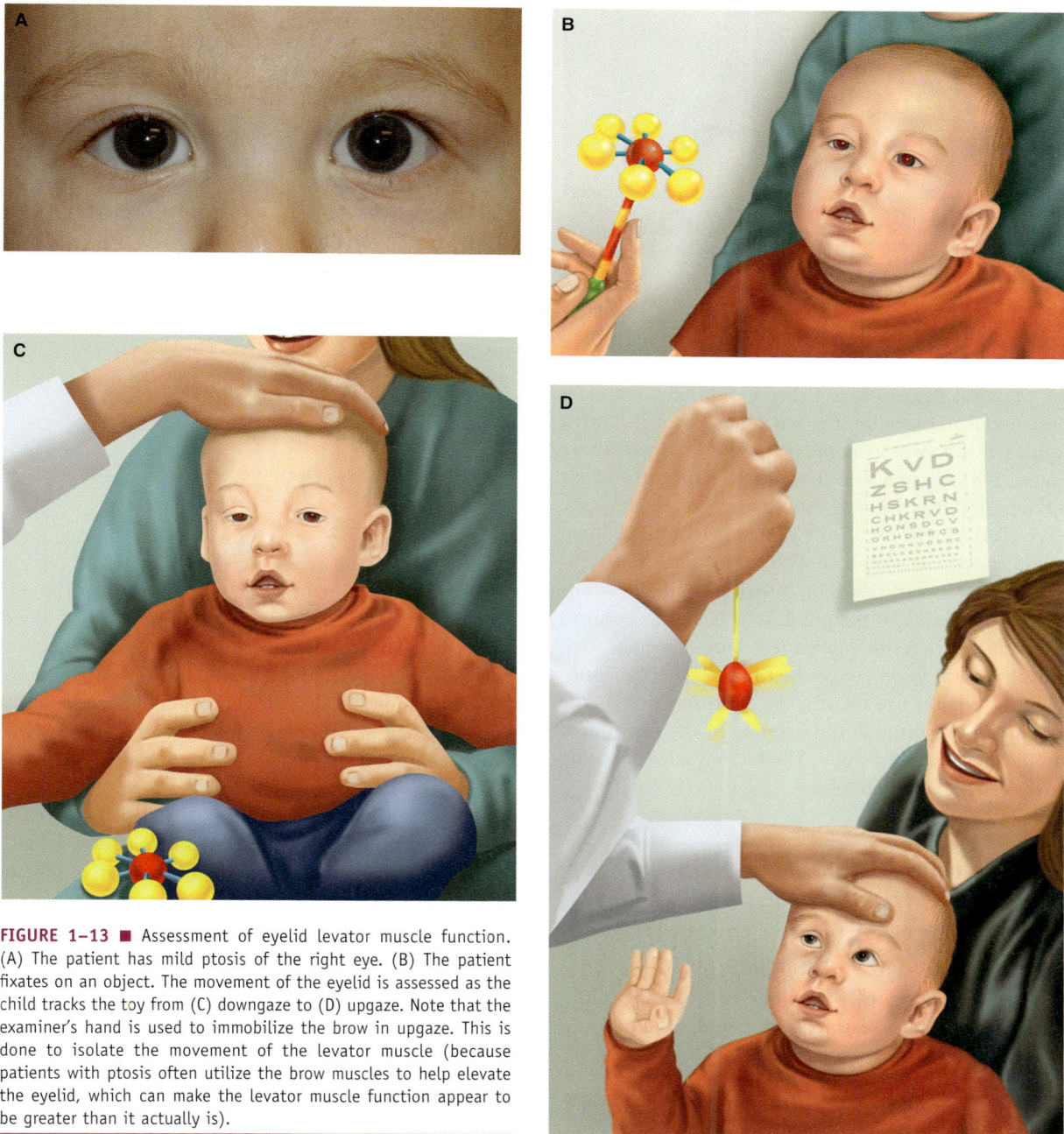

FIGURE 1–13 ■ Assessment of eyelid levator muscle function. (A) The patient has mild ptosis of the right eye. (B) The patient fixates on an object. The movement of the eyelid is assessed as the child tracks the toy from (C) downgaze to (D) upgaze. Note that the examiner's hand is used to immobilize the brow in upgaze. This is done to isolate the movement of the levator muscle (because patients with ptosis often utilize the brow muscles to help elevate the eyelid, which can make the levator muscle function appear to be greater than it actually is).

children to look toward the fingers, which is why they should only be held up briefly while watching the eyes to be sure they do not move. Frequently, this needs to be done repeatedly to be sure the test is done properly. One, 2, or 5 fingers should be held up because these are most easily distinguished. The test is performed separately with each eye, keeping the nontested eye covered.

Eyelid Function

If a child has ptosis, the function of the eyelid levator muscle should be assessed. This is performed by watching the movement of the eyelid as it moves from down-

gaze to upgaze (Figure 1–13A–D). In normal individuals the eyelid should move 12 mm or more. In children with marked congenital ptosis, the movement is often less than 5 mm.

Proptosis

Proptosis refers to anterior displacement of the eye. This occurs most commonly due to mass lesions within the orbit. Proptosis is most readily appreciated by viewing the two eyes from above the patient, looking to see if one eye appears more prominent than the other (Figure 1–14).

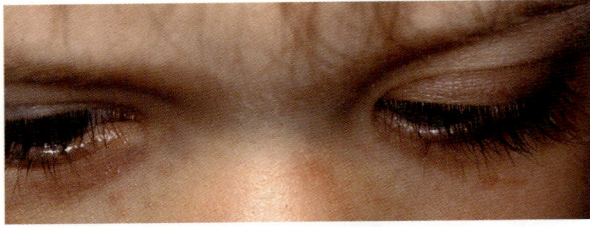

FIGURE 1–14 ■ Proptosis of left eye secondary to left optic nerve glioma. The proptosis is often most easily noticed when the patient is viewed from above.

Direct Ophthalmoscopy

For practical purposes, the direct ophthalmoscope is most useful in assessing the red reflex when it is used from a few feet away from the patient, as discussed above (Figure 1–8). It can also be used to get a magnified view of the posterior portion of the eye, particularly the optic nerve. This cannot usually be done easily until children are old enough to cooperate with the examination, typically after age 5 years. The light from the ophthalmoscope causes constriction of the pupil, so it is best to perform the test in a dark room. The patient should be instructed to fixate on an object across the room. The ophthalmoscope is brought toward the eye from the side as the examiner looks through the opening in the instrument and moves toward the pupil. The focus is adjusted using the dial on the ophthalmoscope (Figure 1–15A–C).

THE OPHTHALMOLOGIST'S EXAMINATION

The examination in the ophthalmologist's office involves evaluation of a number of different items, including careful assessment of visual function and

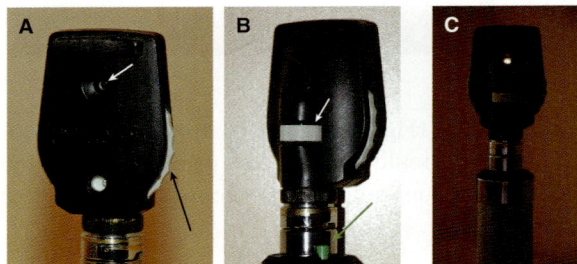

FIGURE 1–15 ■ Direct ophthalmoscope. (A) Examiner's view of instrument. When using to evaluate the retina and optic nerve the examiner looks through the small opening (short arrow). The pupil is visualized and the instrument is moved close to patient's eye. The side dial (large arrow) is used to focus on the retina. (B) The other side of the instrument has a dial that can be used to adjust the size of the light spot (small arrow) and the intensity is adjusted with the knob indicated by the long arrow. (C) Patient's view of the indirect ophthalmoscope.

physical inspection of the various ocular structures. The ability of children to cooperate is quite variable, and some portions of the examination are potentially more bothersome than others. Therefore, flexibility during the examination is important. Depending on the age and demeanor of the patient, in some cases the least bothersome portions of the examination are performed first, leaving the more invasive portions (such as indirect ophthalmoscopy, which may require that the child be briefly restrained) until the end. Because much of the assessment of visual function is based on behavior, this is usually checked first, preferably while the child is calm.

The following tests are performed during examinations in an ophthalmologist's office.

VISUAL ACUITY

Infants and Toddlers

The initial assessment of acuity is based on the same type of behavioral responses to toys and objects described above. The examiner moves an object and sees whether the child tracks equally well with both eyes. If so, this indicates that the child does not have a marked vision deficit in either eye. However, children may track surprisingly well even with moderately decreased vision.

To check for more subtle visual deficits, the examiner looks for a *fixation preference.* This assesses whether the child prefers to use one eye or the other, or whether the child will fixate with either eye without a preference. The test is fairly simple to perform if the patient has strabismus. The examiner watches the child while he or she is in the parent's lap. The child may display spontaneous *alternate fixation.* This is most commonly seen in children with infantile esotropia. When the child is viewing out of the right eye, the left eye is crossed, and vice versa. If the child spontaneously alternates crossing one eye and then the other, it means that the two eyes see equally well or nearly equally well. The test cannot reliably detect a slight difference between the eyes.

If a child with strabismus always has one eye deviated, this suggests the child may be amblyopic in the deviated eye. However, some children simply prefer to fixate with one eye, even if the vision is equal. To determine whether the child is amblyopic, the straight eye is covered. The behavior of the deviated eye is then assessed, and a judgment can be made about the vision based on the response of this eye:

■ If the eye is densely amblyopic, the child will object to having the good eye covered and will not use the strabismic eye to fixate.

- If the vision is moderately decreased, the child may fixate with the strabismic eye temporarily, at least until the normal eye is uncovered. The child will then immediately revert to the normal eye.
- If the two eyes see equally, the child will maintain fixation with the strabismic eye after the normal eye is uncovered. This is usually determined by whether the child holds fixation with the strabismic eye through a blink.
- The caveat discussed above regarding children who are averse to having objects held in front of their eyes applies to this test also. Some children get upset when either eye is covered. This is not necessarily because the vision is decreased in the opposite eye, but because the child does not like having something held in front of their face. This can be fairly easily determined by placing a hand in front of the deviating eye (which the child is not using). If the child gets upset, this indicates that the child simply does not like objects near his or her eyes. If the child does this repeatedly, the test cannot give accurate information.

If a child does not have strabismus, vision can still be assessed based on the same concept, using the *induced tropia test*. This test utilizes a small prism that bends light rays coming through it. When viewed through a prism, the apparent image is displaced toward the apex of the prism (Figure 1–16). In the induced tropia test, the prism is placed with its base down before one of the eyes (both eyes are open during the test). The image is shifted upward in the eye viewing through the prism, and the patient sees two images. Because the eyes move together, one can determine which eye the child is using by watching the direction of the eye movement:

- If the eyes stay straight, the child is using the eye that does not have the prism in front of it.
- If the eyes move up, the child is using the eye with the prism in front of it.

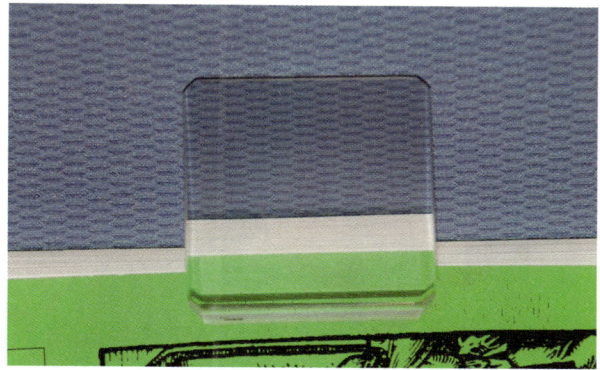

FIGURE 1–16 ■ Image displacement by prism. The base of the prism is down. The image is displaced superiorly by the prism.

- If the child's gaze shifts spontaneously between the two eyes, it means the visual acuity is equal or nearly equal in both eyes.
- If the child's eyes don't move, the examiner must be sure that the child has noticed the image in the eye with the prism. A hand is held in front of the other eye, and the eye behind the prism should move up. The hand is removed, and the child should then alternate spontaneously (Figure 1–17A–C).
- Because the prism blurs the vision slightly, some children prefer to use the eye without the prism. To determine whether the child is amblyopic, the test is performed with the prism in front of each eye. If the child always uses the eye without the prism, the vision is near equal. If the child is amblyopic, they will always prefer the better-seeing eye, regardless of which eye has the prism in front of it.

Common abbreviations used for denoting vision in young children based on the above tests are as follows:

- CSM, which stands for "central" (meaning when the child fixates the eye is straight), "steady" (meaning

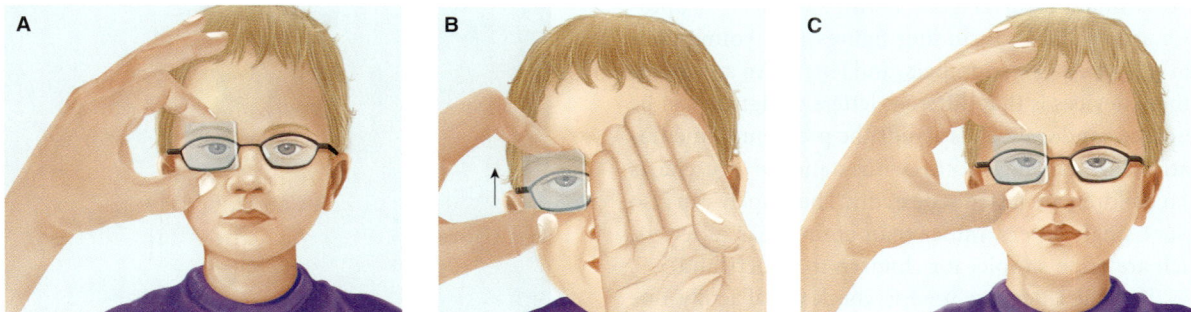

FIGURE 1–17 ■ Induced tropia test for assessing visual acuity. (A) A prism is held with its base down in front of the right eye. This shifts the image in this eye superiorly. In this photograph the patient is continuing to view through the left eye. (B) A hand is placed in front of the left eye, and the right eye moves up to fixate on the image, which has been shifted superiorly by the prism. (C) After the hand is removed, the right eye remains up, indicating that this eye continues to maintain fixation. If both eyes behave in a similar fashion, the vision is equal or nearly equal between the two eyes.

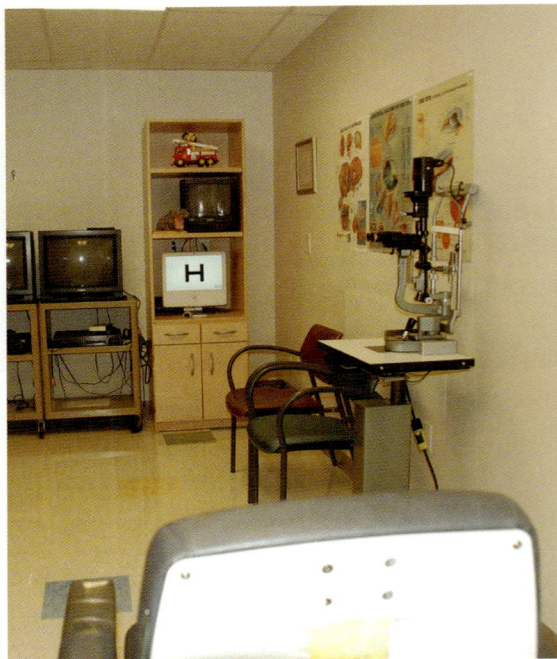

FIGURE 1–18 ■ Typical pediatric ophthalmology examination room. The video monitor with the "H" has a remote control that allows the examiner to adjust the optotypes used to measure visual acuity.

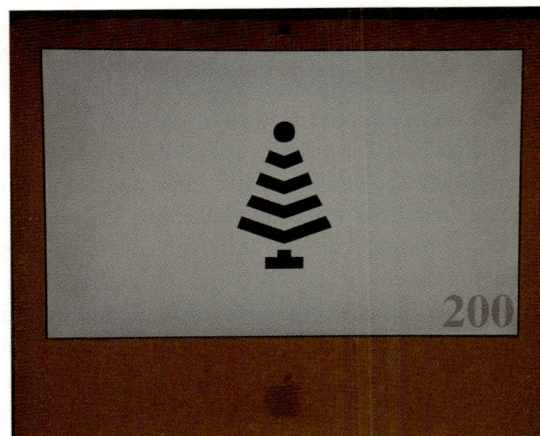

FIGURE 1–19 ■ Figures such as this tree can be used to assess visual acuity in children who are too young to recognize letters.

there is no nystagmus), and "maintained" (meaning the eye maintains fixation through a blink).

■ FFM, which stands for "fix" (meaning the child will fixate on a target), "follow" (meaning the child will follow the target as it is moved) and "maintained" (same meaning as above).

Older Children

Testing with *optotypes* (letters, numbers, or pictures on an eye chart) is performed when children are old enough to cooperate. Most ophthalmology offices now use video monitors to perform this test. The monitors have a standard luminance and are placed at a fixed distance from the examining chair (Figure 1–18). A variety of optotypes are available, including figures (for young children) (Figure 1–19), numbers, and letters. An advantage of these devices is that different letters or figures can be presented randomly. This avoids the problem of memorization, which may occur with standard eye charts when children are tested repeatedly. The display can also present single letters, rather than entire lines of letters, which are often simpler for children to understand.

If single letters are used to check visual acuity, one must be aware of the *crowding phenomenon*. The crowding phenomenon occurs in children with amblyopia. When presented with a line of letters, the visual acuity in an amblyopic eye is usually worse than if a letter of the same size is presented individually. For example, a child may not be able to read better than the 20/60 line when they are

required to identify all of the letters on the line, but might be able to read a letter on the 20/30 line if it is presented alone. The monitors can be used to assess this using *crowding bars*. Letters are presented individually, but they have black lines on their sides (Figure 1–20). In amblyopic eyes, the acuity is worse when the bars are present.

REFRACTION

One of the most common reasons that patients seek the services of an ophthalmologist is because their vision is blurred. This is usually due to a *refractive error*, which means that the eye is not focusing light correctly. When the vision is normal, light rays converge properly on the retinal surface. If the images are focusing behind the retina, the patient is *hyperopic (farsighted)* and the eye is essentially too short. If the images focus in front of the

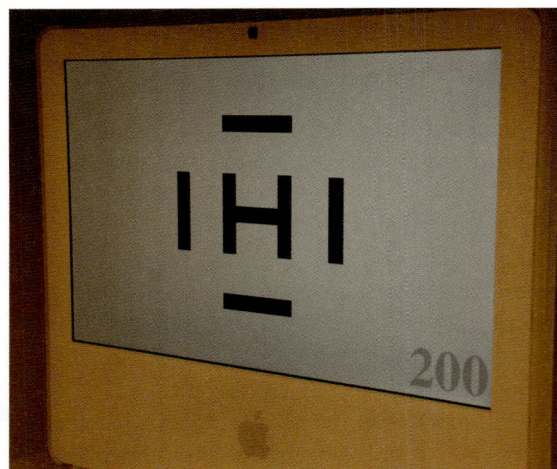

FIGURE 1–20 ■ Crowding bars used in the assessment of amblyopia. In patients with amblyopia, the visual acuity is decreased when the letter is surrounded by bars. In normal patients, the acuity is the same with or without the bars.

Normal eye   **Myopia**   **Hyperopia**
                   (nearsightedness)   **(farsightedness)**

Light focused   Light focused in   Light focused
at the retina   front of retina   behind the retina

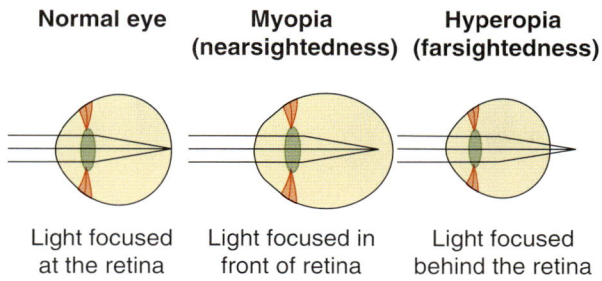

FIGURE 1–21 ■ Refractive errors. In a normal eye, light rays converge and focus on the retina. In a myopic (nearsighted) eye, the light rays converge in front of the retina; in a hyperopic eye they converge behind the retina.

retina, the patient is *myopic (nearsighted)*, in which case the eye is too long (Figure 1–21). *Astigmatism* occurs when the light rays are focused differently in different planes (rather than being symmetric like a basketball, the eye with astigmatism is shaped more like a football).

If decreased vision is noted on the initial testing, the child can be checked with a *pinhole test*, in which the child views the chart through a small, pinhole-sized opening. If the child's decreased vision is due to a refractive error, the visual acuity will improve when viewing through a pinhole. This is because the pinhole eliminates the peripheral light rays that are out of focus, leaving only the central ray, which can be seen clearly regardless of the type of refractive error (Figure 1–22).

The pinhole effect is the reason that people with refractive errors often squint when trying to see things when they aren't wearing glasses. The squinting eliminates the peripheral rays in the same manner that the pinhole does. Occasionally, young children with refractive errors will turn their head to improve vision, achieving a pinhole effect by viewing through the edge of the eyelid. If the vision does not improve with the pinhole tests, it suggests that there is some other reason for decreased vision, rather than a refractive error.

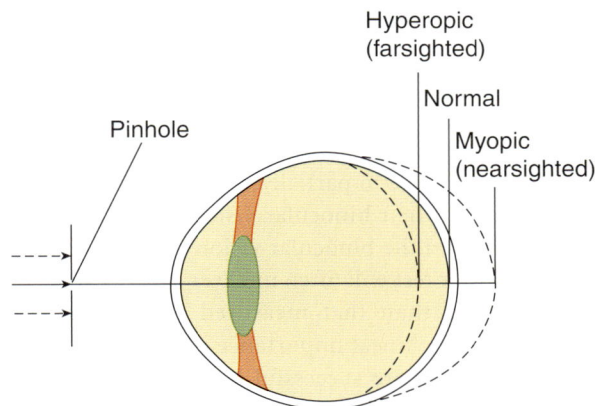

The refractive error is measured manually using a *retinoscope*, which analyzes the bending of light rays by the eye. This is analogous to looking at a reflection in mirrors at a carnival fun house. In a flat mirror the reflection is accurate. If the mirror is curved, the reflection may appear long and thin or short and fat. Similarly, the reflection from the retina can be assessed objectively. By normalizing the reflection with lenses, a very accurate measurement of the refractive error can be obtained (even in uncooperative infants and young children). Automated instruments can measure refractive errors quite accurately and quickly, provided the child is old enough to understand and cooperate with testing (Figure 1–23A and B).

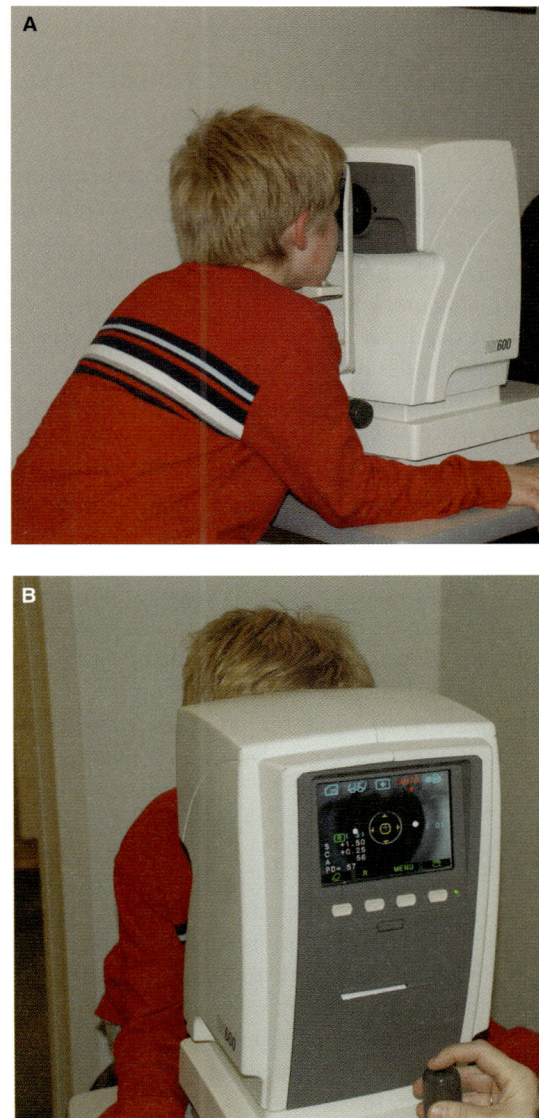

A

B

FIGURE 1–23 ■ Autorefractor. This instrument measures the refractive error in children who are old enough to cooperate. (A) The child sits at the instrument and looks at a small target within the machine. (B) The display shows the patients pupil and a digital readout of the patient's refractive error.

Hyperopic
(farsighted)

Normal

Pinhole

Myopic
(nearsighted)

FIGURE 1–22 ■ Pinhole effect. The central light ray moves straight through the eye. If the peripheral rays are blocked by a pinhole, the central ray will create a clear image regardless of the refractive error.

Almost all children in the first few years of life are moderately farsighted. The reason that very few farsighted infants and young children need to wear glasses is because the lens in the eye can change shape to adjust for farsightedness, automatically bringing the image into focus. To account for this involuntary focusing of the lens, *cycloplegic drops* must be placed in children's eyes to obtain an accurate refraction. These drops cause the ciliary muscle to relax, which allows the lens to assume its natural shape. If cycloplegic drops are not used and the refraction is performed while the child's lens is focusing, this creates an artificial increase in measured myopia. This is a common cause of incorrect glasses prescriptions in children.

In addition to the effect on the lens, the cycloplegic drops also dilate the pupils, which facilitates evaluation of the retina and optic nerve.

BINOCULAR VISION (STEREOPSIS, DEPTH PERCEPTION)

The eyes must be aligned and working together in order for binocular vision to function. There are several methods to assess binocular vision. The primary ones used by the ophthalmologist are the same as described in the earlier section on more detailed tests in the pediatric office—measuring depth perception using stereoscopic glasses.

If the child is too young to perform these tests, the presence of binocular vision can be assessed using the *prism vergence response*. In this test a prism is placed over one eye with the apex toward the nose. If the patient does not have strabismus and the binocular vision is intact, this will produce diplopia, with the image shifted toward the nose in the eye behind the prism. To eliminate the double image, a normal eye will shift inward to align itself with the image from the prism. Therefore, if the prism is held with its apex pointing inward in front of one eye and then the other, and both eyes make inward movements while the other eye stays straight, this indicates that the binocular vision is intact.

STRABISMUS

Strabismus is one of the most common problems encountered in a pediatric ophthalmology practice, and a large portion of the examination is usually devoted to it. The evaluation begins by watching the child during the history-taking portion of the evaluation. Strabismus may be constant or intermittent, and fixation may vary. In some patients the strabismus spontaneously alternates between the eyes, whereas in others only one eye remains deviated.

Most children with strabismus are able to move their eyes freely in all directions, but in some forms

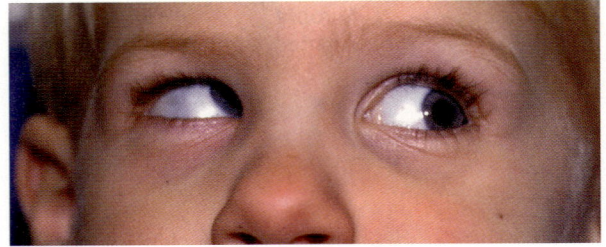

FIGURE 1–24 ■ Inferior oblique muscle overaction. The right eye is more elevated than the left eye when the patient looks to the left.

of strabismus the extraocular movements are limited. Eye movements are assessed by watching the child's eyes as they follow a target. In young children this is usually a small toy; older children can be asked to follow a finger. The target is moved horizontally from side to side, straight up, straight down, and up and down in side gazes. The eye movements are graded as normal, limited, or overacting. The most common overaction involves the inferior oblique muscle. This muscle normally elevates the eye when it is turned toward the nose. In overaction, the in-turned eye elevates more than the corresponding eye (Figure 1–24).

If eye movements are limited, the examiner checks to see whether the limitation is the same when both eyes are open (*versions*) and when one eye is covered (*ductions*). If a muscle is restricted, the limitation will be the same under each condition. If a muscle is palsied, a greater effort will be made to move the eye when it is viewing alone, and the movement will be greater with ductions than with versions.

The main method for assessing strabismus is the cover test. This can be performed in different ways to obtain information about the type of strabismus. As discussed above, the *single cover test* is performed by covering one eye and watching the movements of the opposite eye. If the uncovered eye is strabismic, it will move to a central position when the normal eye is covered. The measurement is usually made with a variant of the test known as the *alternate cover test,* in which the cover is moved alternately between the eyes (Figure 1–25). This is performed quickly so that the two eyes are not allowed to work together. The test is performed in this manner because many patients with strabismus are able to partially control their eye deviation by using their binocular vision when both eyes are open. When the binocular vision is disrupted, the alternate cover test will often uncover a larger angle of misalignment than that measured with the single cover test. The clinical importance of this is that surgery is usually more successful if the full amount of deviation is corrected.

The angle of strabismus is quantified using prisms, which are calibrated to bend light to different degrees. The unit of measurement is the *prism diopter*, which is defined as a 1-cm deflection of light measured at 1 m. The prism is held over the eye with the apex of the prism in the direction of the deviation (e.g., if the eye is exotropic the prism is held with the base toward the nose and the apex toward the ear). When held this way, the prism shifts the light so that it enters the eye from a lateral position. The cover test is repeated with different prisms until neither eye moves, indicating that the prism has aligned the light with the angle of eye deviation. These measurements are made with the eye in various positions of gaze, and when looking straight ahead at distance and near targets.

Pupils

The basic pupil examination is performed in the same manner described in the earlier section on more detailed tests in the pediatric office. The pupils are first measured to be sure that they are the same size. A difference of 0.5 mm or less is normal. Anisocoria is the term used when the pupils are unequal. The evaluation of anisocoria is discussed in Chapter 29 (Iris).

To test the pupil reaction a bright light is directed into each eye separately. The pupils should constrict briskly, and the response of each should be similar. In assessing the pupil reactions, it is important to understand that the signals that control pupil diameter come from both eyes. Normally this input is symmetric, and the diameter of the two pupils is the same. This is true even if one optic nerve is not functioning normally. Although the pupil will not react as well when a light is directed into it (it may not react at all in cases of severe optic nerve damage), the two pupils will still be of equal size because signals from the normal eye are sent to the pupil in the eye with the abnormal optic nerve.

A more sophisticated method of assessing the pupillary light reaction, used to detect optic nerve damage, is the *swinging flashlight test*, which looks for a *relative afferent pupillary defect (RAPD)* (Figure 1–26). This is an excellent test that provides an objective measure of optic nerve function. It is particularly useful in evaluating children who are too young to cooperate with other forms of testing. The test is based on the pupil reaction resulting from input from both eyes. The light is swung back and forth at regular intervals (a few seconds) between the eyes. The pupil of the eye in which the light is shined will receive a constricting signal. At the same time, it receives a dilating signal from the eye in which the light has just been removed (the opposite pupil is dilating because the bright light has been removed). In normal eyes the constricting signal is much stronger, and each pupil constricts initially as the light is shined into it. When an eye has a damaged optic nerve, however, the constricting signal is weaker when the light is shined into it. If it is weak enough, the dilating signal from the opposite eye will overcome it, and

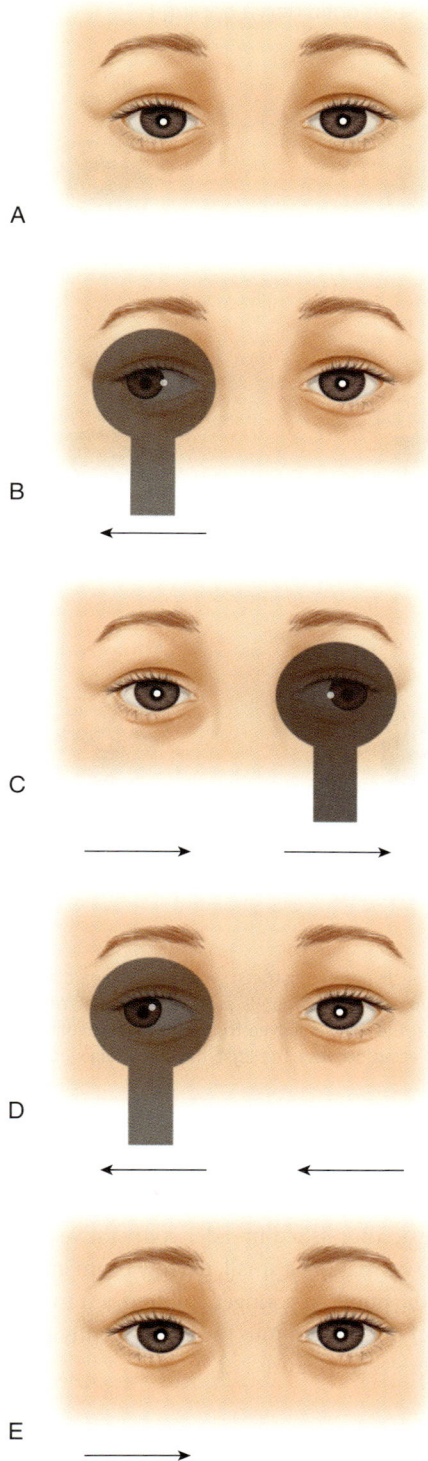

FIGURE 1–25 ■ Alternate cover test, used to detect latent strabismus (phorias). In this test the cover is moved back and forth between the eyes. (A) The eyes are normally straight. (B) When the cover is placed over the right eye, the eye drifts outward. (C) When the cover is moved to the left eye, the right eye moves inward to fixate, and the left eye makes an equal movement to the left. (D) When the cover is moved back to the right eye, the left eye moves inward to fixate, and the right eye makes an equal movement to the right. (E) When the cover is removed, binocular vision is restored. The right eye moves back to the center and the left eye remains straight.

A. Normal response   B. Left optic nerve damage

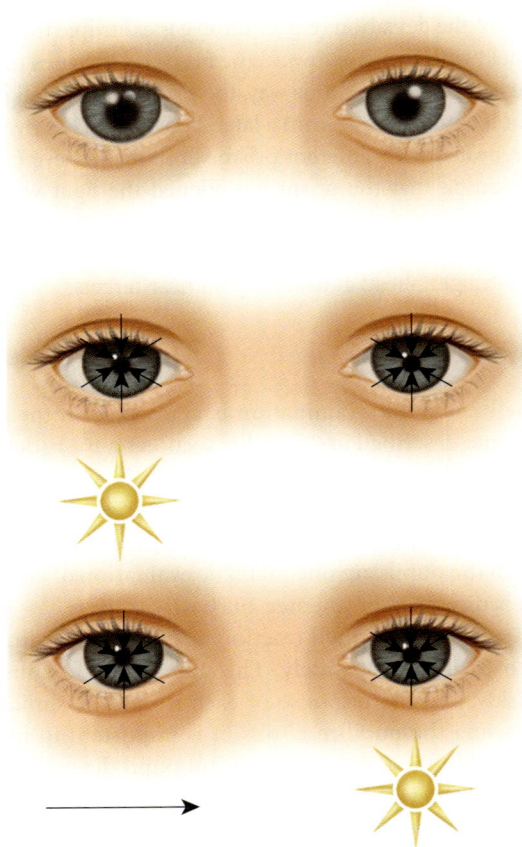

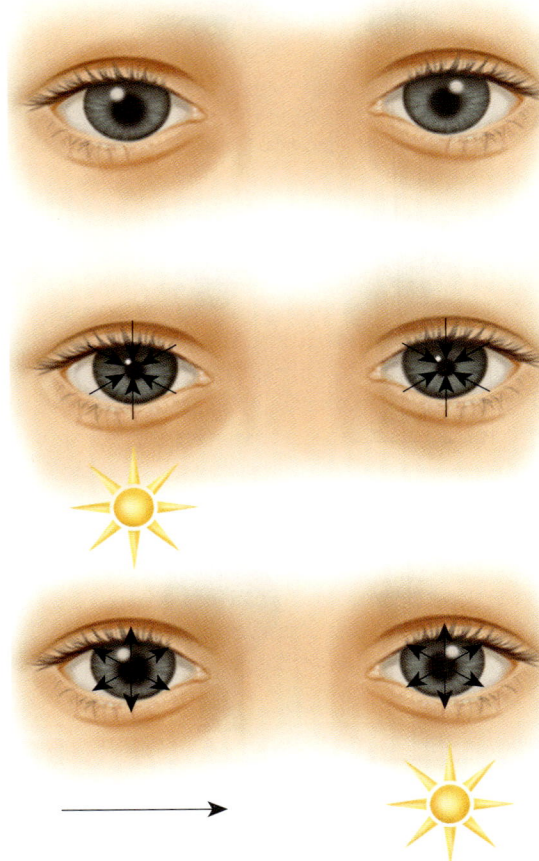

FIGURE 1–26 ■ Relative afferent pupillary defect (RAPD) testing. (A) Normally, each pupil constricts symetrically regardless of which eye is illuminated. (B) Optic nerve damage, left eye. Top: Under normal illumination both pupils are equal. Middle: When a light is shined into the normal right eye, both pupils constrict equally. Bottom: When the light is moved to the left eye, the impulse to constrict is diminished because of the optic nerve damage. The right pupil is dilating because the light has been removed, and this dilation effect is also seen in the left eye.

the pupil will actually dilate as the light is swung to it. The RAPD can be quantified using neutral density filters, which are placed in increasing degrees of opacity over the normal eye until the pupil reactions are balanced.

Some rare retinal abnormalities are associated with a *paradoxical pupil* reaction. In this condition, the pupil dilates in bright light and constricts in dim light. In practice, this is often difficult to measure because many patients with these disorders are photophobic and have nystagmus. Paradoxical pupil reactions are best assessed in a dim room, using a bright light shined into the eyes. The light is then dimmed, and the pupils are seen to constrict as the light intensity decreases.

Transillumination iris defects may occur in ocular conditions such as albinism or traumatic iris injury. These are focal areas of decreased pigment or thinning within the iris. They are not usually visible with a penlight because the light reflects off the front of the iris. They can be visu-

alized if the iris is transilluminated, meaning the light is directed into the eye without shining on the iris surface. This can be accomplished in older cooperative patients at the slitlamp by making a small, narrow beam and shining it through the pupil. In younger children, a transilluminator light can be directed into the eye by gently pressing it on the lower eyelid (Figure 1–27).

Visual Fields

The peripheral visual fields are usually assessed using the evoked saccade and confrontation tests described in the earlier section on more detailed tests in the pediatric office.

The central visual field may be affected in some optic nerve and retinal diseases. Optic nerve disorders often cause a localized defect in the visual field (a *scotoma*). Some retinal disorders cause an abnormality in which objects appear wavy or distorted

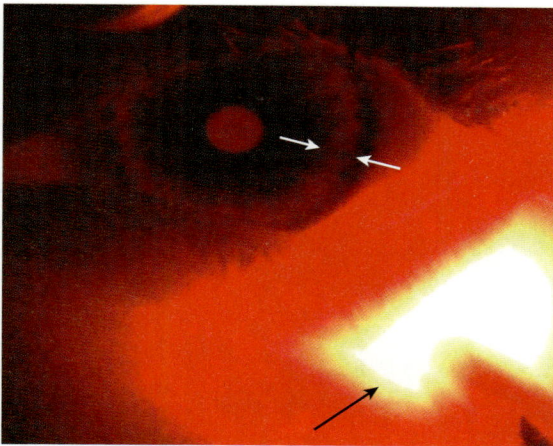

FIGURE 1–27 ■ Transillumination defects of the iris in a patient with ocular albinism. A light pipe is placed gently against the lower eyelid (long arrow), and the peripheral transillumination iris defects are seen as glowing areas for 360° in the iris periphery (short arrows).

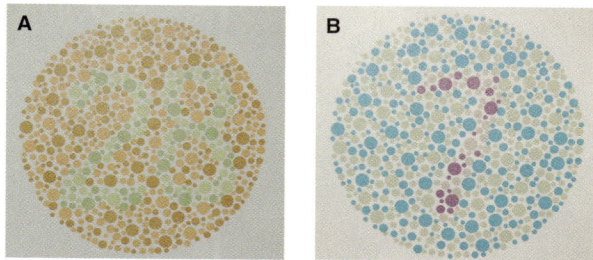

FIGURE 1–29 ■ Color plates to assess for defects in color vision. Normal patients can detect (A) the number 28 and (B) the number 7.

(*metamorphopsia*). These can be assessed using an *Amsler grid* (Wilson Ophthalmic Corp., Mustang, OK) (Figure 1–28). This is a checkerboard pattern that is held a few feet in front of the patient. The patient closes one eye and fixates on the dot in the center of the grid. Patients with scotomas of their central visual fields will describe areas in which the grid is missing or blurred. Patients with metamorphopsia will describe a wavy appearance of the lines.

Color Vision

Several tests are available to assess color vision. Most of these are designed using a pattern of colors with a figure or letter present within the pattern. Patients with normal color vision can see the number, whereas people with deficient color vision cannot (Figure 1–29A and B). For younger children, plates are available in which the patient is asked to trace the line, rather than read a number (Figure 1–30). The most common color vision problem is red:green deficiency, which affects approximately 8% of males. This can be assessed using the Ishihara color test.

Slitlamp Examination

The slitlamp is a biomicroscope with a light beam that is directed into the eyes using a mirror (Figure 1–31). The anterior portions of the eye (the cornea, anterior chamber, iris, and lens) are viewed under high magnification. The diameter of the light beam can be adjusted vertically and horizontally. A broad beam gives illumination similar to a flashlight. When a narrow beam is used, it produces a slit of light that can be directed obliquely into

Amsler recording chart

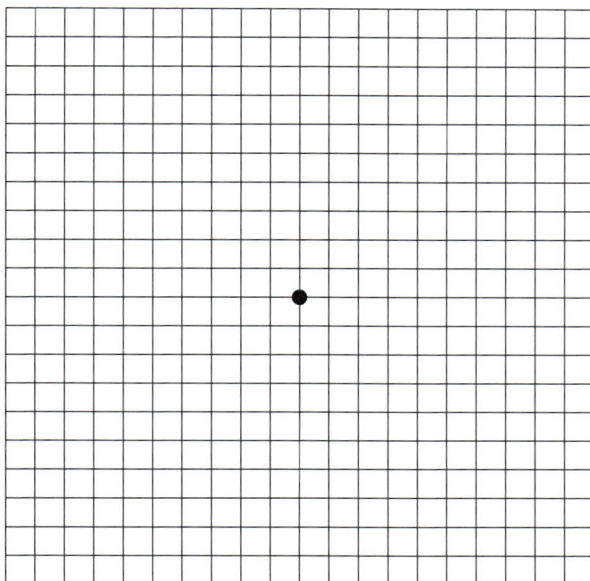

FIGURE 1–28 ■ Amsler grid to check for central visual field abnormalities. The patient looks at the dot in the center of the grid and reports whether the checkerboard pattern looks normal. Metamorphopsia is present if the lines appear wavy. This may occur if the retina is distorted. Scotomas are present if the checkerboards are not visible in a section of the grid.

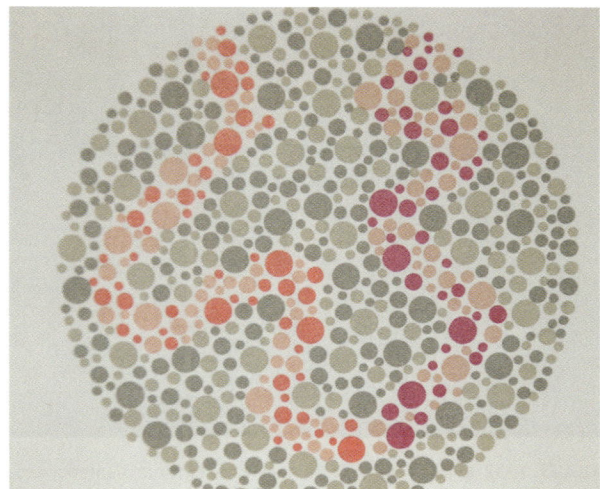

FIGURE 1–30 Color vision test for younger children. The patient is asked to trace the line.

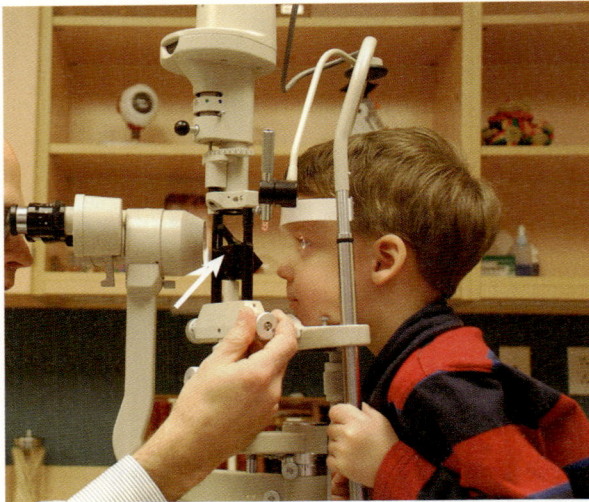

FIGURE 1–31 ■ Slitlamp for examining the anterior portion of the eyes. A light is produced in the top portion of the machine, then reflected through a mirror (arrow) onto the patient's eye. The height, width, and angle of the beam can be adjusted to evaluate different portions of the eye.

the eye. This beam can help localize opacities or defects within different layers of the cornea based on where they interfere with the beam (Figure 1–32).

When evaluating patients with corneal trauma or other abnormalities of the corneal epithelium (such as could occur in patients with poor tear films), fluorescein dye can be placed in the eye. If the corneal epithe-

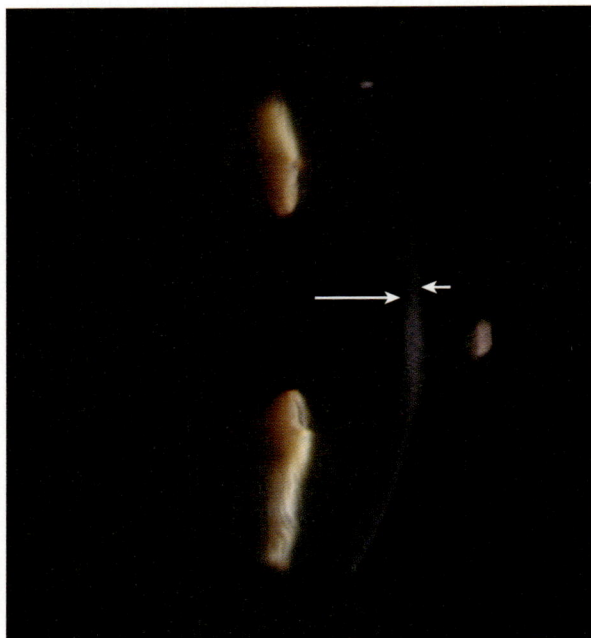

FIGURE 1–32 ■ High-magnification view of cornea and anterior segment through a slitlamp. The light beam is coming obliquely from the right side. The thickness of the cornea is visualized between the beam on the right (short arrow) and the beam on the left (long arrow).

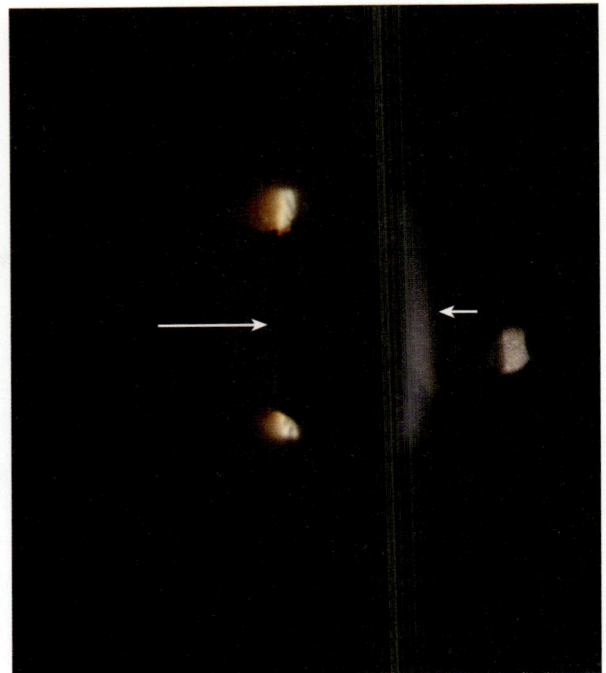

FIGURE 1–33 ■ When evaluating a patient with iritis or a hyphema, a narrow beam of light is directed through the slitlamp. In this normal patient, nothing is present between the beam on the cornea (short arrow) and the anterior lens (long arrow). If iritis or a hyphema is present, small individual cells can be visualized floating in the anterior chamber (similar to seeing particles in the light beam from a movie projector).

lium is absent, the fluorescein will adhere to the cornea in the area of the defect, and this area will fluoresce when viewed with a blue light. This test is best performed by wetting a paper fluorescein strip with a drop of liquid and gently touching it to the everted lower eyelid. Paper strips are usually more effective than fluorescein drops, for 2 reasons. First, the paper strip disturbs young children less than a drop. Second, the amount of fluorescein in a drop is much greater than that in a strip, and the excess fluid may obscure mild corneal irregularities.

When evaluating for iritis, attention is directed toward the beam as it passes through the anterior chamber. In normal people, the fluid in the anterior chamber is clear and the beam of light is not visible (Figure 1–33). In iritis, patients may have circulating inflammatory cells in the anterior chamber, in which case individual cells can be visualized in the beam of light from the slitlamp. Similarly, in patients with hyphemas individual red blood cells can be visualized floating in the anterior chamber. Patients with iritis may also have *flare*, which results from leakage of proteinaceous fluid. This imparts a slightly cloudy appearance to the fluid, which is similar to that seen in a movie theater when one looks at the beam of light from the projector.

Handheld portable slitlamps are available, which are used for evaluating infants and young children, or

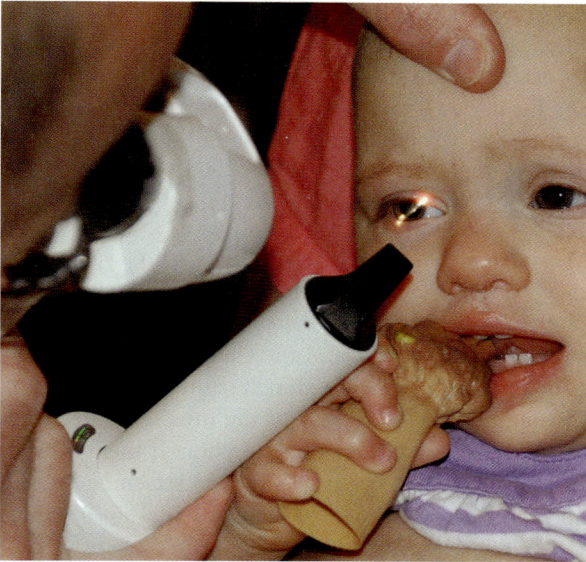

FIGURE 1–34 Portable slitlamp.

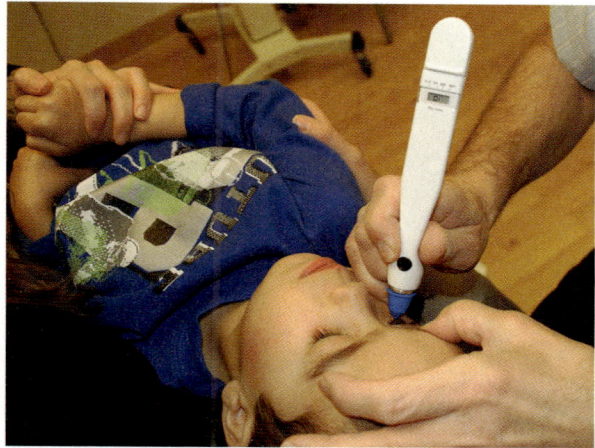

FIGURE 1–35 ■ Tonometer is used to measure intraocular pressure. A drop of topical anesthetic has been placed in the eye and the instrument gently touches the cornea to obtain readings. Children are often much less cooperative for this test than the patient seen here.

older children who are unable to sit at the regular slit-lamp (Figure 1–34).

Intraocular Pressure

The normal intraocular pressure (IOP) ranges from 10 to 21 mm Hg. If the IOP is elevated, damage to the optic nerve may occur, which can lead to vision loss. This occurs in glaucoma. Glaucoma is relatively common in older adults, and IOP measurement is part of a standard adult ophthalmic examination. In young children, however, IOP measurements are usually not made unless there is some reason to suspect that the child may have elevated IOP. This is primarily because IOP measurement is usually performed using a *contact tonometer*. The instrument gently indents the cornea, and the amount of pressure required to do so is used to calculate the IOP (Figure 1–35).

Because tonometry requires contact with the cornea, it is difficult to perform in young children. Although topical anesthetics are used and the measurement is not painful, the anxiety invoked by having an instrument brought close to the eye causes most children (and many adults) to squeeze their eyelids shut. The eyelids must then be separated by the examiner to access the cornea. This squeezing causes the IOP to temporarily elevate, in which case it is not possible to measure the true IOP. In infants this can sometimes be overcome by having the baby take a bottle before the measurement. As the baby falls asleep, the eyelids can often be gently opened and a measurement taken. This is usually not possible in older toddlers and young children. For this reason, children with glaucoma often require examination under anesthesia to accurately measure the IOP.

Gonioscopy

Intraocular fluid is created in the ciliary processes, flows around the lens and iris into the anterior chamber, and drains into the trabecular meshwork in the anterior chamber angle. This angle cannot be viewed directly, but is visible with a *goniolens* (Figure 1–36A–C). This is

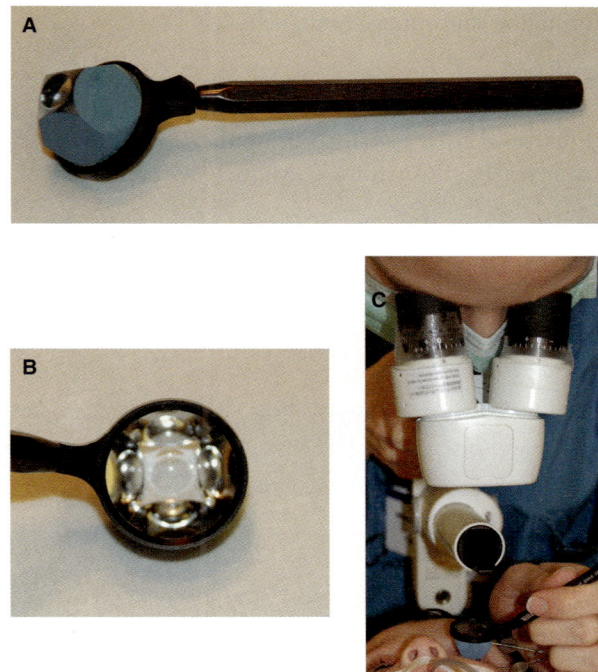

FIGURE 1–36 ■ Gonioscopy used to examine the trabecular meshwork. (A) The instrument is a small, handheld, 4-sided mirror. (B) Viewed from above. The center portion rests on the cornea and the mirrors on the side are used to visualize the trabecular meshwork. (C) A magnified view is obtained by using the goniolens with a portable slitlamp.

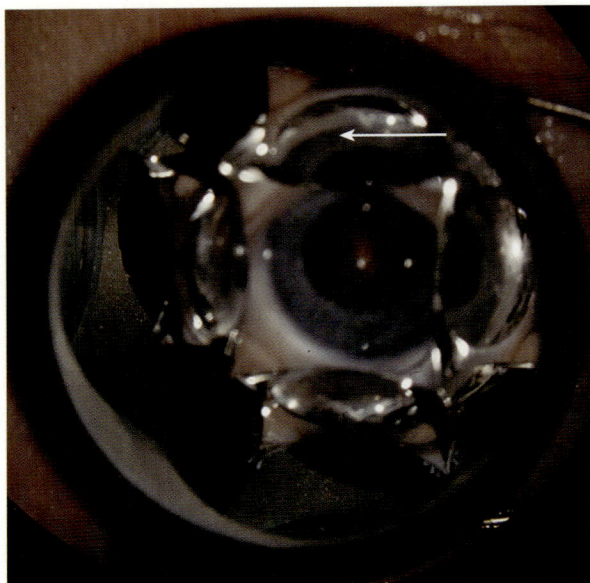

FIGURE 1–37 ■ View of gonioscopy through a slitlamp. The peripheral iris and trabecular meshwork are seen (arrow) in the reflection through a mirror.

a lens that comes into direct contact with the cornea. It has mirrors on its sides. When the mirrors are viewed with a slitlamp, the trabecular meshwork is visible (Figure 1–37). Gonioscopy can be performed in older cooperative children at the slitlamp with the use of topical anesthetic. Examination under anesthesia is required for infants and young children.

Proptosis

Proptosis can be measured using the *Hertel exophthalmometer* (G. Rodenstock, Munich, Germany). This instrument is held to the patient's face and rests on the lateral orbital bones. Mirrors in the instrument reflect the cornea. A millimeter ruler is present on the instrument, and the degree of proptosis can be assessed by measuring how far the cornea protrudes (Figure 1–38A–C).

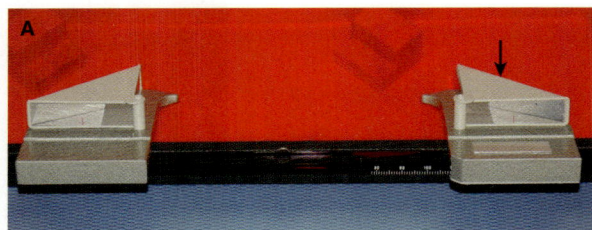

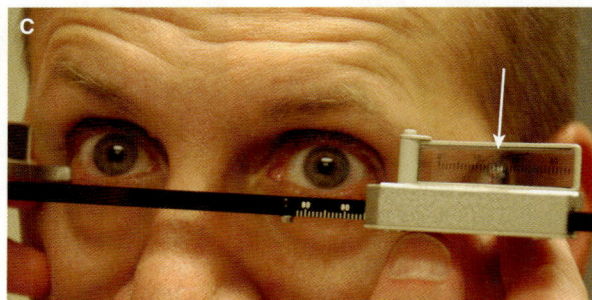

Eyelid Levator Muscle Function

Measurement of the function of the eyelid levator muscle is an important component of the ptosis evaluation. Most ptosis in children results from decreased function of the levator muscle, and the choice of surgical treatment depends on how much function is present. Tightening (strengthening) of the muscle is effective if the muscle has some residual function. If there is minimal function, surgery is performed by attaching the eyelid to the brow muscles, which provides an alternate source of eyelid elevation.

Levator muscle function is quantified by measuring the excursion of the eyelid from maximal downgaze to maximal upgaze, using a handheld ruler next to the eyelid (Figure 1–39A–C). In normal individuals the eyelid will move 15 mm or more during this maneuver. In moderate ptosis the function is usually in the 6 to 10 mm range. In infants with marked congenital ptosis, the function is usually 5 mm or less.

This measurement can be made in older children by asking them to follow a finger or simply asking them to look up and down. In young children, an interesting target needs to be presented so that the patient will track as it moves from downgaze to upgaze (Figure 1–13).

Particular attention must be paid to 2 things during evaluation of levator muscle function:

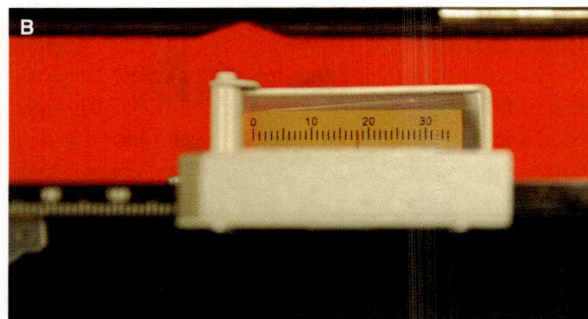

FIGURE 1–38 ■ (A) Hertel exophthalmometer. The instrument is used to measure proptosis. Mirrors are present in the casings (arrow), which reflect an image of the eye when the instrument is held in place. (B) A millimeter gauge is used to measure the location of the anterior cornea. (C) Exophthalmometer in place. The reflection of the eye and the ruler are visible (arrow).

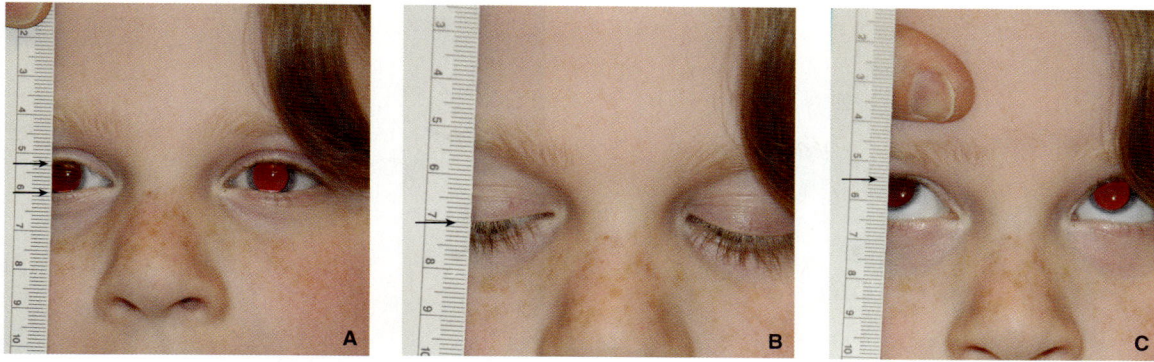

FIGURE 1–39 ■ Measurement of eyelid levator muscle function. The ruler is placed next to the patient's eye and is used to measure movement of the eyelid. (A) When looking straight ahead, the space between the edges of the upper and lower eyelids is 8 mm (normal) (arrows). (B) The patient looks down and the location of the upper eyelid margin is noted (at the 7-cm mark in this photograph [arrow]). (C) The patient looks up while the ruler is held in place. The upper lid margin is now at the 5.4-cm mark (arrow), indicating that the eyelid has moved 16 mm (normal). Note that the examiner's thumb is used to immobilize the brow in upgaze. This is done to isolate the movement of the levator muscle because patients with ptosis often recruit the brow to help elevate the eyelid, which can make the levator muscle function appear to be greater than it actually is.

- Children with ptosis that occludes the eye usually adopt a chin-up head posture to view beneath the obstructing eyelid. The child's head should be held straight when making the measurement. This sometimes causes difficulty because the children object to holding their head in a position that decreases their vision.
- Children with visually significant ptosis usually recruit the brow muscles of the forehead to assist in elevating the eyelid, which causes arching of the eyebrow and furrowing of the brow. To eliminate the effect of the brow muscles and isolate the eyelid levator muscle during measurement, a finger is held over the eyebrow (Figures 1–13D, 1–39C).

Tear Drainage

In most children with lacrimal disorders delayed tear drainage is obvious. Patients have a thick layer of tears on the lower eyelid margin, and often there is frank epiphora (overflow of tears onto the cheeks). In some cases the parents may report intermittent epiphora, but the eyes appear fairly normal on examination. In this case, a *dye disappearance test* can be performed. A drop of fluorescein is placed in each eye and the eyes are gently dabbed with a tissue to remove excess dye. After 1 to 2 minutes a blue light is shined into the eyes. In normal patients, there will only be a thin layer of fluorescein-stained fluid remaining in the lower tear lake (between the eyelid and the eyeball). In patients with lacrimal obstruction, a thicker layer is present in the obstructed eye, reflecting the delayed drainage of tears (Figure 1–40). This test is also useful in children who present with decreased tearing. Most such children have normal basal tear formation, which can be verified by noting a normal tear layer. At the same time, the cornea can be examined with a slitlamp to check for signs of microscopic irritation.

Tear Production

The production of tears can be assessed using the Schirmer test, which measures basal tear production. In this test, a drop of topical anesthetic is placed in the eye to decrease the production of reflex tears due to ocular irritation. The lower conjunctival fornix is gently swabbed with a cotton-tipped applicator to remove the tears that are present. A standardized strip of absorbent blotter paper is placed over the lower eyelid and the patient holds their eyes closed gently for 5 minutes. Tear production is assessed by measuring the length of fluid that accumulates on the blotter paper (Figure 1–41). In normal patients, tears travel 5 to 10 mm or more along the paper. The Schirmer test requires a good deal of cooperation, and cannot be performed accurately in young patients.

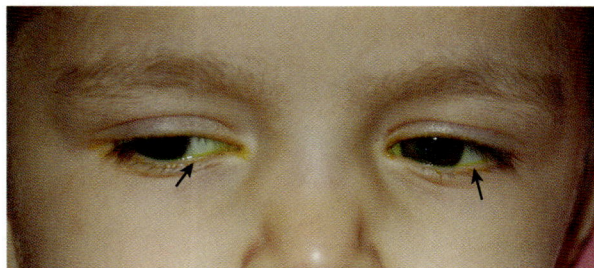

FIGURE 1–40 ■ Dye disappearance test in a patient with mild right lacrimal obstruction. A drop of fluorescein has been placed in each eye, and the patient is assessed 1 to 2 minutes later. The examiner notes how much dye is present in the tear lakes between the eyelid and the eyeball. Note the thicker layer of yellow dye in the right tear lake (arrow) compared to the minimal amount remaining on the left (arrow).

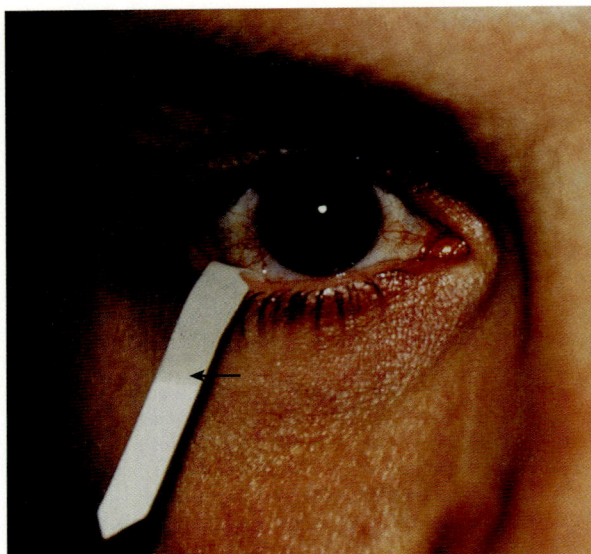

FIGURE 1–41 ■ Schirmer's testing. The patient's eyes are anesthetized with topical drops and a strip of standardized blotter paper is placed on the lower eyelid for 5 minutes. Tear production is assessed by measuring the length of paper that is moistened (arrow).

Evaluation of the Retina and Optic Nerve

The most common method used by ophthalmologists to examine the *posterior* pole (the retina and optic nerve) in children is the *indirect ophthalmoscope*. A lens is held in front of the patient's eye, which produces an image that is viewed through the indirect ophthalmoscope, which is worn on the examiner's head (Figure 1–42). The direct ophthalmoscope is sometimes used, but it requires a cooperative patient who can fixate a distant target while the examiner shines the light into the

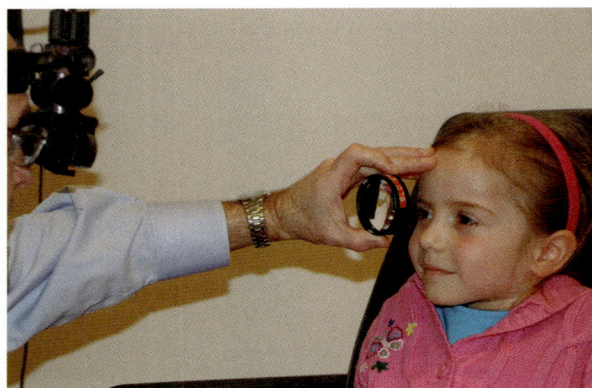

FIGURE 1–42 Indirect ophthalmoscopy in the office.

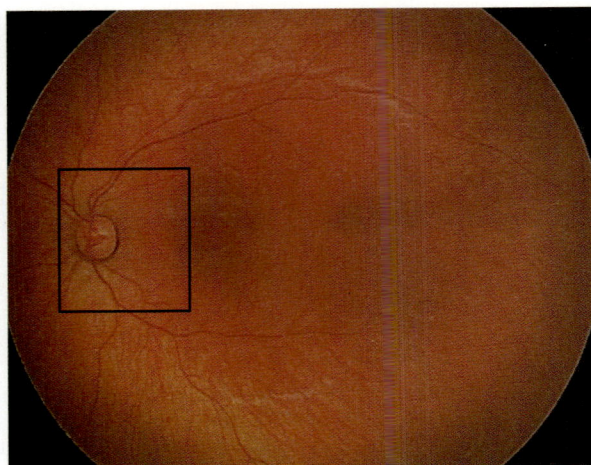

FIGURE 1–43 ■ View of normal retina with an indirect ophthalmoscope. The box indicates the much smaller field of view with the direct opthalmoscope.

patient's eye. There are several advantages of the indirect ophthalmoscope:

- The field of view is much wider than that of the direct ophthalmoscope. This not only allows a view of the optic nerve and the macula (the posterior portion of the retina) (Figure 1–43), but also can be used to evaluate the peripheral retina (which cannot be seen with the direct ophthalmoscope).
- Evaluation of the far peripheral retina may be indicated in children with retinal tumors or diseases that predispose to retinal detachments. Using the indirect ophthalmoscope, the entire peripheral retina can be examined by gently pressing on the eye with a *scleral depressor*. This brings portions of the retina into view that could not otherwise be visualized (Figure 1–44A–C). This test can be performed in adults using topical anesthetic drops, but usually requires examination under anesthesia in children.
- Although indirect ophthalmoscopy is usually performed after pharmacological dilation of the pupil, the instrument can be adjusted to view through small pupils. This may allow evaluation of patients who have abnormal pupils (e.g., if they are scarred due to intraocular inflammation), or patients in whom dilation is not desired (e.g., a patient with trauma whose pupils are being monitored for signs of intracranial herniation).
- Because the instrument is binocular a 3-D view of the retina is achieved. This can be used to assess elevated lesions within the retina, such as tumors or retinal detachments (in which fluid accumulates beneath the retina).

Lens

Pupil

Edge of retina

Can see this far without indentation

Optic nerve

Indenter

Lens

Pupil

Can see this far with indentation

Optic nerve

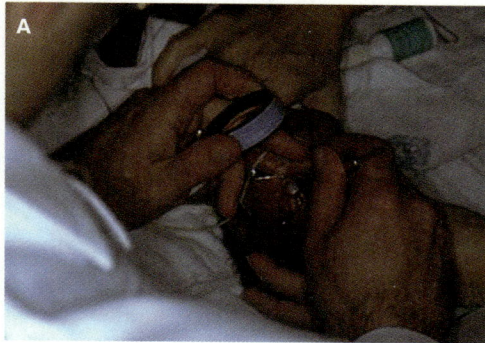

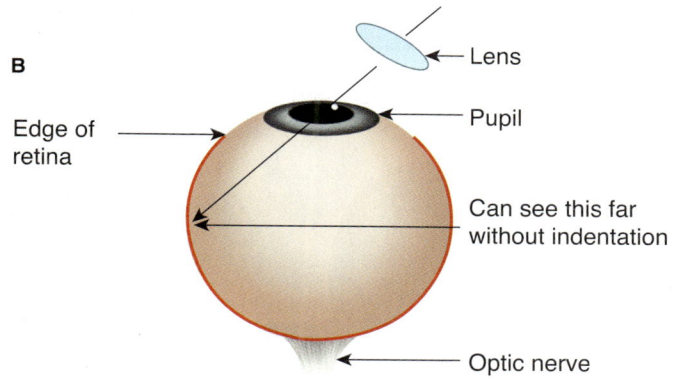

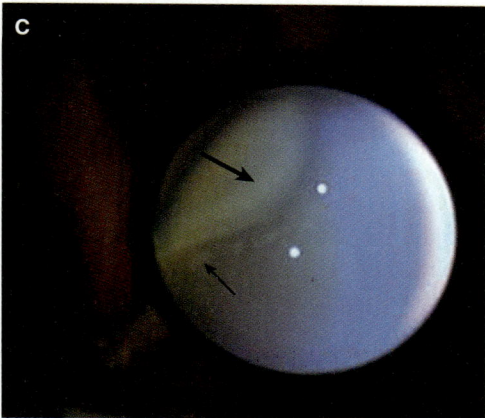

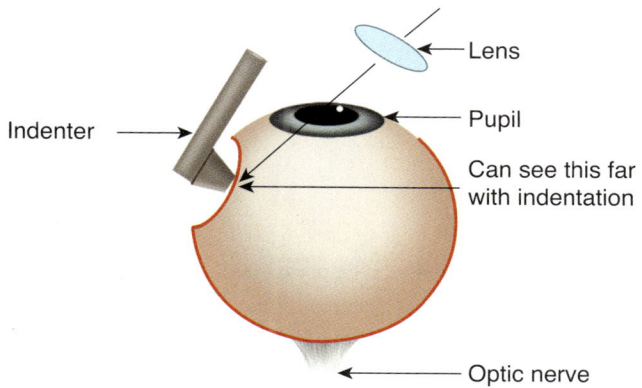

FIGURE 1–44 ■ Examination of peripheral retina using indirect ophthalmoscope and scleral depression. (A) The eye is gently depressed with a scleral depressor. (B) Top: Without indentation, the midperiphery of the retina can be viewed with the indirect ophthalmoscope. Bottom: To examine the far peripheral retina, the eye must be indented with a scleral depressor, which brings the peripheral retina into view. (C) View of the retina through the indirect ophthalmoscope lens. The elevated area of retina is brought into the field of view by the depression (the indented retina is marked by a thick arrow). This patient has retinopathy of prematurity, with tufts of extraretinal fibrovascular tissue (thin arrow).

CHAPTER 2

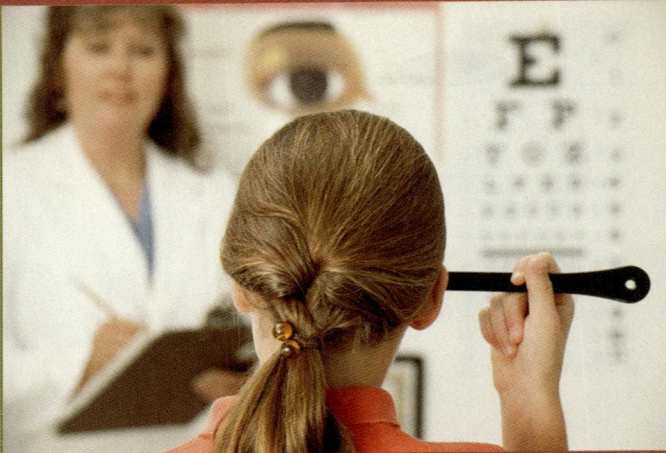

Ancillary Tests in Pediatric Ophthalmology

INTRODUCTION

A number of additional tests can be performed in the ophthalmologist's office. They are generally reserved for specific indications, as described in the following sections.

ASSESSMENT OF VISUAL ACUITY IN PREVERBAL CHILDREN

Infants and young children obviously cannot perform subjective visual acuity testing by asking them to read an eye chart. In many cases, the behavioral methods of assessing vision discussed in Chapter 1 are adequate. However, these methods are not quantitative, and more precise evaluation of visual acuity is sometimes desired. This information may be useful in determining whether an intervention is needed (cataract surgery, for example), or to monitor improvement in vision while a patient is being treated.

Two useful methods for quantifying visual acuity in preverbal children are described:

Forced preferential looking tests. These tests are based on the normal instinct for children to look at interesting objects. In one form of this test, drawings placed on one end of a card, and the opposite end is blank (Figure 2–1A–C). When the card is held in front of the infant, their attention will naturally turn to the picture. The examiner watches the child's eyes from behind the card. If the child's eyes consistently turn and look in the direction of the picture, one infers that the infant can see it. The cards come in a set with gradually smaller pictures. As the size decreases the eye eventually cannot distinguish the figure from the background. At this point, the infant will no longer make consistent eye movements in the direction of the picture. The size of the smallest identified picture is used as a measure of acuity. The eyes are tested independently (Figure 2–2).

Spatial-sweep visual-evoked potentials (SSVEPs). Visual acuity in nonverbal children can be assessed in a more sophisticated manner by measuring SSVEPs. In this test, electrodes are placed on the occipital lobe and the child sits in the parent's lap. The infant watches a series of bar patterns on a monitor (Figure 2–3). When the bars are large enough to see, a visual impulse is created and this is transmitted from the eye to the occipital lobe, where the scalp electrodes record the activity. The bar width gradually decreases. A threshold is reached at which the bars cannot be distinguished from the background, and the cortical activity stops. This endpoint can be converted into a measure of visual acuity.

VISUAL FIELD TESTING

If children are old enough to cooperate, computer-based visual field testing can be performed (*automated perimetry*). The patient's head is positioned so that he looks into a large bowl-shaped machine, and he is asked to look straight ahead. The computer then generates a series of brief light flashes in the peripheral visual field. The patient pushes a button when he notices the light (Figure 2–4A and B). The computer tracks the responses and gradually dims the lights in each portion of the field until the patient can no longer see them, and these thresholds are recorded.

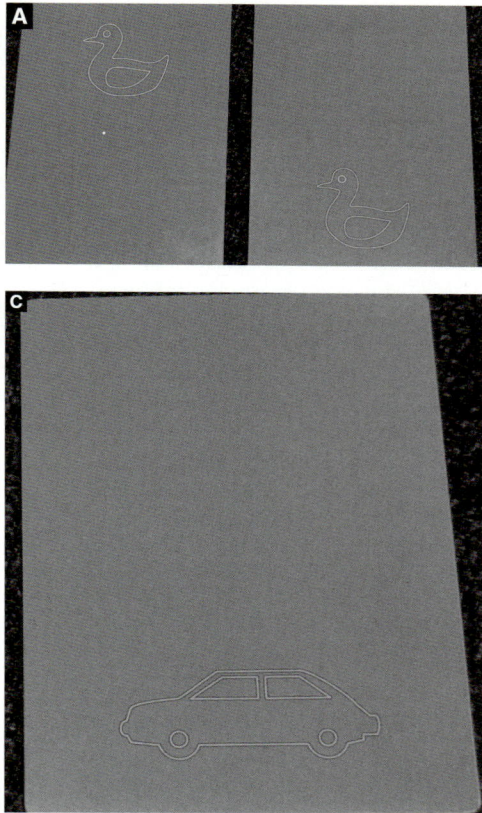

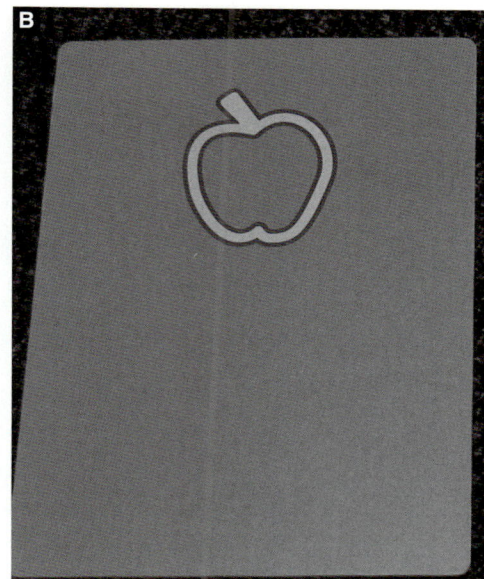

FIGURE 2–1 ■ Forced preferential looking testing cards. (A) A picture is present on either the top or the bottom of the card. One of the cards is held in front of the infant. If the child's eyes turn to the picture, this indicates the child is able to see it. (B) and (C) The cards come with various sizes of pictures. Vision is measured by determining the smallest figure the infant consistently responds to.

This type of testing requires a fair amount of cooperation and concentration. The examiner must monitor the patient's fixation to be sure he is staring straight ahead, because the natural inclination for most people taking the test is to move the eyes toward the light targets. The computer randomly checks for false-negative and false-positive responses. False negatives are recorded when the patient fails to respond to bright light in the center of fixation. False positives occur when the patient indicates that he sees a dim light that is intentionally placed in the blind spot.

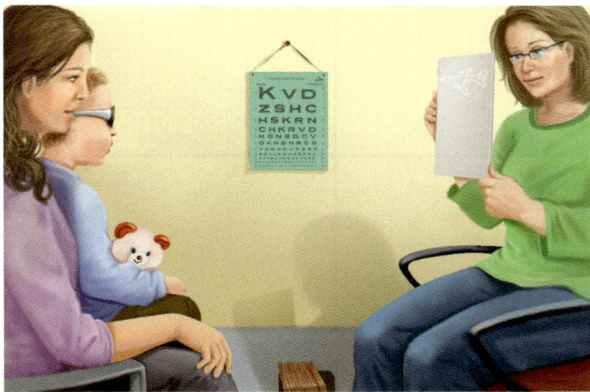

When the test is completed, the computer generates a printout of the results (Figure 2–5A and B). In addition to the graphical representation, a great deal of other statistical information regarding the patient's performance is recorded, including whether the test appears to be abnormal and what specific defects are present. This information is stored, and can be statistically compared on future tests to monitor for changes.

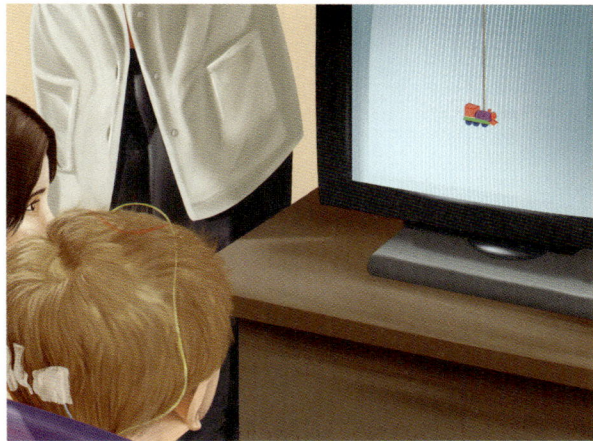

FIGURE 2–2 ■ Forced preferential looking test. The glasses on the child have an occluder on one side and are open on the other, so the eyes can be tested independently. The examiner (right) watches the child's eye movements to see whether they move consistently toward the picture.

FIGURE 2–3 ■ Spatial sweep visual evoked potential (SSVEP). The child's attention is drawn to the monitor with a small toy. The vertical bars stimulate an occipital lobe response, which is measured by the scalp electrodes. The size of the bars is decreased until they cannot be distinguished, at which point the occipital lobe response stops. This endpoint is converted to a measure of visual acuity.

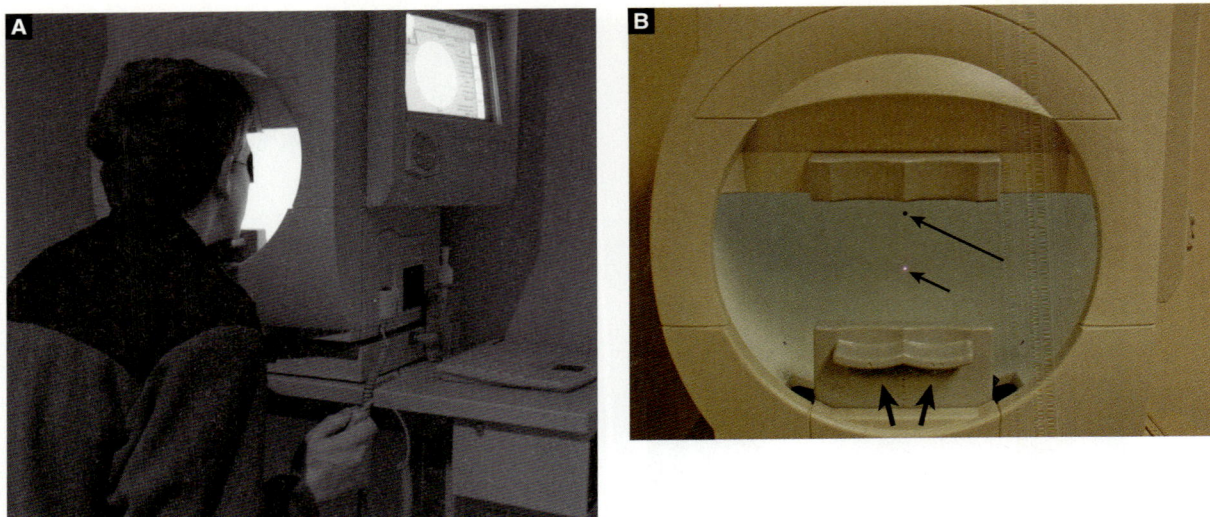

FIGURE 2–4 ■ Automated visual field testing. (A) The patient sits at the machine and looks at a target in the center of a lighted bowl. Lights are flashed in the peripheral field and the patient presses the button when they are seen. The examiner watches the patient's fixation with the monitor on the side of the machine. (B) View inside the testing bowl. The patient fixates on the bright white light (short arrow). The dark spot above this light (long arrow) is the camera that allows the examiner to monitor the patient's fixation. The patient's chin rests in a different chin rest for each eye (thick arrows).

For younger patients, visual fields may be measured manually using a *Goldmann perimeter*. The patient is seated in front of a white bowl, similar to that used for automated perimetry. The examiner monitors the patient's fixation and projects light of various intensities and sizes in the peripheral visual field. The lights is slowly moved centrally until the patient indicates that they see it. Manual perimetry is less precise than automated perimetry, but it is easier for many younger patients to perform (Figure 2–6).

Visual field testing provides information about the central and peripheral vision. The retinal area of central vision, particularly the fovea, is most sensitive to fine visual discrimination. The peripheral retina is less sensitive, and the sensitivity decreases with increasing distance from the center of vision. Therefore, brighter lights are required to be detected in the periphery. Each eye is tested independently. The area where the optic nerve penetrates the back of the eye produces a *blind spot*. This is not noticed during normal viewing because the 2 visual fields overlap, but it can be mapped when the eyes are tested individually (Figures 2–5 and 2–6).

Specific visual field abnormalities may suggest certain diagnoses. For instance, lesions that affect the

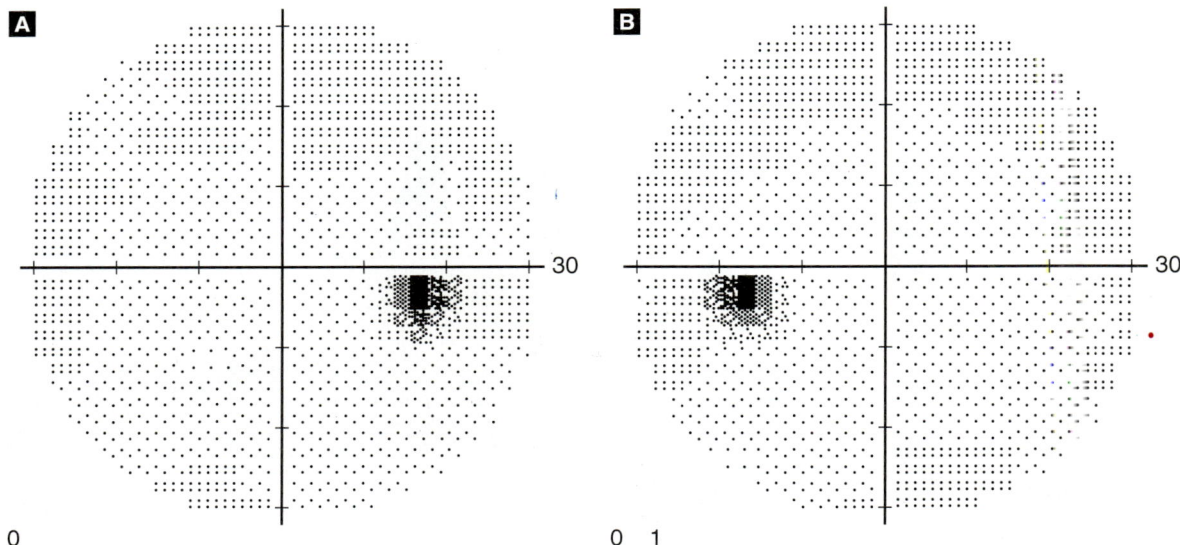

FIGURE 2–5 ■ Normal automated visual fields of (A) right eye and (B) left eye. The "30" represents the number of degrees from central fixation. The black areas represent the normal blind spots, due to the lack of photoreceptors overlying the optic nerve.

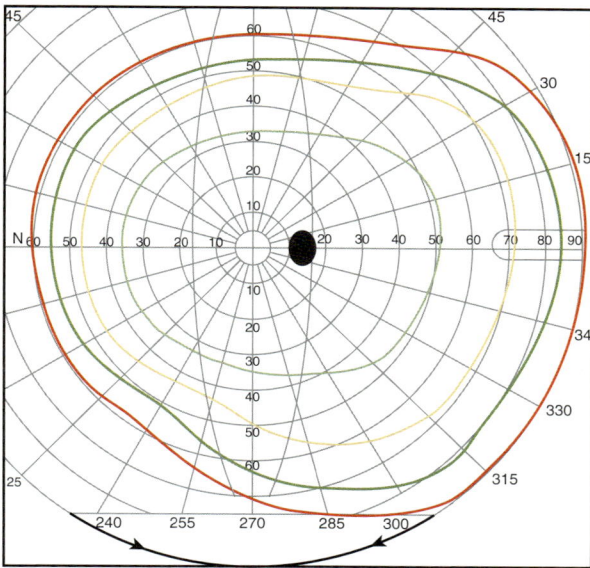

FIGURE 2–6 ■ Goldmann visual field. The blind spot is in its normal location, approximately 15° from the center of fixation. Goldmann visual field testing is performed manually, which is often easier for young children. The different colored lines indicate varying light intensities used for testing. The farther from the center, the brighter the light must be for the patient to detect it.

optic nerve often cause central or paracentral defects; glaucoma causes defects in an arcuate pattern emanating from the blind spot. Central nervous system abnormalities may produce specific visual field loss that can help localize the site of the lesion. These defects are discussed further in Chapter 33.

PUPILLOGRAPHY

Very sophisticated measurements of the pupillary responses can be made with pupillography. This is performed in a darkened room using infrared lights and video cameras to monitor and measure the pupil reactions. The amount of light shined into the eyes is controlled, and image analysis software is used to record the pupil responses (Figure 2–7). This test is particularly useful for measuring subtle relative afferent pupillary defects, which provides an objective measure of visual dysfunction.

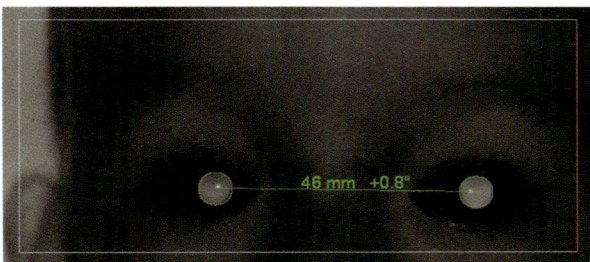

FIGURE 2–7 ■ Pupillography, performed by computer analysis of pupil images as they respond to light.

PACHYMETRY

Pachymetry measures the thickness of the cornea. The tip of a small portable device is brought into contact with the cornea and rapidly obtains a measurement. The test is performed using topical anesthetic drops. In young children it may require an examination under anesthesia. The corneal thickness may be affected in certain corneal disorders. Thickening due to edema frequently occurs in infantile glaucoma.

VISUAL EVOKED POTENTIALS

In addition to the spatial sweep test discussed above, other forms of visual evoked potentials can be performed to assess different aspects of visual function.

Flash Visual Evoked Potentials (FVEPs)

This test is used primarily to measure optic nerve function. Using electrodes overlying the occipital lobe to measure cortical activity, a bright light is flashed into each eye independently. The *amplitude* of the response measures the amount of cortical activity produced by the stimulus. The *latency* of the response measures the delay between the onset of the light flash and the recording of activity in the occipital lobe (Figure 2–8). In general, compressive, ischemic, or toxic optic nerve lesions cause a decrease in the amplitude of the response, and defects in myelinization cause an increase in the latency.

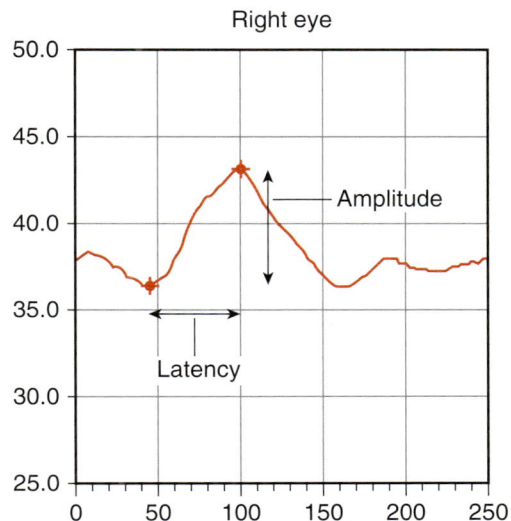

FIGURE 2–8 ■ Normal flash visual evoked potential. The *y*-coordinates measure voltage and the *x*-coordinates measure time (milliseconds). The amplitude is the voltage between the trough and the peak. The latency is the time between the trough and peak.

Lateralization Visual Evoked Potentials (LVEPs)

This is a specialized form of VEP that measures how light is transmitted to the different occipital lobes. It is used primarily as a diagnostic test for albinism. In normal individuals approximately half of the visual information in each eye is transferred to one occipital cortex and half to the other. The temporal retinal impulses project to the ipsilateral cortex, and nasal retinal impulses cross the optic chiasm and project to the contralateral occipital cortex. In a normal individual, a bright light shined into one eye produces symmetric responses on each side (Figure 2–9A).

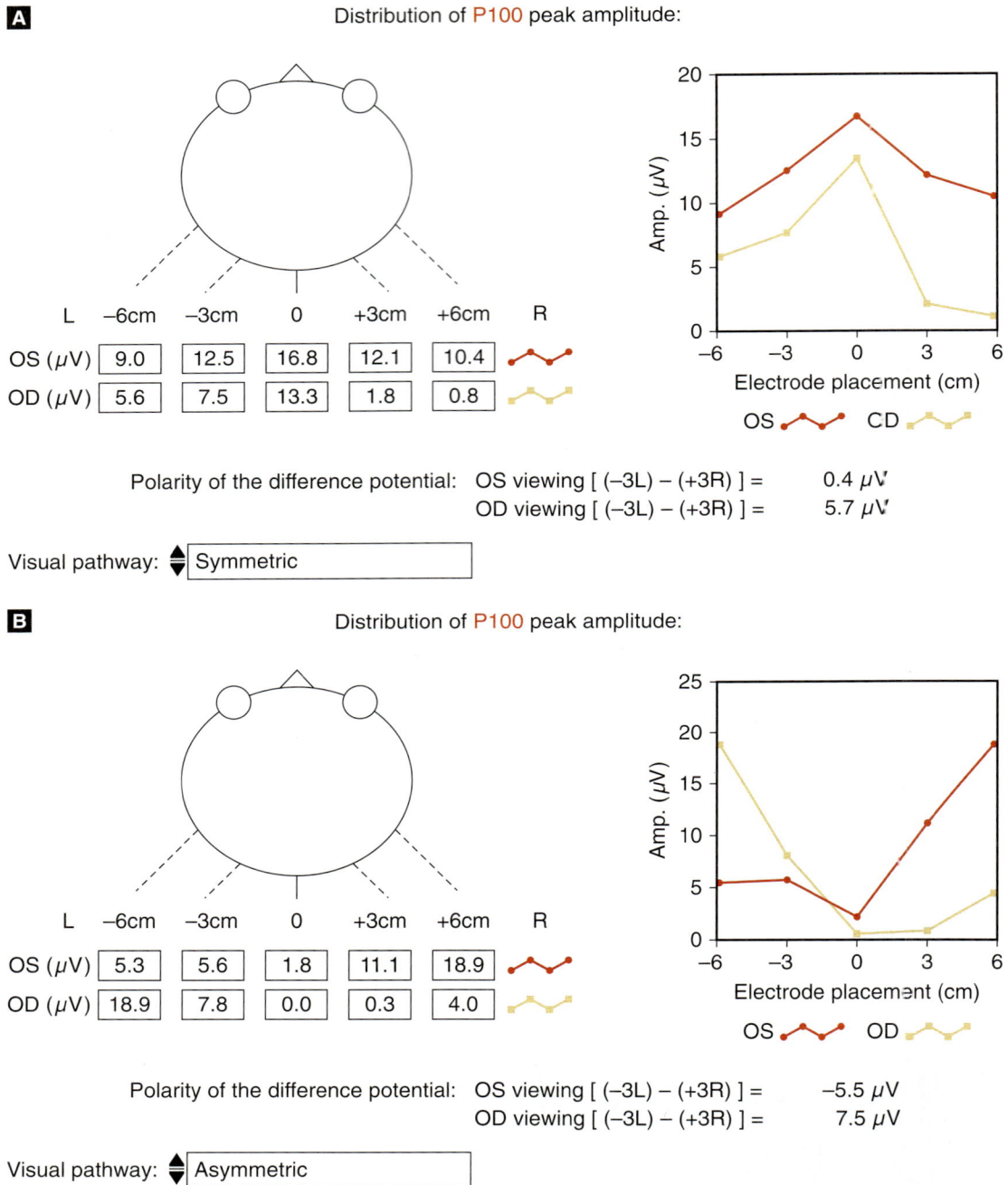

A Distribution of P100 peak amplitude:

	L	−6cm	−3cm	0	+3cm	+6cm	R
OS (μV)		9.0	12.5	16.8	12.1	10.4	
OD (μV)		5.6	7.5	13.3	1.8	0.8	

Polarity of the difference potential: OS viewing [(−3L) − (+3R)] = 0.4 μV
OD viewing [(−3L) − (+3R)] = 5.7 μV

Visual pathway: Symmetric

B Distribution of P100 peak amplitude:

	L	−6cm	−3cm	0	+3cm	+6cm	R
OS (μV)		5.3	5.6	1.8	11.1	18.9	
OD (μV)		18.9	7.8	0.0	0.3	4.0	

Polarity of the difference potential: OS viewing [(−3L) − (+3R)] = −5.5 μV
OD viewing [(−3L) − (+3R)] = 7.5 μV

Visual pathway: Asymmetric

FIGURE 2–9 ■ Lateralization visual evoked potentials. (A) Normal results. The graphical representation at the upper left shows the position of the eyes (top) and the locations of the occipital lobe electrodes. Beneath this are the voltage recordings at the various positions. OS refers to lights flashed in the left eye and OD to the right eye. On the right is a graphical representation of the response. In normal patients approximately half of the visual input from each eye goes to each occipital lobe. (B) Results in a patient with albinism, showing characteristic abnormal decussation of the visual pathways. When a light is flashed in each eye, a larger response is generated in the contralateral occipital lobe. The graph at right reflects this asymmetry.

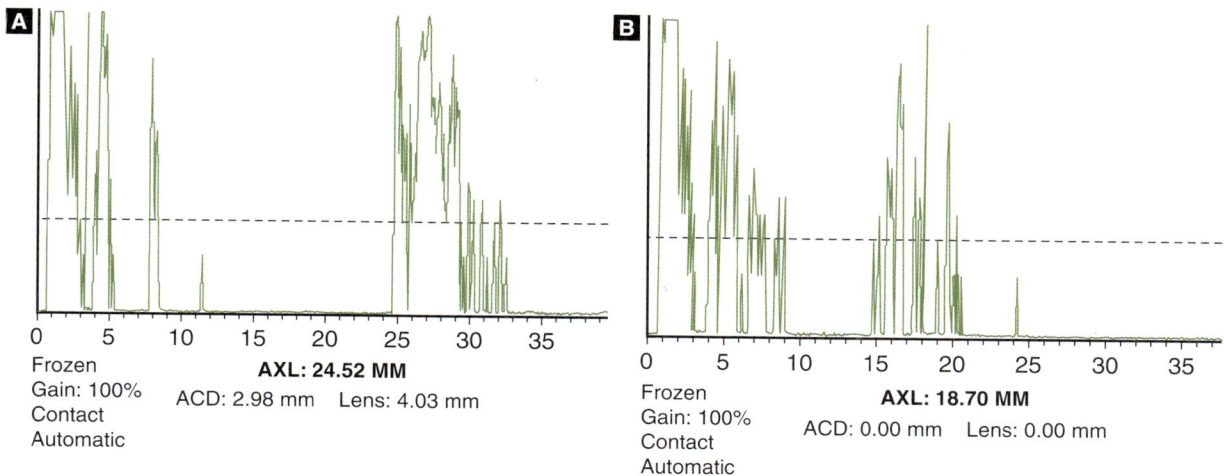

FIGURE 2–10 ■ A-scan ultrasonography. (A) Normal left eye. "AXL" refers to axial eye length, which is 23.76 mm in this patient. "ACD" refers to anterior chamber depth (2.98 mm), and the thickness of the lens is 4.03 mm. The peaks represent different structures in the eye. The central space between peaks represents the optically empty vitreous cavity (normal on this scan). (B) The patient's right eye is microphthalmic due to a retinal detachment. The axial eye length is considerably shorter (18.70 mm). The anterior chamber depth and lens thickness cannot be measured due to noise from the abnormal retinal tissue.

In albinism, a characteristic finding is an increase in the percentage of decussating fibers, such that 70% to 80% of the visual information from one eye will be projected to the contralateral occipital cortex, and the remaining 20% to 30% to the ipsilateral occipital cortex. When a light is shined into an albino's eye, the response from the contralateral cortex will therefore be greater than the response over the ipsilateral cortex. This is a very specific abnormality (Figure 2–9B). It is particularly useful in diagnosing *ocular albinism*, in which affected patients do not have the characteristic marked decrease in skin, hair, and iris pigmentation that occurs in *oculocutaneous albinism*.

ULTRASONOGRAPHY

Ultrasonography is a very useful test that can be performed even in awake young children with little difficulty. In ultrasonography, ultrasound impulses are projected into the eye. By measuring the characteristics of the reflected waves, important information can be obtained. There are 2 main types of ultrasonograpy:

A-Scan Ultrasonograpy

A-scan ultrasonograpy is used primarily to measure the length of the eye, and sometimes to monitor the size of lesions within the eye (Figure 2–10A and B). The measurements are very precise. Clinically, the eye length is most important in calculating intraocular lens power in patients undergoing cataract surgery with intraocular lens implantation, and in monitoring for abnormal eye growth in patients with glaucoma.

B-Scan Ultrasonography

B-scan ultrasonography provides a cross-sectional view of the inside of the eye (Figure 2–11). It has several important clinical applications.

■ In some patients the retina cannot be directly visualized, such as those with cataracts or vitreous hemorrhage. The retina can be imaged with ultrasonography to look for retinal detachment or other abnormalities in these patients (Figure 2–12A and B).
■ The characteristics of the ultrasound image may provide diagnostic information in patients with retinoblastoma or other retinal lesion. The response

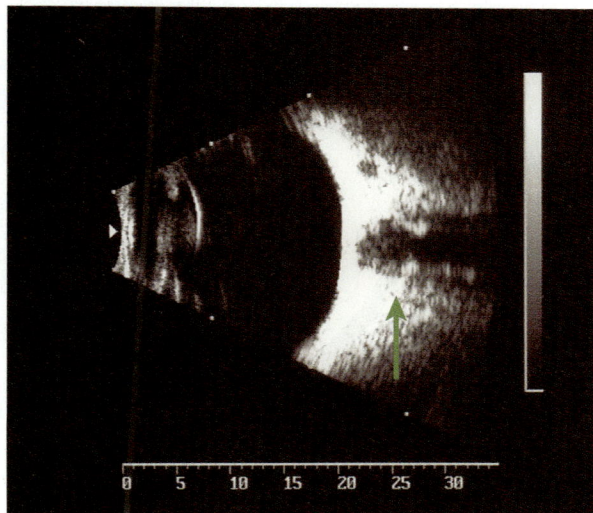

FIGURE 2–11 ■ Normal B-scan ultrasonogram. The anterior portion of the eye is on the left and the posterior retina on the right. The black portion behind the eye (arrow) is the optic nerve.

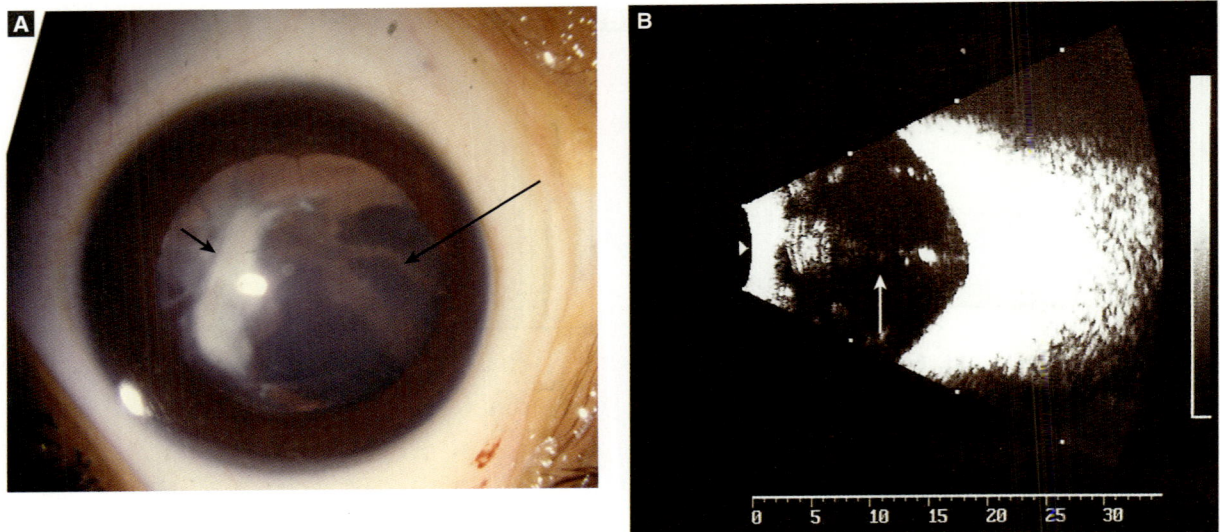

FIGURE 2–12 ■ (A) Persistent fetal vasculature with cataract (small arrow) and central contraction of ciliary processes (long arrow). The retina cannot be directly visualized due to these abnormalities. (B) B-scan ultrasound shows stalk of tissue extending between optic nerve and lens (arrow), a common finding in persistent fetal vasculature (discussed in Chapter 30).

of tumors to treatment can be monitored with serial examinations.

■ Some patients with pseudopapilledema have optic nerve head drusen. These are calcified lesions that can often be identified ultrasonographically by bright reflections from the optic nerve head (see Chapter 33).

Ultrasound Biomicroscopy

This is a specialized form of ultrasonography in which high-resolution images of the anterior segment structures in the eye can be obtained. It is useful in evaluating abnormalities of the cornea, iris, lens, and outflow paths in glaucoma.

ELECTRORETINOGRAM (ERG)

ERGs are used to measure the function of the retina. They are employed primarily in the assessment of inherited retinal disorders. Lights with different characteristics are shined into the eyes, and a special contact lens measures the electrical responses generated by the rods, cones, and other cells within the retina. In children, the testing usually requires sedation (Figure 2–13A and B).

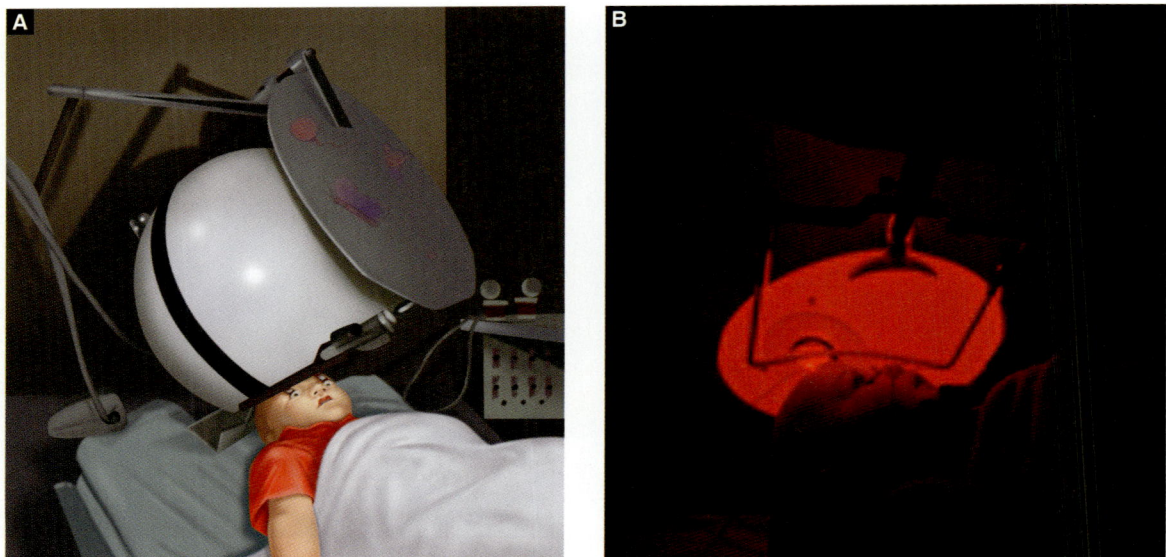

FIGURE 2–13 ■ (A) Patient undergoing sedated ERG. (B) Different colors and intensities of light are shined into the patient's eyes, and the electrical response generated by the retina is recorded.

The contribution of the rods and cones can be isolated by changing the type of light stimulus. To measure rod function, the patient is placed in a dark room for approximately 30 minutes; then a dim white light is flashed into the eyes. To measure cone function, the test is performed in an illuminated room with a bright light, and by using a high-frequency stimulus that only cones can respond to. The normal ERG response has an initial negative A-wave, which is generated by the photoreceptors, than a positive B-wave, which is generated by the retinal cells that transmit information between the photoreceptors and the ganglion cells. By analyzing the responses to the various test conditions, one can determine what type of retinal disorder is present.

ELECTROOCULOGRAM

This test is similar to an ERG in that it measures electrical potentials within the eye. It primarily assesses the function of the retinal pigment epithelium. It is not widely used, but may be diagnostic in patients with Best vitelliform dystrophy.

OPTICAL COHERENCE TOMOGRAPHY (OCT)

OCT is a relatively new technology that has not been used widely in children. It is similar to ultrasonograpy in that images are produced by analysis of reflected light within the retina. OCT is used primarily to obtain very fine images of the macula, with resolution approaching that of histological sections (Figure 2–14). It can also measure the nerve fiber layer, which can be used to monitor ganglion cell loss in patients with glaucoma. The use of this technology in pediatric patients will likely increase as the portability of the instruments improves.

RETINAL IMAGING

Retinal Fundus Photography

Various instruments are available to image the retina. Such images are useful for documenting findings and monitoring changes. A widely used instrument in pediatrics is the RetCam (Massie Labratories, Pleasanton, CA). This is a portable system with specially designed lenses that can be used to capture images. It is very useful in documenting retinal findings in children with suspected abuse, and in monitoring tumors in patients

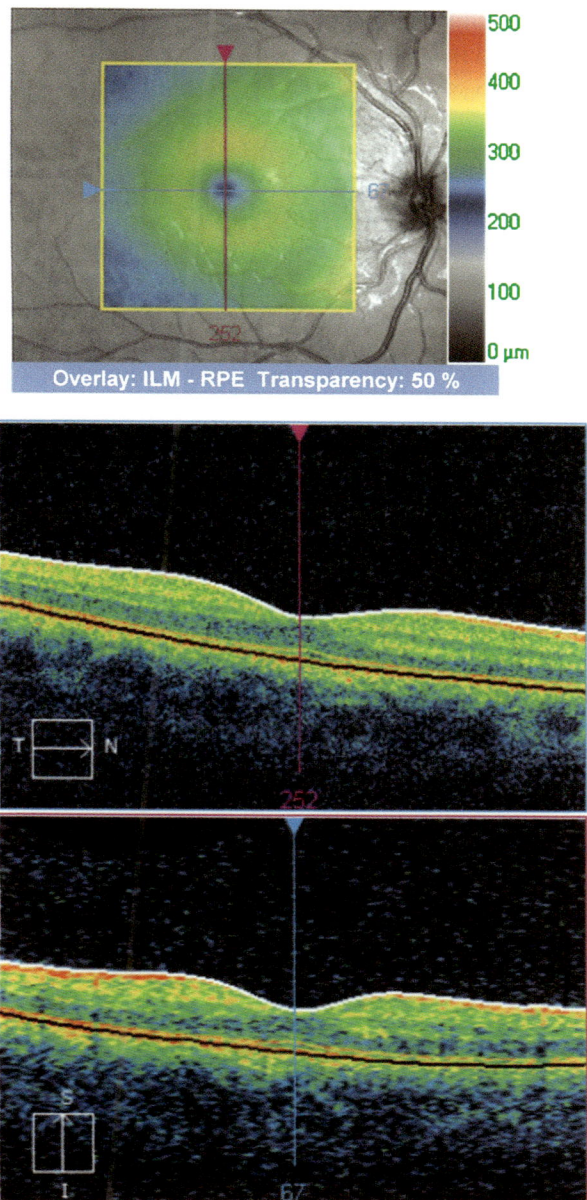

FIGURE 2–14 ■ Optical coherence tomography (normal). The top portion is an image of the posterior retina, centered on the fovea. The bottom images represent the vertical and horizontal axes through the fovea. The central depressions represent the normal foveal pit, and the different colors represent the various layers of the retina.

with retinoblastoma. Remote acquisition of images in neonatal intensive care units, with central reading by an ophthalmologist, is being evaluated as a possible alternative method of screening for retinopathy of prematurity.

Fundus Fluorescein Angiography

This test is performed by injecting intravenous fluorescein dye into a patient, then photographing the retina as the dye circulates. The patient sits at a slitlamp during the imaging process. Special filters are used to stimulate fluorescence and image the response. The test is particularly useful for documenting leakage of fluid from retinal blood vessels, such as occurs with diabetic retinopathy. In practice, the test is rarely used in children due to the necessity of injection and cooperation during acquisition of images. This imaging technique is an alternative method for diagnosing optic nerve head drusen, which demonstrate autofluorescence (which does not require dye injection) (Figure 2–15).

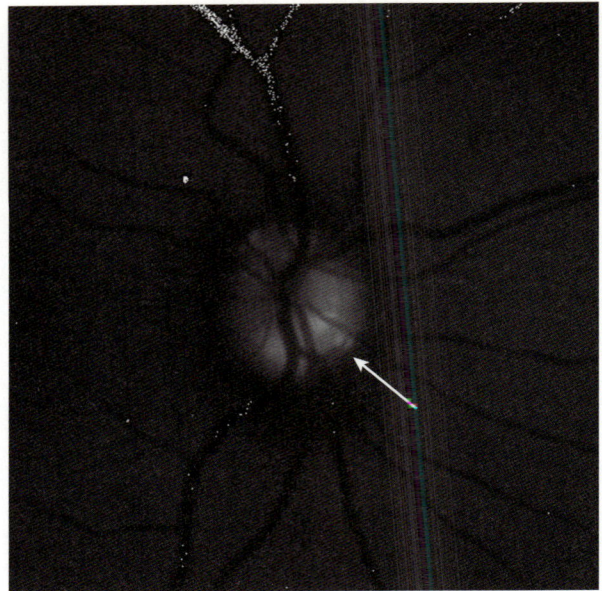

FIGURE 2–15 ■ Autofluorescence of optic nerve head (arrow) due to drusen, imaged using the same filters used for fluorescein angiography.

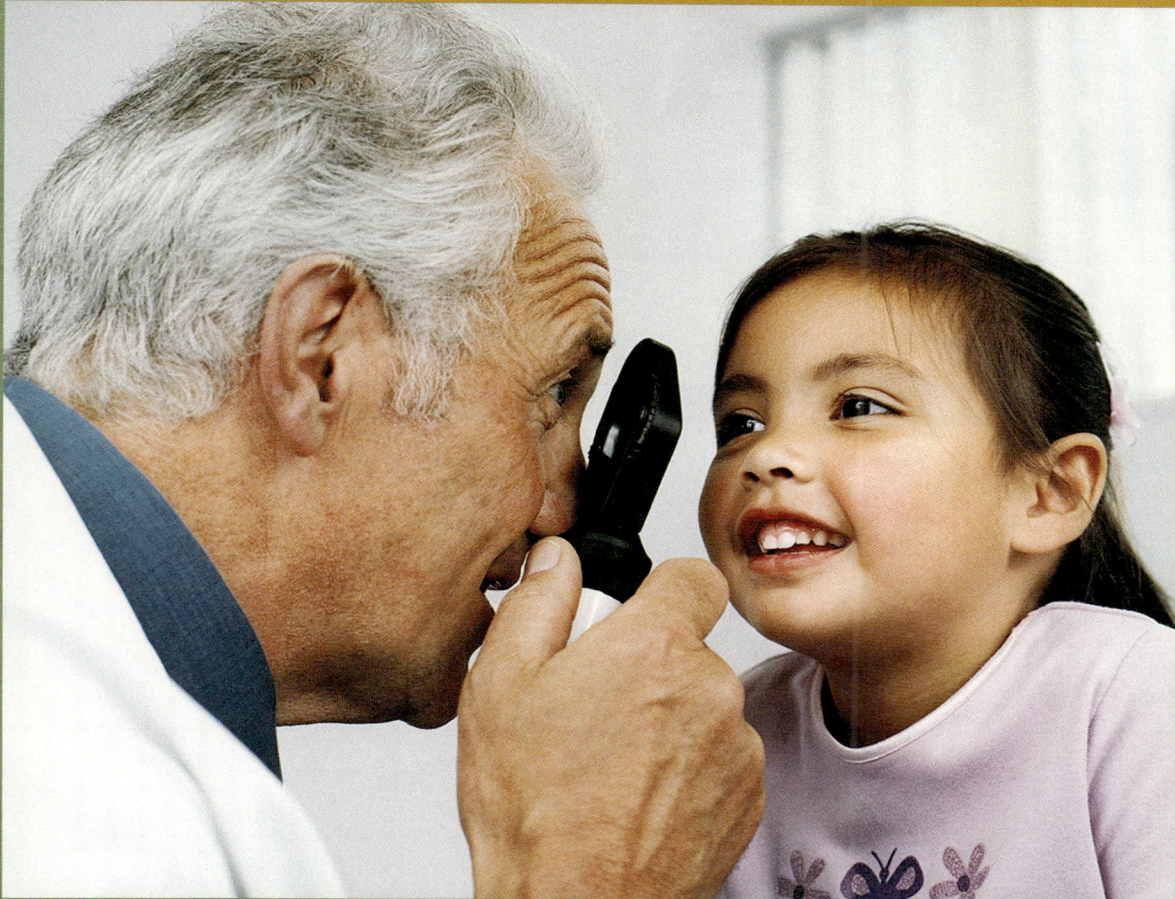

Symptoms

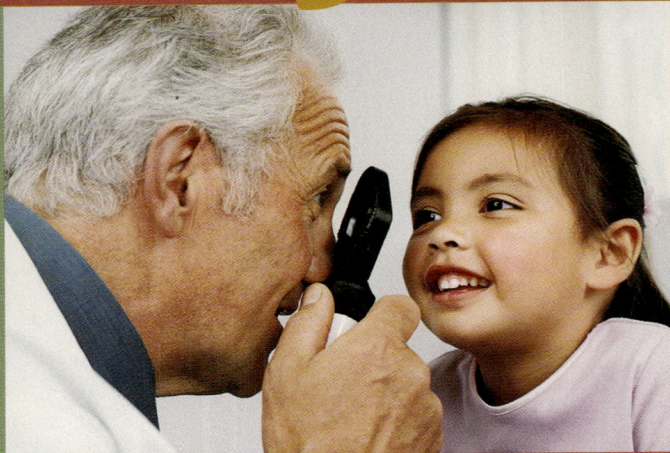

CHAPTER 3

The Infant Who Does Not Appear To See

The Problem
"My baby doesn't see."

Common Causes
Otherwise normal baby:
  delayed visual maturation
Central nervous system problems:
  cortical visual impairment
Underlying eye problem with
  decreased vision

KEY FINDINGS

History
Other medical problems?
Family history of vision loss in young children?

Examination
Any response to light
Nystagmus
Pupil reactions

WHAT SHOULD YOU DO?

If history and examination are otherwise normal, wait 2 months to refer.

If nystagmus or abnormal pupils are present, refer.

What Shouldn't Be Missed

Septo-optic dysplasia should not be missed owing to the potential for pituitary dysfunction.

COMMON CAUSES

During the first 1 to 2 months of life, visual behavior in infants varies widely. Some babies fixate immediately after birth, whereas others take several weeks to begin tracking. At the 1-month well-child examination parents may specifically express concern if their baby is not fixating. Others may not be aware of any problems, but you will notice poor tracking on your examination. If everything else is normal (see the following sections), an appropriate plan is to wait until 2 months of age to see whether the tracking spontaneously improves, which will occur in most cases.

By 2 months of age, the absence of fixation does not necessarily mean that there is an underlying problem, but the level of concern is raised. Referral to a pediatric ophthalmologist is appropriate at this time. Items from the history and ocular examination can help determine what additional steps are indicated.

There are 3 main categories for infants who are not fixating by 2 months of age:

1. *Infants who are otherwise normal, and have no other ocular abnormalities.*
   These children most commonly have *delayed visual maturation* (DVM) (also known as *cortical inattention*). The eyes themselves are fine in these babies, but the cortical connections that allow the brain to perceive images and make appropriate behavioral responses are underdeveloped. Most of these children will improve by 4 to 6 months of age, and further

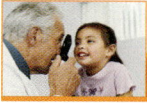

Table 3–1.

Systemic Diseases That May Cause Visual Tracking Delay

- Prematurity (<32 weeks gestation)
- Perinatal hypoxia
- Hydrocephalus
- Seizure disorder
- Trisomy 21
- Any serious medical illness (e.g., cardiac disease, pulmonary disease)
- Any disorder associated with developmental delay

workup by the ophthalmologist is not indicated early in life, unless other abnormalities are found on the eye examination. If the infants continue to demonstrate poor fixation when they return for their follow-up examination with the ophthalmologist, additional testing will be necessary.

2. *History of serious systemic disease.*

Any significant illness, particularly one that affects the central nervous system, may cause a delay in visual tracking in infants (Table 3–1). Common diseases include prematurity (especially less than 30 weeks gestation), perinatal hypoxia, hydrocephalus, and seizure disorders. Children with other severe systemic diseases, such as cardiac or pulmonary disorders, may also not track well initially.

Children with developmental delay, regardless of the etiology, also frequently take longer than usual to begin tracking normally. However, because of the wide variability in normal development in the first few months of life, and because isolated poor visual tracking may be confused with general developmental delay, it may be difficult to determine whether children are delayed until they are several months old.

Children with these other medical problems may have DVM, but it frequently takes more time to improve than similarly affected normal infants described above. If the vision does not improve, *cortical visual impairment* (CVI) may be present. Unlike DVM, in which normal cortical connections eventually form, children with CVI are assumed to have structural abnormalities in the visual processing portions of the brain. Although the vision in affected patients usually improves with age, it may not reach normal levels.

3. *Children with primary vision disorders.*

If an infant has an ocular problem that seriously affects vision, a pattern of abnormalities typically develops by 2 to 3 months of age. Depending on the severity of the underlying disorder, the infants may have no or minimal reactions to light, even when very bright lights are shined directly into the eyes. The absence of pupil reactions to light is another manifestation of severe vision loss. Although this is an excellent objective measure of visual function, the pupil reaction may be difficult to assess in a newborn. If infants do not have normal vision, nystagmus usually develops around 2 months of age. The combination of these 3 findings (abnormal pupil reactions, no or minimal fixation, and nystagmus) suggests a serious underlying problem, and further investigations are warranted. The list of potential etiologies is very long, including congenital retinal dystrophies (e.g., Leber's congenital amaurosis), cataracts, optic nerve hypoplasia, severe retinopathy of prematurity, and multiple other disorders.

The presence of nystagmus alone, in an otherwise normal infant who seems to be fixating and tracking well, may be due to congenital motor nystagmus (infantile nystagmus syndrome). In this condition the eyes themselves are normal. The nystagmus is caused by abnormalities of the visual motor system. The visual prognosis for these children is good (see further Chapter 34).

An unusual eye movement disorder that may simulate poor vision in an infant is congenital ocular motor apraxia (COMA). In this condition the eyes themselves are normal, but patients cannot generate normal eye movements. The assessment of normal infant vision is based on behavior, particularly noting that the baby moves their eyes to look at objects. In COMA, the inability to make these movements may be mistaken for poor vision. These infants will respond to bright lights and smile appropriately when they are looking at faces, but they cannot track objects that are moved back and forth in front of them. When the infants get older, they learn to move their heads to generate eye movements, creating an unusual head thrusting when they want to localize an object in their peripheral field of vision.

APPROACH TO THE PATIENT

History

The presence of poor fixation in a 1- to 2-month-old baby may be brought to your attention by the child's parents, or you may notice it during your examination. Because you will likely have been caring for the patient since birth, you will be aware of any significant systemic illnesses that could contribute to poor tracking (e.g., prematurity, serious cardiac disease). The parents should be asked about any family history of ocular problems in infants (inherited retinal disorders, cataracts, etc.).

General questions about development will be a routine part of your well-child examination. In the first 1 to 2 months of life, however, normal development varies widely. Because of this, it is often difficult to identify with certainty whether an infant is delayed. The presence of poor fixation may further confuse the issue: Is the baby truly delayed, and therefore not tracking well, or is the baby otherwise normal, but appears delayed because of poor visual tracking? The answer will usually become more clear by 4 to 6 months of age.

Parent's intuitive impressions of their infant's vision are usually quite accurate. They should be asked whether they have any concerns about their baby's vision, whether the baby responds to bright lights, and whether the baby "locks in" on their faces. They should also be asked whether they have noted any abnormal eye movements.

Examination

The examination should include an age-appropriate assessment of vision. Does the baby fixate on your face? Will the baby track your face as you move from side to side? If the baby does not track, you should assess whether the baby responds to lights. Watch the baby in a dark room when you turn on the room lights, or shine a bright light into the eyes. If the baby squints, then at least some visual connections must be present. A good objective measure of visual response is the *eye-popping reflex* (Figure 3–1A and B). Watch the baby when the room lights are dimmed suddenly. Normal awake babies will often open their eyes widely when this occurs, indicating the presence of some vision.

Assessment of the pupils is useful when evaluating infants with poor fixation, but it may be difficult in a baby, for several reasons. First, even in normal infants the iris may not be fully developed, and may respond sluggishly. Second, infants often squint their eyes when exposed to sudden bright lights, which makes it hard to see the pupil response. Third, the pupil will constrict normally with accommodation (focusing at near). Infants often spontaneously do this, so it may be difficult to determine whether a pupil response is due to a bright light or accommodation. Finally, some rare conditions (e.g., achromatopsia) may have a paradoxical pupil response—the pupils constrict in dim light and dilate in bright light.

The red reflex should be carefully evaluated in babies who are not fixating well. Abnormal red reflexes may result from many abnormalities that cause decreased vision, including opacities of the cornea or lens (cataracts), retinal detachments or tumors, and large colobomas.

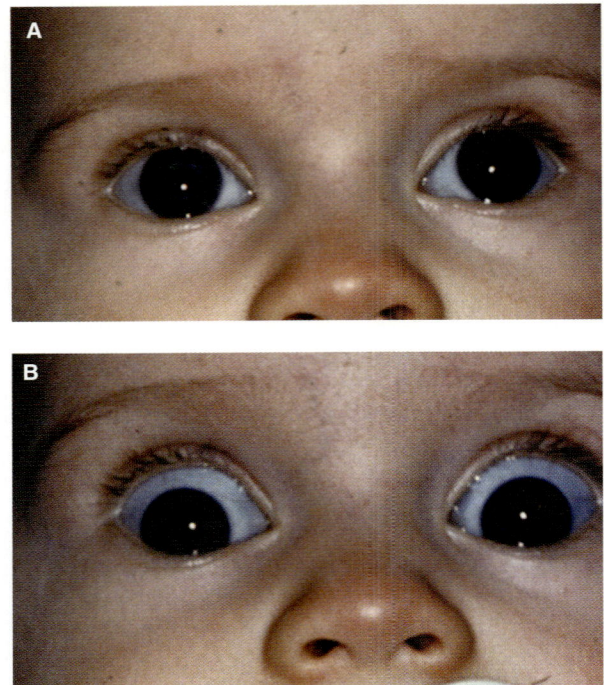

FIGURE 3–1 ■ Eye-popping response: (A) Baby in room light and (B) baby opens eyes widely when room light turned off, indicating that the baby is able to perceive the change in room illumination.

The presence of abnormal eye movements should also be noted. A wide variety of eye movement abnormalities may occur transiently in the first 1 to 2 months of life. Occasional brief eye crossing, tonic up- or downgaze, and brief nystagmus may be normal. The presence of constant strabismus (most commonly eye crossing in infants), nystagmus, or wandering eye movements is not normal, and may indicate a more serious problem (Table 3–2).

PLAN

1. If the infant is otherwise healthy, there is no family history of early eye diseases, and the examination is normal except for poor fixation, it is appropriate to recommend waiting until the baby is 2 months old and reassess the vision. The family can be told that the vision will likely improve, but that the presence of an abnormality cannot be excluded with certainty at this young age. If the baby is still not fixating by age 2 months, referral to a pediatric ophthalmologist is appropriate.
2. At age 1 month or older, if the baby has other examination findings that suggest poor vision (no response to light at all, nystagmus or wandering eye movements, no pupil reaction), then referral to a pediatric ophthalmologist is indicated.

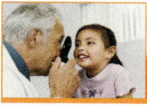

Table 3–2.

Worrisome Versus Less Worrisome Signs and Symptoms of Vision Problems in a Newborn

	Worrisome	Less worrisome
Parents' report of visual responses	None	At least some
Response to light on examination	None	At least some
Nystagmus or wandering eye movements	Yes	No
Pupil reactions to light	Poor or absent	Normal
Red reflex	Abnormal	Normal

WHAT SHOULDN'T BE MISSED

One of the frequent causes of poor vision in infants is *septo-optic dysplasia*. In this disorder, underdevelopment of the optic nerves (*optic nerve hypoplasia*) is associated with central nervous system abnormalities, which may include an *ectopic pituitary gland*. Endocrine function is abnormal in infants with ectopic pituitary glands, and the dysfunction may include *adrenocorticotropic hormone deficiency*. Affected children may not be able to mount a normal stress response, and are at risk of serious problems should they become ill. These children normally present in the first few months of life with minimal fixation and abnormal eye movements. The diagnosis is made by examination of the optic nerves, magnetic resonance imaging, and evaluation of the child by a pediatric endocrinologist. If the diagnosis is suspected, the baby's family should be warned of this possibility while the workup is in progress, emphasizing the need for prompt evaluation should the infant become ill (Figure 3–2).

When to Refer

- Infant not tracking normally by 2 months of age
- Infant not tracking at any age with nystagmus or abnormal pupil reactions

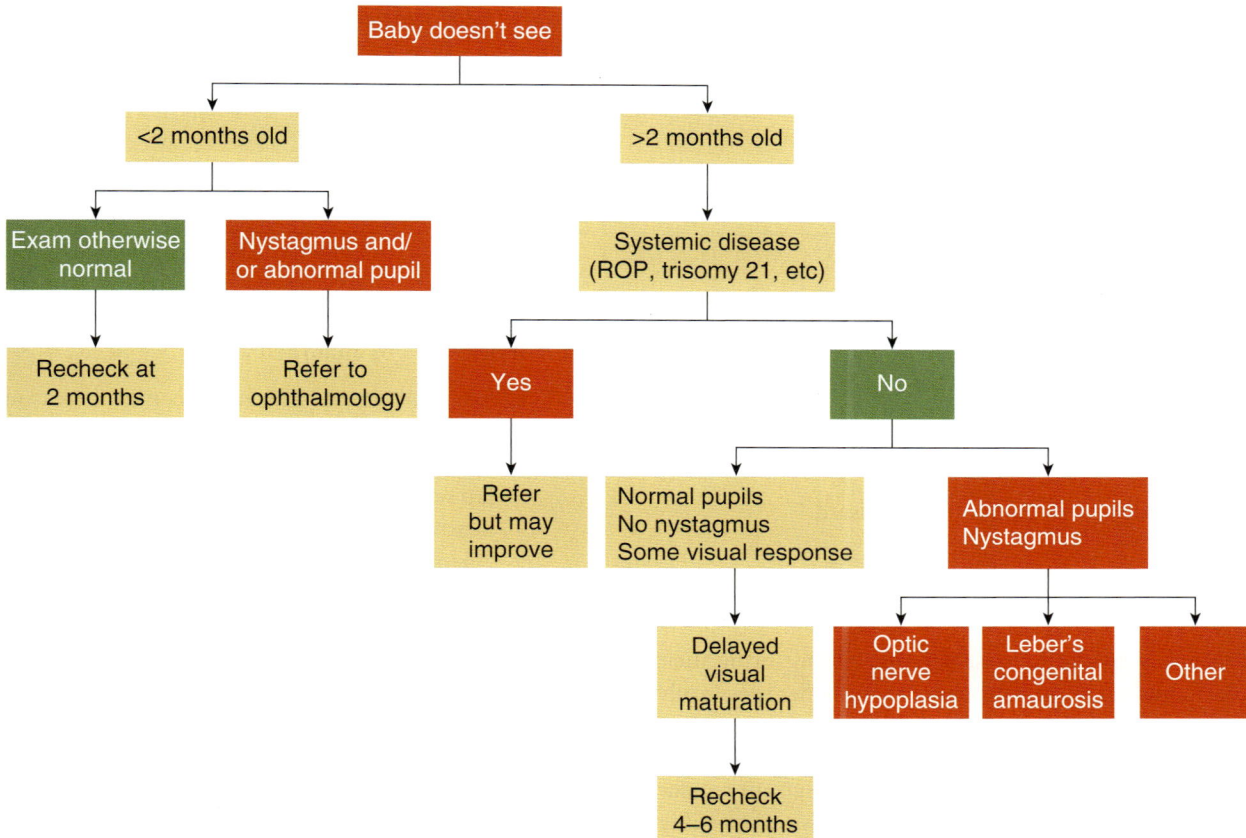

FIGURE 3–2 ■ Algorithm for evaluation of an infant who does not appear to see.

CHAPTER 4

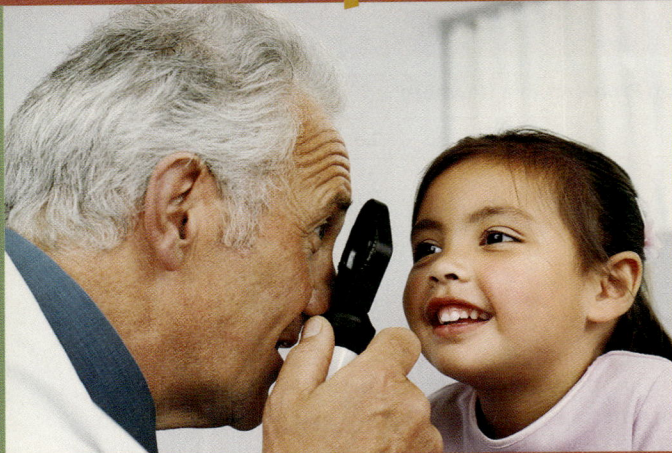

Decreased Vision in Older Children

The Problem

"My child is having trouble seeing."

Common Causes

Needs glasses
Learning disorder
Wants glasses
Dry eyes
Colored spots
   Physiological after-images
   Migraine

KEY FINDINGS

History

Needs glasses:
   Trouble seeing board at school, squinting

Learning disability:
   Trouble reading, normal visual acuity
Wants glasses:
   Peer at school recently got "cool" glasses
Dry eyes:
   Trouble after reading for several minutes, eye irritation
Colored spots:
   Physiological: No other complaints
   Migraine: Associated headache

Examination

Check vision on eye chart
Check for papilledema

WHAT SHOULD YOU DO?

Refer to an ophthalmologist.

What Shouldn't Be Missed

Learning disorders should not be missed.

COMMON CAUSES

Practically speaking, most parents will not bring their older children to their primary care provider specifically because of complaints of decreased or abnormal vision. Vision problems will usually come to attention either by your specific questions about vision during your regular well-child history, or if the child fails a vision screening test in the office.

There are several reasons older children may complain of decreased or abnormal vision:

1. *Need for glasses.* The most common reason children and young adults need glasses is myopia (nearsightedness). Patients with myopia can see things at near, but have difficulty seeing clearly in the distance. Myopia usually begins during grade school and typically worsens gradually. It is not uncommon for children with myopia to be unaware that they have a vision problem until it is specifically brought to their attention. This may occur either during a vision screening test or if the child is with someone who notes a distant object that the child cannot see (Table 4–1).

2. *Learning disorders.* Children with learning disabilities frequently complain that they are

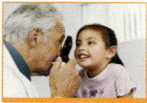

Table 4–1.

Signs and Symptoms of Myopia

- Can't see things other family members or friends can see
- Squinting when viewing distant objects
- Sitting close to television (but this is also common in children without vision problems)

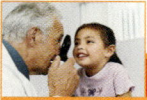

Table 4–3.

Signs and Symptoms of Dry Eyes

- Blurred vision begins after a period of concentration (reading, watching TV, etc.)
- Complaints of eye irritation
- Symptoms worse in cold, dry weather

Table 4–2.

Signs and Symptoms of Learning Disorder

- Complaint of difficulty reading
- Often does well in subjects that require less reading (e.g., math)
- Normal eye examination
  - Normal visual acuity
  - Normal accommodation
  - No strabismus

having trouble seeing. However, the problem for the vast majority of children with reading problems is not the eyes, but the processing of written information in the brain. It is important that these children be evaluated to verify that they do not have an underlying visual problem. If the eyes are fine, these children are best served with additional educational assistance (Table 4–2).

3. *The child wants glasses.* Some children, typically in early elementary school, may feign vision problems due to a desire to wear glasses. Most commonly, this occurs after someone in their class has received glasses that bring them

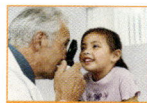

positive attention (such as glasses with a cartoon character theme). Such children are often visibly disappointed when told they do not need to wear glasses.

4. *Dry eyes.* Problems with the tear film in children are not uncommon, and they are a frequently overlooked cause of blurred vision. A stable tear film is necessary to form crisp visual images. Children with dry eyes usually complain that things become blurry after they have been reading for a while. They may also complain of eye irritation (Table 4–3).

5. *Colored spots.* There are 2 common etiologies for children who describe colored spots. The first is physiological after-images. These are natural phenomena that occur after looking at lights. They can be demonstrated by looking at a bright light (such as a flashlight) in a dark room. When the light is turned off, persistent images can be appreciated. A striking example is illustrated in Figure 4–1. Physiological after-images occur in adults, but are usually ignored. Children may spontaneously report them, typically around age 5 or 6 years. The second common cause of seeing colored spots is migraine-associated phenomena. Classic migraines may be preceded by various visual symptoms, including colored spots, jagged streaks, sparkling lights, visual field loss,

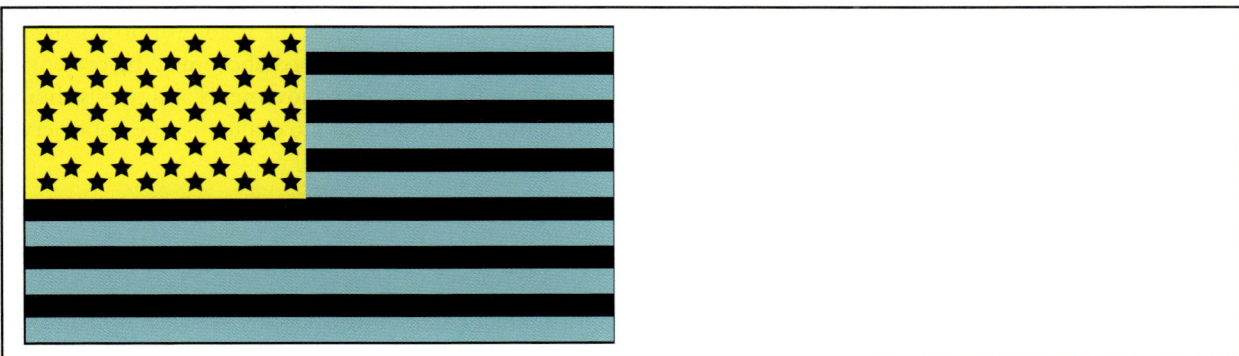

FIGURE 4–1 ■ Flag after image illusion. To experience this effect, stare at the center of the flag for 30 seconds, then look at the white area to the right of the picture. You should see an image of the flag with the normal red, white, and blue coloring. If you have trouble appreciating the image, try blinking a few times as you look at the white page.

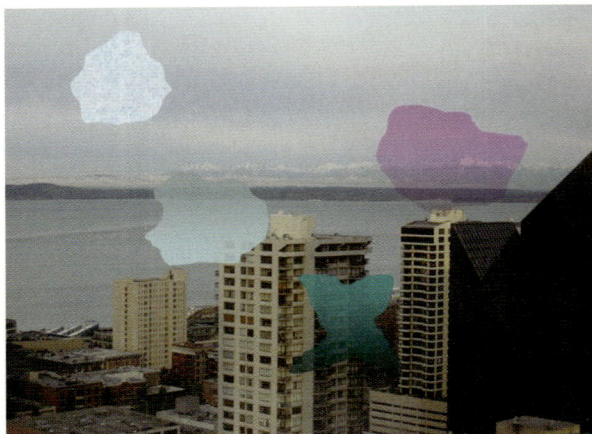

FIGURE 4–2 ■ Migraine phenomenon. Patients with prodromal symptoms may report seeing colored spots before the onset of the headache.

or a sensation similar to looking through jet flumes (Figure 4–2).

APPROACH TO THE PATIENT

History

A focused history is very helpful in sorting out the various causes for decreased vision. Most myopia (nearsightedness) begins in about third or fourth grade. Children may spontaneously complain of difficulty seeing the board at school, and they sometimes squint when trying to view distant objects. It is not uncommon, however, for children to be unaware of a vision problem. This is why vision screening is important. Sitting close to the television set and holding books closely when reading may also raise a suspicion of myopia, but these are common behaviors in children younger than 4 to 5 years, most of whom have no vision problems. There is a genetic component to myopia, so one should ask whether other family members wear glasses.

Children with learning disorders are usually identified in early-grade school, when the child is noted to lag behind his or her peers in school. Some patients have other developmental delays, and the learning problems can be ascribed to these. However, many children with specific reading problems are of normal or above-normal intelligence. They have specific difficulty processing written information. They often do better in subjects that do not require reading, such as math, and worse in subjects that rely on written information. They sometimes specifically complain about having trouble seeing, even if the visual acuity and eye examination are normal. The combination of these complaints and normal examination is often what brings the diagnosis of a reading disorder to light.

If one suspects that the child's agenda is to get glasses, most will answer direct questions honestly. Asking if someone in the child's class has gotten glasses, if the child likes the glasses, and if the child is hoping to get similar glasses will usually be answered affirmatively.

The presence of vision difficulties due to dry eyes can also be strongly suspected based on history. The rate of blinking normally decreases when visually concentrating, such as while reading or watching a movie. If the tear film is unstable, this will produce blurring as the tears evaporate. Therefore, one should ask the child whether things are blurry immediately when they start reading, or whether they become blurry after reading for a few minutes. If the latter is reported, dry eyes are likely. Children with dry eyes may also complain of intermittent eye irritation and increased sensitivity to bright lights.

The differentiation between physiological colored spots and migraine-associated visual phenomena is usually straightforward. Children with physiological afterimages are usually not bothered by them.[1] They are brought to attention when they tell their parents they are seeing them, often in casual conversation. They report no other visual problems. Children who present for evaluation of this problem are typically bright and articulate. It is most common in kindergarten or first grade.

Children with colored spots associated with migraine will usually have associated headaches, typically shortly after the visual symptoms begin. Some patients, however, may experience the visual changes without the headaches (*acephalgic migraine*). The presence of headache, particularly accompanied by photophobia and nausea and/or vomiting, supports this diagnosis. Most patients have a family history of migraine.

Examination

Older children who present with complaints of vision problems should have their visual acuity checked with an eye chart. If the vision is decreased, a need for glasses is the most likely reason. If the vision is normal, one of the other problems discussed above may be present. A brief examination of eye movements and pupils should be performed, in addition to evaluating the optic nerves for papilledema.

PLAN

Most older children with specific visual complaints will require referral to an eye specialist. If the acuity is decreased on the eye chart, and the child is older than 5 years, evaluation with either an optometrist or ophthalmologist is indicated to check for glasses. If one of

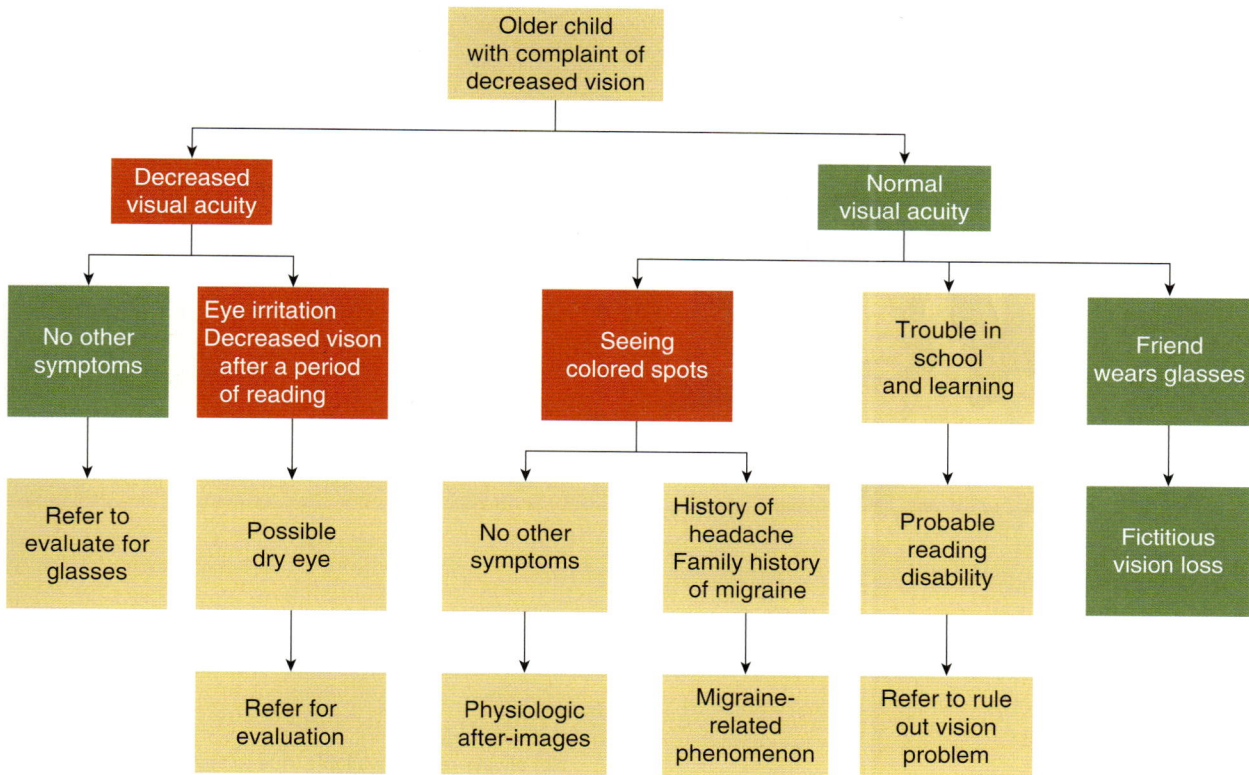

```
                    Older child
                    with complaint of
                    decreased vision
                          │
        ┌─────────────────┴─────────────────┐
  Decreased                              Normal
  visual acuity                          visual acuity
        │                                     │
   ┌────┴─────┐                    ┌───────────┼────────────┐
 No other   Eye irritation       Seeing      Trouble in    Friend
 symptoms   Decreased vison      colored     school        wears glasses
            after a period       spots       and learning
            of reading
    │            │           ┌────┴────┐         │             │
 Refer to    Possible     No other   History of  Probable   Fictitious
 evaluate    dry eye      symptoms   headache    reading    vision loss
 for                                 Family      disability
 glasses                             history of
                                     migraine
                 │            │          │           │
              Refer for   Physiologic  Migraine-  Refer to rule
              evaluation  after-images related    out vision
                                       phenomenon problem
```

FIGURE 4–3 ■ Algorithm for evaluation of complaints of decreased vision in older children.

the other problems discussed above is suspected, referral to a pediatric ophthalmologist is most appropriate.

WHAT SHOULDN'T BE MISSED

To be an effective patient advocate, it is important for the pediatrician to recognize that vision abnormalities are rarely the cause of learning difficulties. These patients should be evaluated by an ophthalmologist to be sure that they do not have an underlying eye problem that could affect reading, such as strabismus or a refractive error, but this is rarely found.

The families of children with learning problems may be referred to optometric vision therapists by well-meaning, but poorly informed, acquaintances, therapists, or teachers. Vision therapists purport to improve reading by a series of expensive and time-consuming eye exercises, which can cost several thousand dollars, and which the family often has to pay for directly. There is no scientific evidence that supports the use of vision therapy for these children.[2,3]

It is helpful for the pediatrician to suggest a second opinion with a pediatric ophthalmologist before commencing this expensive and ineffective treatment (Figure 4–3).

When to Refer

- Most children with complaints of decreased vision should be referred to an ophthalmologist or optometrist
- Urgent referral is indicated with sudden marked vision loss, or vision loss accompanied by pain
- If vision therapy is recommended for a child with learning problems, referral to a pediatric ophthalmologist for a second opinion is recommended

REFERENCES

1. Wright JD Jr, Boger WP 3rd. Visual complaints from healthy children. *Surv Ophthalmol.* 1999;44:113–121.
2. Barrett BT. A critical evaluation of the evidence supporting the practice of behavioural vision therapy. *Ophthalmic Physiol Opt.* 2009;29:4–25.
3. American Academy of Pediatrics, Section on Ophthalmology, Council on Children with Disabilities; American Academy of Ophthalmology; American Association for Pediatric Ophthalmology and Strabismus; American Association of Certified Orthoptists. Joint statement—learning disabilities, dyslexia, and vision. *Pediatrics.* 2009;124:837–844.

CHAPTER 5

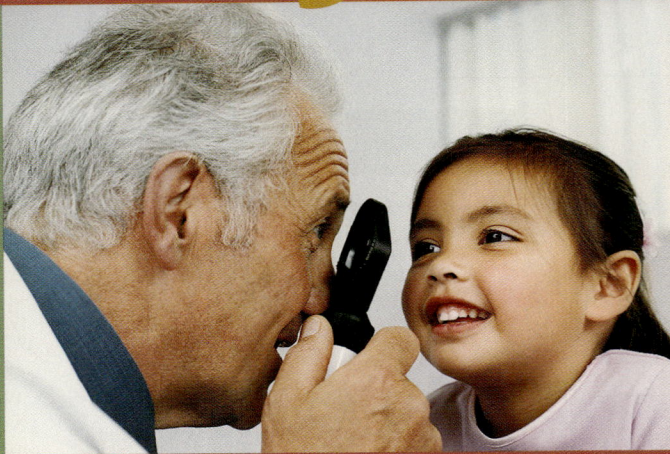

Red Eye

The Problem
"My child's eye is red."

Common Causes
Conjunctivitis
  Infectious
  Allergic
Trauma
  Corneal abrasion/foreign body
  Blunt trauma
Contact lens related
  Poor fit
  Infection

Other Causes
Episcleritis
Iritis
Acute glaucoma

KEY FINDINGS

History
Conjunctivitis
  Infectious
    Exposure to other infected children
    Recent upper respiratory infection
  Allergic
    Itching
    Atopic history

Trauma
  History of incident
    Not always readily available (due to age, attempting to
      hide story due to fear of punishment, etc.)
Contact lens related
  History of contact lens wear
  Poor lens hygiene
  Continued wear despite discomfort

Examination
Conjunctivitis
  Infectious
    Watery (viral) or purulent (bacterial) discharge
    Conjunctival swelling
    Cornea usually clear
  Allergic
    Mild conjunctival swelling
    Watery discharge
Trauma
  Corneal abrasion or corneal foreign body
  Hyphema
  Subconjunctival hemorrhage
Contact lens related
  Conjunctival inflammation
  Corneal clouding

WHAT SHOULD YOU DO?

The main decision in evaluating a patient with a red eye is whether the disorder is likely to recover without sequela or whether there is a potentially serious problem. If the patient has bacterial conjunctivitis, the cornea is clear, and the patient is not significantly uncomfortable, then they should be treated with topical antibiotics. A culture is usually not necessary unless the discharge is hyperpurulent. Patients with allergic conjunctivitis can be treated with topical medication, although oral allergy medication is often better tolerated in children.

If a patient has a corneal abrasion, the cornea is otherwise clear, and there is no suspicion of an intraocular foreign body, then treatment with topical antibiotics is indicated. Small foreign bodies can sometimes be removed with topical anesthetic and gentle manipulation with a cotton-tipped applicator. If a foreign body cannot be removed, or if there is any clouding of the cornea, referral is indicated.

Patients with direct ocular injuries, such as from a ball or fist, should be evaluated for a hyphema, corneal damage, and orbital fracture. Referral is indicated for most patients with nontrivial blunt ocular trauma.

Patients with red eyes who wear contact lenses should be instructed to stop wearing the lenses immediately. There is an increased risk of corneal infections in these patients, and they should be referred promptly to their eye care provider.

For any of these conditions, patients with marked pain that cannot be readily explained (e.g., from an uncomplicated corneal abrasion), or whose vision is significantly decreased, should be referred to a pediatric ophthalmologist.

What Shouldn't Be Missed

If a patient has a corneal abrasion that does not heal in 1 to 2 days, this raises the possibility of a foreign body. Small fragments of items such as clear plastic or glass may be difficult to visualize. If the cornea becomes cloudy in any patient with a red eye, prompt referral is indicated.

Although it is rare, meninogoccal conjunctivitis may present with hyperpurulent discharge. This organism has the potential for rapid dissemination, which may progress to meningitis and sepsis. Prompt treatment is indicated to minimize this risk.

COMMON CAUSES

1. *Infectious conjunctivitis.* Viral conjunctivitis ("pink eye") is the most common form of infectious conjunctivitis. It usually develops in association with a systemic viral illness, and there is frequently a history of exposure to other infected individuals. Patients with viral conjunctivitis usually have follicles on the inner lower eyelid (Figure 5–1). Bacterial conjuncitivitis is less common, though potentially more severe, than viral conjunctivitis. The discharge in viral conjunctivitis tends to be watery. It is purulent in bacterial conjunctivitis.

2. *Allergic conjunctivitis.* A hallmark of allergic conjunctivitis is the specific symptom of itching. If the patient is old enough to reliably articulate this symptom, it is highly likely that allergic conjunctivitis is the cause of the red eye. The conjunctiva may be mildly edematous and injected, but often the symptoms are out of proportion to the examination findings. These

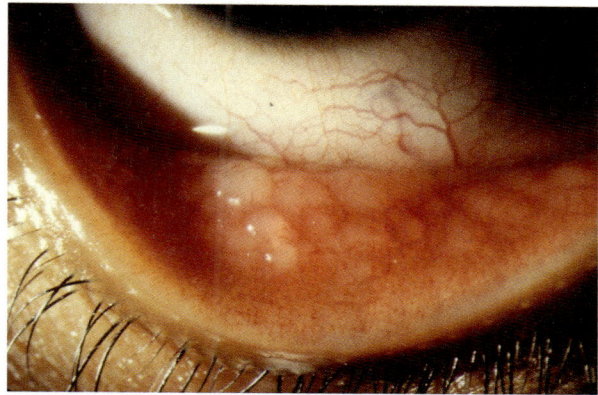

FIGURE 5–1 ■ Viral conjunctivitis with follicular reaction on inner lower eyelid (the follicles are the elevated bumps).

patients frequently have a history of other atopic disease.

3. *Trauma.* Mild trauma may produce a subconjunctival hemorrhage. These are benign, but may have a striking appearance of bright red blood against the white scleral background (Figure 5–2). More severe trauma may produce corneal abrasions, hyphemas, intraocular damage, and damage to the orbit and periocular structures (Figure 5–3). Corneal foreign bodies or abrasions are usually visible with a penlight, but are sometimes difficult to see.

APPROACH TO THE PATIENT

The goal of the evaluation of the patient with a red eye is to determine which patients can be safely managed in the primary care setting, and which have potentially serious problems that require referral.

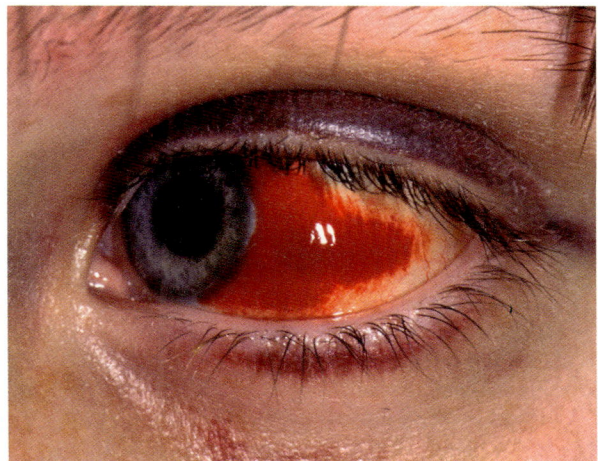

FIGURE 5–2 ■ Subconjunctival hemorrhage. Bright red blood against a white scleral background.

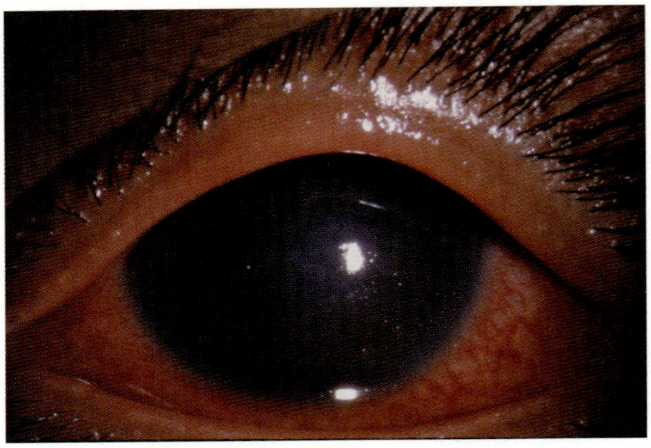

FIGURE 5–3 ■ Diffuse conjunctival edema and injection, and central corneal clouding, in a patient with an air-bag injury.

History

The history is very helpful in evaluating patients with red eyes. The most common causes of this disorder are infectious conjunctivitis, allergic conjunctivitis, and trauma (Table 5–1). A likely diagnosis can be established by the history. One of the most common etiologies is viral conjunctivitis. These patients typically report watery discharge, and frequently have had a preceding viral upper respiratory infection. Viral conjunctivitis is quite contagious. Many patients will have been exposed to other infected individuals at home or at school. Patients with bacterial conjunctivitis typically report purulent discharge, and may have an associated febrile illness.

Allergic conjunctivitis is characterized by itching. This specific symptom is highly diagnostic, and is very helpful in patients who are old enough to reliably report it. Many, but not all, patients with allergic conjunctivitis will have other allergic problems, such as seasonal rhinitis, asthma, and eczema.

In most patients with trauma, the history will match the physical findings. However, a specific history may not be available in toddlers who develop acute eye symptoms during unwitnessed play. Similarly, some older children may be hesitant to report specific incidents if they fear disciplinary reprisals. If available, the history is useful in assessing the risk of intraocular injury, retained foreign bodies, or infection. If there was a significant impact (from a fist or baseball, for example), the risk of intraocular injury is heightened. If the patient was injured by shattered glass or some other material, small portions may remain in the eye and be difficult to detect. If a child develops a corneal abrasion from vegetable material (e.g., a plant), or while playing in a lake, the risk of potentially serious infection is increased.

If the patient has a history of contact lens use, the patient should be questioned about the onset of the red eye in relation to lens wear. If the patient does not take proper care of their lenses, or wears them for longer periods than recommended, there is an increased risk of corneal infection. The risk of complications is greatly increased with overnight wear, even with lenses that are marketed for extended wear.[1]

The absence of any symptoms in a patient with red eye is most suggestive of either a subconjunctival hemorrhage or episcleritis (Table 5–2).

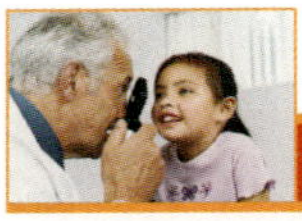

Examination

Before performing the examination, one should assess the level of suspicion for viral conjunctivitis. If the history and description of the symptoms are typical, appropriate precautions should be used to decrease the risk of viral transmission. The examination is usually limited to that necessary to confirm the diagnosis and rule out associated serious problems. Using gloves, an assessment of vision and a penlight examination to be sure the corneas are clear may be all that is necessary. If the diagnosis is in question, the inner lining of the lower eyelid should be examined. The presence of a follicular reaction (elevated mounds of tissue) strongly suggests viral conjunctivitis (Figure 5-1).

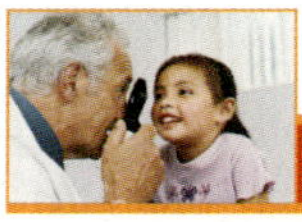

Table 5–1.

Important Signs and Symptoms of Common Causes of Red Eye

- Bacterial conjunctivitis
  - Purulent discharge
  - May have febrile illness
- Viral conjunctivitis
  - Watery or mucoid discharge
  - Conjunctival follicles
  - Often history of upper respiratory infection
- Allergic conjunctivitis
  - Specific complaint of *itching*
  - History of atopic disease
  - Mild conjunctival injection or edema
- Corneal abrasion or foreign body
  - Acute onset of symptoms
  - Corneal abnormality visible on examination

Table 5–2.

Causes of Red Eye With No Other Symptoms

- Subconjunctival hemorrhage (bright red blood)
- Episcleritis (wedge-shaped erythema)

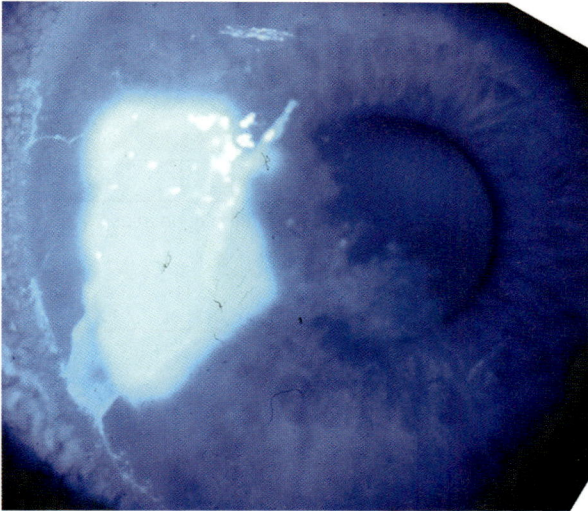

FIGURE 5–4 ■ Corneal abrasion. The eye has been stained with fluorescein and is examined with a blue light. The area of the corneal epithelial abrasion is demarcated by the fluorescence.

FIGURE 5–5 ■ Five-year-old girl with 2-week history of red eye. The patient has a corneal foreign body that is difficult to visualize with a penlight. (A) Examination of the cornea using the red reflex is suspicious for a foreign body (arrow). (B) Detailed examination reveals a clear plastic corneal foreign body.

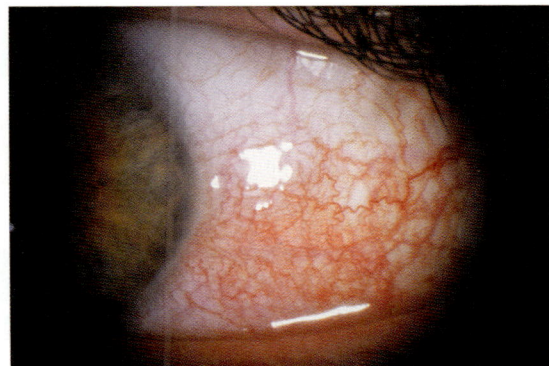

FIGURE 5–6 ■ Episcleritis. Sectoral edema and dilation of blood vessels. The patients are otherwise asymptomatic.

For patients in whom transmission of infection is not a concern, a standard eye examination is indicated. The vision in patients with bacterial or allergic conjunctivitis should be normal or near-normal. The cornea should be clear and the anterior segment structures readily visible. The pupils should react normally and the red reflex should be clear.

The examination of patients with trauma will be directed by the nature of the injury. Depending on the severity, injuries may occur to the eye itself or to the bones and soft tissue surrounding the eye (Figure 5–3). If a corneal abrasion is suspected, the use of fluorescein dye and a fluorescent light can confirm the diagnosis (Figure 5–4). The cornea should be inspected carefully for a retained foreign body. Clear foreign bodies, such as plastic, may be difficult to visualize. They may be easier to see by viewing the red reflex (Figure 5–5A and B). If a hyphema is present, the patient should be referred to a pediatric ophthalmologist. *If other serious ocular injuries are found, such as an ocular laceration, it is often best to stop the examination and refer the patient, due to the risk of further damage due to manipulation of the eye.*

Two entities deserve mention due to their striking appearance, yet benign prognosis. Subconjunctival hemorrhages can develop from either direct injury or due to increased venous pressure, typically associated with a Valsalva maneuver (from lifting a heavy weight, for example). These produce a striking appearance of bright red blood within the conjunctiva (Figure 5–2). The second entity is episcleritis. This is uncommon, but very distinctive. It presents with a wedge-shaped area of episcleral erythema medially or laterally (Figure 5–6).

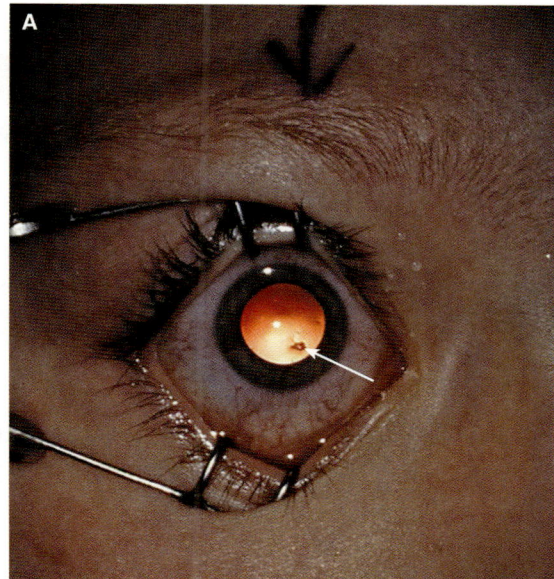

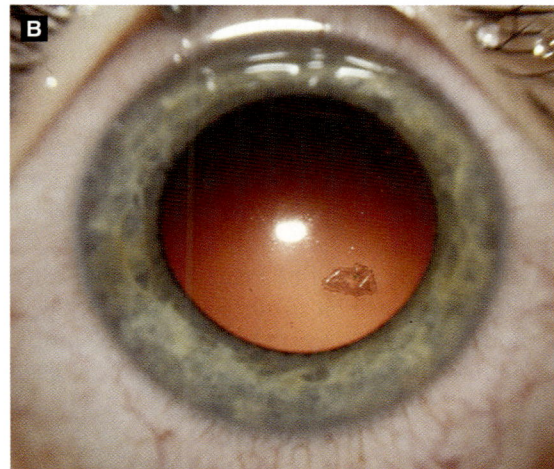

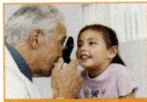

Table 5–3.

Worrisome Versus Less Worrisome Signs and Symptoms in a Patient With Red Eye

	Worrisome	Less worrisome
Vision	Decreased	Normal or minimally decreased
Pain/discomfort	Moderate or severe	None or mild
Corneal examination	Foreign body, abrasion, or clouding (possible infectious infiltrate)	Clear

With both of these conditions, the patients have a notable lack of symptoms, and their vision is normal.

PLAN

For viral conjunctivitis, supportive therapy is indicated. Cool compresses or lubricating drops may be helpful. Bacterial conjunctivitis should be treated with topical antibiotics. Cultures are usually not necessary, unless the discharge is hyperpurulent. Allergic conjunctivitis may be treated with either systemic or topical medication. Oral medications may be less effective in treating specific ocular symptoms, but are often better tolerated in young children.

Minor trauma can be managed by the pediatrician, if the examination is otherwise normal. Corneal abrasions should be treated with topical antibiotics. Ointment is often more soothing than drops. Patch-ing is not necessary.[2] Patching does not improve healing, and is often bothersome to young children. If an abrasion does not heal in 24 to 48 hours, or if progressive pain or corneal clouding develops, referral is indicated.

The management of other trauma depends on the severity of the injury. Subconjunctival hemorrhages are benign and self-limited. Children with hyphemas or other serious injury should be referred.

Patients with red eyes who wear contact lenses should be told to stop wearing their contact lenses and should be referred promptly to their eye care provider due to the potential risk of serious complications.

In general, for most patients with red eyes, if the vision is normal, there is not significant discomfort, and the corneas are clear, then management by the pediatrician is appropriate. Patients with marked pain, significant decreased vision, corneal clouding, or other progressive problems should be referred (Table 5–3).

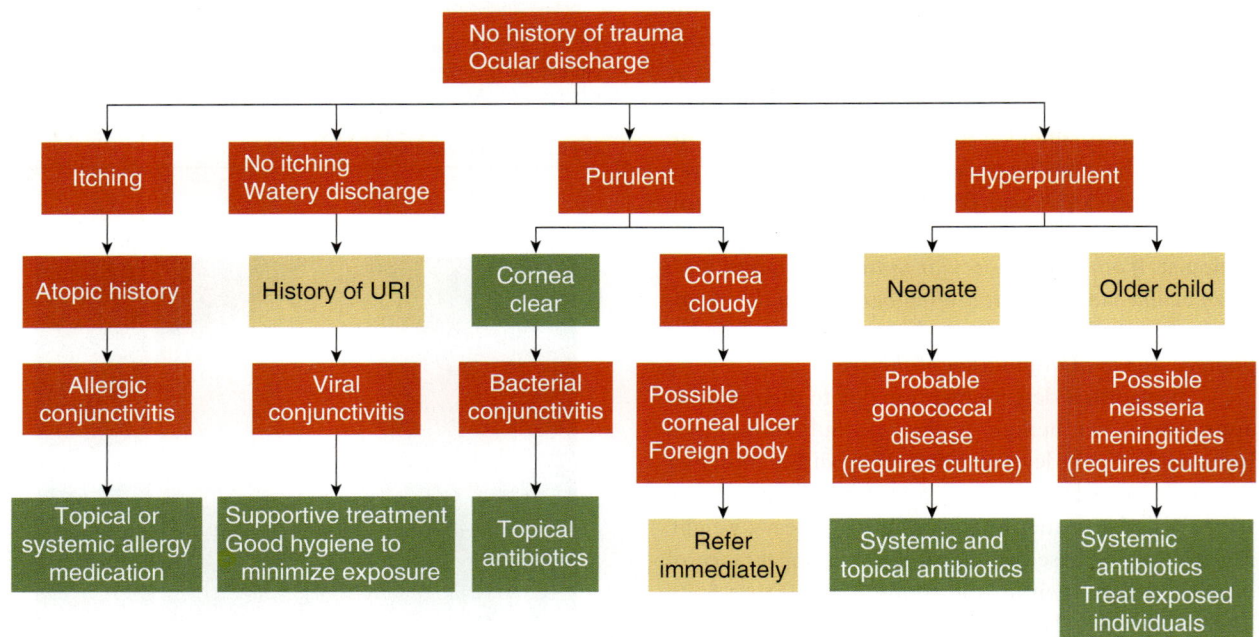

FIGURE 5–7 ■ Algorithm for evaluation and management of a child with a red eye with ocular discharge and no history of trauma.

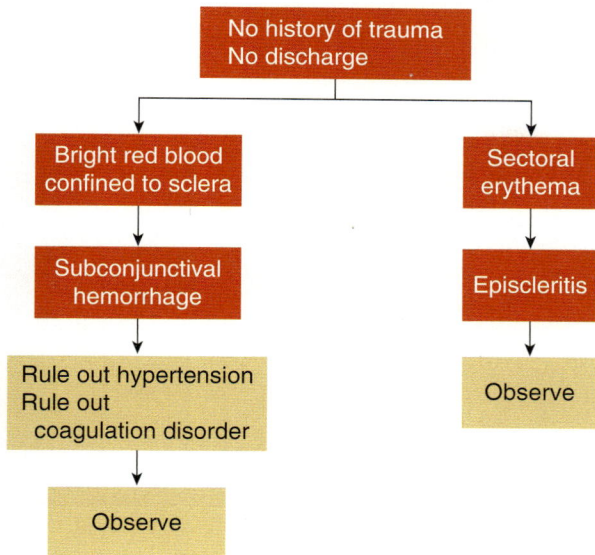

FIGURE 5–8 ■ Algorithm for evaluation and management of a child with a red eye without ocular discharge and no history of trauma.

WHAT SHOULDN'T BE MISSED

Occult foreign bodies may result in nonhealing corneal abrasions or ocular infection. Patients with corneal abrasions that do not heal in 1 to 2 days should be referred for slitlamp examination.

Meningococcal disease is a rare cause of conjunctivitis, characterized by hyperpurulent discharge. *Neisseria meningitidis* can spread systemically, causing meningitis and sepsis. Systemic antibiotic treatment is therefore necessary. Although cultures are not necessary for the majority of patients with conjunctivitis, they are indicated if hyperpurulent discharge is present (Figures 5–7, 5–8, and 5–9).

REFERENCES

1. Schein OD, Buehler PO, Stamler JF, Verdier DD, Katz J. The impact of overnight wear on the risk of contact lens-associated ulcerative keratitis. *Arch Ophthalmol.* 1994;112:186–190.
2. Kaiser PK. A comparison of pressure patching versus no patching for corneal abrasions due to trauma or foreign body removal. Corneal Abrasion Patching Study Group. *Ophthalmology.* 1995;102:1936–1942.

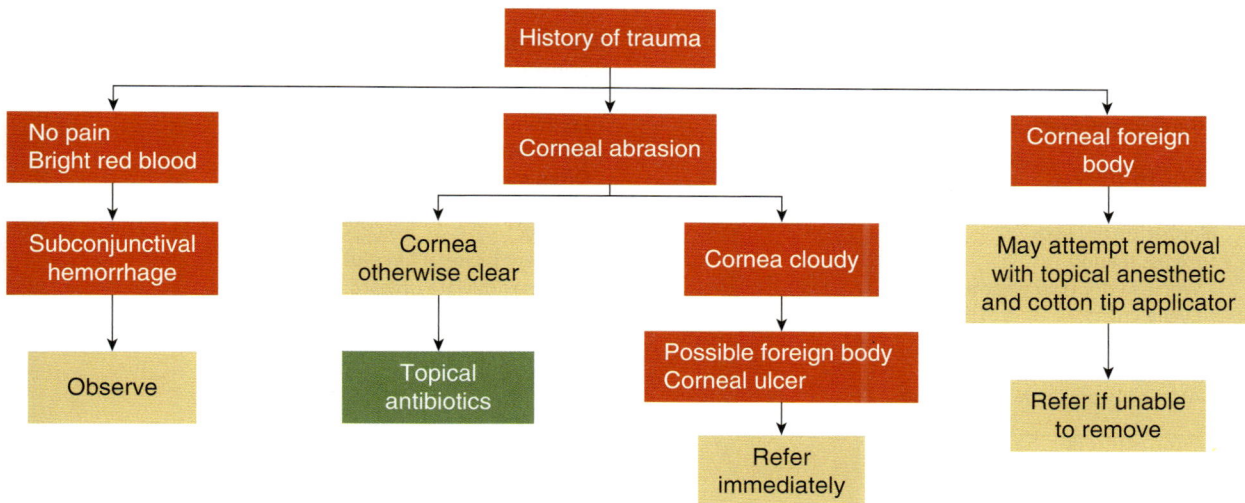

FIGURE 5–9 ■ Algorithm for evaluation and management of a child with a red eye and a history of trauma.

CHAPTER 6

Irritated Eyes (But not Red)

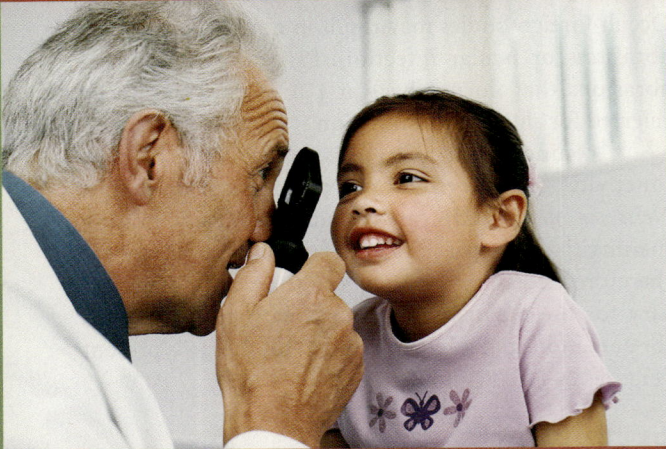

The Problem

"My child's eyes are irritated" *but not red (bloodshot).*

Common Causes

Idiopathic (general light sensitivity)
Blepharitis/dry eyes
Ocular allergy
Pseudo:
   Ocular tic (blepharospasm)
   Squint from strabismus

KEY FINDINGS

History

Blepharitis/dry eyes
   Excess tearing
   Worse in dry, cold weather
   Eyelid crusts
Ocular allergy
   Itching
   Atopic history (asthma, eczema)

Ocular tic
   Frequent forceful blinking
   No eye redness, discharge
   Possible other vocal, motor tics
   History of attention deficit hyperactivity disorder

Examination

Blepharitis
   Crusts on eyelashes
   Erythema of eyelid margin
Ocular allergy
   Often minimal or no visible changes
   May have mild conjunctival swelling
Ocular tic
   Frequent bilateral forceful blinking
   Eyes may deviate upward and laterally

WHAT SHOULD YOU DO?

The etiology of eye irritation (or pseudoirritation) in a child whose eyes are not red (bloodshot) can often be identified by history. The examination in most such children is relatively unremarkable. Most of the disorders associated with this symptom are not dangerous. If the etiology can't be identified with reasonable certainty, referral to a pediatric ophthalmologist is indicated.

What Shouldn't Be Missed

Ocular tics are fairly common in childhood, and may present as bilateral frequent forceful blinking. Hemifacial spasm is rare, and is characterized by contraction of the periocular *and* facial muscles on only half of the face. This may be associated with brainstem or posterior fossa lesions. Imaging is indicated in these patients.

COMMON CAUSES OF EYE IRRITATION (WITHOUT A RED EYE)

1. **Idiopathic.** Some children are generally more light sensitive than others. They squint in bright light and may want to wear sunglasses or avoid bright situations. These patients tend to have fair skin and light-colored irises.

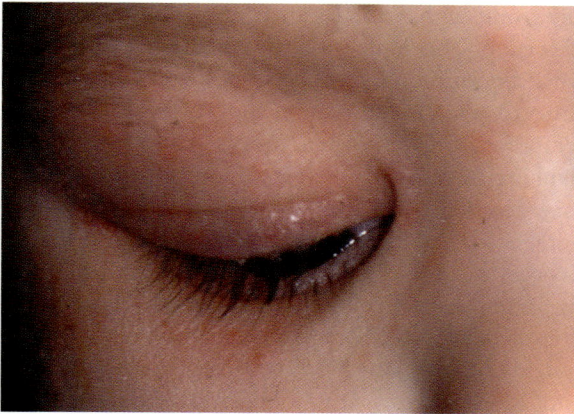

FIGURE 6–1 ■ Blepharitis. Note erythema of eyelid skin and crusts in eyelashes.

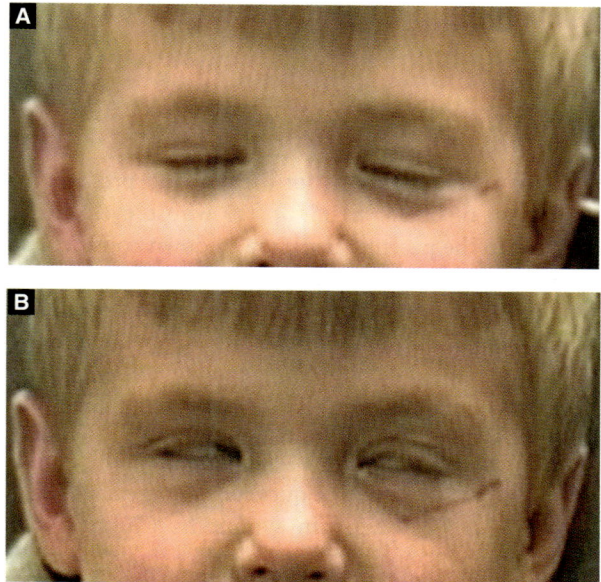

FIGURE 6–2 ■ Ocular tic (images obtained from video). (A) The patient blinks more frequently and forcefully than normal. (B) Upward and lateral deviation of the eyes in association with the blinking is not always present, but is a specific sign of an ocular tic.

2. **Blepharitis/dry eyes.** Blepharitis is a condition in which the meibomian glands of the eyelids do not function normally. The eyelid margins are usually erythematous and crusts are present (Figure 6–1). This results in an unstable tear film. The tears tend to evaporate rapidly, creating symptoms of eye irritation and frequent blinking. Blepharitis is a common cause of dry eyes, although not all patients with dry eyes have blepharitis. *Paradoxically, some patients with dry eyes may have symptoms of excess tearing.* This is because there are 2 types of tears: basal tears that keep the eyes moist and comfortable, and reflex tears that are produced in response to irritation. Patients with dry eyes have abnormal basal tears, so they tend to have cyclic symptoms of eye irritation, reflex tears that temporarily improve the symptoms, and then recurrent irritation as the reflex tears evaporate.

3. **Ocular allergy.** The key historical feature of ocular allergy is itching. If the child is old enough to reliably articulate this symptom and differentiate it from nonspecific ocular irritation, the diagnosis of allergy is very likely. Many patients with ocular allergies will have other atopic problems, such as reactive airway disease or eczema.

4. **Ocular tics.** Tic disorders are frequent during childhood, occurring in approximately 10% of children. Ocular tics present with frequent bilateral forceful blinking, sometimes associated with upward and lateral deviation of the eyes (Figure 6–2A and B). These children do not complain of eye irritation and the eyes are not red. They may, however, be bothered by the symptom, which they cannot control. Most ocular tics are benign and self-limited, but Tourette syndrome should be considered if the child has other associated vocal or motor tics.

Ocular tics need to be distinguished from hemifacial spasm. This condition is unilateral, and the eyelid contractions are accompanied by facial and perioral contractions (Figure 6–3). Hemifacial spasm may be caused by central nervous system mass lesions.[1]

5. **Squint from strabismus.** Unilateral squinting in bright light is a common symptom of strabismus, particularly intermittent exotropia. This is not associated with eye pain or redness.

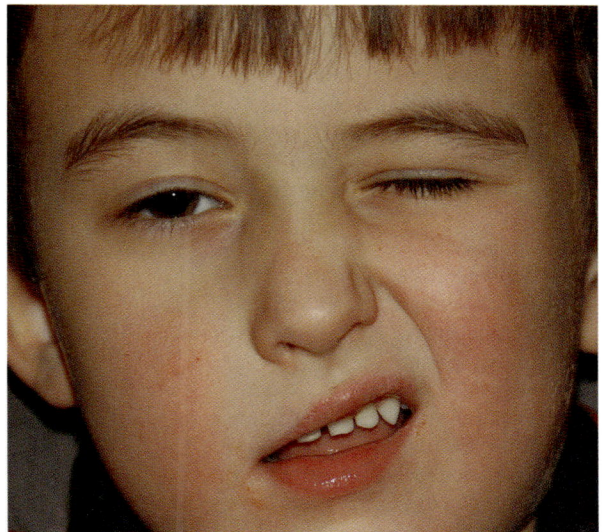

FIGURE 6–3 ■ Hemifacial spasm. Unilateral contraction of the eyelid and facial muscles.

Intermittent exotropia is not always easy to elicit on examination.

APPROACH TO THE PATIENT

The differential diagnosis for a child who presents for evaluation of ocular irritation (or whose eyes appear irritated to the parents) is narrowed down considerably if the eyes are not red (Table 6–1). A careful history is very useful, and can often accurately identify a diagnosis. Many such patients can be managed without referral.

History

A key point in the history is whether the child is symptomatic. If so, then specific questions are useful in identifying a likely cause for the symptoms. Children with idiopathic light sensitivity typically like to avoid bright lights or wear sunglasses when outside. They do not develop eye redness or discharge. Many will have fair complexions, and may sunburn easily. If the symptoms are severe, such as the child not wanting to leave the house or wanting the lights turned off indoors, one should suspect another ocular problem, and referral to a pediatric ophthalmologist is warranted.

Children with blepharitis or dry eyes usually complain of eye irritation or a foreign-body sensation ("There's something in my eye."). This symptom is usu-

Table 6–1.

Differentiating Signs and Symptoms of Irritated Eyes

■ Blepharitis
  □ Eyes feel scratchy, dry
  □ Eyelid crusts (worse on awakening)
  □ May have increased tearing
  □ Crusts and erythema of eyelids
■ Ocular allergy
  □ Specific symptom of itching
  □ May have other atopic disease
■ Ocular tics
  □ Bilateral
  □ Frequent forceful blinking
  □ Eyes may deviate up and out
  □ No complaints of eye redness or irritation
■ Hemifacial spasm
  □ Unilateral
  □ Forceful contraction of eyelids *and* facial, perioral muscles
■ Squinting due to strabismus
  □ Usually due to exotropia (but strabismus often not visible due to eyelid closure)
  □ Worse when viewing at distance
  □ Worse in bright light

ally worse with activities such as reading or watching television. This is because the blinking rate decreases with concentration, and the tears therefore have more time to evaporate. Tear evaporation may produce temporary blurred vision that is relieved with extra blinking or resting the eyes. Children with blepharitis may describe crusting of the eyelashes, which is most notable on awakening. Blepharitis is a common cause of dry eyes, but not all patients with dry eyes have blepharitis. In the absence of blepharitis, most dry eyes in children are idiopathic. They may occur, however, with other systemic diseases, such as arthritis, Sjögren syndrome, and Riley-Day syndrome (familial dysautonomia). Therefore, the review of systems should include questions about joint pain or difficulty eating (which may occur due to decreased salivation).

The key historical feature of ocular allergies is itching. If the patient is old enough to reliably articulate this symptom, then the diagnosis is highly likely. These patients will usually, but not always, have other allergic disorders.

The onset of ocular tics is usually fairly abrupt. The parents describe bilateral exaggerated eyelid blinking, which they may mistake for ocular irritation. The children do not have specific symptoms of pain or irritation. They sometimes complain of their eyes "bothering them," but on careful questioning it is their inability to control the symptoms that is bothersome, rather than the blinking itself. Ocular tics are often worse in stressful situations. They are usually self-limited, lasting a few weeks to months.

Squinting in bright lights is a fairly common symptom of strabismus, especially intermittent exotropia. The children's vision is not affected, and they do not complain of eye irritation. The key historical element is that the squinting is unilateral.

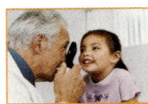

Examination

The examination in most children with the disorders discussed in this chapter is fairly unremarkable. The vision is normal, except for possible temporary blurring in patients with dry eyes. Children with blepharitis usually have crusts on the eyelashes, and the margin of the eyelid may be erythematous (Figure 6–1). Children with active allergic conjunctivitis may have mild swelling of the conjunctiva and increased tearing. Strabismus may be noted in patients with unilateral squinting, but it may be difficult to detect. This is because intermittent exotropia is usually most noticeable when the child is fixating on a distant object, but in the pediatrician's office, eye movements are usually assessed while the child is fixating at near.

In patients with blepharospasm, it is important to distinguish benign ocular tics from hemifacial spasm.

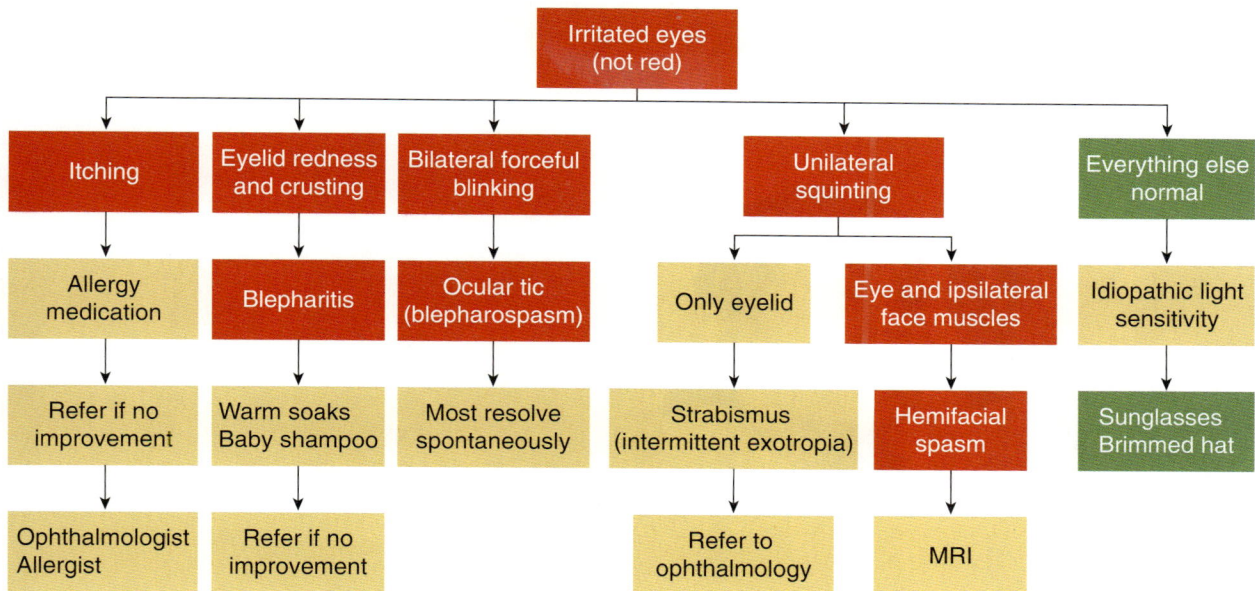

FIGURE 6–4 ■ Algorithm for evaluation of irritated eyes that are not red.

Patients with ocular tics will have frequent forceful blinking of both eyelids, which is confined to the orbicularis muscle. Hemifacial spasm is distinctly different. It occurs on only half of the face, and the periocular spasm is accompanied by facial and periocular contractions.

PLAN

If the disorders listed above can be reliably identified based on the history and examination, and the symptoms are fairly mild, then referral to a pediatric ophthalmologist may not be necessary. If the diagnosis is uncertain, or the symptoms are more marked, then referral is indicated (Figure 6–4).

Children with mild idiopathic light sensitivity can be managed with sunglasses or brimmed hats. If the child is markedly averse to light, referral for evaluation of a more serious disorder is indicated.

Blepharitis often improves with warm soaks to the eyes and gentle scrubbing with baby shampoo. This is most conveniently performed during baths or showers. Because the symptoms of dry eyes are often worse during reading, intermittent eye rest or lid closure may be beneficial. Older children may benefit from artificial tear drops.

Children with ocular allergies are often best treated with systemic medication. Although there are several very effective topical medications, most young children are averse to having drops put in their eyes, and the use of the drops themselves may be more bothersome than the underlying disorder.

If an ocular tic is suspected, and the ocular examination is otherwise normal, a period of observation is appropriate. Most ocular tics will resolve within 1 to 2 months. If the child has other vocal or motor tics, evaluation by a pediatric neurologist for Tourette syndrome may be indicated.

WHAT SHOULDN'T BE MISSED

Patients with hemifacial spasm should not be mistaken for benign ocular tics. Due to the association of posterior fossa and cerebellar disorders associated with hemifacial spasm, central nervous system imaging is indicated.

When to Refer

- Any child with marked light sensitivity (photophobia)
- Patients with hemifacial spasm
- Patients with blepharitis who do not improve with warm soaks or baby shampoo scrubs
- Other conditions that do not respond to treatment

REFERENCE

1. Flüeler U, Taylor D, Hing S, Kendall B, Finn JP, Brett E. Hemifacial spasm in infancy. *Arch Ophthalmol.* 1990;108: 812–815.

CHAPTER 7

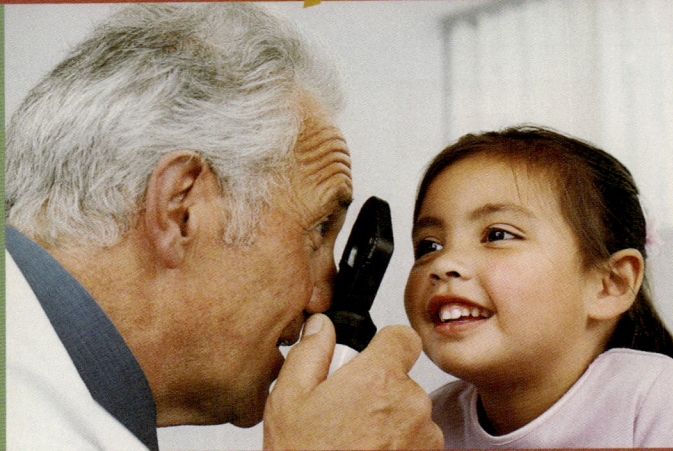

Excess Tearing in Infants

The Problem
"My baby looks like she is crying all the time."

Common Causes
Nasolacrimal duct obstruction

Other Causes
Other anatomic abnormalities of the lacrimal system
- Absent lacrimal puncta
- Lacrimal fistula

Misdirected eyelashes
Glaucoma
Corneal problems
Retinal dystrophies

KEY FINDINGS

History
Nasolacrimal obstruction (by far most common)
  Overflow tearing
  Periocular crusting, worse in morning
  Child otherwise fine, does not appear bothered by problem
  Other anatomic problems
    Absent lacrimal puncta
      Excess tearing only
      No crusting
    Lacrimal fistula
      Excess tearing
      Tears emanate from fistula tract between the eye and
        the nose
Misdirected eyelashes
  Parents note in-turning of lower eyelid
  Excess tearing, mucoid discharge
Cornea problems
  Child is light sensitive
  Frequent blinking
  Eye rubbing
Glaucoma
  One or both eyes larger than normal
  Glassy or cloudy appearance to cornea

Tearing only, not crusting
  Photophobia (light sensitivity)
Retinal dystrophies
  Photophobia
  Usually markedly decreased vision
  Nystagmus

Examination
Nasolacrimal obstruction
  Increased tear lakes, periocular crusts
  Child usually otherwise normal
  Conjunctiva white, no inflammation
  Cornea clear
Other anatomic abnormalities
  Punctal atresia
    Same except no ocular discharge
  Lacrimal fistula
    Excess tears (arise from fistula)
Eyelid malposition
  Same except mucoid discharge
  Lower eyelashes turned inward against
    cornea (epiblepharon)
Corneal problems
  Photophobia
  Cloudy cornea
Glaucoma
  One or both eyes enlarged
    (buphthalmos)
  Cloudy or glassy appearance
    to cornea
  Clear tears only
  Photophobia
Retinal dystrophies
  Photophobia
  Decreased vision
  Nystagmus

WHAT SHOULD YOU DO?

In case of a lacrimal obstruction, lacrimal massage and topical antibiotics as needed are indicated. If no improvement occurs with age, refer to an ophthalmologist.

If corneal problems or glaucoma are suspected, refer immediately to an ophthalmologist.

What Shouldn't Be Missed

Glaucoma should not be missed. Early treatment of glaucoma is critical to optimizing vision. *If a child with excess tearing has corneal clouding or eye size asymmetry, immediate referral to an ophthalmologist is indicated.*

COMMON CAUSES

Excess tearing in infants is one of the most common eye problems that pediatricians encounter. Approximately 6% of infants have some symptoms of excess tearing. Most of these spontaneously improve. Because this symptom is so common, however, it is possible to overlook much rarer but potentially serious disorders that present with the same clinical picture.

1. *Nasolacrimal duct obstruction (NLDO).* This is by far the most common cause of excess tearing in infants. It results from incomplete opening of the tear ducts, with symptoms of overflow tearing (epiphora), periocular crusting, or both (Figure 7–1). Most symptoms of NLDO resolve within the first 1 to 2 months of life.
2. *Other anatomic abnormalities of the lacrimal system.*
   a. *Absent lacrimal puncta.* Much less frequently, infants are born with absent or imperforate lacrimal puncta (the site on the eyelid where the tears enter the lacrimal system) (Figure 7–2A and B). These children present with overflow tearing only. Unlike most children with NLDO, these patients do not get periocular crusts or other symptoms of infection.

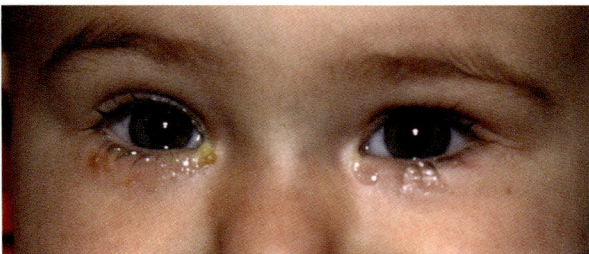

FIGURE 7–1 ■ NLDO. Bilateral overflow tearing (ephiphora) and periocular crusting.

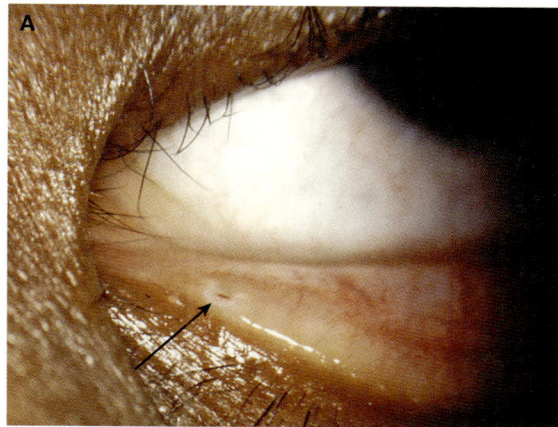

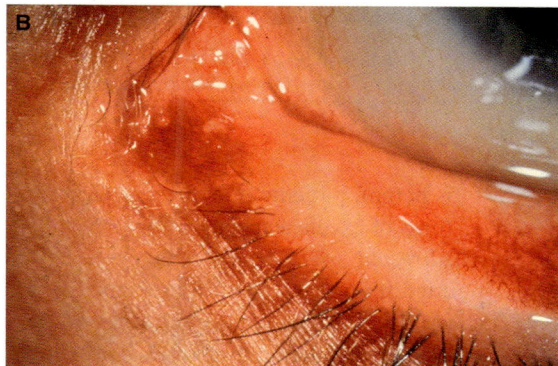

FIGURE 7–2 ■ (A) Normal lacrimal punctum (arrow). (B) Absent lacrimal punctum. (Figure B is reprinted with permission from *Semin Ophthalmol*. 1997;12(2):109–116. Copyright Informa Medical and Pharmaceutical Science.)

b. *Lacrimal fistula.* This is a rare anatomic abnormality in which an accessory lacrimal duct extends to the skin, usually nasal and inferior to the eye (Figure 7–3). If the fistula

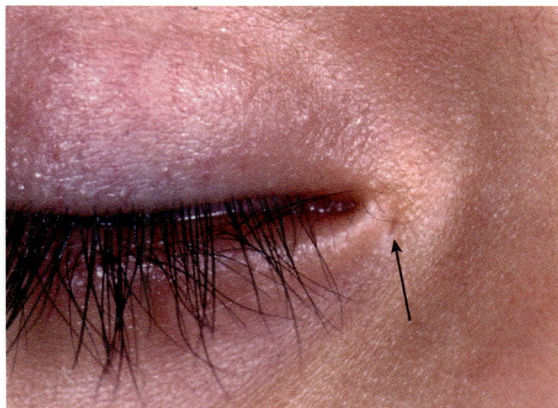

FIGURE 7–3 ■ Lacrimal fistula. These usually present as small dimples medial to the eyelids (arrow), which may be difficult to detect. (Reprinted with permission from *Semin Ophthalmol*. 1997;12(2):109–116. Copyright Informa Medical and Pharmaceutical Science.)

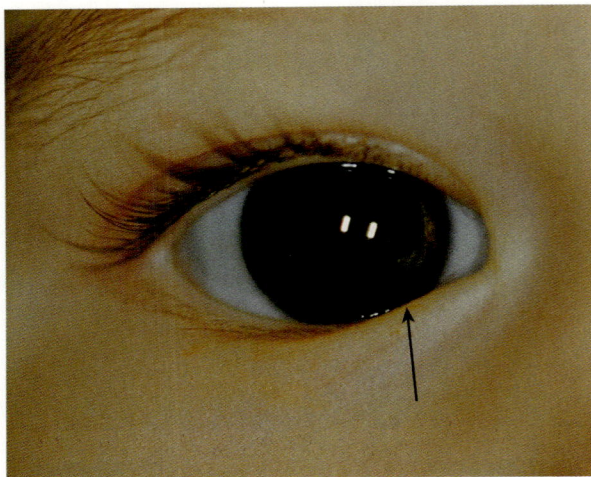

FIGURE 7–4 ■ Epiblepharon (extra fold of skin on lower eyelid) causing inward turning of lashes (arrow), which rub against cornea.

is patent, patients may present with symptoms of excess tearing.

3. *Misdirected eyelashes.* If the eyelashes are pointed toward the cornea, they may produce chronic irritation, with symptoms of excess tearing and mucoid discharge. These symptoms are similar to those of NLDO. The most common cause of misdirected eyelashes is *epiblepharon,* an extra fold of skin on the lower eyelid, which causes the eyelashes to turn in toward the cornea (Figure 7–4).

4. *Other corneal problems.* Corneal abnormalities are uncommon in infants. Potential etiologies include inherited disorders, infection, foreign bodies, and dry eyes.

5. *Glaucoma.* Glaucoma results from increased pressure in the eye. In many infants the cornea enlarges and becomes edematous, which causes ocular irritation and light sensitivity. Many affected infants therefore have symptoms of excess tearing (Figure 7–5).

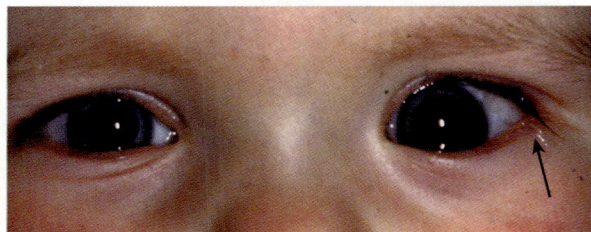

FIGURE 7–5 ■ Overflow tearing (arrow), left eye, secondary to infantile glaucoma. Note left eye appears larger than right: the corneal diameter is greater and the lower eyelid crease is less distinct due to forward displacement of the eye.

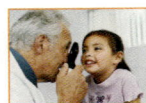

Table 7–1.

Signs and Symptoms of Nasolacrimal Obstruction

- Increased tear lake
- Overflow tearing onto cheek
- Periocular crusts
- Conjunctiva white
- Baby usually not bothered by problem
- If severe—periocular skin erythema

6. *Retinal dystrophies.* Increased light sensitivity occurs in some inherited retinal dystrophies, which may result in excess tearing, particularly in bright light. Most of these disorders have profound effects on vision, and concern about the abnormal vision is usually what brings these patients to medical attention.

APPROACH TO THE PATIENT

Because NLDO is so common, and the other causes of excess tearing are rare, it is possible that potentially serious problems can be overlooked. The following approach can help make this distinction (Table 7–1).

History

NLDO affects approximately 6% of infants. Therefore, this abnormality will be found on many well-child visits, particularly during the first 1 to 2 months of life. If the symptoms are mild, the parents may not mention it. If the baby has frequent obvious overflow tearing, or recurrent ocular discharge that requires wiping of the eyes, most parents will express specific concerns and have questions about the problem.

The symptoms of NLDO are quite variable. Overflow tearing may be constant or intermittent. If intermittent, it is often worse in windy conditions or if the patient has an upper respiratory infection. Periocular crusting usually results from low-grade infection of the lacrimal system. Some children have mild intermittent crusting. Others have marked discharge, usually worse on awakening. In these children, the parents sometimes need to wipe the eyelashes with a washcloth before the eye will open. In severe cases, patient may develop erythema and maceration of the eyelid skin due to the constant exposure to moisture (Figure 7–6).

A key differentiating factor in the history is whether other symptoms are present. Children with NLDO typically present with excess tearing and

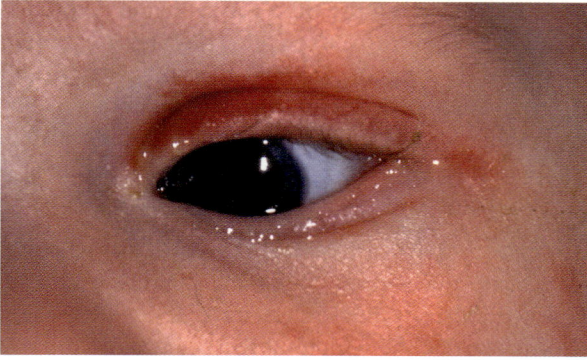

FIGURE 7–6 ■ Nasolacrimal obstruction with periocular erythema due to chronic exposure to excess moisture.

recurrent ocular discharge. However, the eyeballs themselves are not directly affected, and the children are otherwise asymptomatic. The excess tearing in most other disorders results from ocular irritation (Table 7–2). Children with these disorders are sensitive to light and blink more frequently and forcefully than normal (Table 7–3). *If the baby does not appear bothered by the symptoms of excess tearing, NLDO is by far the most likely etiology.* Similarly, NLDO has no effects on vision. If the parents have concerns about vision, one of the other disorders should be suspected.

Examination

The presence of excess tearing should be verified. If the obstruction is marked, there may be frank overflow

Table 7–2.

Conditions Causing Epiphora Due To Ocular Irritation

- Glaucoma
- Cornea abnormality
- Misdirected eyelashes (epiblepharon)
- Retinal dystrophy (rare)

Table 7–3.

Signs and Symptoms Suggesting Disorder Other Than Nasolacrimal Obstruction

- Light sensitivity (photophobia)
- Conjunctival redness
- Corneal clouding
- Decreased vision

tears on the cheeks. More subtle obstruction may produce enlargement of the lower tear lake between the eyelid and the eyeball. This gives the appearance that the baby is about to start crying. Subtle obstruction is more easily assessed if the patient has unilateral NLDO, because the normal eye can be compared to the abnormal eye.

The presence of periocular discharge should be noted. This may range from mild crusts on the eyelashes to frank purulent material that overflows onto the cheeks. Pressing on the lacrimal sac between the eye and the nose may produce reflux of mucopurulent material from the sac. This finding, though not always present, confirms a diagnosis of NLDO.

It is critical on examination to verify the normal size and clarity of the cornea and absence of light sensitivity. The position of the eyelids and eyelashes should be examined for misdirection against the cornea. As with any eye examination, the baby's vision and eye movements should be assessed. If these findings are normal, it is very likely that the child has NLDO, rather than any of the potentially serious disorders discussed in this chapter.

PLAN

After a diagnosis of NLDO is established, the treatment plan depends on the patient's age and severity of symptoms. Most NLDO will spontaneously resolve in the first 1 to 2 months of life. If the patient has mild symptoms, no treatment is necessary. If the symptoms are more marked, the periocular discharge is usually more bothersome than the excess tearing. Two treatments may be offered to such patients:

1. *Lacrimal massage.* The purpose of lacrimal massage is to produce pressure within the tear sac that forces fluid down the lacrimal duct to the site of obstruction. The hydraulic pressure may therefore cause the obstruction to open. *If lacrimal massage is recommended, proper technique should be demonstrated.* The only site where the lacrimal sac can be palpated is between the eye and the nose. By pushing at this site, the sac is compressed (Figure 7–7). This can be verified by noting expression of tears and mucopurulent material onto the eye through the tear ducts. Moving the finger down the side of the nose is not effective because the tear duct is covered by bone at this site and cannot be compressed.

2. *Topical antibiotics.* If the infant has marked periocular discharge, topical antibiotics can be used. These will often improve the symptoms, but they do not cure the underlying obstruction. It

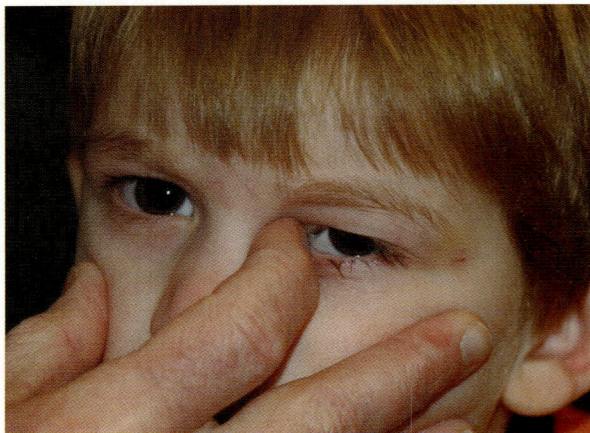

FIGURE 7–7 ■ Lacrimal massage. Pressure should be applied directly over the lacrimal sac between the medial eye and nose.

is common for symptoms to recur when antibiotics are discontinued. This will continue until either the NLDO spontaneously resolves, or the patient has surgery. Unlike most other infections for which antibiotics are prescribed for a specific duration, parents of patients with NLDO may use the topical antibiotics intermit-

tently when the child is symptomatic, and discontinue them when the symptoms improve. In most instances, lacrimal infection will be due to common bacteria, rather than significant pathogens. Most topical antibiotics will produce some improvement, and cultures are usually not necessary.

For patients with NLDO, it is particularly helpful to educate the parents about the condition and its expected course. If they understand that it will probably resolve, but that the symptoms will often vary from day to day until resolution occurs, they will be less worried when this occurs. They should also understand that antibiotics will not cure the problem, but will be a temporizing measure while waiting for the duct to open.

Spontaneous improvement in NLDO occurs in over 90% of patients during the first 6 to 12 months of life. If patients remain symptomatic beyond this age, referral to a pediatric ophthalmologist is indicated for consideration of nasolacrimal duct probing. Some ophthalmologists prefer to perform NLD probing in young infants (before age 6 months) while awake in the office, whereas others wait until the children are older and perform the procedure in the operating room. Both

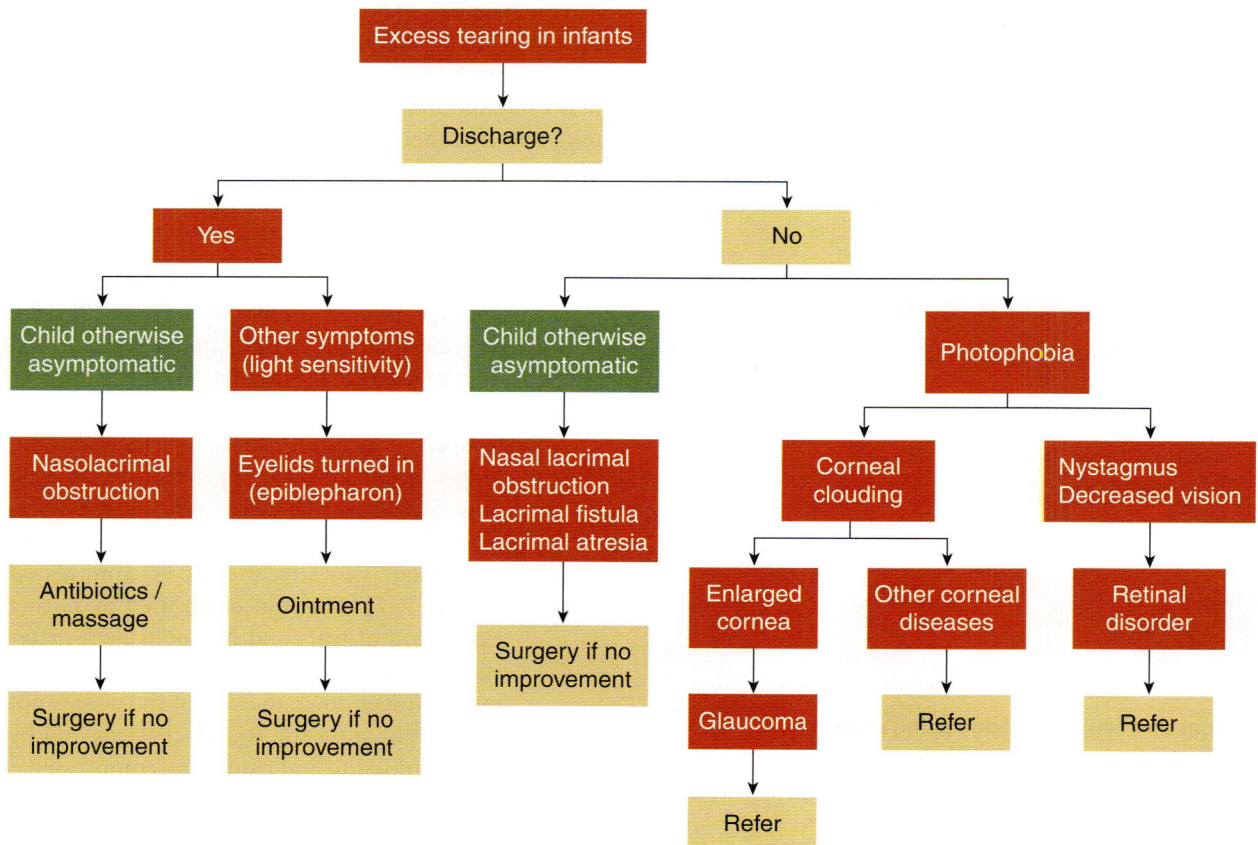

FIGURE 7–8 ■ Algorithm for evaluation and management of infants with excess tearing.

of these approaches are reasonable, and the age at which you refer the patient will depend on local practices. The surgical treatment of NLDO is discussed further in Chapter 24. Earlier surgery is sometimes considered if children have marked periocular erythema and breakdown of the skin surface (Figure 7–6).

Epiblepharon with in-turning eyelashes often spontaneously improves during the first 6 to 12 months of life. Surgery to evert the eyelashes may be indicated if it does not. The other disorders noted in the differential diagnosis will not spontaneously improve. If one of these is suspected, referral to a pediatric ophthalmologist is indicated (Figure 7–8).

WHAT SHOULDN'T BE MISSED

Glaucoma is a progressive disease that may cause irreversible vision loss. Early diagnosis and treatment greatly improves the prognosis. Glaucoma in infants is rare. Many pediatricians will only see 1 or 2 patients with this during their careers, whereas they will see hundreds of patients with NLDO. It is important to recognize the features that distinguish these disorders, including light sensitivity, corneal clouding, and corneal enlargement. If in doubt, it is better to refer a patient to a pediatric ophthalmologist early to have the diagnosis excluded, rather than waiting until the child is older. The diagnosis is confirmed if the child is found to have increased intraocular pressure and evidence of optic nerve damage due to the pressure.

When to Refer

- Refer infants with enlarged or cloudy corneas promptly to an ophthalmologist
- Refer patients with typical NLDO to an ophthalmologist if the problem does not resolve by 6 to 12 months of age
  - Earlier referral may be considered if the child develops maceration and breakdown of the periocular skin

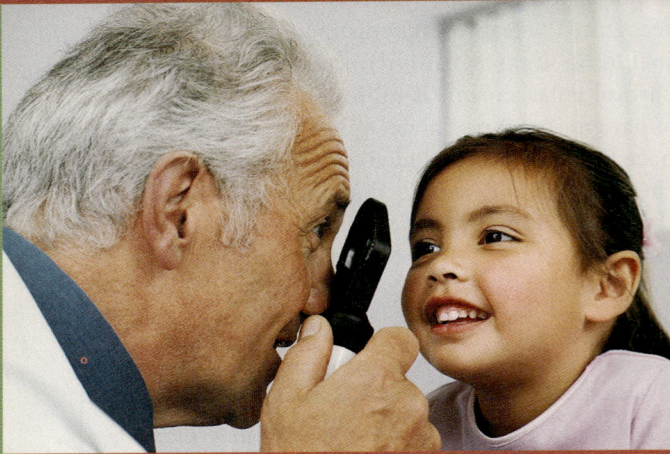

CHAPTER 8

Absent Tearing in Infants

The Problem
"My baby doesn't cry."

Common Cause
Absent reflex tears

Other Causes
Dry eyes (*alacrima*)
- Isolated
- Associated with other systemic diseases

KEY FINDINGS

History
Absent reflex tears
 Baby doesn't make tears when crying
 Otherwise completely normal
Dry eyes
 Decreased tears
 Glassy appearance to eyes

Increased light sensitivity
*Paradoxically, some patients with dry eyes have
 symptoms of excess tearing (see text)*

Examination
Absent reflex tearing
 Eyes otherwise appear normal
 Cornea and conjunctiva crisp and clear
 Normal tear lakes
Dry eye
 Photophobia
 Conjunctival redness
 Possible visible corneal scars
 Other systemic abnormalities
 Sometimes excess tearing

WHAT SHOULD YOU DO?

If there are no other symptoms are present and the examination is otherwise normal (including a clear cornea), reassurance is usually all that is necessary.

If the patient has symptoms of ocular irritation and photophobia, referral is indicated.

What Shouldn't Be Missed

Riley-Day syndrome (familial dysautonomia) causes markedly decreased tear production, which increases the risk of vision loss due to corneal scarring and infection. Early treatment with aggressive lubrication is indicated.

COMMON CAUSES

In children, underproduction of tears is much less common than excess tearing. There are 2 types of tears. *Basal tears* are continuously secreted. They are necessary to keep the eye lubricated and healthy. *Reflex tears* occur in response to either external or emotional stimulation, such as increased tearing in a brisk wind or crying when upset. They are not necessary for ocular health.

1. *Decreased reflex tears.* This is much more common than true dry eyes. These children have normal basal tears (Figure 8–1) and their eyes are otherwise normal.

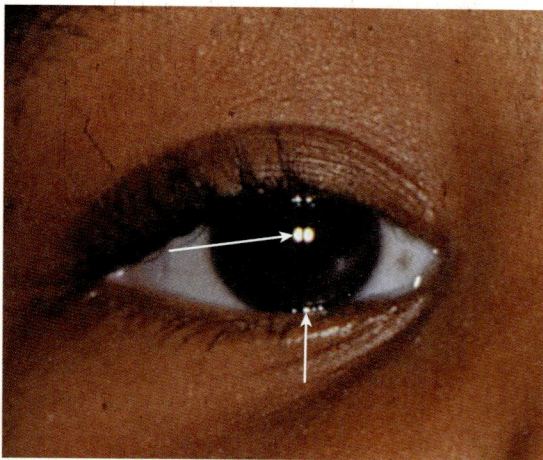

FIGURE 8–1 ■ Normal tear lake. This is most easily visualized with a penlight as a thin layer of fluid between the lower eyelid and the eyeball (arrow). Note that the cornea is clear and the corneal light reflex (long arrow) is crisp.

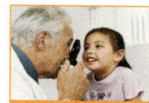

Table 8–1.

Systemic Diseases Associated With Dry Eye

- Sjögren syndrome
- Riley-Day (familial dysautonomia)
- Graft versus host disease
- Sarcoidosis
- Other autoimmune disease

2. *Dry eyes.* Dry eyes occur frequently in adults as part of the aging process. They are less common in infants and children. Patients with dry eyes have decreased or unstable basal tear layers. This usually results in chronic ocular irritation. This may be an isolated finding, or it may occur in association with other systemic problems (Table 8–1). *Paradoxically, some patients with dry eyes may have symptoms of excess tearing* (Figure 8–2).

This occurs because the decreased basal tears predispose the patient to ocular irritation. If the patients have normal reflex tears, they will produce a bolus of tears in response to the irritation, often enough to overflow and produce epiphora. As this bolus wears off, the irritation recurs, and the patients go through a repetitive cycle of decreased tears, irritation, and excess tears.

APPROACH TO THE PATIENT

History

The key historical finding for patients with absent reflex tears is the absence of other ocular symptoms. Parents usually note within the first few months of life that their

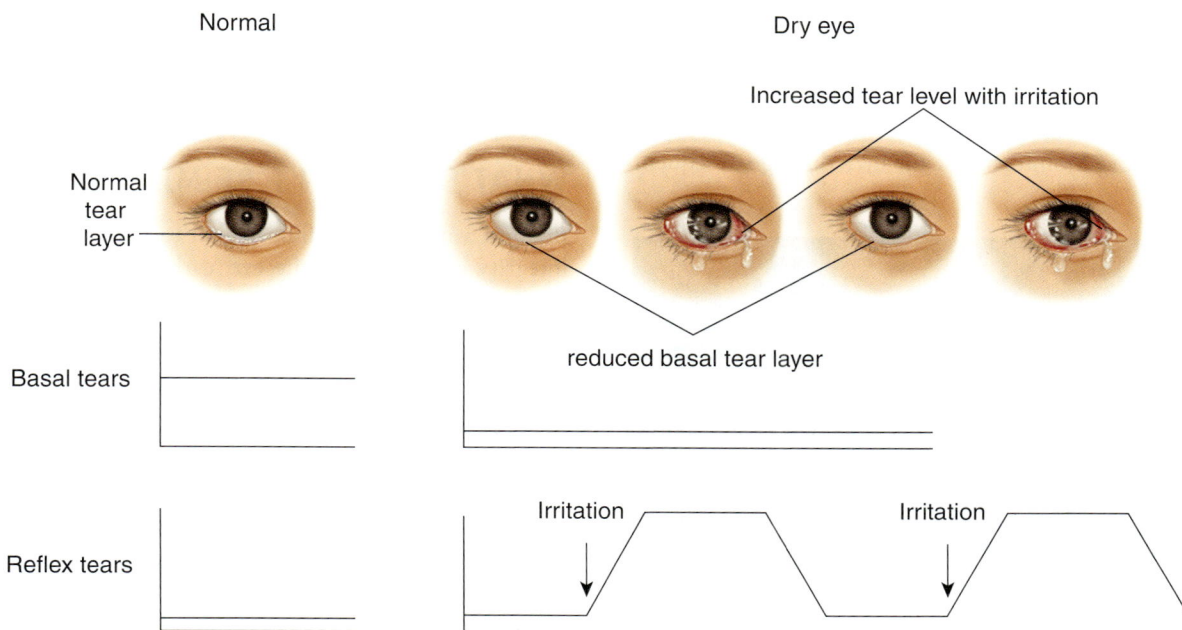

FIGURE 8–2 ■ Figure 8-2 Paradoxical intermittent excess tearing in patients with dry eyes. In normal patients (left) there is a continuous production of basal tears that keep the eyes healthy and comfortable. In patients with dry eyes (right), the decreased tears result in ocular irritation, which causes a bolus of reflex tears that temporarily improves the symptoms. The symptoms recur as the reflex tears evaporate.

child does not produce tears when he or she is crying, but otherwise is normal.

The combination of decreased tears with increased light sensitivity and frequent blinking suggests that the patient has alacrima (dry eyes). The history should include questions about systemic diseases associated with dry eyes (Table 8–1).

Examination

If the child with absent reflex tearing demonstrates crying behavior during the examination, but no tears are produced, the absence of reflex tearing can be verified. In these patients, the cornea otherwise appears crisp and clear and the child is not light sensitive. The tear lake is the normal thin layer of fluid that forms between the lower eyelid and the eyeball. It can be visualized with a penlight, and is normal in patients with absent reflex tears (Figure 8–1). The conjunctiva is also normal.

Patients with true dry eyes will be sensitive to light, demonstrated by aversion to examination lights and frequent blinking. The conjunctiva may be injected. In marked cases, corneal scarring may be visible on penlight examination. A slitlamp examination is often necessary to demonstrate microscopic corneal irritation (Figure 8–3). As discussed above, some patients with dry eyes will have intermittent excess tears and epiphora. It is difficult to make this distinction without an ophthalmic evaluation.

PLAN

Because of the striking difference in history and examination between patients with absent reflex tears and patients with true dry eyes, the distinction can often be made with reasonable certainty. If so, reassurance of the parents and monitoring of the eyes during subsequent

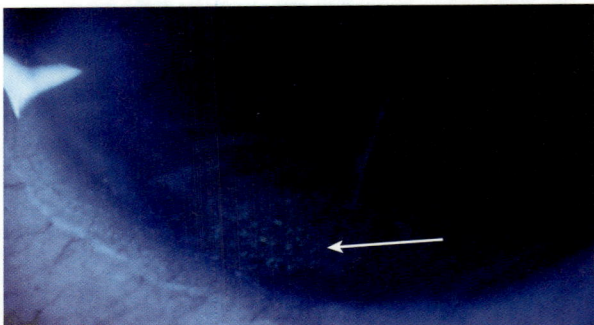

FIGURE 8–3 ■ Slitlamp photograph of microscopic irritation spots (superficial punctate keratopathy) of peripheral cornea (arrow), stained with fluorescein and viewed through cobalt blue light. (Photograph contributed by Anthony Lubniewski, MD.)

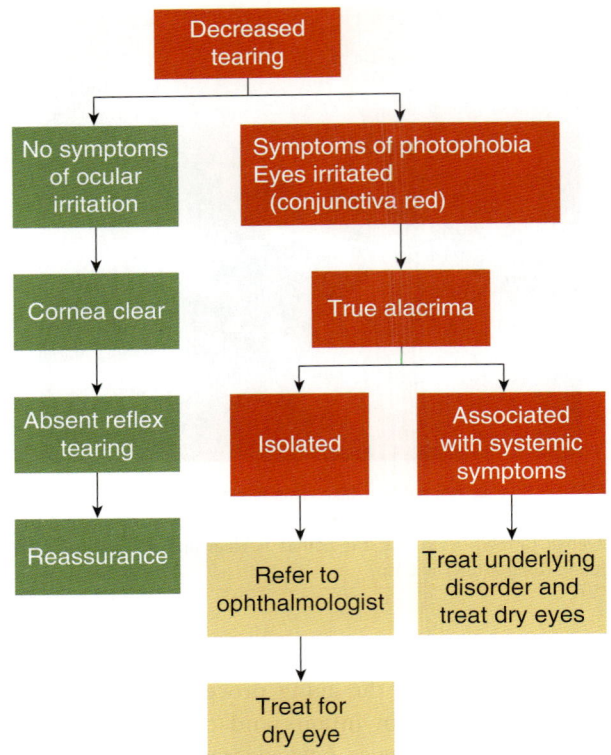

FIGURE 8–4 ■ Algorithm for evaluation and management of an infant with decreased tearing.

well-child examinations is the recommended course of action. Frequently, parents will be concerned enough about the absent tears that referral to an ophthalmologist for confirmation is warranted.

Patients with dry eyes accompanied by ocular irritation and photophobia should be referred to a pediatric ophthalmologist (Figure 8–4).

WHAT SHOULDN'T BE MISSED

Because a normal tear film is vital to maintaining the integrity and health of the eye, early identification of severe problems is essential to improve the prognosis. Riley-Day syndrome (familial dysautonomia) results in markedly decreased tear production, with concomitant increased risk of scarring and infection. It is much easier to avoid these complications with aggressive ocular lubrication, rather than treat them once they have occurred.

When to Refer

- If the patient has symptoms of light sensitivity
- If corneal abnormalities are seen on examination

CHAPTER 9

Strabismus in Infants

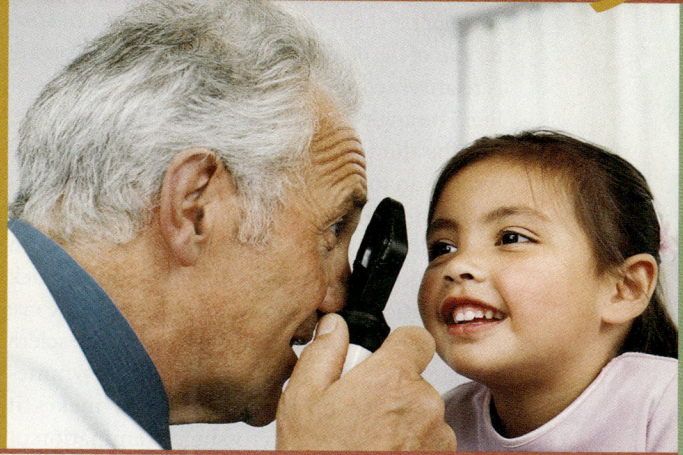

The Problem
"My baby's eyes aren't straight."

Common Causes
Normal newborn
Pseudostrabismus
Infantile esotropia
Strabismus secondary to decreased vision

Other Causes
Other strabismus (see Chapters 10 and 34)
  Duane syndrome
  Cranial nerve palsy
  Möbius syndrome

KEY FINDINGS

History
Normal newborn
  Child otherwise normal
  Brief, occasional crossing during first 1 to 2 months
Pseudostrabismus
  Occasional appearance of mild crossing
  Often noticed in photographs
  Worse in side gaze
Infantile esotropia
  Prolonged periods of crossing
  Worse when tired
  May have family history of strabismus
  More common in children with neurological problems
Decreased vision
  Frequent strabismus
  More variable than infantile esotropia

Examination
Normal newborn
  Esotropia lasts a few seconds
  Child less than 2 months old
  Eye examination otherwise normal
Pseudostrabismus
  Epicanthal folds/wide nasal bridge
  Appears worse in side gaze
  Corneal light reflex symmetric
  Eyes straight with cover test
Infantile esotropia
  Large angle crossing
  Asymmetric corneal light reflex
  Prolonged or constant crossing
  Possible amblyopia
Strabismus secondary to decreased vision
  Strabismus usually variable, both in duration and in angle
  Possible abnormal red reflex

WHAT SHOULD YOU DO?

If the child is less than 2 months old and the eyes cross occasionally, and there are no visible abnormalities of the eyes, the child should be rechecked after 2 months of age. *Patients with constant crossing at any age, or intermittent crossing that persists after 2 months of age, should be referred to a pediatric ophthalmologist.*

What Shouldn't Be Missed

Although uncommon, abnormalities of the eye such as cataract or retinoblastoma may initially present with strabismus (secondary to decreased vision). The prognosis for these disorders is greatly improved with prompt treatment. *Any child with strabismus and an abnormal red reflex should be referred immediately.*

COMMON CAUSES

1. *Normal newborn (physiological intermittent strabismus of the newborn).* Intermittent eye crossing is relatively common in the first 1 to 2 months of life. The angle of eye crossing may be quite large, but the duration is brief (a few seconds). This resolves in most infants by 2 months of age.

2. *Pseudostrabismus.* Normal infants have a wider and flatter nasal bridge than adults. When an infant looks to the side, this tissue may block visualization of the white nasal sclera in the eye that is turned toward the nose, while the sclera remains visible in the other eye. This asymmetry creates an optical illusion that makes it appear as if one eye is crossing. Examination of the corneal light reflex reveals that the eyes are straight (Figure 9–1).

3. *Infantile esotropia.* True eye crossing (esotropia) is usually not present at birth. It most often begins around age 2 months. Initially it may occur intermittently, but usually progresses rapidly to constant crossing. When the infant's eye crosses, the brain stops paying attention to the visual information from the eye. This may cause amblyopia if one eye is constantly crossed. Some children spontaneously alternate fixation between the eyes (alternate fixation) (Figure 9–2A and B). Binocular vision cannot develop in children with infantile esotropia unless the crossing is corrected. Early surgical realignment of the eyes improves the outcome. Infantile esotropia is more common in children with developmental delay (Table 9–1).

4. *Decreased vision.* Any condition that causes decreased vision, particularly if it affects only one eye, may cause a secondary strabismus. In infants, the strabismus in the poorly seeing

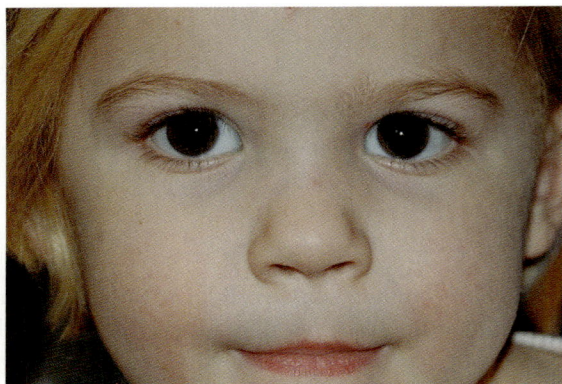

FIGURE 9–2 ■ Infantile esotropia with alternate fixation. The child spontaneously switches between (A) the right eye crossing and (B) the left eye crossing. Note that the light is deflected laterally from the pupil in the crossed eye.

eye is most commonly esotropia. The list of possible causes includes virtually any ocular disorder that affects vision. Some of these are incurable (such as optic nerve hypoplasia or large retinal colobomas), but some are amenable to treatment (such as cataracts or retinoblastoma). For the latter, early diagnosis and treatment may dramatically improve the prognosis.

APPROACH TO THE PATIENT

History

During a well-child evaluation, the patient's parents may raise concern about strabismus, or the examiner may note possible ocular misalignment during the examination. If the parents have noted eye misalignment, the history should include the parents' perception

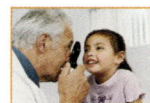

FIGURE 9–1 ■ Pseudostrabismus. The left eye appears to be crossed because less sclera is visible nasally in the left eye compared to the right. The corneal reflexes are symmetric, *indicating that no true esotropia is present.*

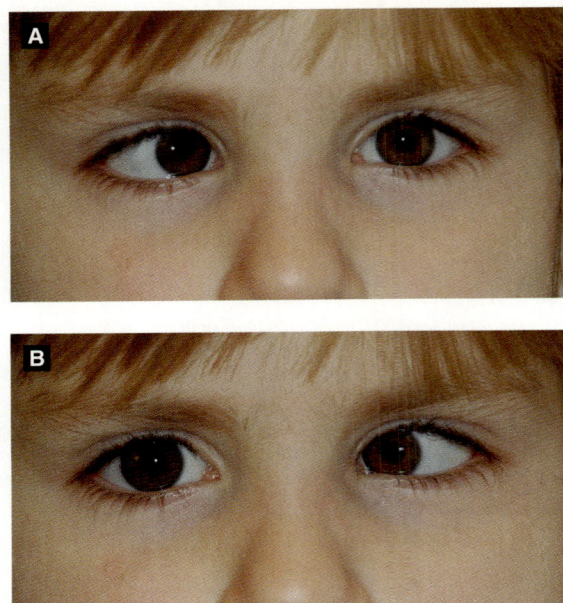

Table 9–1.

Disorders Associated With Esotropia

- Prematurity
- Birth asphyxia/perinatal hypoxia
- Developmental delay
  - Syndromes associated with delay
  - Trisomy-21
  - Hydrocephalus

of their child's vision. Does the baby fixate on their faces? Does the baby respond to lights? Are other abnormal eye movements present, especially nystagmus? If you notice strabismus during your examination, the parents should be asked whether they have seen this at home. Experienced parents may recognize that occasional brief crossing is fairly common in newborns, and may not have bothered to mention it. However, some parents may mistakenly believe that more severe strabismus, such as constant large-angle crossing or crossing that persists beyond 2 months of age, is also normal. This can be determined by specific questioning.

The amount and frequency of the eye crossing should be determined. If the parents see only brief crossing during the first 1 to 2 months of life, and the baby is otherwise developing well, this is likely normal. If they see constant crossing at any age, even in the first 2 months of life, this is usually not normal. An important caveat is that true infantile esotropia may initially present with intermittent crossing, typically worse when the child is tired. It usually progresses to constant crossing by 3 to 4 months of age (unlike normal occasional infant crossing, which should resolve by this age) (Table 9–2).

If the parents see only mild crossing, and it seems worse when the baby looks to the side, this is probably pseudostrabismus. This condition is often noted in photographs, the inspection of which may confirm the diagnosis if the corneal light reflexes are symmetric (Figure 9–1).

The baby's medical history is part of the well-child evaluation by the pediatrician. Many conditions that cause developmental problems are associated with a higher incidence of infantile esotropia. Examples include prematurity, perinatal hypoxia, Trisomy-21, and hydrocephalus (Table 9–1).

Infantile esotropia is not inherited in a mendelian fashion, but there is a genetic predisposition to the disease. If children have first-degree relatives with strabismus, they should be monitored carefully for the onset of eye misalignment. Other potentially heritable causes of decreased vision that may initially present with strabismus include infantile cataracts and retinoblastoma.

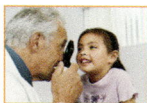

Examination

In addition to a regular well-child examination, infants whose parents report eye crossing or in whom this is noted during the examination should have their vision carefully checked. *It is important to recognize that a child who has decreased vision in one eye, but normal vision in the other, will appear to see normally when both eyes are open.* In a child with strabismus and decreased vision, the vision loss may be secondary to the strabismus (amblyopia) or the strabismus may be secondary to the decreased vision. In either case, the infant will ignore the eye with decreased vision, and usually functions well using only the good eye.

To check the vision in an infant with strabismus, watch to see whether the strabismus spontaneously alternates between the eyes (Figure 9–2). If it does, this indicates that the vision is equal or nearly equal in both eyes. If one eye is constantly crossed, the examiner should cover the eye that is straight and see whether the child fixates on a toy or the examiner's face with the strabismic eye. If the child uses this eye well and is not bothered by having the normally straight eye covered, the vision is probably equal or nearly equal in both eyes.

The type of strabismus should be noted, including the degree and frequency of the crossing. The corneal light reflection test is a good way to assess this. If the child is esotropic, the light reflection will be centered in the eye that is looking at the penlight, and it will be displaced onto the temporal cornea in the crossed eye (Figure 9–2).

Children with pseudostrabismus appear esotropic on initial examination. These children usually have epicanthal folds or a wide nasal bridge. The corneal light reflex is symmetric, indicating esotropia is not present (Figure 9–1).

As noted above, brief episodes of crossing, which can be quite marked, are often normal in the first 1 to 2 months of life. If an infant's eyes are constantly crossed, referral to an ophthalmologist is indicated.

Examination findings that indicate there may be other ocular problems in addition to the strabismus include bilateral poor visual fixation, nystagmus, and/or an abnormal red reflex (Table 9-3).

Table 9–2.

Signs and Symptoms Suggesting True Esotropia (Versus Physiological Intermittent Esotropia or Pseudostrabismus)

- Large-angle crossing
- Constant crossing
- Worse when tired
- Family history of strabismus
- Developmental delay

Table 9–3.

Signs Suggesting Other Problems in Addition to Esotropia

- Poor visual fixation
- Nystagmus
- Decreased red reflex

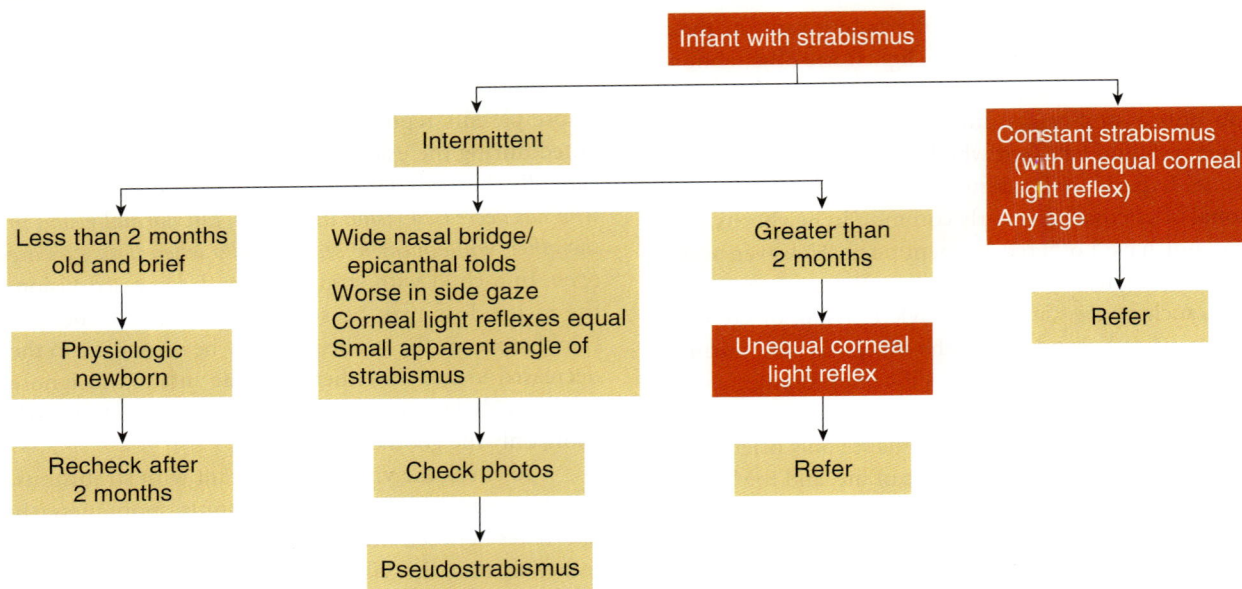

FIGURE 9–3 ■ Algorithm for evaluation and management of an infant with strabismus.

PLAN

In a healthy child who has only occasional brief eye crossing in the first 1 to 2 months (whether by parents' history, your examination, or both), and whose vision and eye examination are otherwise normal, reexamination at 2 to 3 months of age is appropriate.

If the examiner suspects a child has pseudostrabismus, it should be kept in mind that true esotropia may initially be intermittent, and therefore may not be present during an office examination. A question that may help in distinguishing true estropia from pseudostrabismus is whether the parents note the crossing is worse when the baby is tired. If so, true esotropia is more likely. In addition, if there are other concerning historical features, such as developmental delay or a family history of strabismus, referral for verification should be considered (Table 9–2).

An infant with constant eye crossing at any age, an abnormal red reflex, or in whom decreased vision is suspected should be referred to an ophthalmologist (Figure 9–3).

WHAT SHOULDN'T BE MISSED

Esotropia may be the presenting sign of serious ocular conditions such as infantile cataracts and retinoblastoma. The red reflex examination will usually be abnormal in such patients. Because the prognosis for vision (and life, in the case of retinoblastoma) is largely dependent on early diagnosis and treatment, these patients should be referred to an ophthalmologist and seen within a few days.

For less serious disorders, including strabismus and amblyopia, early diagnosis is also very beneficial. *In general, if the examiner cannot be certain whether true ocular misalignment is present, it is preferable to err on the side of caution and refer such patients for a full evaluation. It is better to have a child evaluated by an ophthalmologist and found to be normal, rather than risk delay in diagnosing a potentially serious condition.*

When to Refer

■ Any infant with constant strabismus
■ Intermittent esotropia that persists after 3 to 4 months
■ An infant with strabismus and other abnormalities
    □ Nystagmus
    □ Poor vision
    □ Abnormal red reflex

CHAPTER 10

Strabismus in an Older Child

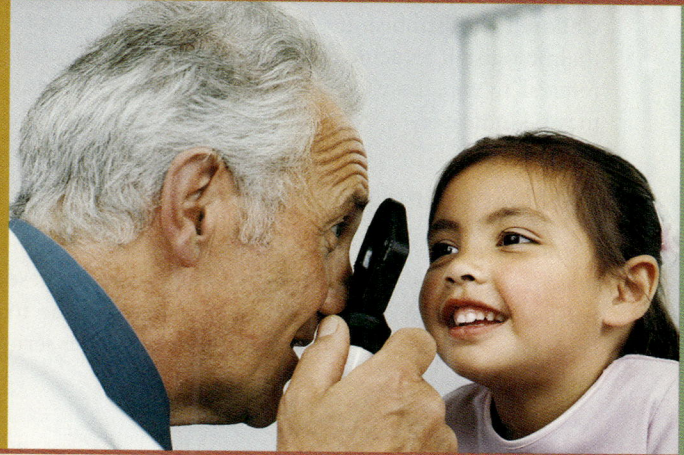

The Problem

"My (older) child's eyes aren't straight."

Common Causes

Accommodative esotropia (crossing due to farsightedness)
Exotropia
Recurrent strabismus following treatment for
  infantile infantile esotropia
Acute comitant esotropia

Other Causes

Duane syndrome
Cranial nerve palsies (third, fourth, sixth)

KEY FINDINGS

History

Accommodative esotropia
  Onset usually about 3 to 5 years
  Initially intermittent, rapid increase over few months
  Worse when viewing at near
Acute comitant esotropia
  Sudden-onset esotropia, usually ages 3 to 5 years
  No diplopia
  No other neurological symptoms
  Often family history strabismus
Exotropia
  Usually intermittent
  Worse with fatigue
  Worse when viewing at distance
Recurrent strabismus after treatment for infantile esotropia
  History of surgery for esotropia when younger
  May be esotropia, exotropia, or vertical strabismus
Duane syndrome
  Present at birth, but often not noted until older
  Most commonly appear esotropic
  Worse in side gaze
  Affected eye may appear "smaller" (due to narrow lid fissure)
Cranial nerve palsy
  Strabismus dependent on which cranial nerve involved
  Diplopia

Other symptoms dependent on etiology of cranial
  nerve problem

Examination

Accommodative esotropia
  Variable eye crossing, worse when fixating at near
  Otherwise normal
Acute comitant esotropia
  Full extraocular movements
  Examination otherwise normal
Exotropia
  May not see anything abnormal on examination
  Eye alignment often normal when viewing object at near
  Cover test may reveal exotropia when patient fixates
    at distance
Recurrent strabismus after treatment for infantile esotropia
  May be any type: esotropia, exotropia, or vertical
    strabismus
Duane syndrome
  Horizontal gaze abnormality
  Most commonly limited outward movement of eye
  Small or moderate esotropia
    May appear similar to sixth cranial nerve palsy
  Eyelids narrow when eye turned toward nose
Cranial nerve palsy
  Third cranial nerve
    Eye out and down
    Ptosis (droopy eyelid)
    Dilated pupil
  Fourth cranial nerve
    Affected eye higher
    Worse when head tilted to side of palsy
    Eye moves up when turned toward nose
  Sixth cranial nerve
    Large-angle esotropia
    Limited outward movement of eye

WHAT SHOULD YOU DO?

Children with strabismus should be referred to an ophthalmologist. If an acute cranial nerve palsy is suspected, referral to a pediatric neurologist and brain imaging may be indicated.

What Shouldn't Be Missed

Third, fourth, and sixth cranial nerve palsies may initially present with strabismus. Although some causes of these palsies are benign or self-limited, they may be due to central nervous system infections, tumors, or other serious diseases.

COMMON CAUSES

1. *Accommodative esotropia.* Accommodative esotropia is a form of eye crossing due to farsightedness. The majority of children in the first several years of life are farsighted. Few young children need to wear glasses, however, because the lens is able to change its shape to focus (accommodation), as if the children have a built-in pair of glasses. When children are more farsighted than normal, the effort to focus is greater, and this effort may induce esotropia. The esotropia usually resolves when the farsightedness is corrected with spectacles. Bifocal glasses are sometimes used if the eye crossing is worse when viewing near objects (Figure 10–1A and B).

2. *Acute comitant esotropia.* Esotropia that is not due to farsightedness may occasionally develop rapidly in children after infancy. These children often have a family history of strabismus, and they do not experience diplopia. It is felt that many of these children have had a strabismic tendency that was never noticed, and that

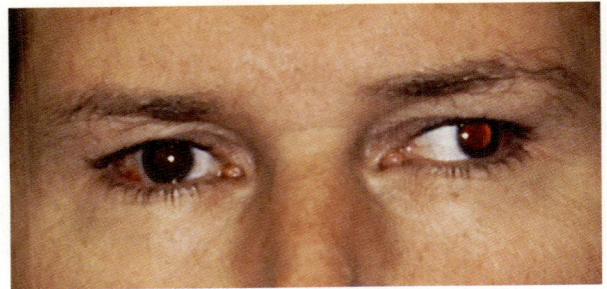

FIGURE 10–2 ■ Large left exotropia. Note marked asymmetry of corneal light reflexes.

at some point they lose the ability to control this and develop manifest strabismus. These children are usually otherwise healthy, but the acute onset may warrant evaluation to rule out other abnormalities.

3. *Exotropia.* Exotropia usually presents in older children, but may develop in infancy. In most patients it is intermittent, and the vision is usually normal in both eyes. It is more noticeable when children are tired, ill, or daydreaming, and it is worse when viewing distant objects (Figure 10–2).

   Older children with exotropia are usually otherwise healthy. It is unusual for exotropia to present before 1 year of age, and infantile exotropia may be associated with developmental delay. If the exotropia is constant at any age, there may be an underlying ocular disorder causing decreased vision (i.e., the exotropia is a secondary effect of the decreased vision).

4. *Recurrent strabismus following infantile esotropia.* Infantile esotropia usually appears by 3 to 4 months of age. It is treated by surgically weakening or strengthening the horizontal extraocular muscles. Patients with any form of strabismus may require more than 1 surgery to

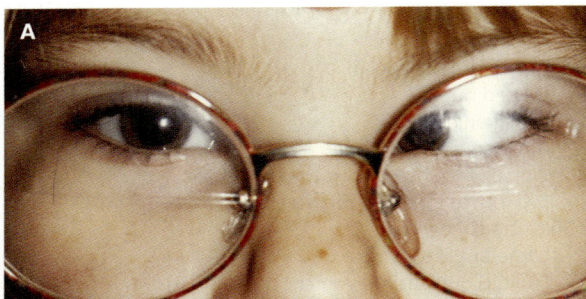

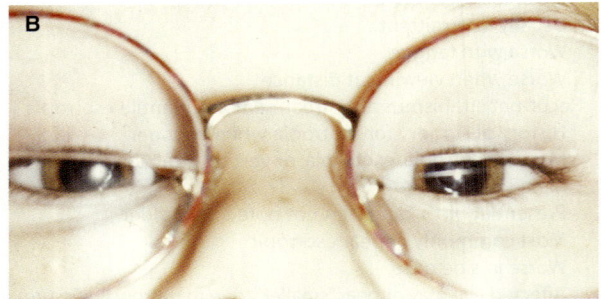

FIGURE 10–1 ■ Accommodative esotropia with eye crossing greater when viewing near objects. (A) Large esotropia when viewing at near through top portion of glasses. (B) Eyes straight when viewing through bifocals.

attain adequate ocular alignment, and the need for additional surgeries is more common in children with infantile esotropia. Recurrent strabismus may manifest as eye crossing (*recurrent esotropia*), outward drifting (*consecutive exotropia*), or vertical eye misalignment (*dissociated vertical deviation or inferior oblique muscle overaction*).

5. *Duane syndrome.* Duane syndrome results from a congenital miswiring of the cranial nerves that control the extraocular muscles. In the most common form, the nerve that innervates the lateral rectus muscle gets crossed with the nerve that innervates the medial rectus muscle. When the patient attempts to look to the side of the affected eye, there is no innervation to the lateral rectus muscle. The opposite eye moves normally (toward the nose), but the affected eye does not move out. Therefore, the patient appears esotropic. When the patient attempts to look toward the side of the normal eye, both the medial and lateral rectus muscles in the affected eye contract and the eye is pulled posteriorly (*globe retraction*), which narrows the space between the eyelids and may give the appearance of ptosis or the affected eye appearing smaller than normal (Figure 10–3).

6. *Cranial nerve palsies.* Cranial nerves III, IV, and VI innervate the extraocular muscles.

    a. *Cranial nerve III* innervates the medial rectus muscle, inferior rectus muscle, inferior

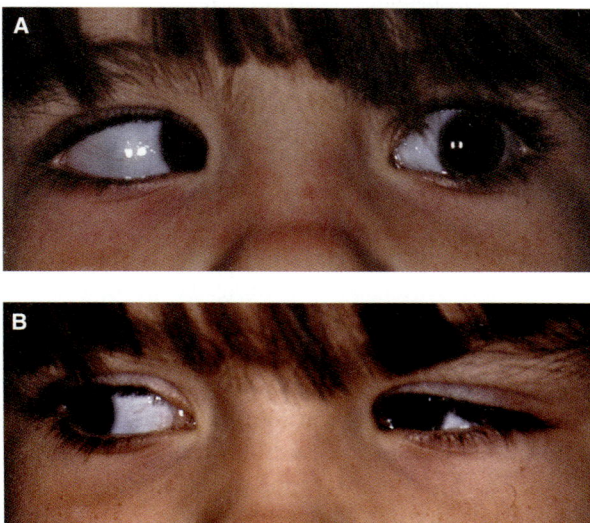

FIGURE 10–4 ■ Partial third nerve palsy, left eye. The left eye is exotropic (out) and hypotropic (down), and the left eyelid is ptotic.

oblique muscle, and superior rectus muscle, as well as the eyelid levator muscle, and the iris sphincter muscle. In patients with third cranial nerve palsies the only functioning extraocular muscles are the superior oblique and lateral rectus muscles. Therefore, the affected eye is out and down, and the patient has ptosis and a dilated pupil on the affected side (Figure 10–4). Of the 3 cranial nerve palsies discussed here, third nerve palsies are the most likely to be associated with significant intracranial disorders.

    b. *Cranial nerve IV* innervates the superior oblique muscle. This muscle moves the eye down when it is turned toward the nose. In fourth nerve palsies the affected eye is elevated. This elevation is worse when the eye is turned toward the nose or when the patient tilts his or her head toward the side of the palsy. Therefore, patients often present with a head tilt to the opposite side, which is adopted to keep the eyes aligned (Figure 10–5A–C). Fourth nerve palsies may result from intracranial pathology, but they are most commonly considered congenital and otherwise benign. They usually are not present in infancy, but become noticeable later in childhood (sometimes not until adulthood).

    c. *Cranial nerve VI* innervates the lateral rectus muscle. Patients with sixth nerve palsies cannot turn their eyes outward, and they present with esotropia of the affected eye (Figure 10–6). Unlike most other forms of childhood strabismus, patients with sixth nerve palsies often complain of diplopia. Sixth nerve palsies may occur following viral illness, in which case they are usually benign and self-limited, but they may also occur due to increased intracranial pressure.

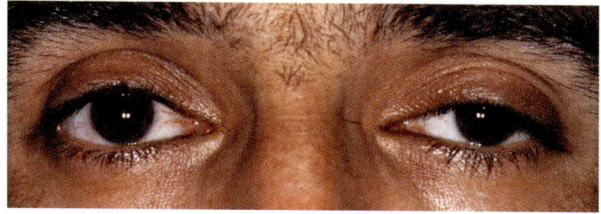

FIGURE 10–3 ■ Duane retraction syndrome, left eye. (A) The left eye cannot move fully outward when the patient looks to the left. (B) When the patient looks to the right, the space between the eyelids narrows on the left (due to retraction of the eyeball).

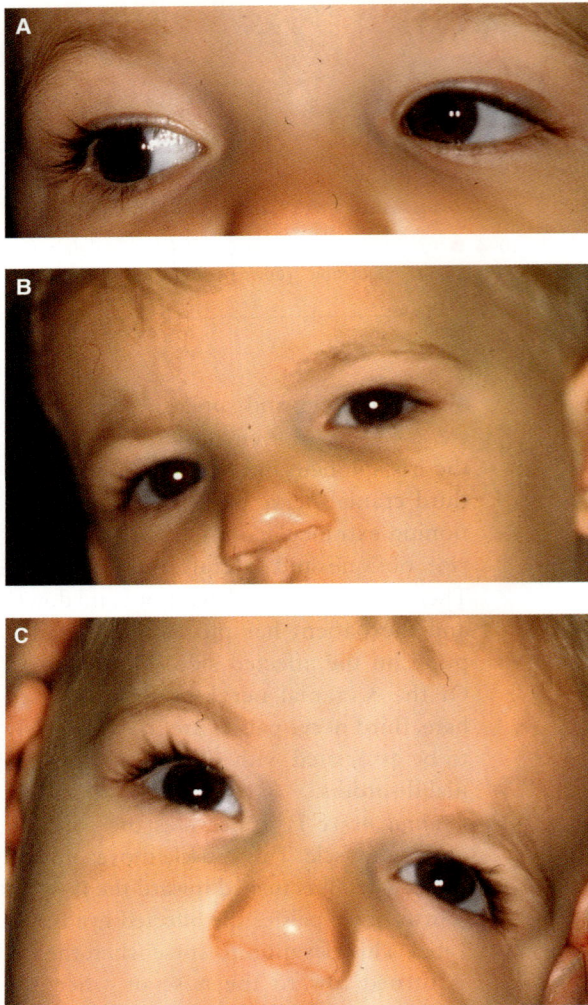

FIGURE 10–5 ■ Congenital left fourth nerve palsy. (A) Left eye has limited downgaze when attempting to look to right and down (right eye is moving normally). (B) Patient adopts compensatory right head tilt to keep eyes aligned. (C) Left eye moves up when patient's head is tilted to left.

APPROACH TO THE PATIENT

Strabismus is a relatively common problem in childhood, affecting approximately 3% to 4% of children. The majority of children with strabismus are otherwise normal, but there are 2 important exceptions. First,

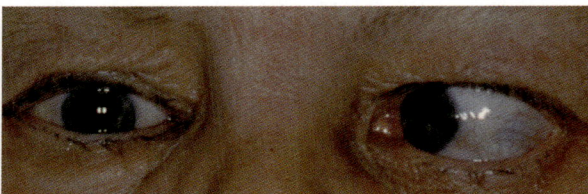

FIGURE 10–6 ■ Acute left sixth cranial nerve palsy. Large-angle esotropia due to inability of left eye to move outward.

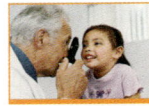

Table 10–1.

Worrisome Signs in Older Child With Strabismus

	Worrisome	Less worrisome
Diplopia	Yes	No
Family history strabismus	No	Yes
Other neurological abnormalities	Yes	No
Limited eye movements	Yes	No
Abnormal red reflex	Yes	No

strabismus in children may be the presenting sign of unilateral decreased vision from any cause. Although rare, entities such as retinoblastoma need to be considered in any patient with strabismus. Second, strabismus could be the presenting sign of a neurological illness, particularly in patients who have new-onset cranial nerve palsies. *As almost all children with strabismus will be referred to an ophthalmologist, the pediatrician's role is to screen for problems that require urgent evaluation* (Table 10–1).

History

The history in children with new-onset strabismus should be focused on 2 things: the strabismus itself and any associated systemic problems. Because most children with strabismus do not have diplopia, they are often unaware that a problem exists. Family members are usually the first to notice eye misalignment, but sometimes other caregivers or teachers initially detect it.

Questions should be asked about the characteristics of the ocular deviation. In older children strabismus usually is intermittent initially. It is often most noticeable when the children are tired. Accommodative esotropia is typically worse at near, and exotropia at distance. *Because intermittent exotropia is usually most noticeable when children are looking at things far away, it is not uncommon for parents to be unaware of it when it first develops.* This is because most visual interactions between parents and young children occur at relatively close distances, such as during meals or while reading books. Families tend to view things at distance together, such as when they are watching television or looking at things while driving. Because of this, parents do not often look at their child's eyes when the child is looking far away. This is why teachers or other nonfamily members may be the first to notice intermittent exotropia. For instance, a teacher may notice it in school when the child is across the classroom.

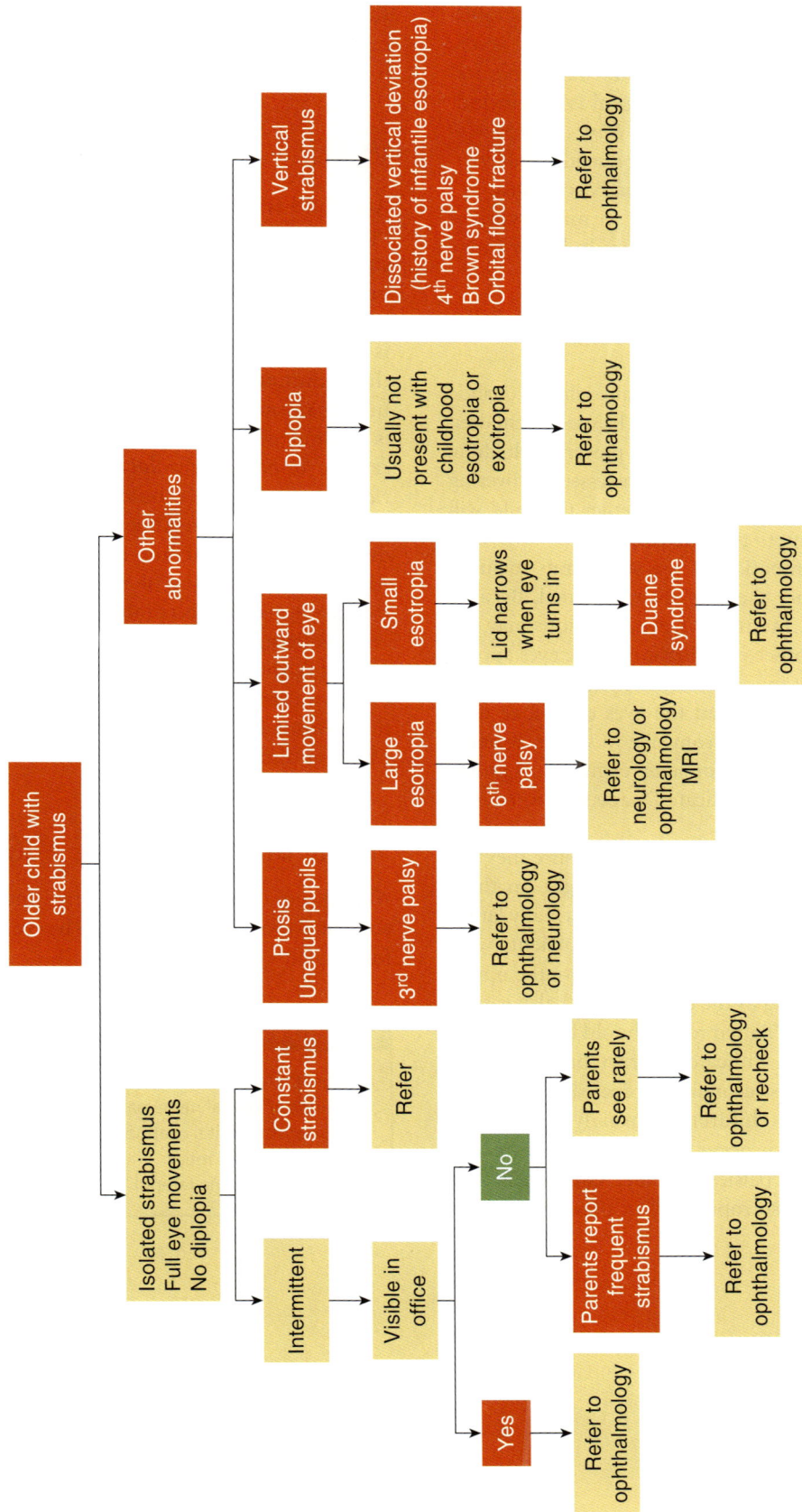

FIGURE 10–7 ■ Algorithm for evaluation and management of an older child with strabismus.

Some systemic problems associated with strabismus may be obvious, such as meningitis or severe trauma. In the absence of other abnormalities, questions should be focused on neurological issues, including a neurological review of systems. *Most children with strabismus do not have diplopia. Its presence is concerning, indicating the possibility of a cranial nerve palsy.*

There is a genetic component to many types of childhood strabismus. A positive family history may suggest a diagnosis.

Examination

The examination of a child with strabismus should include testing the vision. An eye chart should be used in children who are old enough to cooperate. In preverbal children, the vision in the strabismic eye can be assessed by covering the straight eye and determining whether the child will use the strabismic eye to track objects.

Specific examination of the strabismus includes determining whether the eyes are misaligned. Because strabismus may be intermittent, eye deviations may not be present during office examination. If the eyes appear straight, a cover test may sometimes elicit the deviation. It is important to verify that the eyes can move normally. The eyes move fully from side to side in patients with accommodative esotropia or exotropia. Limitations of movement may indicate Duane syndrome or a cranial nerve palsy.

The pupils should be checked to be sure they are equal in size and respond normally to light. In third cranial nerve palsies the affected pupil is normally larger than the unaffected eye (an exception is patients with congenital third nerve palsies, who may have the opposite finding). Drooping of the eyelid (ptosis) also is seen in third nerve palsy. The red reflex should be examined. Abnormalities could indicate cataract or retinoblastoma, with strabismus secondary to decreased vision.

Strabismus in children is usually horizontal. Vertical strabismus may occur in patients with third and fourth cranial nerve palsies, in older children with a history of infantile esotropia, and in other conditions such as Brown syndrome or orbital floor fractures. The examination findings in these conditions are discussed in detail in Chapter 34.

PLAN

Any child with strabismus should be referred to an ophthalmologist (Figure 10–7). Patients with presumed accommodative esotropia or exotropia should be seen relatively soon, but an urgent evaluation is not required. The acute onset of comitant esotropia is similar to that of accommodative esotropia, and the 2 cannot be differentiated without an ophthalmic examination to determine whether the child is farsighted. *If the history and examination are concerning for possible cranial nerve palsy, prompt evaluation is indicated.* This could be accomplished by referring the patient to an ophthalmologist, who can determine what further evaluation is appropriate. Alternatively, imaging or referral to a pediatric neurologist is also an acceptable approach.

Patients with a history suspicious for intermittent exotropia should be referred to an ophthalmologist, even if no strabismus is detected during your examination. This is because it may be difficult to elicit in the office (as discussed above).

WHAT SHOULDN'T BE MISSED

A child with the acute onset of strabismus, diplopia, and abnormal eye movements should be evaluated promptly for possible cranial nerve palsy.

When to Refer

- Urgent referral if other abnormalities
  - Signs of cranial nerve palsy
  - Proptosis, orbital changes
  - Abnormal red reflex
- Otherwise routine referral

CHAPTER 11

Diplopia

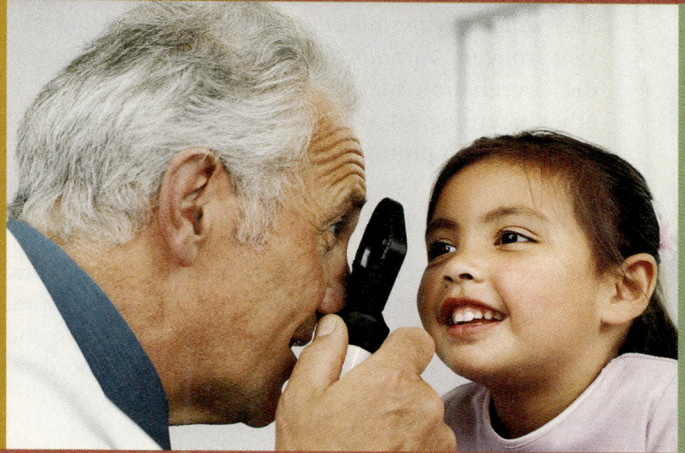

The Problem
"I see two of things."

Common Causes
Physiological diplopia
Breakdown of phoria
Cranial nerve palsy
  Third nerve palsy
  Fourth nerve palsy
  Sixth nerve palsy

Other Causes
Decompensated childhood strabismus
Duane syndrome
Myasthenia gravis (discussed in ptosis chapter)

KEY FINDINGS

History
Physiological diplopia
  Usually noticed about ages 5 to 6 years
  Most common in bright, observant children
  Not bothered by symptoms
Breakdown of phoria
  Often no known history of strabismus
  Develop strabismus and diplopia during severe illness
  Resolves after recovery of illness
Cranial nerve palsies
  Third nerve palsy
    Horizontal and vertical diplopia
    Ptosis
    Unequal pupils (anisocoria)
  Fourth nerve palsy
    Usually gradually worsening vertical diplopia
    Head tilt
  Sixth nerve palsy
    Horizontal diplopia
    Recent viral illness

Idiopathic intracranial hypertension
  Headache
  Brief episodes of vision loss (transient visual
    obscurations)
  Recent medication change
    Corticosteroids, isotretinoic acid, others

Examination
Physiological diplopia
  Normal ophthalmic examination
  Normal physical examination
Breakdown of phoria
  Variable esotropia or exotropia
  No limitation of extraocular movements
Cranial nerve palsies
  Fourth nerve palsy
    Usually head tilt
    Eyes straight when head tilted to
      unaffected side
    Vertical misalignment when tilted to
      affected side
  Sixth nerve palsy
    Esotropia
    Inability to move affected eye outward
    Idiopathic intracranial hypertension
      Obesity
      Papilledema
  Third nerve palsy
    Eye out and down
    Ptosis on affected side
    Anisocoria (affected pupil larger in acquired
      third nerve palsy)
    Possible other neurological signs

WHAT SHOULD YOU DO?

Most children with strabismus do not *experience diplopia. This symptom warrants referral to an ophthalmologist.* If the examination suggests a cranial nerve palsy, or if other neurological symptoms are present, the child should be seen promptly.

What Shouldn't Be Missed

Acute cranial nerve palsies may be due to idiopathic intracranial hypertension or other intracranial diseases. Prompt evaluation and treatment may improve the prognosis for both vision and the underlying disorder.

COMMON CAUSES

1. *Physiological diplopia.* This is a normal phenomenon that is most commonly noted by bright and observant children around ages 5 to 6 years. The eyes normally focus on objects in a single plane, and these are seen as single images. Objects in front of or behind the object of attention appear to be double, but most people do not notice this. The diplopia can be demonstrated by holding one finger up at arm's distance in front of your face, with another object (e.g., something on the wall) in the background in line with your finger. If you focus on your finger but pay attention to the object in the background, the background object will appear double. Conversely, if you focus on the background object but pay attention to your finger, the finger will appear double (Figure 11–1). Most of the time these double images are ignored, but children may become aware of them and report them to their parents.

2. *Breakdown of a phoria.* Many normal individuals have a phoria. A phoria is a tendency for the eyes to become misaligned when one eye is covered. The eyes are straight during normal viewing conditions with both eyes open. With a phoria, when one is covered it drifts off center (either inward or outward). The eye returns to its normal position when the eye is uncovered (Figure 11–2). In some patients, usually in association with severe illness or trauma, the ability to control the phoria is temporarily lost, and they develop manifest strabismus (esotropia or exotropia) and diplopia. This usually resolves in conjunction with recovery from the underlying problem.

3. *Fourth nerve palsy.* This is most often congenital and not associated with other neurological problems.

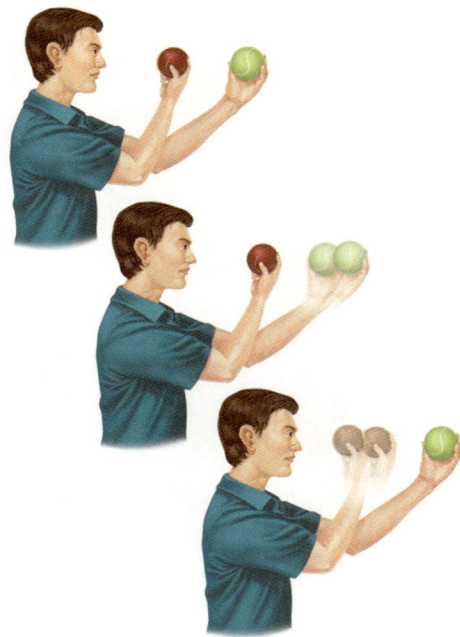

FIGURE 11–1 ■ Physiological diplopia. (Top) This can be demonstrated by holding two objects in line with each other in front of the eyes. (Middle) If the eyes focus on the near object, the far object will appear double. (Bottom) If the eyes focus on the far object, the near object will appear double (bottom figure).

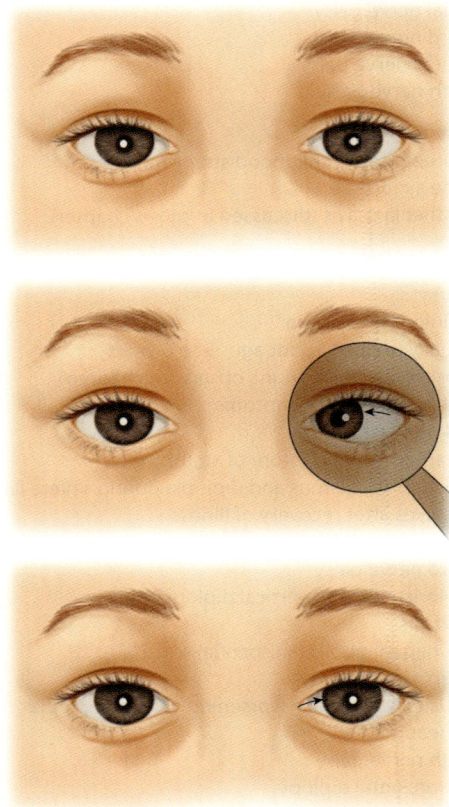

FIGURE 11–2 ■ Left esophoria. (Top) The eyes are normally straight. (Middle) If a cover is placed in front of the left eye, the eye moves inward behind the cover. (Bottom) When the cover is removed, the left eye returns to its normal position.

4. *Third nerve palsy.* Acquired third nerve palsy may result from many different neurological problems.
5. *Sixth nerve palsy.* Most common causes are transient sixth nerve palsy of childhood (often associated with preceding viral illness) and increased intracranial pressure.

APPROACH TO THE PATIENT

Strabismus in childhood is most commonly due to the disorders discussed in Chapters 7 and 8. In these forms of strabismus it is unusual for children to complain of diplopia because the child's visual system typically suppresses (ignores) the image from the misaligned eye. When a child complains of diplopia, prompt investigation may be warranted if there is evidence of an acute cranial nerve palsy.

History

The primary concern in a child who reports diplopia is whether a cranial nerve palsy is present. Cranial nerve palsies may result from trauma, which is usually severe. In this case a history of injury would be easily identified. In the absence of trauma, other neurological signs or symptoms, such as headache, lethargy, nausea, and vomiting, should raise concern. A complete neurological review of systems should be obtained in these patients.

Cranial nerve palsies need to be differentiated from a breakdown of a phoria, which may also occur in association with a severe illnesses or trauma. Both may cause diplopia, and they are differentiated from one another by the examination and history (Table 11–1).

Some cranial nerve palsies in children are benign, particularly congenital fourth nerve palsies. These produce a vertical strabismus that is worse when the head is tilted to the side of the palsy. The patients typically develop a compensatory head tilt to the opposite side to minimize the strabismus. In some families, this occurs so frequently that the family no longer notices it. Evaluation of old photographs may show that a head tilt has been present since early childhood. These children often do not complain of diplopia when they are young, but when they are older they may describe vertical diplopia when their head is tilted to side of the palsy or when they look to the side.

Children may develop transient sixth nerve palsies in the absence of other neurological problems. If the children are old enough to verbalize symptoms, they usually complain of horizontal diplopia. These patients often have a history of a viral illness in the few weeks before the onset of the palsy.

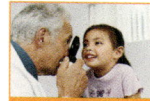

Table 11–1.

Differentiating Breakdown of a Phoria From a Cranial Nerve Palsy

Associated illness
- Phoria: Symptoms occur during acute illness or after trauma
- Cranial nerve palsy: May have neurological symptoms, often normal

History
- Phoria: Usually no history of strabismus
- Cranial nerve palsy
  - Sixth nerve palsy: often after viral illness
  - Fourth nerve palsy: often long history of head tilt

Examination
- Phoria
  - Esotropia or exotropia
  - No limitation of extraocular movements
  - Examination usually normal after illness resolves
- Cranial nerve palsy
  - Fourth nerve
    - Head tilt to side opposite palsy
    - Vertical strabismus when head tilted to side of palsy
  - Third nerve
    - Eye out and down
    - Ptosis
    - Pupil smaller on affected side
  - Sixth nerve
    - Esotropia
    - Limited outward movement of eye
    - If increased intracranial pressure: papilledema

Children with physiological diplopia usually describe seeing double at approximately 5 to 6 years of age. They are usually not bothered by this phenomenon, and often it is first brought to attention during casual conversation with their parents. These children are otherwise healthy, have no neurological symptoms, and are often described as bright and observant.

Examination

The evaluation of a child with diplopia should include a complete neurological examination. Direct ophthalmoscopy should be performed to look for papilledema. Children with diplopia due to breakdown of a phoria usually have visible esotropia or exotropia during the illness that precipitates the diplopia. Their extraocular movements are otherwise normal, with no limitation, which differentiates this problem from a cranial nerve palsy. The ocular findings that occur in third, fourth, and sixth cranial nerve palsies are described in Chapter 10. Children with physiological diplopia have normal examinations.

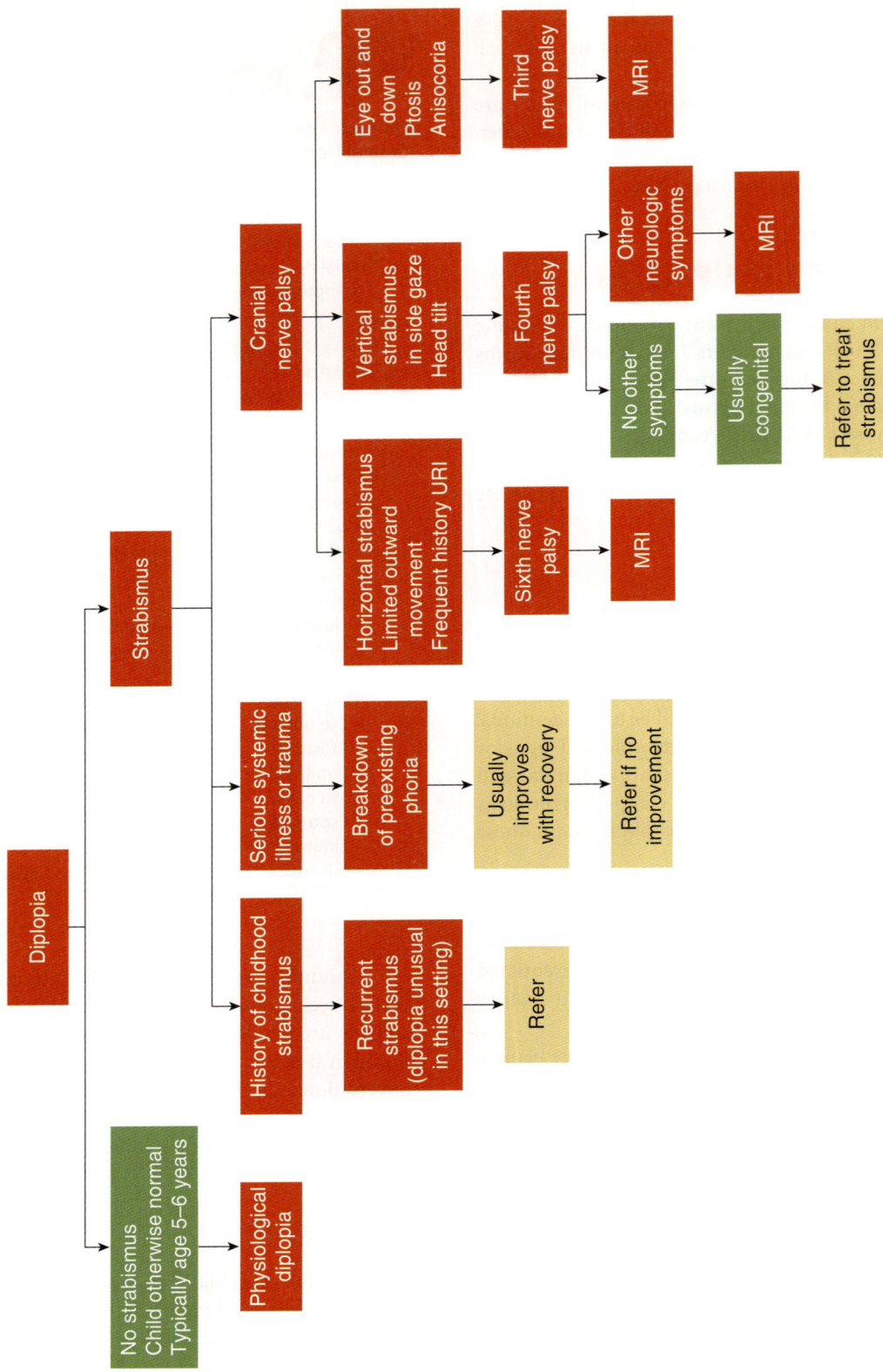

FIGURE 11–3 ■ Algorithm for evaluation and management of a patient with diplopia.

PLAN

If an acute cranial nerve palsy is suspected, children should be referred promptly for further studies. These usually include central nervous system imaging and ophthalmology and neurology consultations. If a congenital fourth nerve palsy is suspected (based on a long-standing head tilt), referral to a pediatric ophthalmologist is recommended. Most of these children do not require imaging. If physiological diplopia is suspected, referral to a pediatric ophthalmologist is indicated to verify the diagnosis (Figure 11–3).

WHAT SHOULDN'T BE MISSED

Children with the new onset of diplopia may have *cranial nerve palsies*, which may be due to central nervous system lesions.

When to Refer

■ Urgent referral if other abnormalities
  □ Signs of cranial nerve palsy
  □ Signs of orbital abnormality
■ Otherwise regular referral

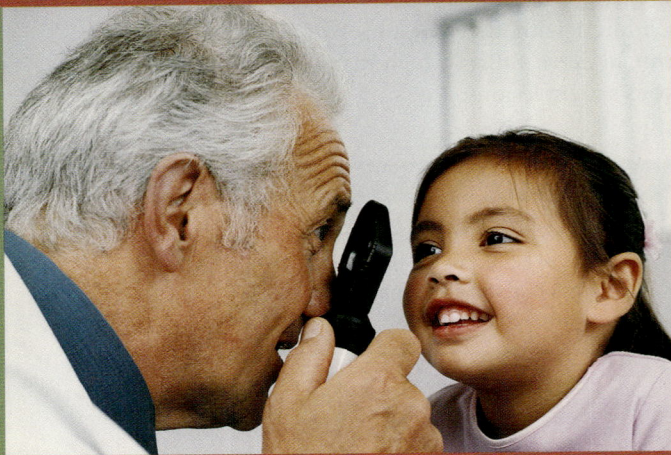

CHAPTER 12

Nystagmus

The Problem
"My child's eyes jiggle back and forth."

Common Causes
Congenital motor nystagmus (vision otherwise normal)
Sensory nystagmus (nystagmus secondary to decreased vision)

Other Causes
Latent nystagmus (associated with infantile strabismus)
Voluntary nystagmus
Central nervous system tumors, malformations
Pharmacological

KEY FINDINGS
History
Congenital motor nystagmus (infantile nystagmus syndrome)
   Onset in first few months of life
   Vision otherwise seems normal
   May be hereditary

Sensory nystagmus
   Onset in first few months of life
   Variable vision—profoundly impaired to near-normal
   Possible family history (depending on diagnosis)
   Other problems affecting development

Examination
Congenital motor nystagmus
   Horizontal nystagmus
   Vision seems normal
   Pupils react normally
   Possible abnormal head posture (to decrease nystagmus)
Sensory nystagmus
   Usually horizontal, possible vertical or rotary
   Vision variable (very poor to near-normal)
   Poor pupil reactions
   Possible abnormal head posture (to decrease nystagmus)
   Other findings depending on underlying diagnosis

WHAT SHOULD YOU DO?

Children with nystagmus should be referred for further evaluation. This is usually done most efficiently by initially referring the child to an ophthalmologist. Nystagmus that presents in infancy and early childhood is usually due to either congenital motor nystagmus or is secondary to an underlying ocular disorder. Acquired nystagmus in older children is more likely to be associated with an underlying neurological disorder. Older children with nystagmus may need to be evaluated by both an ophthalmologist and a neurologist.

What Shouldn't Be Missed

Sensory nystagmus in infants may be due to septo-optic dysplasia. This is often associated with pituitary gland dysfunction. Affected infants may not be able to mount a normal stress response and are therefore at risk for decompensating with minor illnesses. If this diagnosis is suspected, the infant's family should be warned of this

Table 12–1.

Signs and Symptoms of Congenital Motor Nystagmus (Infantile Nystagmus Syndrome)

■ Visual acuity near normal
■ Child otherwise healthy with normal development
■ May have family history
■ Horizontal nystagmus
■ Nystagmus remains horizontal in up- and downgaze (uniplanar)

possibility while waiting for an endocrinological evaluation.

COMMON CAUSES

1. *Congenital motor nystagmus (infantile nystagmus syndrome)*. In congenital motor nystagmus, the eyes themselves are fine. The nystagmus results from abnormalities of the ocular motor system. Despite the nystagmus, most children see surprisingly well (Table 12–1).

2. *Sensory nystagmus*. Any disorder that affects the vision in both eyes during infancy may present with nystagmus in the first few months of life. The prognosis for vision depends on the underlying disorder. Common etiologies include albinism, optic nerve hypoplasia (septo-optic dysplasia), and Leber's congenital amaurosis (Table 12–2).

3. *Acquired nystagmus in older children*. Acquired nystagmus is relatively rare in childhood. Unlike infantile nystagmus, older children with acquired nystagmus may complain of oscillopsia, the sensation of the world moving back and forth. Acquired nystagmus may result from central nervous system lesions or as a side effect of medication (Table 12–3).

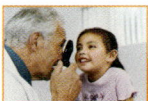

Table 12–2.

Conditions Associated With Decreased Vision and Nystagmus in Infancy

■ Bilateral cataract
■ Bilateral retinoblastoma
■ Optic nerve hypoplasia
■ Leber's congenital amaurosis
■ Ocular or oculocutaneous albinism
■ Other retinal or ocular disorders

4. *Voluntary nystagmus*. Some patients are able to voluntarily elicit nystagmus. This is a high-frequency horizontal oscillation. It cannot be sustained longer than a few seconds.

5. *Latent nystagmus (fusion maldevelopment nystagmus)*. Patients with infantile esotropia develop nystagmus when one of their eyes is covered. The nystagmus is usually not visible when both eyes are opened. It is the strabismus, rather than nystagmus, that usually brings the patient to medical attention.

6. *Normal newborn*. Occasionally, normal infants may have episodes of abnormal eye movements, including nystagmus or tonic gaze deviations, during the first 1 to 2 months of life. This is uncommon, and usually such infants require ophthalmic evaluation to rule out other problems.

APPROACH TO THE PATIENT

Most nystagmus in pediatric patients appears in early infancy. This can be classified as either primary nystagmus (congenital motor nystagmus), in which everything else is normal and the visual prognosis is good, or secondary nystagmus (sensory nystagmus), in which the nystagmus develops as a result of poor vision. The vision in sensory nystagmus varies from mildly to profoundly impaired. In both types of nystagmus, children may discover that the nystagmus decreases in a certain field of gaze (*null zone*). This is usually in right or left gaze, but may also occur in up- or downgaze or with a head tilt. These patients frequently adopt an abnormal head posture to keep their eyes in the null zone to decrease the nystagmus and improve vision.

History

The appropriate history will depend on the age of presentation. For infants with nystagmus, general questions should address the child's birth history and development. The age of onset and characteristics of the nystagmus should be ascertained. Questions should include how well the child appears to see, whether any other ocular abnormalities have been noticed, and whether there is a family history of nystagmus or early visual problems.

In older children with acquired nystagmus, questions should include how well the child appears to see, whether the child experiences oscillopsia, whether other neurological abnormalities have been noted, and whether the child is on any medication (Table 12–3).

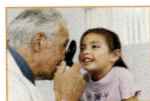

Table 12–3.

Medications Associated With Nystagmus

- Anticonvulsants
- Sedatives
- Alcohol
- Furosemide
- Aminoglycoside antibiotics
- Carboplatin
- Cisplatin
- Reported as potential side effect with many other medications

Examination

Because most pediatric nystagmus develops in early infancy, the examination will be limited by the young age. The examination should include an assessment of the child's visual behavior (Does the child respond to lights?, track objects? smile at their mother?). The pupils should be checked for reactivity. The eye movements should be evaluated for strabismus. The characteristics of the nystagmus should be noted—is it horizontal or vertical? Does it change in different directions of gaze?

Examination of the iris and pupil reactions is important, but this is often difficult in infants. Abnormalities of the iris associated with decreased vision

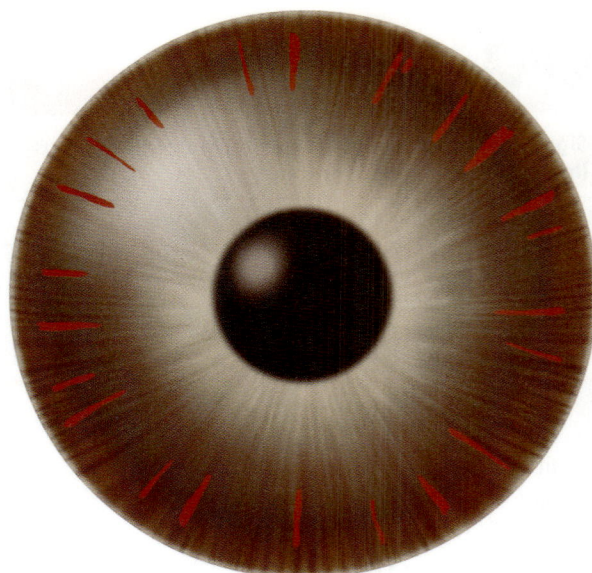

FIGURE 12–1 ■ Transillumination defects of the iris, most commonly seen in albinism. The defects appear as linear, spoke-like, red areas in the peripheral iris when the eye is retroilluminated.

and nystagmus include aniridia and albinism. Patients with oculocutaneous albinism have generalized decreased pigment, with white hair, very fair skin, and minimal iris pigment. Patients with ocular albinism, however, may have nearly normal generalized pigment. The iris may look fairly normal under direct

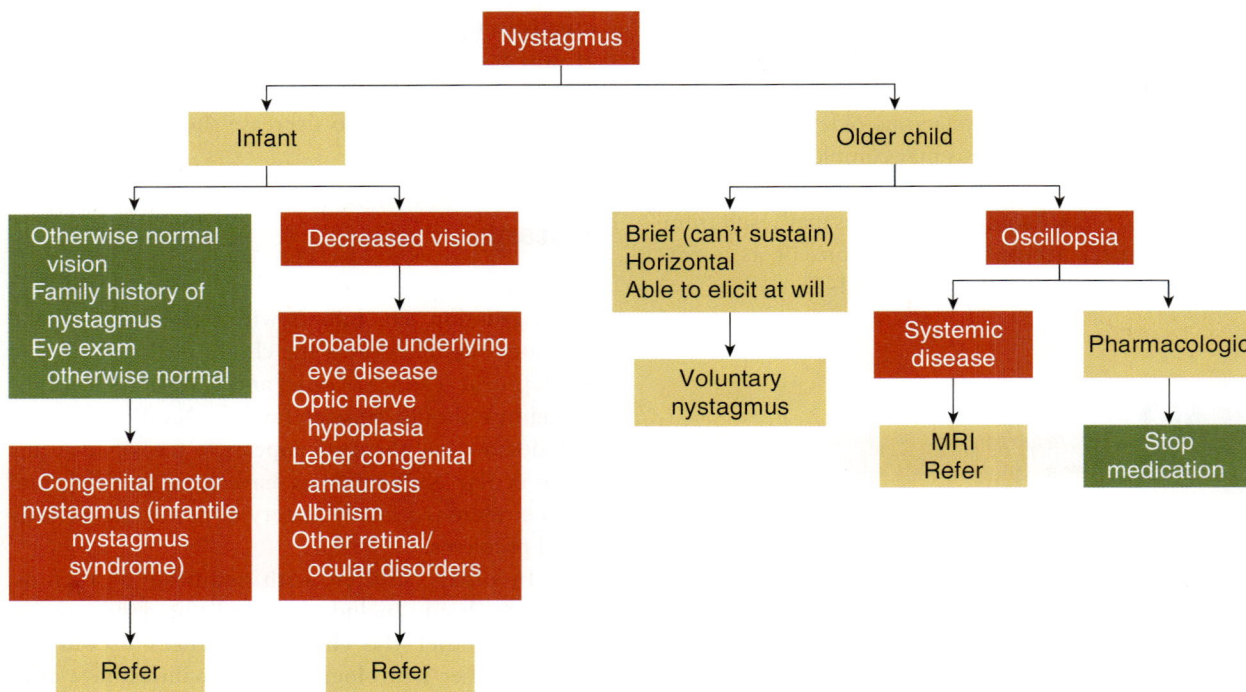

FIGURE 12–2 ■ Algorithm for evaluation and management of a patient with nystagmus.

light, but transillumination defects are present when the eye is retroilluminated (Figure 12–1). Examination of the pupil reactions may also provide clues to a diagnosis. If the pupils react only minimally or not at all, this suggests a serious vision problem, such as Leber's congenital amaurosis or severe optic nerve hypoplasia. Rare retinal problems (e.g., rod monochromatism) may produce a paradoxical pupil reaction, in which the pupil constricts in darkness and dilates with illumination.

Examination of the red reflex may detect cataracts, which can result in nystagmus if the vision is decreased. Retinal abnormalities such as retinoblastoma, large retinal colobomas, and retinal detachments may cause leukocoria.

If an older child presents with acquired nystagmus, a general neurological evaluation should be performed. Evaluation for papilledema is important, though often difficult with the direct ophthalmoscope due to the nystagmus.

PLAN

Infants with nystagmus should be referred to a pediatric ophthalmologist. This should be done promptly due to the possible association with vision- or life-threatening conditions (cataracts, retinoblastoma, etc.). The results of the ophthalmic examination will determine what additional investigations, such as imaging studies or referral to a neurologist, are indicated.

Due to the much higher concern with neurological disease in older children with acquired nystagmus, these patients will often require evaluation by both pediatric ophthalmologists and neurologists. Depending on the findings, either of these may be appropriate for the initial referral.

WHAT SHOULDN'T BE MISSED

Nystagmus may be the initial abnormality noted in infants with poor vision. There are many causes for this finding, including life-threatening disorders such as retinoblastoma and septo-optic dysplasia (which may be associated with adrenocorticotropic hormone deficiency). In older children, acquired nystagmus may be the initial sign of neurological diseases. Therefore, any child with nystagmus should be referred promptly for further evaluation (Figure 12–2).

When to Refer

- Any infant or child with constant nystagmus
- An infant with intermittent nystagmus persisting after 3 to 4 months
- Urgent referral if other neurological abnormalities

CHAPTER 13

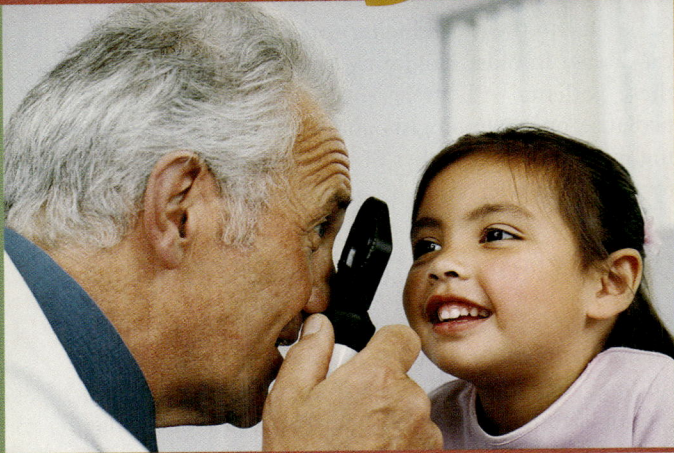

Bumps Around the Eyes

The Problem
"My child has a bump on (or near) his eye."

Common Causes
Newborns
  Hemangioma
  Dermoid
  Mucocele
Older children
  Stye/chalazion

Other Causes
Newborns
  Conjunctival dermolipoma
  Encephalocele
Older children
  Molluscum contagiosum
  Keratin cysts
  Pilomatrixoma
  Conjunctival nevus

KEY FINDINGS

History
Infantile capillary hemangioma
  Initially noted in first few weeks of life
  Grows rapidly in first 1 to 2 months
Orbital dermoid
  Present at birth (though may not be noticed until later)
  Most commonly located at superolateral orbit
Mucocele
  Present at or shortly after birth

Mass on medial canthus
May have symptoms of lacrimal obstruction
If large, associated nasal cyst may cause respiratory
  difficulties
Stye/chalazion
  Initial eyelid erythema (may mimic cellulitis)
  Usually evolves into discrete nodule

Examination
Infantile capillary hemangioma
  Vascular-appearing lesion
  If subcutaneous, vascular character may not be visible
  May have hemangiomas elsewhere on the body
Dermoid
  Smooth, firm, subcutaneous nodule
  Most commonly located at superotemporal orbital rim
Mucocele
  Usually blue-tinged mass overlying lacrimal sac
  If infected, becomes erythematous
  May have periocular crusts, discharge
Stye/chalazion/hordeolum
  Initially may have diffuse eyelid swelling and erythema
    (may mimic cellulitis)
  Usually develop erythematous nodule, often with
    white center
  May drain spontaneously
  If chronic, usually firm nodule
  May have multiple, recurrent lesions
  Blepharitis common (crusts of lashes, erythematous
    lid margin)

WHAT SHOULD YOU DO?

Infants with noninfected mucoceles should be treated with warm compresses and topical antibiotics. If the lesion does not resolve, or if the mucocele becomes infected, referral to a pediatric ophthalmologist is indicated.

Infants with hemangiomas involving the eyelids or periocular structures should be referred to a pediatric ophthalmologist due to the risk of amblyopia.

Styes and chalazia should be treated initially with warm compresses. Topical antibiotics may also be used. Most resolve with conservative treatment in 1 to 2 months. If they do not, referral for incision and drainage may be indicated.

What Shouldn't Be Missed

Infantile mucoceles are almost always associated with nasolacrimal duct cysts. If these are large, they may cause respiratory difficulties. These patients require prompt nasal endoscopy and removal of the cysts.

COMMON CAUSES

1. *Hemangioma.* Hemangiomas are vascular lesions that develop within the first few weeks of life. They usually go through a fairly rapid growth phase over the next few months, then slowly involute. The lesions themselves are benign, but periocular hemangiomas can cause amblyopia, either due to obstruction of vision or by inducing astigmatism (Figure 13–1).

2. *Orbital dermoids.* Orbital dermoids are benign lesions that arise from entrapment of ectodermal tissue between the growth plates during the embryological development of the skull. They are most commonly located along the superolateral orbital rim (Figure 13–2). They may rupture, which can incite a marked inflammatory response.

3. *Mucocele (dacryocele, dacryocystocele, amniotocele).* These lesions result from dilation of the lacrimal sac in newborns with lacrimal

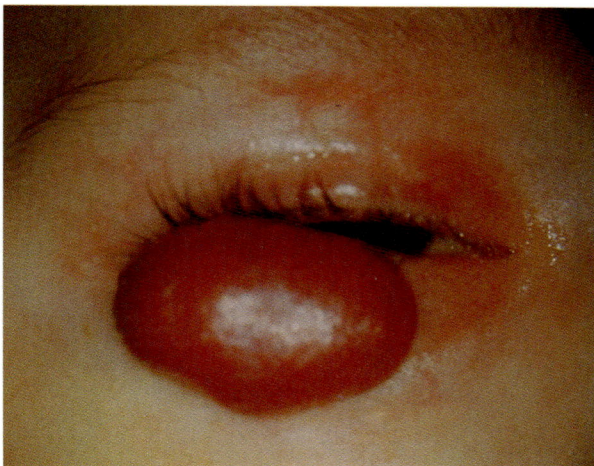

FIGURE 13–2 ■ Dermoid cyst at superolateral orbital.

obstruction. They present as blue-tinged masses overlying the lacrimal sac between the eye and the nose (Figure 13–3). They may become infected and produce an abscess within the lacrimal sac, in which case prompt treatment is warranted.

4. *Chalazion/stye/hordeolum.* Styes result from blockage of the oil glands of the eyelids. The initial inflammatory phase may be associated with diffuse erythema and swelling of the eyelid, which can appear similar to preseptal cellulitis (Figure 13–4). If the lesions do not resolve, they may transform into firm nodules (chalazia) (Figure 13–5). Some patients are prone to recurrent styes.

5. *Other.* A wide variety of lesions may present as bumps around the eyes. The most common

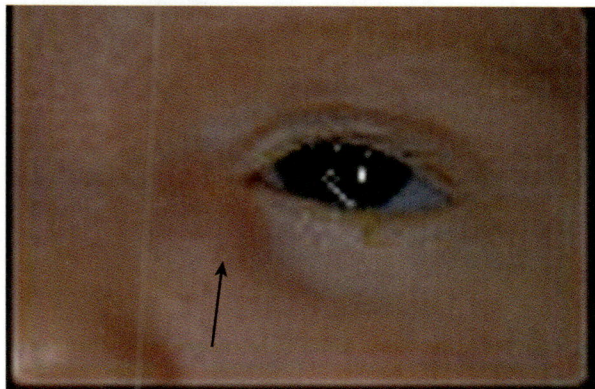

FIGURE 13–1 ■ Large lower eyelid hemangioma, with high risk of amblyopia.

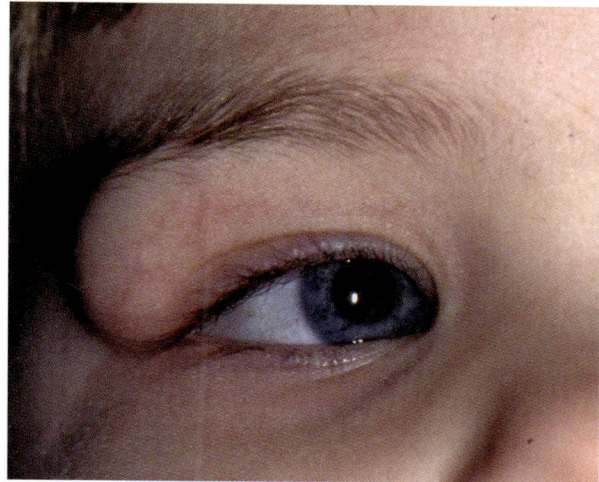

FIGURE 13–3 ■ Neonatal mucocele causing swelling (arrow) over left lacrimal sac. (Reprinted with permission from *Semin Ophthalmol.* 1997;12(2):109-116. Copyright Informa Medical and Pharmaceutical Science.)

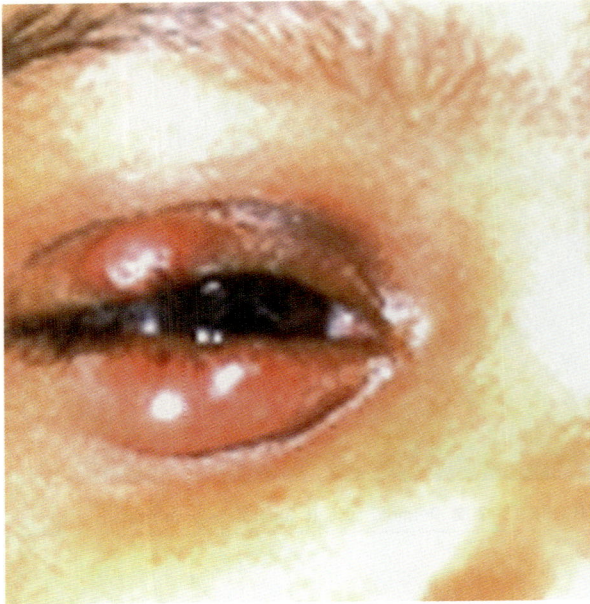

FIGURE 13–4 ■ Erythema and swelling of eyelids secondary to multiple chalazia.

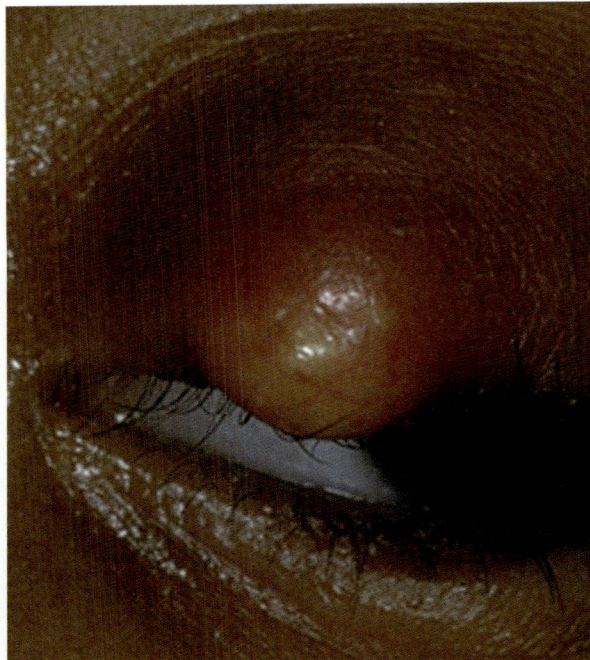

FIGURE 13–6 ■ Conjunctival dermolipomas present as fleshy masses of the lateral conjunctiva.

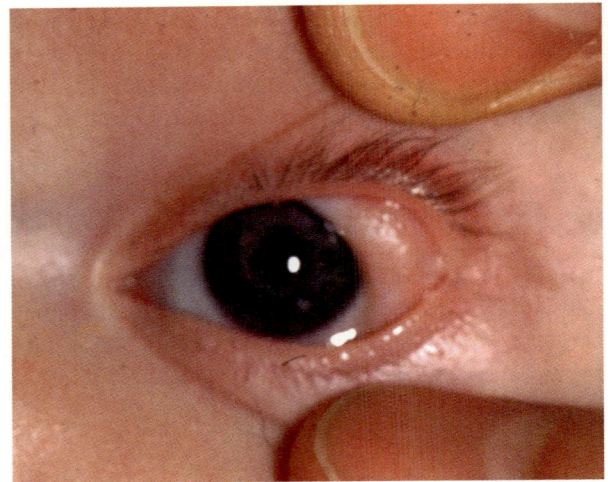

FIGURE 13–5 ■ Chronic chalazion.

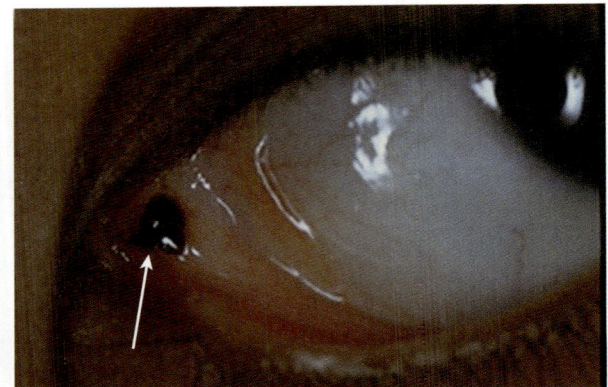

FIGURE 13–7 ■ Darkly pigmented nevus (arrow) of the conjunctival caruncle.

are discussed above. Examples of other eyelid lesions include conjunctival dermolipomas (Figure 13–6), conjunctival nevi (Figure 13–7), pilomatrixoma (Figure 13–8), and papillomas (Figure 13–9). These lesions are discussed in more detail in Chapters 25, 26, and 27.

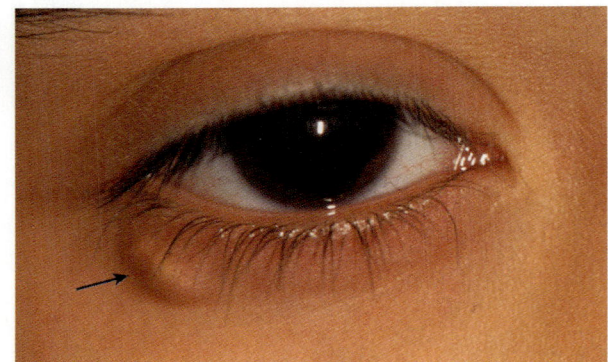

FIGURE 13–8 ■ Pilomatrixomas (arrow) present as firm eyelid nodules, often with a whitish center.

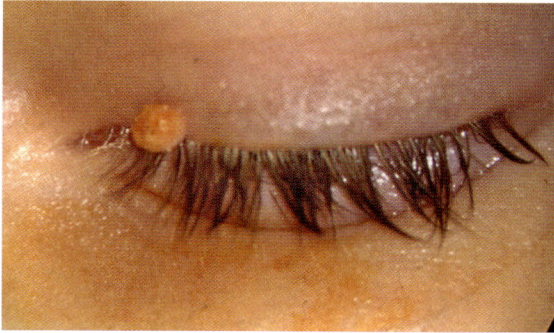

FIGURE 13–9 ■ Papillomatous lesion of upper eyelid.

APPROACH TO THE PATIENT

Most lesions that develop around the eyes in children are benign, although some may have secondary effects that can affect vision. Pediatricians can treat many of these lesions successfully, but some may require referral (Figures 13–10 and 13–11).

History

The differential diagnosis for periocular lesions is quite different between infants and older children. Therefore, the age of onset of the lesion is important. Hemangiomas are usually not present immediately at birth, but are typically noted within the first few weeks of life. They typically grow rapidly during the first few months. Orbital dermoids are present at birth, although they may not be noticed if they are small. They may be stable or grow slowly. If they rupture, an inflammatory reaction may occur. Mucoceles are usually noted within the first week of life. Affected infants may have periocular crusting due to associated nasolacrimal duct obstructions. Mucoceles are almost always associated with nasolacrimal duct cysts. If the nasal cyst is large, it may interfere with breathing. This is worse during feeding because the mouth is occluded and the infant cannot breathe through the obstructed nasal passage.

In older children, styes are the most common periocular lesion. These usually initially develop as red nodules on the eyelid, which may be moderately painful. Occasionally they may produce diffuse erythema and swelling of the lid, which can be difficult to distinguish from preseptal cellulitis. Styes may spontaneously rupture and drain. If they do not resolve, they may transform into a firm, noninflamed eyelid nodule (chalazion).

Examination

The location and appearance of periocular lesions in infants are useful in establishing a diagnosis. Capillary hemangiomas are usually elevated and have a distinctive vascular appearance, which may be smooth or lobular (Figure 13–1). An exception to this is a subcutaneous hemangioma. These lesions must grow for some time before they produce visible changes on the skin surface, and they may not appear vascular initially. Hemangiomas of the eyelid and periocular region may produce mechanical ptosis or physically obstruct the visual axis. Subcutaneous orbital hemangiomas may present as proptosis (bulging of the eye).

Orbital dermoids are most commonly located along the superolateral orbital rim (Figure 13–2), but may also occur superomedially. They are subcutaneous, firm, and slightly mobile to palpation. They are not painful.

Mucoceles develop in newborns between the eye and the nose, slightly below the medial canthus (Figure 13–3). They initially may have a bluish tinge. They are slightly firm. Gentle pressure on the lesion may produce reflux of mucoid material onto the eyes. If these lesions become infected, they may appear erythematous and purulent drainage may develop. A cyst is sometimes visible in the nares beneath the inferior turbinate.

Hordeola most commonly present as localized erythematous nodules of the eyelid (Figure 13–4), although they may present with diffuse erythema and edema. They are usually located along the half of the upper or lower eyelid closest to the eyelid margin. They may have a white center and can spontaneously drain, either on the skin surface or on the internal surface of the eyelid. Styes are occasionally associated with pyogenic granulomas, which have a pink, fleshly, lobulated appearance on the inner eyelid at the site of the sty. Chronic chalazia are palpable as firm, nontender nodules within the eyelid (Figure 13–5).

PLAN

Most capillary hemangiomas will spontaneously regress, but periocular lesions may cause amblyopia. Infants with hemangiomas involving the eyelids or other areas near the eye should be referred to a pediatric ophthalmologist. Because these lesions grow rapidly, early referral (even for small eyelid lesions) can allow prompt treatment to minimize the risk of visual problems.

Most pediatric ophthalmologists recommend surgical excision of orbital dermoids due to the risks of continued growth and potential rupture with inflammation. This is not urgent.

Infants with mucoceles should be evaluated for respiratory problems due to nasal cysts. If respiratory difficulties are present, urgent treatment is indicated. If there are no breathing problems and the mucocele is not infected, initial conservative treatment with warm compresses, topical antibiotics, and gentle massage may induce resolution of the mucocele. If the lesion does not resolve, or if it becomes acutely infected, referral to a pediatric ophthalmologist is indicated.

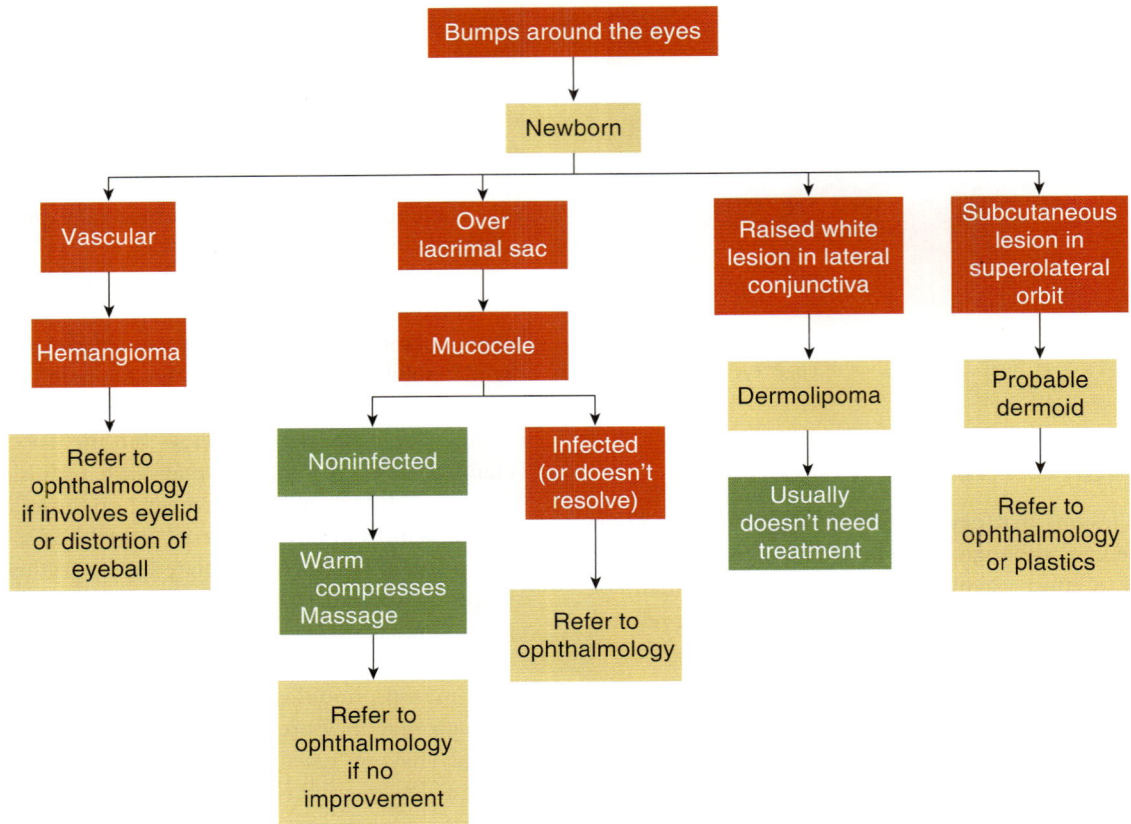

FIGURE 13–10 ■ Algorithm for evaluation and management of a newborn with bumps around the eyes.

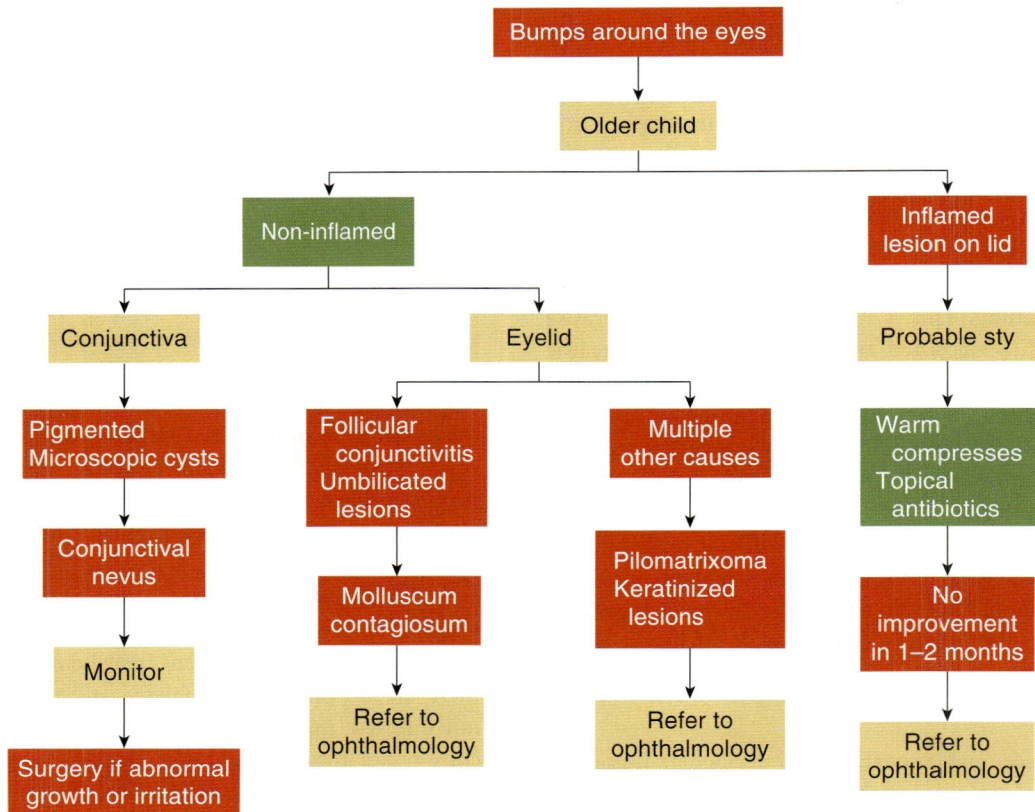

FIGURE 13–11 ■ Algorithm for evaluation and management of an older child with bumps around the eyes.

WHAT SHOULDN'T BE MISSED

Capillary hemangiomas involving the eyelids and surrounding tissue may cause amblyopia. Early referral may allow treatment to minimize growth and improve the visual outcome. Infants with mucoceles may have associated nasal cysts that obstruct the airways and cause respiratory compromise. This can be effectively treated with rapid recognition of the problem and removal of the nasal cysts.

When to Refer

- Infants with mucoceles that do not resolve within 1 to 2 weeks or that become infected
- Infants with hemangiomas that affect the eyelids or orbit
- Older children with styes that do not resolve after 1 to 2 months with conservative treatment
- Infants with orbital dermoids

Droopy Eyelids

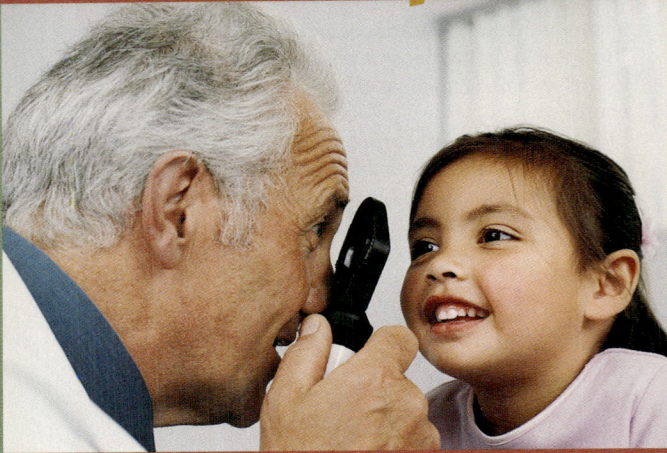

The Problem
"My child's eyelid is droopy."

Common Causes
Congenital ptosis

Other Causes
Myasthenia gravis
Horner syndrome
Third nerve palsy
Eyelid or orbital mass
Pseudoptosis
  Eyelid retraction of opposite eye
  Eyebrow skin overhanging normal eyelid

KEY FINDINGS

History
Congenital ptosis
  Present from birth
  Isolated, familial, or syndromic
  Often worse with fatigue
  Chin-up head posture
Myasthenia
  Variable ptosis, worse with fatigue
  Often have strabismus/diplopia
Horner syndrome
  Congenital or acquired
  Unequal pupils
  Decreased sweating on affected side
  Unequal iris colors (if congenital)
Third cranial nerve palsy
  Strabismus/diplopia
  Unequal pupils
  Other symptoms depending on etiology
Eyelid or orbital mass
  Eyelid lesion or proptosis
  Possible limited eye movement
  Other symptoms depending on etiology

Pseudoptosis
  Mild appearance of ptosis due to excess skin
    overhanging eyelid
  Squinting of eyelid due to other ocular disorder
    History of light sensitivity
    Foreign body sensation or ocular discomfort
  Eyelid retraction on opposite side
    Alternates between eyelid retraction of one
      eye and ptosis of the other
    Proptosis of opposite eye
    Other symptoms depending on etiology
      of proptosis

Examination
Congenital ptosis
  Unilateral or bilateral drooping of eyelids
  Varies from mild to almost complete occlusion
  Decreased ability to elevate eyelid
  Decreased eyelid crease
  Brow lift and chin-up posture if
    marked ptosis
Myasthenia gravis
  Variable ptosis
  Eyelid twitch (Cogan's sign)
  Increased eyelid opening after rest,
    ice test
  Often have strabismus
Horner syndrome
  Usually mild-to-moderate ptosis
  Pupil smaller on affected side
  Decreased sweating/facial flushing on
    affected side
Third nerve palsy
  Usually moderate to marked ptosis
  Strabismus (eye out and down)
  Unequal pupils (pupil larger on affected side,
    except may be smaller in congenital third
    nerve palsy)

(continued)

Examination (continued)

Eyelid or orbital mass
  Visible lesion on eyelid
  Proptosis
  Limited extraocular movements
Pseudoptosis
    Extra eyebrow skin
      Eyelid height and function normal
    Strabismus
      Appearance of ptosis due to strabismic
        eye being lower

Voluntary closure due to other ocular problems
    Corneal foreign body, abrasion
    Other ocular inflammatory disorders
Eyelid retraction on opposite side
    If child fixes with retracted eye, opposite eye
      appears ptotic
    If child fixes with normal eye, retraction worse
      in opposite eye
    Possible proptosis on side with eyelid
      retraction

WHAT SHOULD YOU DO?

Children with congenital ptosis may develop amblyopia, particularly if the ptosis is unilateral and occludes the pupil. These children should be referred to a pediatric ophthalmologist to determine whether surgical treatment is indicated. Mild-to-moderate ptosis usually is not an immediate threat to vision, but evaluation is important due to its possible association with systemic diseases. Children with new onset of acquired ptosis, particularly if associated with signs of third nerve palsy or orbital mass, should be referred promptly for further evaluation.

What Shouldn't Be Missed

Acquired ptosis may be the initial sign of a serious underlying disorder, such as a third nerve palsy or an orbital tumor. Prompt diagnosis improves the outcome of most of these disorders (Table 14–1).

COMMON CAUSES

1. *Congenital ptosis.* Congenital ptosis is present at birth. It may be unilateral or bilateral, and varies in severity from mild to severe. Congenital ptosis may be familial or associated with an underlying syndrome, but is often an isolated finding in an otherwise healthy child. Severe congenital ptosis requires early repair due to the risk of amblyopia (Figure 14–1A and B).

2. *Myasthenia gravis.* Myasthenia gravis is rare, but ptosis is often the presenting complaint. It may be present at birth due to transplacental maternal antibodies, or may be acquired. The hallmark of myasthenia gravis is variability. It is worse when the child is fatigued. Variable strabismus is also commonly present.

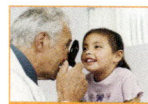

Table 14–1.

Causes of Ptosis With Potential Serious Systemic Implications

■ Third nerve palsy
  □ Intracranial tumor
  □ Trauma
■ Orbital tumor
  □ Primary
  □ Metatstatic
■ Horner syndrome
  □ Neuroblastoma

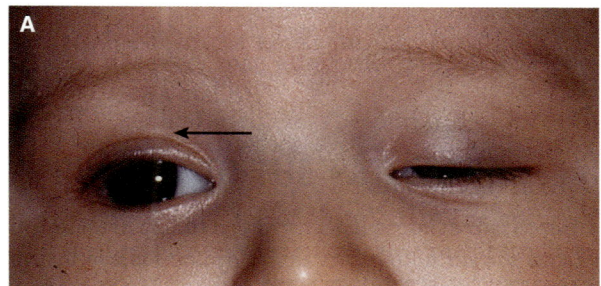

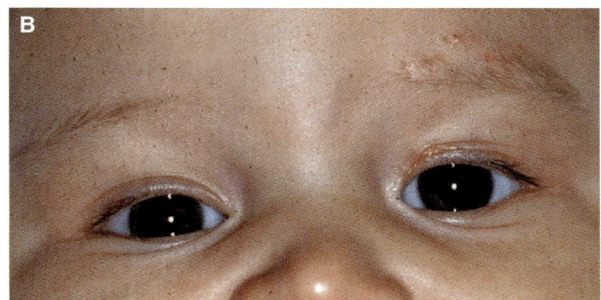

FIGURE 14–1 ■ Severe congenital ptosis, left eye. (A) High risk of amblyopia because eyelid completely covers pupil. Note normal right upper eyelid crease (arrow) and absence of left upper eyelid crease. (B) After surgery, patient can see normally.

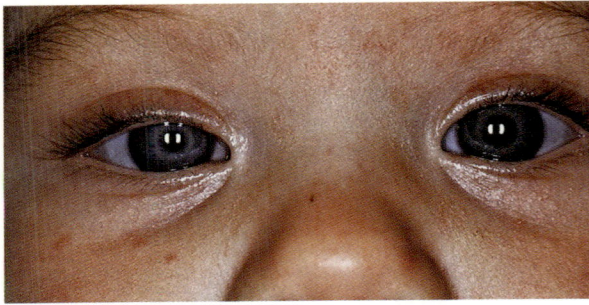

FIGURE 14-2 ■ Horner syndrome, right eye. Note mild right ptosis and anisocoria (right pupil smaller than left).

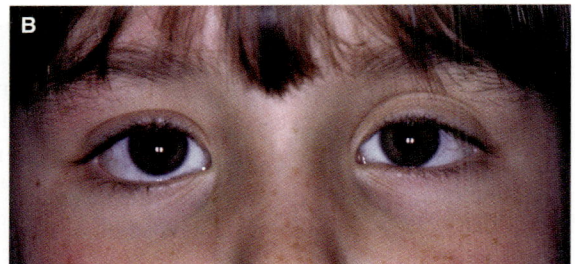

Table 14-2.

Causes of Pseudoptosis

- Excess eyelid skin overhanging eyelid margin
- Eyelid retraction of opposite eye
- Voluntary lid closure
  - Eye irritation
  - Strabismus (especially exotropia)
- Vertical strabismus

3. *Horner syndrome.* The ptosis in patients with Horner syndrome is usually mild to moderate. Patients have unequal pupils (smaller on the affected side), and may demonstrate decreased sweating of the brow on the affected side (Figure 14–2). Horner syndrome itself does not cause vision problems. Its importance lies in possible associations with systemic diseases, such as neuroblastoma.

4. *Third nerve palsy.* Patients with complete third nerve palsies usually have marked ptosis on the affected side, severe strabismus with the eye out and down, and a larger pupil on the affected side (although the pupil in some patients with congenital third nerve palsy may be smaller) (Figure 14–3). Severe ptosis from a third nerve palsy may cause amblyopia in young patients. The presence of an acquired third nerve palsy requires prompt evaluation.

5. *Eyelid or orbital mass.* A large number of eyelid and orbital lesions may cause secondary ptosis. In most eyelid lesions, this is a mechanical effect due to the increased weight of the eyelids, and the etiology is obvious on examination. Early orbital lesions may cause ptosis without marked

proptosis, and this possibility should be kept in mind in patients with acquired ptosis.

6. *Pseudoptosis.* This may occur for a variety of reasons (Table 14–2).
   a. Excess brow skin on the affected side may produce mild apparent eyelid asymmetry. This is benign.
   b. Eyelid retraction of the opposite eye. This may be an isolated finding, or a secondary effect of proptosis (usually due to an orbital mass).
   c. Voluntary closure of the eye due to ocular irritation or light sensitivity.
   d. Vertical strabismus, in which the eyelid on the side with the lower eye appears to have ptosis (Figure 14–4A and B).

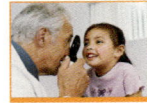

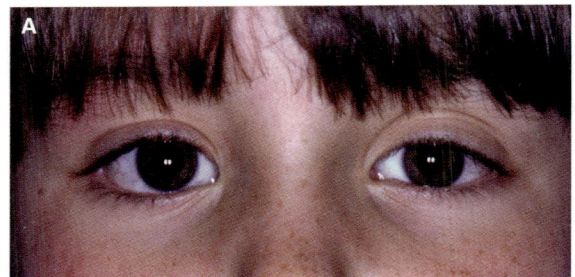

FIGURE 14-4 ■ Pseudo-ptosis due to vertical strabismus. The left eye is hypotropic (lower than the right eye). (A) When the patient fixates with the right eye, the left eyelid appears to have ptosis because the left eye is lower than the right. (B) The left eyelid elevates when the patient fixates with the left eye. Note the visible sclera beneath the right iris due to associated upward movement of right eye.

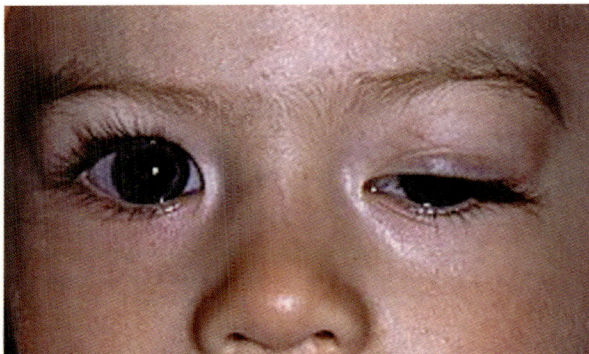

FIGURE 14-3 ■ Third nerve palsy, left eye. Marked ptosis of left eye. Note that the eye is also displaced downward and outward.

Table 14–3.

Ptosis—Associations With Other Eye Findings

- Ptosis + strabismus
  □ Third nerve palsy (eye out and down)
  □ Myasthenia gravis (variable strabismus)
  □ Orbital mass
- Ptosis + unequal pupils (anisocoria)
  □ Horner syndrome (pupil smaller on affected side)
  □ Third nerve palsy (pupil usually larger on affected side)

APPROACH TO THE PATIENT

The primary factors in the evaluation of a patient with ptosis are the age of onset and the presence of associated signs and symptoms, such as strabismus or unequal pupils (Table 14–3). Ptosis that is present at birth is usually due to isolated congenital ptosis, and the need for treatment is based on severity. Acquired ptosis at any age is usually not an immediate vision problem, but important primarily due to the possible presence of an underlying serious disorder.

History

The first important point in assessing patients with ptosis is identifying the age of onset. If present at birth, it is very likely isolated congenital ptosis. Horner syndrome may also be congenital, and is accompanied by unequal pupils (smaller on the affected side). Third nerve palsies and myasthenia rarely present at birth. Third nerve palsies are associated with unequal pupils and strabismus. Most congenital myasthenia is due to the transplacental transmission of maternal antibodies, with a maternal history of myasthenia gravis.

Congenital ptosis may be isolated, familial, or associated with numerous syndromes. Questions should be asked about other affected family members and systemic problems that could indicate a specific syndrome. Birth trauma may cause ptosis due to swelling of the eyelids. This is usually temporary and resolves as the edema improves, but more severe injury (e.g., due to forceps) may cause permanent ptosis. Congenital ptosis is typically somewhat variable, worse when the child is tired. If the ptosis is moderate or severe, parents may describe a chin-up head posture or excessive elevation of the brow, which the child uses to see beneath the drooping eyelid.

Isolated acquired ptosis in older children is rare. The presence of acquired ptosis raises concern for underlying systemic disorders. Most acquired ptosis

will be associated with other signs or symptoms that help identify an etiology. Myasthenia gravis patients have variable ptosis that is worse with fatigue. They often also have strabismus and diplopia. Patients who have eyelid retraction may present with a complaint of ptosis of the opposite eye, when it is actually the retracted eye that is abnormal. Other disorders in the differential diagnosis are discussed in greater detail elsewhere (Horner syndrome—Chapter 29; third cranial nerve palsy—Chapter 34; orbital mass—Chapter 26; eyelid lesions—Chapter 25).

Examination

Children who present with ptosis at birth should be examined for signs of birth trauma or other ocular disorders. In the absence of anioscoria or strabismus to suggest congenital Horner syndrome or third nerve palsy, most patients will have isolated congenital ptosis. This can vary from mild to severe. If the eyelid is obstructing the pupil, the patient may arch their brow to recruit the forehead muscles to help lift the eyelid (Figure 14–5), or use a chin-up head posture to look beneath the eyelid.

Eyelid function is measured by holding the patient's head straight and moving a toy or other target from below the patient to above the patient. The normal eyelid will move 12 mm or more with this maneuver. Patients with severe ptosis typically have less than 5 mm of movement. In normal patients, small fibers of the levator muscle attach to the eyelid skin to form the upper eyelid crease. Because this muscle is underdeveloped in congenital ptosis, patients often have decreased upper eyelid creases (Figure 14–1A). The muscle may be stiff in patients with severe ptosis, which may cause incomplete eyelid closure.

The ptosis associated with myasthenia gravis is variable, and worse with fatigue. A characteristic sign of myasthenia gravis is Cogan's lid twitch. When the patient looks rapidly from down to up, there is an initial

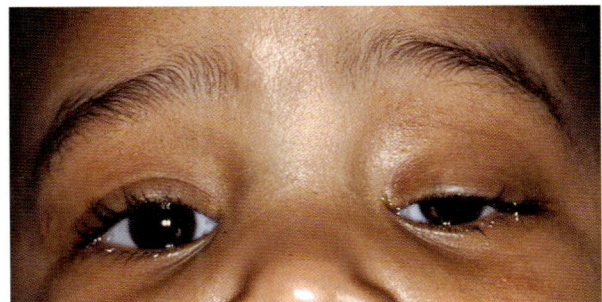

FIGURE 14–5 ■ Compensatory brow left due to congenital ptosis, left eye. The patient is elevating the brow to help lift the eyelid above the pupil.

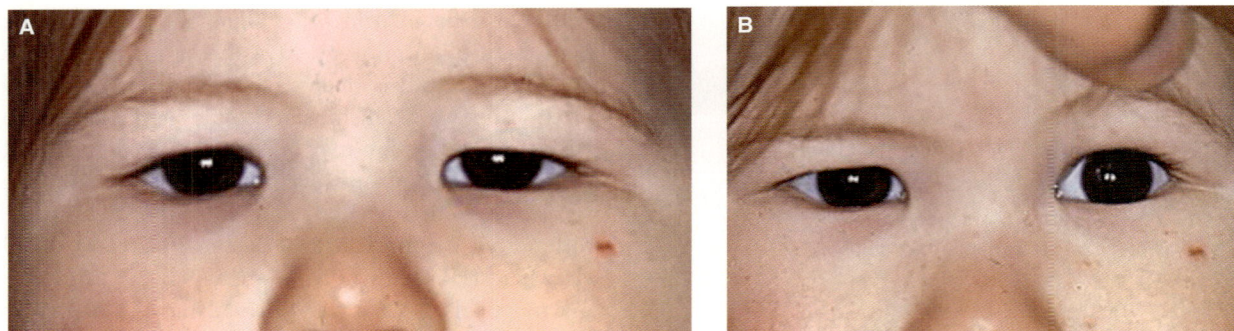

FIGURE 14–6 ■ Pseudo-ptosis. (A) Excess upper eyelid skin (left greater than right) blocks visualization of upper eyelid margin, creating the false appearance of ptosis. (B) When the excess skin is elevated, the actual eyelid margin is found to be in normal position.

overshoot of the lid, which then returns to its normal position. If the patient rests for a few minutes, the eyelid can usually be opened to a greater degree. Applying an ice pack to the eyelids can result in temporary normalization of the lid function. This often cannot be performed in young children due to their aversion to the cold temperature. Variable strabismus, which can mimic cranial nerve palsies, is also often present in patients with myasthenia gravis.

The findings associated with Horner syndrome, third nerve palsy, and orbital and eyelid masses are discussed in further detail elsewhere in this book.

Patients with a complaint of droopy eyelid may have pseudoptosis. In some patients this is because they have excess brow skin that hangs over the lid (Figure 14–6A and B). When this tissue is lifted by the examiner, the underlying eyelid height and function are found to be normal. Pseudoptosis may also occur due to ocular irritation, with the patient voluntarily squinting the eyelid closed. Examination of the cornea and other ocular structures should be performed in these patients. Rarely, patients may have the appearance of ptosis on one side that is actually due to eyelid retraction in the opposite eye. If the patient fixates visually with the eye

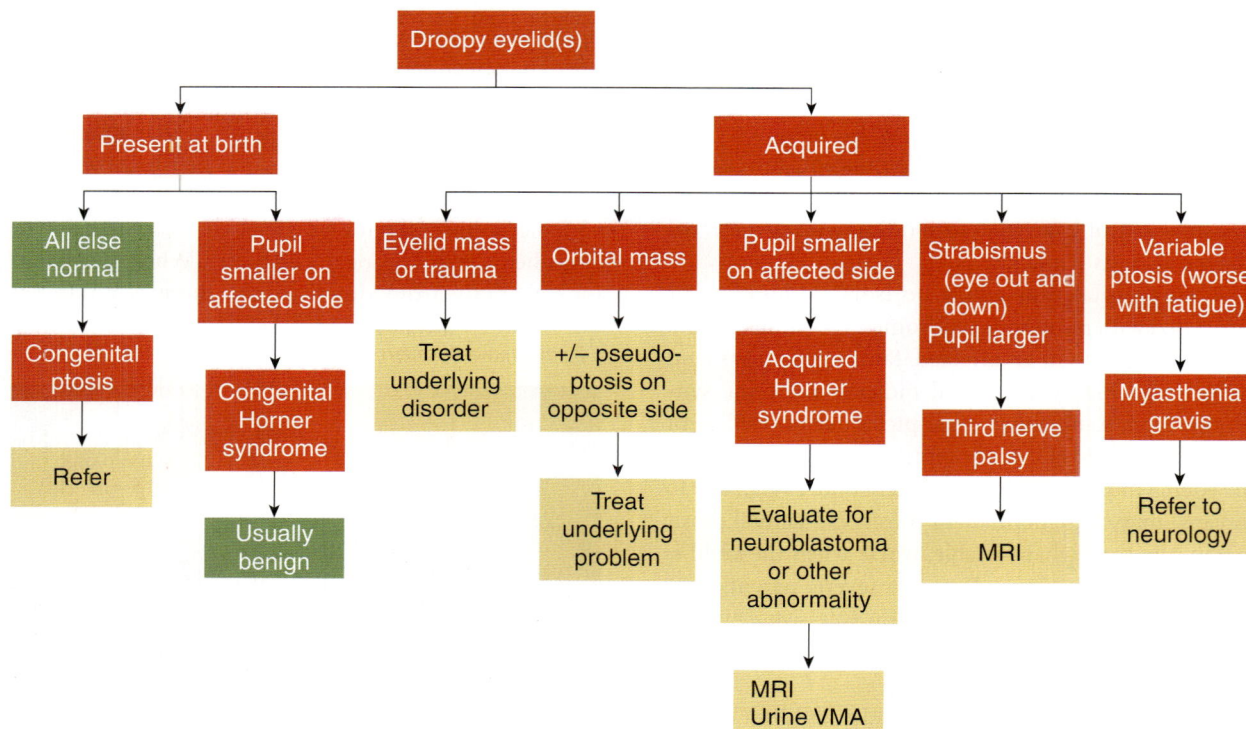

FIGURE 14–7 ■ Etiology and management of ptosis.

CHAPTER 14 Droopy Eyelids ■ 93

with the retracted eyelid, the contralateral eyelid will appear to droop.

PLAN

Infants with congenital ptosis should be referred to a pediatric ophthalmologist. Early referral is indicated if the ptosis is severe (i.e., blocking the pupil) due to the risk of amblyopia.

Patients with acquired ptosis need careful evaluation to look for associated ocular and systemic disorders. Urgent additional investigations are indicated if an acquired third nerve palsy or possible orbital mass is identified (Figure 14–7).

WHAT SHOULDN'T BE MISSED

The sudden onset of ptosis in children is unusual and often associated with other problems. The list of potential diagnoses is long, including orbital and central nervous system tumors.

When to Refer
■ Infants with ptosis
◻ Early referral if severe
◻ Routine referral if mild or moderate
■ Older children with acquired ptosis
◻ Urgent referral if signs of cranial nerve palsy or orbital abnormality

CHAPTER 15

Bulging Eyeball

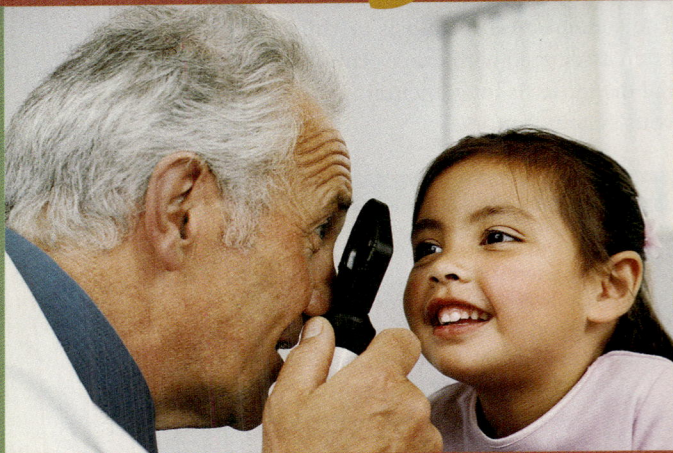

The Problem

"My child's eye is bulging."

Common Causes

Orbital tumors
Orbital cellulitis
Orbital lymphangioma
Orbital pseudotumor
Infantile glaucoma

Other Causes

High myopia
Craniofacial malformations
Thyroid opthalmopathy
Capillary hemangioma

KEY FINDINGS

History

Diplopia may occur with any of these lesions
Decreased vision more common with rapidly
  growing lesions
Orbital tumors
  Rhabdomyosarcoma—rapid painless proptosis
  Optic nerve glioma—may present rapidly
    More common in patients with neurofibromatosis
  Other tumors—gradual proptosis
Orbital cellulitis
  Pain, fever, systemic illness
  Rapid onset
  History of sinus disease

Lymphangioma
  Rapid-onset proptosis if acute bleeding
Orbital pseudotumor
  Pain, worse with eye movement
  Often systemic symptoms (fever, malaise)
Infantile glaucoma
  Excess tearing
  Light sensitivity (photophobia)

Examination

All lesions with proptosis may have limited eye movements,
  decreased vision, and conjunctival swelling
Orbital tumor
  Often nontender proptosis
Orbital cellulitis
  Periocular erythema and edema
  Abnormal pupil reactions
Lymphangioma
  Usually subtle proptosis unless acute hemorrhage
  Acute hemorrhage may produce marked proptosis
    and swelling
Orbital pseudotumor
  Pain with eye movement
  Inflammation over extraocular muscles
Infantile glaucoma
  Cornea enlarged, may be cloudy
  Overflow tearing

WHAT SHOULD YOU DO?

Children with new-onset proptosis should be referred promptly to a pediatric ophthalmologist. The differential diagnosis includes several life- and vision-threatening disorders.

What Shouldn't Be Missed

Proptosis is a serious condition that requires prompt evaluation and treatment. In particular, patients with decreased vision or signs of orbital cellulitis should be referred immediately.

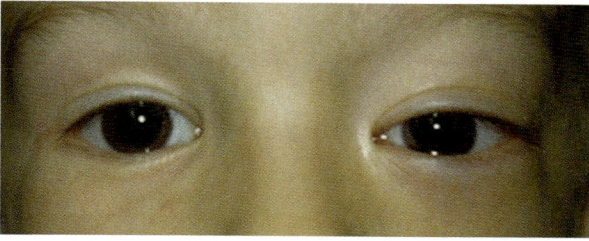

FIGURE 15–1 ■ Rhabdomyosarcoma, left orbit. The left eye is bulging forward. Note stretched appearance of upper and lower eyelids, and decreased left lower eyelid skin crease.

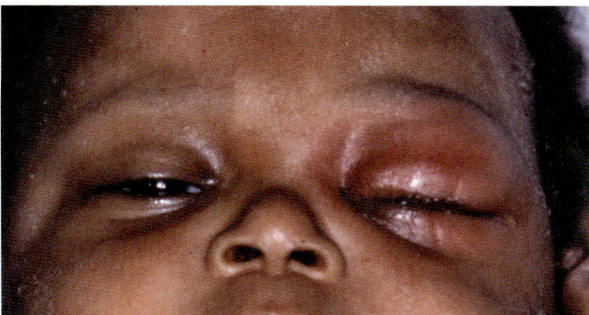

FIGURE 15–3 ■ Proptosis secondary to left orbital lymphangioma with acute hemorrhage. The bulging eye is often more easily noted when viewed from above.

COMMON CAUSES

1. *Orbital tumors.* The most common primary orbital tumor in children is rhabdomyosarcoma, which classically presents with rapid onset of painless proptosis (Figure 15–1). Optic pathway gliomas affecting the optic nerve sometimes present with rapid onset of proptosis due to mucinous degeneration. Metastatic lesions, including neuroblastoma, leukemia, and lymphoma, are less common.

2. *Orbital cellulitis.* Orbital cellulitis is a serious infection that most commonly results from contiguous spread of sinus disease (Figure 15–2). Prompt treatment with intravenous antibiotics is indicated. Orbital cellulitis is frequently associated with subperiosteal orbital abscesses, which may improve with antibiotics and not require surgical drainage.

3. *Lymphangioma.* Lymphangiomas are congenital lesions that may not be noticed initially. These lesions are prone to internal hemorrhage, which presents with the rapid onset of proptosis (Figure 15–3). This may be difficult to distinguish from an orbital tumor without a biopsy.

4. *Orbital pseudotumor.* Orbital pseudotumor is an idiopathic condition characterized by inflammation of the orbital tissue. It is often preceded by a systemic febrile illness, and presents with marked periocular pain. It may be localized to the extraocular muscles (myositis). It characteristically responds very promptly to systemic corticosteroid treatment.

5. *Infantile glaucoma.* Although not an orbital disorder, glaucoma that presents in infancy or early childhood may cause enlargement of the eyeball, with a clinical appearance similar to proptosis (Figure 15–4). Affected children often have cloudy corneas and excess tearing due to corneal irritation.

6. *Other causes.* Apparent proptosis may result from underlying abnormalities of the orbit or eyeball itself. Patients with craniofacial abnormalities or craniosynostosis may have shallow orbits, and patients who are markedly nearsighted (myopic) may have elongated eyes. Orbital hemorrhage due to trauma or bleeding disorders may also cause proptosis (Figure 15–5A and B).

APPROACH TO THE PATIENT

Proptosis in children is an unusual problem that requires urgent evaluation. The signs and symptoms are usually readily apparent (Table 15–1). The differential diagnosis

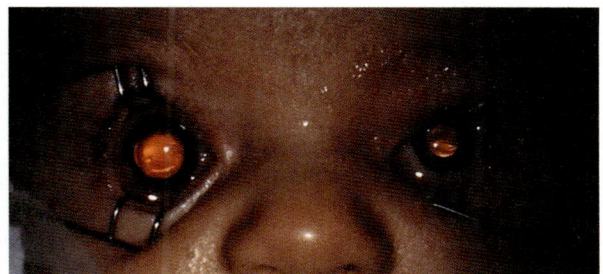

FIGURE 15–2 ■ Left orbital cellulitis. Note edema and erythema of left periocular skin.

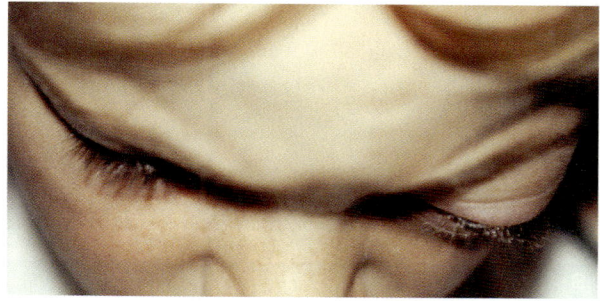

FIGURE 15–4 ■ Infantile glaucoma, right eye. The eyeball and cornea are much larger on the right, which gives an appearance similar to proptosis.

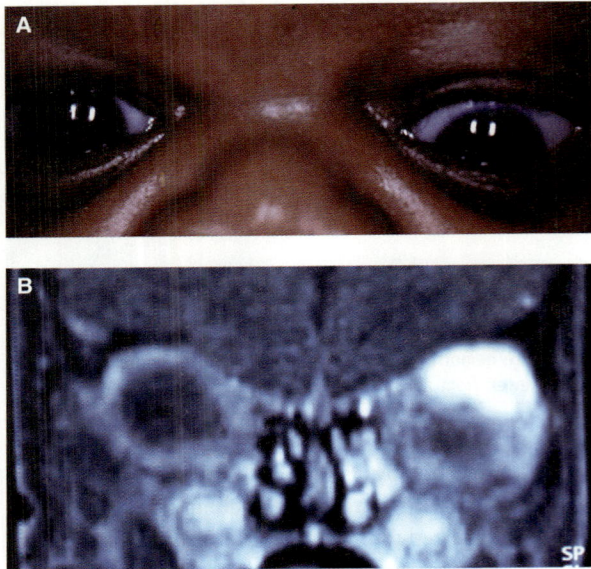

FIGURE 15–5 ■ Orbital hemorrhage, left eye. (A) Left eye is bulging forward and displaced down. (B) Magnetic resonance image of left superior orbital hemorrhage. (Figure A and B are reprinted with permission from SLACK Incorporated: Bart DJ, Lueder GT. Orbital hemorrhage following extracorporeal membrane oxygenation in a newborn. *J Pediatr Ophthalmol Strabismus.* 1997;34(1):65–67.)

for orbital lesions is large, with many rare disorders (Table 15–2). However, a few entities account for the majority of cases.

History

The primary historical considerations are the rapidity of onset and the association of inflammatory signs. Larger lesions may obstruct eye movements and produce diplopia. Lesions that compress the optic nerve may cause decreased vision and abnormal pupil reactions. Although uncommon in children, thyroid ophthalmopathy may occur, and a review of systems for symptoms of hypo- or hyperthyroidism should be included. The orbit may be a site of metastatic disease, which would be a likely etiology for proptosis in patients with a known history of leukemia, lymphoma, or neuroblastoma. Most patients with orbital cellulitis have a

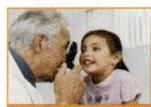

Table 15–1.

Symptoms of Orbital Mass

- Proptosis
- Limited eye movements (diplopia)
- Ocular irritation (due to corneal exposure)
- Decreased vision

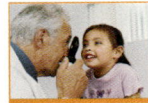

Table 15–2.

Systemic Diseases Associated With Proptosis

- Orbital or optic nerve tumors
  □ Primary orbital tumors
    – Rhabdomyosarcoma
  □ Metastatic orbital tumors
    – Leukemia
    – Neuroblastoma
  □ Optic nerve tumors
    – Optic glioma (neurofibromatosis)
- Thyroid dysfunction (Graves disease)
- Craniofacial malformations

history of sinus disease. Trauma, particularly if associated with an orbital foreign body, may also cause orbital cellulitis. Children with orbital pseudotumor often have a history of preceding systemic illness, including fever and malaise. Bulging eyeballs due to glaucoma usually occur in infancy, and are accompanied by symptoms of excess tearing and light sensitivity.

Examination

The initial examination of patients with proptosis should focus on the vision and whether there are signs of infection. The visual acuity and pupil reactions should be assessed. Examination of extraocular movements may reveal limitation. The presence of periocular erythema and edema should be noted. Patients with rapid proptosis may have conjunctival swelling or corneal irritation due to exposure. Myositis may produce localized inflammation over an extraocular muscle. Infantile glaucoma that causes enlargement of the eye usually also causes clouding of the cornea.

PLAN

All patients with new-onset proptosis require referral for further evaluation(Figure 15–6). The main initial decision is how soon this needs to be performed. Patients with signs and symptoms of orbital cellulitis and patients whose vision is decreased should be referred immediately, either directly to the referring physician's office or through an emergency room. Other patients with proptosis should be seen promptly.

WHAT SHOULDN'T BE MISSED

Rapid treatment of orbital cellulitis is indicated in all patients, but particularly in those who are immunocompromised, due to the risk of cavernous sinus

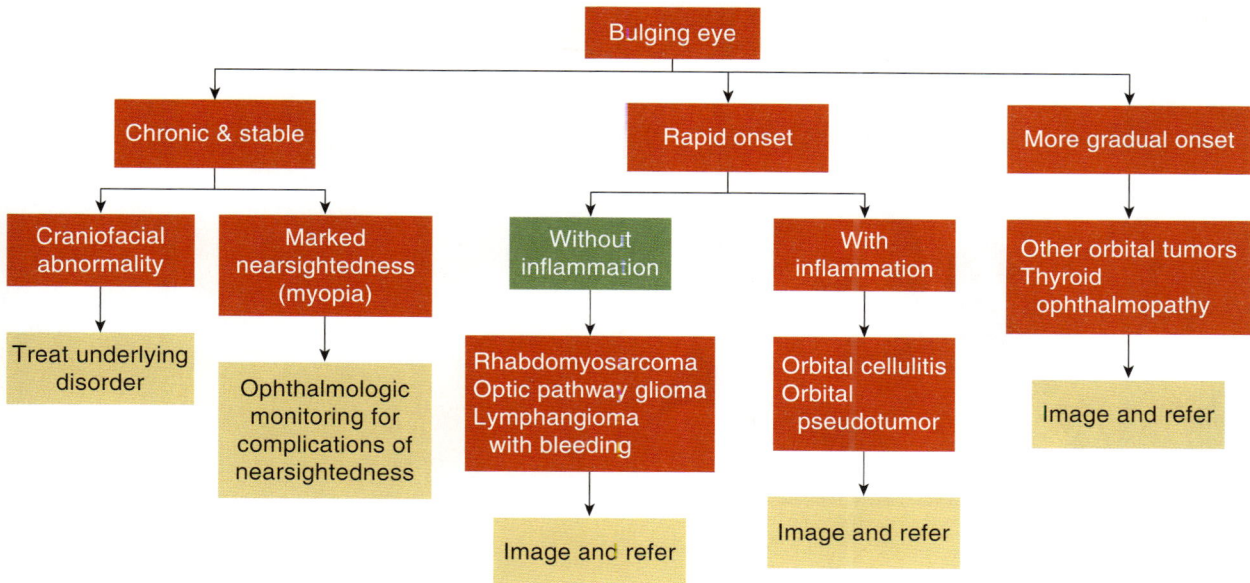

FIGURE 15–6 ■ Algorithm for evaluation and management of a bulging eye (proptosis).

thrombosis or spread of infection to the central nervous system. Patients with proptosis and decreased vision may have optic nerve compression, which requires immediate treatment.

When to Refer

■ Patients with acquired proptosis should be referred promptly for evaluation

CHAPTER 16

Cloudy Cornea

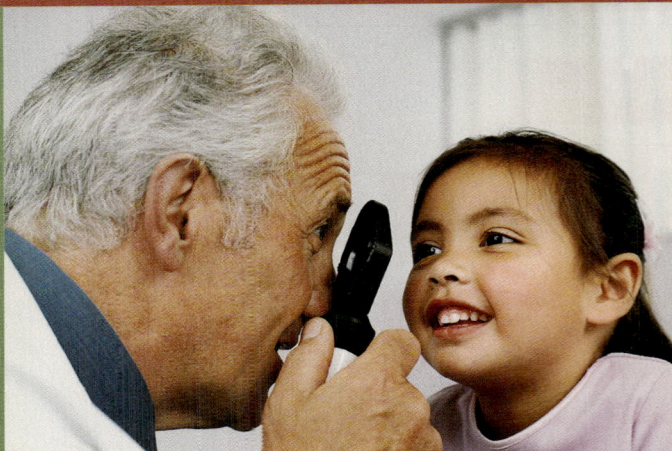

The Problem
"My child's eye looks cloudy."

Common Causes
Infantile glaucoma
Corneal infection
Forceps injury
Peter's anomaly

Other Causes
Sclerocornea
Congenital corneal dystrophy
Mucopolysaccharidosis
Trauma

KEY FINDINGS

History
Infantile glaucoma
  Eye appears larger than normal
  Light sensitivity and excess tearing
Corneal infection
  Most common in older children who wear
    contact lenses
  Usually very uncomfortable
  Possible trauma, foreign body
Forceps injury
  Difficult delivery requiring forceps

Peter's anomaly
  Cloudy central cornea at birth
Other causes
  May be associated with other systemic problems
    (e.g., mucopolysaccharidosis)
  History of trauma

Examination
Infantile glaucoma
  Enlarged cornea
  Ground-glass appearance
  Photophobia, excess tearing
Corneal infection
  Focal areas of increased corneal clouding
  Possible corneal foreign body
  Eye appears bloodshot (conjunctival injection)
  Corneal dendrites (herpes simplex virus infection)
Corneal forceps injury
  Cornea initially usually diffusely cloudy
    Later—oblique scars
  Periocular and facial bruising and swelling
    from forceps
Peter's anomaly
  Central corneal clouding
  Peripheral cornea usually clear

WHAT SHOULD YOU DO?

Children with cloudy corneas should be referred promptly to a pediatric ophthalmologist.

What Shouldn't Be Missed

Corneal infections require prompt treatment to minimize the risk of corneal ulcer and permanent visual damage. Infants with cloudy corneas are at high risk for amblyopia (similar to infants with cataracts), and early treatment may greatly improve the prognosis.

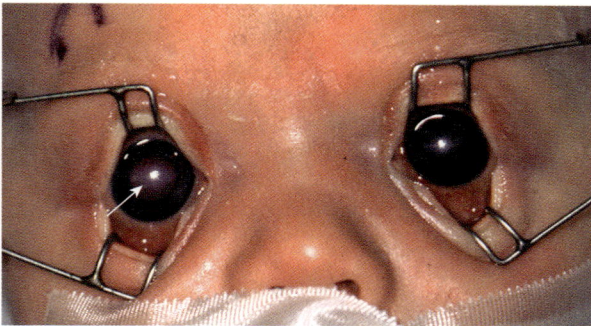

FIGURE 16–1 ■ Infantile glaucoma, right eye. Note right eye is larger than left, and central cornea is cloudy (arrow).

COMMON CAUSES

1. *Infantile glaucoma.* Glaucoma results from increased intraocular pressure. In infants and young children with glaucoma, the pressure may cause abnormal growth of the eye. The affected eye(s) appears larger than normal (Figure 16–1). The pressure interferes with the normal mechanisms that keep the cornea clear, and the cornea often has a ground-glass appearance. Haab striae (curvilinear scars in the corneal endothelium) may develop (Figure 16–2).

2. *Corneal infections.* Corneal infections are a potentially serious problem that may result in permanent visual loss. Bacterial infections are usually associated with a foreign body, either

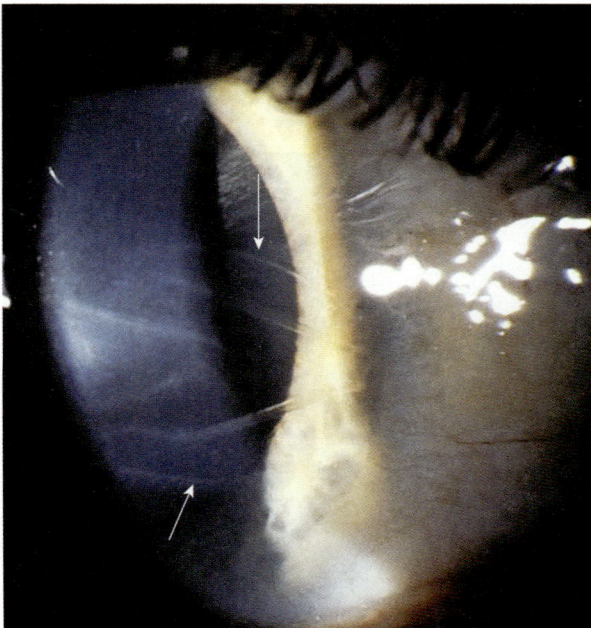

FIGURE 16–3 ■ Central corneal ulcer with focal clouding. The lesion stains with fluorescein, indicating disruption of the corneal epithelium.

accidental or from contact lenses. (Figure 16–3). Herpes simplex virus may also affect the cornea (Figure 16–4).

3. *Forceps injury.* Forceps may be used by obstetricians during difficult deliveries. If the forceps produce direct pressure on the eye, children may develop traumatic opacification of the cornea. The opacification usually improves, but patients often have residual scarring and high astigmatism (Figure 16–5). They are at risk for deprivation amblyopia.

4. *Peter's anomaly.* Peter's anomaly is a congenital corneal abnormality that presents with opacification of the central cornea (Figure 16–6). The peripheral cornea is usually clear. Glaucoma and cataracts may also develop.

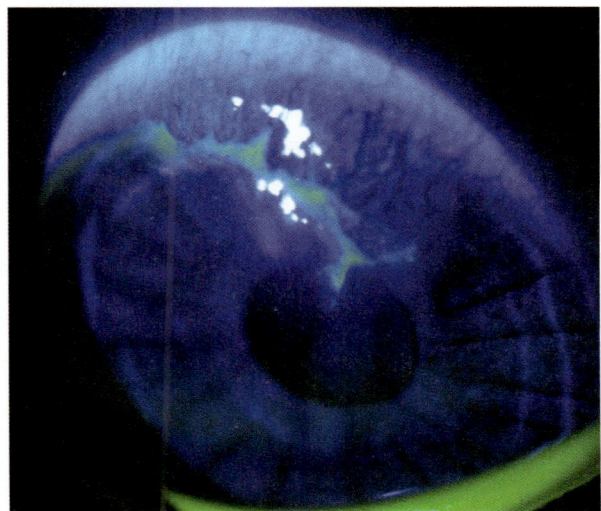

FIGURE 16–2 ■ Curvilinear Haab striae (arrows) in a patient with infantile glaucoma.

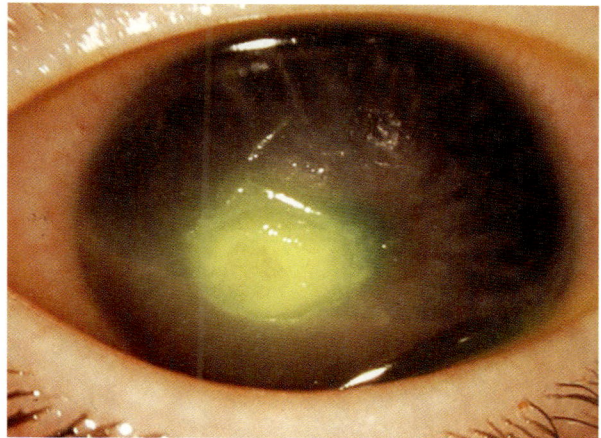

FIGURE 16–4 Peripheral herpes simplex viral corneal infection, stained with fluorescein. The lesion has a dendritic appearance.

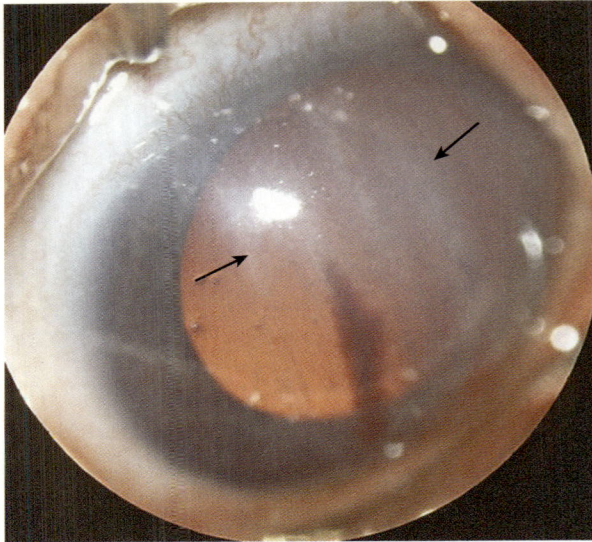

FIGURE 16–5 ■ Corneal forceps injury. Note oblique linear Haab striae (arrows). The blood is on the corneal endothelium.

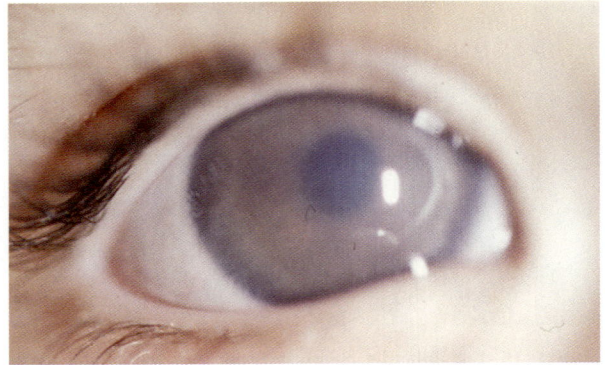

FIGURE 16–7 ■ Diffuse corneal clouding secondary to congenital hereditary endothelial dystrophy.

5. *Other.* Several other rare disorders may cause corneal clouding, including sclerocornea, congenital corneal dystrophies (Figure 16–7), and mucopolysaccharidosis (Figure 16–8). Cystinosis does not cause clouding per se, but patients usually have progressive crystalline deposits in their corneas, which cause light sensitivity (Figure 16–9). Trauma in older children may cause corneal foreign bodies, lacerations, and corneal edema (Figure 16–10).

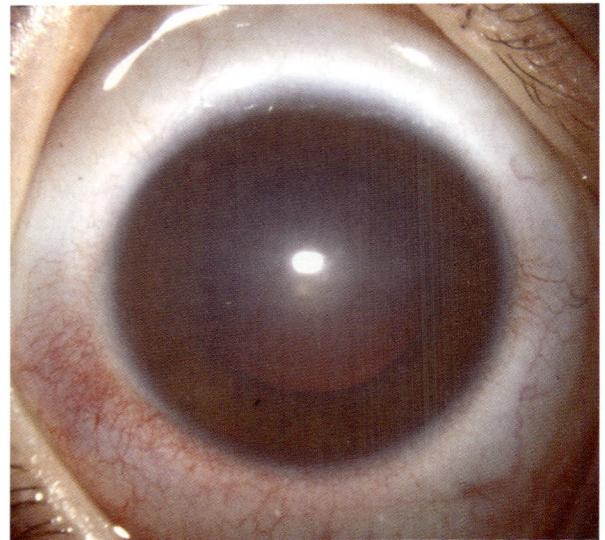

FIGURE 16–8 ■ Diffuse corneal clouding due to Hurler syndrome (mucopolysaccharidosis type 1H).

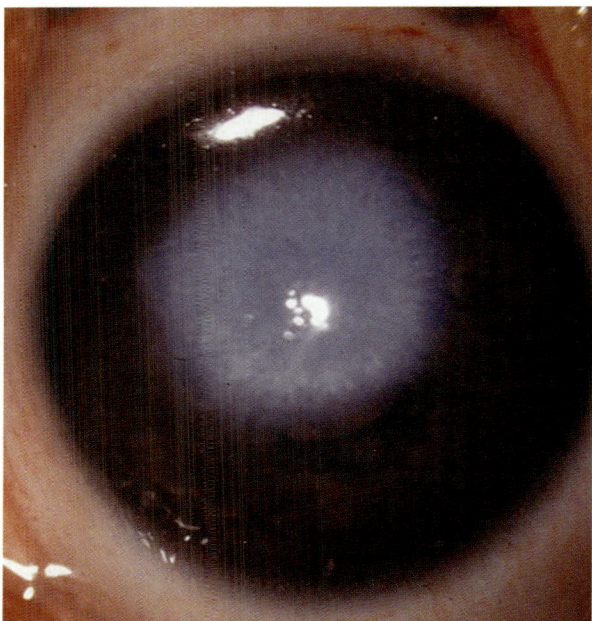

FIGURE 16–6 ■ Peter's anomaly with central area of corneal clouding.

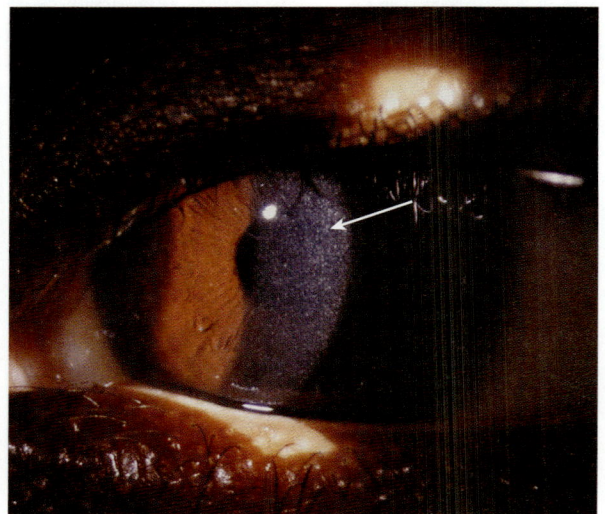

FIGURE 16–9 ■ Cystinosis. Diffuse fine crystals (arrow) are visible in the slitlamp light beam through the central cornea.

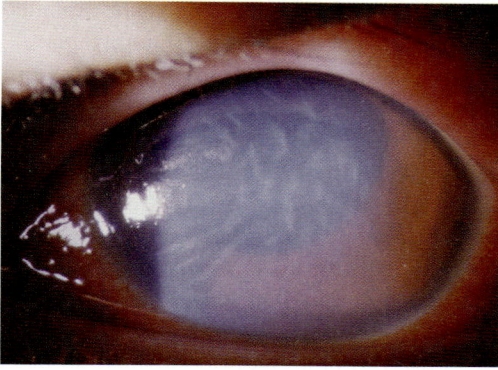

FIGURE 16–10 ■ Diffuse corneal clouding following blunt injury. The linear opacities are caused by folds in the corneal endothelium.

APPROACH TO THE PATIENT

Opacification of the cornea is rare in infancy. It is most commonly secondary to glaucoma, but may also result from primary corneal disorders. In older children, cloudy corneas usually are caused by infection or trauma (Table 16–1).

History

In the absence of trauma (forceps injury), most infants who are born with cloudy corneas have glaucoma. Infantile glaucoma may be familial, and therefore a family history should be obtained. The primary corneal disorders that present in infancy with clouding are usually isolated to the eye, although Peter's anomaly is sometimes associated with other abnormalities.

Cloudy corneas in older children usually result from extraneous causes, rather than primary corneal problems. The cornea has a rich supply of nerves, and corneal disorders are usually very uncomfortable. Light sensitivity and excess tearing are frequent. Corneal foreign bodies may occur at any age, and the foreign body increases the risk of infection, which causes clouding. Foreign bodies usually present with a history of the abrupt onset of eye discomfort, and the cause of the foreign body is usually known. The history may be unclear in toddlers, particularly if the symptoms develop during unwitnessed activities. More severe traumatic corneal injuries usually have a clear history of the inciting incident. Contact lenses, particularly if they are not cared for properly, increase the risk of corneal infection.

A relatively small number of metabolic diseases, mucopolysaccharidosis being the most common, may have corneal clouding as one of their features (Figure 16–8). Affected children usually have several other systemic abnormalities that assist in the identification of these disorders.

Examination

The regular newborn examination should include a penlight evaluation of the cornea and red reflex. If the cornea is cloudy, details of the iris will be obscured and the red reflex will be abnormal. Many corneal disorders will also produce irritation, so the infants may be light sensitive and have increased tearing, which makes the examination more difficult. Congenital glaucoma and Peter's anomaly may be bilateral or unilateral. The corneas are bilaterally affected in congenital corneal dystrophies and systemic diseases that cause corneal clouding.

Older children with corneal infections may be difficult to examine due to discomfort. The eye will usually appear bloodshot, and early infections usually have focal, rather than diffuse, areas of opacification (Figure 16–3). Foreign bodies, particularly wood or metal, may be visible with a penlight (Figure 16–11).

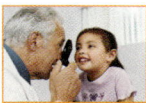

Table 16–1.

Causes of Corneal Clouding

- Infants
  - Glaucoma
  - Trauma (forceps)
  - Congenital corneal abnormality
    - Peter's anomaly
    - Sclerocornea
  - Congenital infection (rare)
    - Herpes simplex virus
- Older children
  - Systemic disease
    - Mucopolysaccharidosis
    - Cystinosis
  - Infection
    - Contact lens
    - Herpes simplex virus
  - Trauma

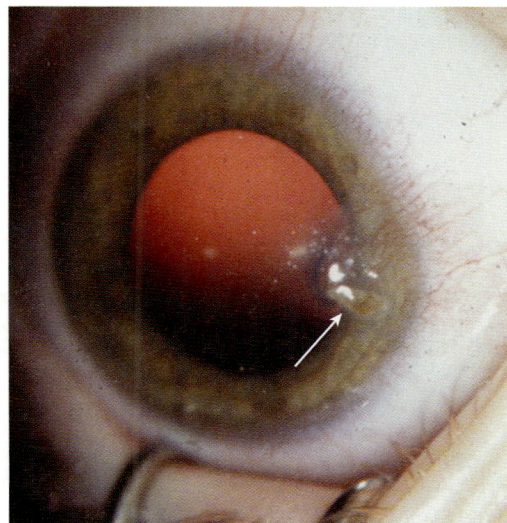

FIGURE 16–11 ■ Peripheral corneal foreign body (arrow).

Clear plastic or glass foreign bodies may be difficult to visualize without a slitlamp and anesthesia (topical or general). Examination of the red reflex may help identify foreign bodies. Herpes simplex virus corneal infections often have a distinctive dendritic appearance (Figure 16–4).

PLAN

If corneal clouding is noted during a routine newborn evaluation, prompt referral to a pediatric ophthalmologist is indicated (Figures 16–12). The prognosis for vision depends on the type of abnormality. Infants with corneal opacities are at high risk for amblyopia.

Older children with corneal infections from any cause should be referred immediately to an ophthalmologist (Figures 16–13). If a child has a superficial corneal foreign body that is not infected, removal may be attempted with the use of topical anesthetic and a cotton-tipped applicator. If the foreign body cannot be removed, or if there are signs of infection, the child should be referred. Children with infected corneas are at risk for progressive opacification and vision loss. Early treatment decreases the risk of permanent problems.

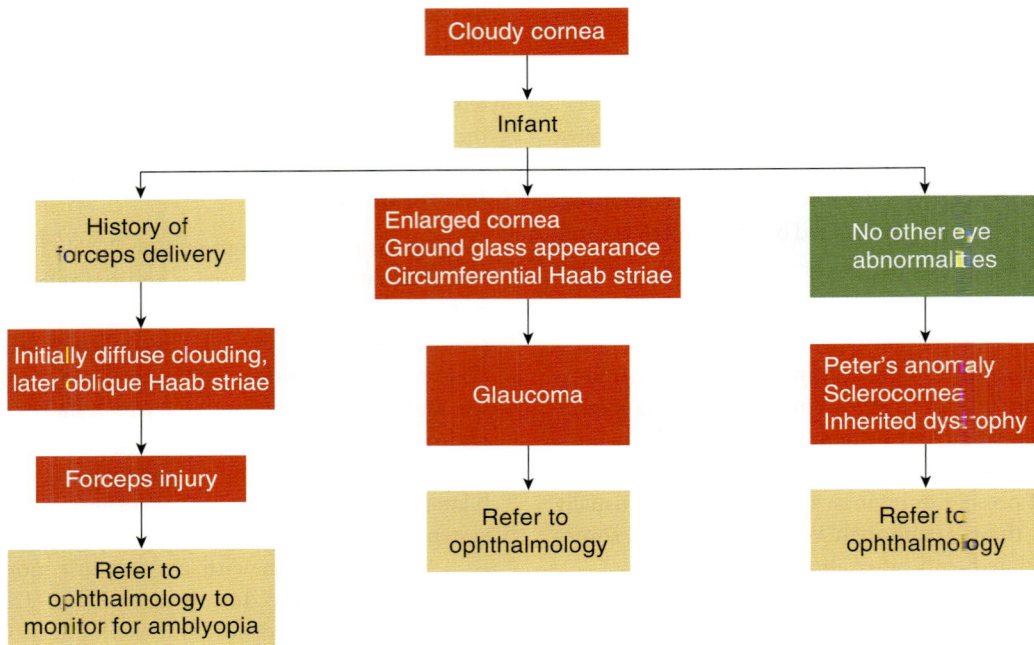

FIGURE 16–12 ■ Algorithm for evaluation and management of an infant with a cloudy cornea.

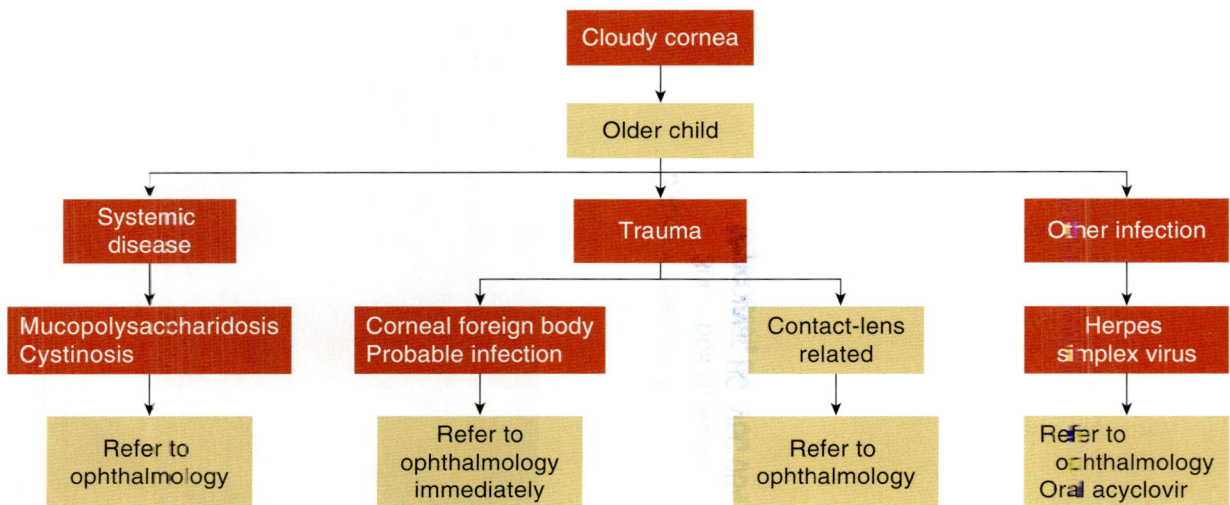

FIGURE 16–13 ■ Algorithm for evaluation and management of an older child with a cloudy cornea

WHAT SHOULDN'T BE MISSED

Similar to infantile cataracts, children with congenital corneal opacities have a very high risk of vision loss due to amblyopia. Early treatment is essential to maximize vision. Older children with corneal clouding also require prompt treatment, particularly for removal of foreign bodies and vigorous treatment of infection.

When to Refer

- Infants with cloudy corneas should be evaluated by an ophthalmologist promptly
- Older children with the acute onset of cloudy corneas should be evaluated promptly

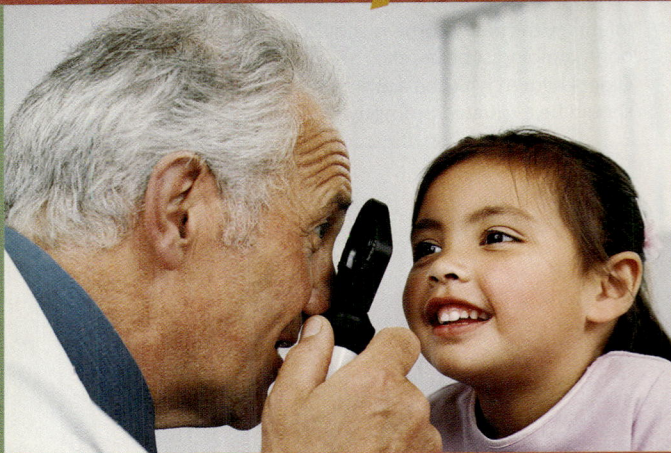

CHAPTER 17

Bumps on the Iris

The Problem
"My child has bumps on the colored part of the eye."

Common Causes
Small iris cysts at the pupillary border
Lisch nodules
Iris nevi

Other Causes
Large iris cysts
Congenital iris ectropion
Intraocular tumor (diktyoma)
Iris mammillations
Juvenile xanthogranuloma

KEY FINDINGS

History
Small lesions on the iris are usually asymptomatic and do not affect vision. A history of eye pain, corneal clouding, or decreased vision suggests a possible tumor. Juvenile xanthogranuloma (JXG) may be associated with small orange-brown papules on the head or face. Iris JXG lesions may bleed, and the resultant hyphema may cause ocular pain.

Examination
Without a slit lamp, evaluation of iris lesions may be difficult, particularly in a noncooperative toddler. Some lesions may be visible with a penlight. Benign iris cysts are often seen best by examining the pupil margin when evaluating the red reflex with a direct ophthalmoscope.

WHAT SHOULD YOU DO?

Small irregular lesions at the pupil margin in an infant do not require further evaluation. Small iris nevi are common and also do not require evaluation unless abnormal growth occurs. Children with other iris abnormalities should be referred to a pediatric ophthalmologist.

Lisch nodules are almost pathognomonic of neurofibromatosis, and evaluation for other abnormalities associated with neurofibromatosis should be performed.

What Shouldn't Be Missed

Although extremely rare, large iris cysts or iris distortion due to intraocular tumors (diktyoma) may cause glaucoma, eye pain, redness, and corneal clouding. This requires immediate evaluation.

COMMON CAUSES

1. *Iris cysts.* Cysts of the iris are not common, but may occur in otherwise normal children. Small, scalloped irregularities at the pupil margin are almost always benign (Figure 17–1). Large iris cysts are very rare. They may cause vision loss (Figure 17–2).
2. *Lisch nodules.* Lisch nodules almost always occur in children with neurofibromatosis. They are usually not present in infancy. The

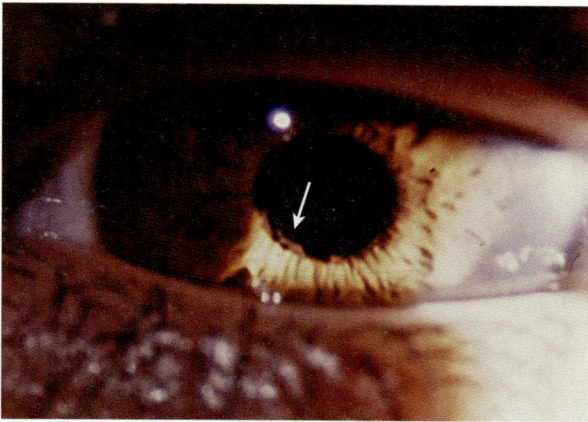

FIGURE 17–1 ■ Small iris pigment epithelial cysts (arrow) at pupil margin. These cause no visual problems.

incidence and number of lesions increase with age. By age 20, more than 95% of patients with neurofibromatosis have Lisch nodules. Lisch nodules are small, tan, and slightly elevated from the iris surface (Figure 17–3A and B). The Lisch nodules do not cause any vision problems. They play an important role in establishing a diagnosis.

3. *Iris nevi.* Iris nevi present as areas of irregular pigment on the surface of the iris. They are most easily noticed when the nevi are brown and the underlying iris pigment is fair (Figure 17–4). These are flat (rather than elevated like Lisch nodules), but this feature cannot be accurately assessed without a slit lamp. Iris nevi in children are almost always benign.

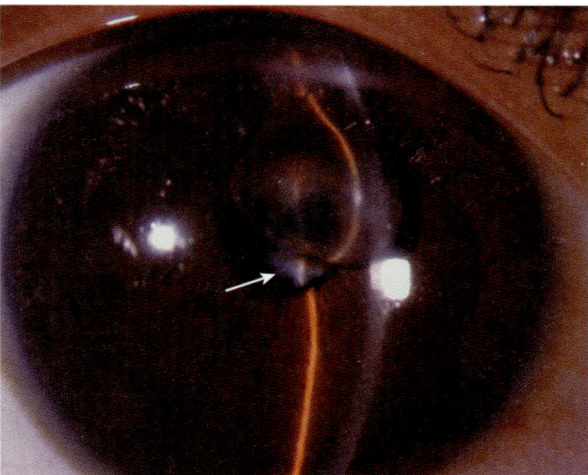

FIGURE 17–3 ■ (A and B) Lisch nodules in patients with neurofibromatosis. They appear as small, tan mounds of tissue on the iris surface. Lisch nodules increase in number with age.

APPROACH TO THE PATIENT

Iris lesions in infants and young children are uncommon, and they are usually benign (Table 17–1). From a practical standpoint, they may be easily missed because of their small size and the difficulty examining an active young child.

History

Bumps on the iris may be brought to your attention by the parents, or may be noticed during a well-child check. If the parents have noticed them, they should be asked when the bumps were first identified, and whether they have changed in size or shape. General questions about vision and any associated ocular symptoms should be asked. If Lisch nodules are suspected, a family history of neurofibromatosis may be present, and

FIGURE 17–2 ■ Large iris cyst obstructing pupil. A cataract is also present (arrow). The irregular vertical line is the slit beam, which is distorted superiorly by the cyst.

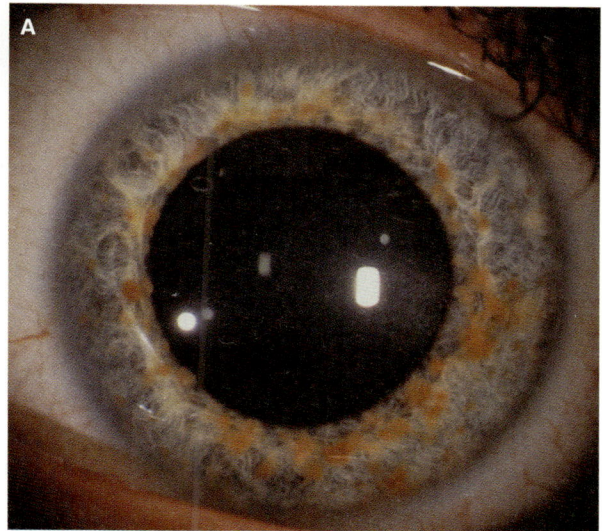

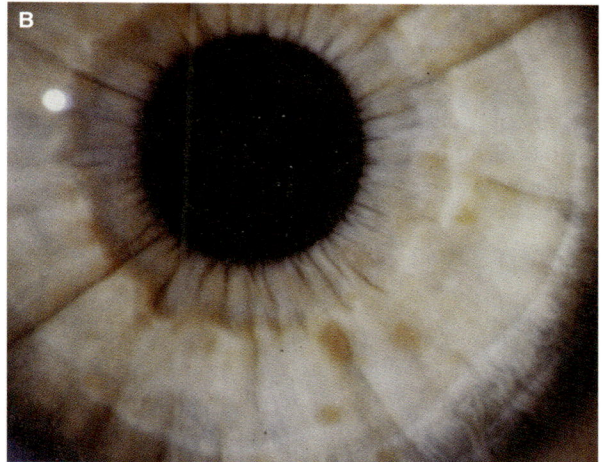

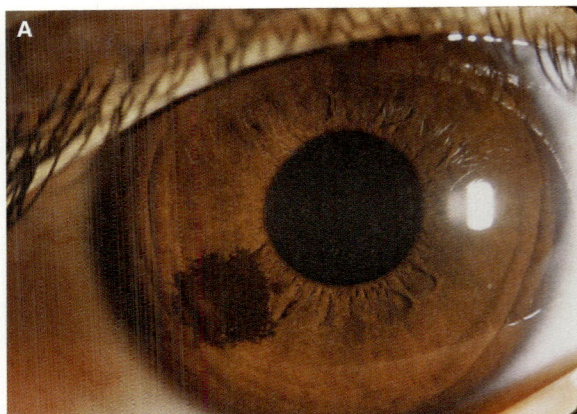

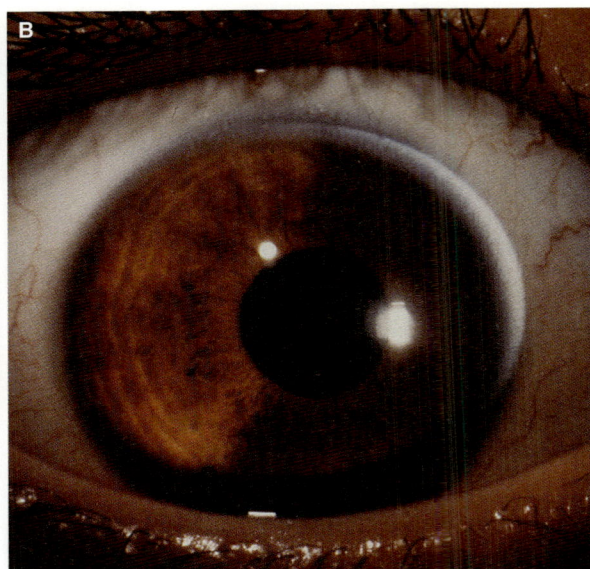

FIGURE 17–4 ■ Iris nevi. (A) Typical hyperpigmented iris nevus. (B) Large iris nevus (the dark portion of the iris), involving just over half of the iris surface. Nevi appear as flat, circumscribed areas of increased pigmentation on the iris. The underlying iris architecture is visible beneath the nevus.

the child's development may be delayed. If an iris nevus is present, questions should be asked about a family history of multiple nevi or skin cancer (e.g., dysplastic nevus syndrome).

Examination

The child's vision should be checked using age-appropriate methods. A penlight should be used to assess the iris. In addition to the lesions themselves, the examiner should check the pupillary reactions and look for irregularities of the iris. Small iris cysts at the pupil margin are often best visualized by examining the red reflex with a direct ophthalmoscope.

Iris nevi are relatively common. They appear as flat areas of pigmentation that are distinct from the underlying iris. They are usually discrete, but sometimes cover a large portion of the iris (Figure 17–4).

Large cysts of the iris are rare, and ciliary body tumors are even rarer. These may appear as elevated iris irregularities. If they produce glaucoma, corneal clouding and light sensitivity may be present.

If Lisch nodules are suspected, the child should be checked for café-au-lait spots, axillary freckling, and other systemic manifestations of neurofibromatosis.

Table 17–1.

Causes of Iris Lesions in Children

- Iris cyst
- JXG
- Lisch nodules
- Iris nevi

JXG may present as an elevated orange-brown lesion of the iris, which may bleed and cause a hyphema. The lesion may be isolated to the iris, or be associated with small papular lesions of the head and neck.

PLAN

Small, scalloped irregularities of the pupil margin in an infant do not require additional evaluation. Infants with other iris lesions should be referred to an ophthalmologist (Figure 17-5). Children with Lisch nodules should be evaluated for other stigmata of neurofibromatosis. Iris nevi are almost always benign in children. However, like skin nevi, they should be monitored for abnormal growth. Large iris lesions are rare, but they should be evaluated by an ophthalmologist (Figure 17-6).

WHAT SHOULDN'T BE MISSED

Patients with significant iris lesions, such as large cysts or possible ciliary body tumor, should be referred for prompt ophthalmic evaluation. The presence of Lisch nodules strongly suggests a diagnosis of neurofibromatosis, and confirmatory evaluation is indicated.

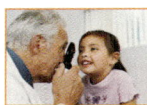

When to Refer

- Small scalloped lesions at the pupil margin do not require referral
- The iris should be evaluated in patients who have other findings suggestive of neurofibromatosis
- Patients with iris nevi should be referred if the lesions are changing
- Patients with large cysts or other iris abnormalities should be referred

```
                        ┌─────────────────┐
                        │   Iris lesions  │
                        └─────────────────┘
                                 │
                                 ▼
                        ┌─────────────────┐
                        │     Infant      │
                        └─────────────────┘
                                 │
        ┌────────────────────────┼────────────────────────┐
        ▼                        ▼                         ▼
┌─────────────────┐    ┌─────────────────┐    ┌─────────────────┐
│ Small scalloped │    │  Orange-brown   │    │ Large iris cysts│
│    lesions      │    │ lesion on iris  │    │                 │
│ at pupil margin │    │                 │    │                 │
└─────────────────┘    └─────────────────┘    └─────────────────┘
        │                        │                         │
        ▼                        ▼                         ▼
┌─────────────────┐    ┌─────────────────┐    ┌─────────────────┐
│  Iris pigment   │    │    Juvenile     │    │    Refer to     │
│ epithelial cysts│    │ xanthogranuloma │    │  ophthalmology  │
└─────────────────┘    └─────────────────┘    └─────────────────┘
        │                        │
        ▼                        ▼
┌─────────────────┐    ┌─────────────────┐
│  No treatment   │    │   May cause     │
│     needed      │    │    hyphema      │
└─────────────────┘    └─────────────────┘
                                 │
                                 ▼
                        ┌─────────────────┐
                        │    Refer to     │
                        │  ophthalmology  │
                        └─────────────────┘
```

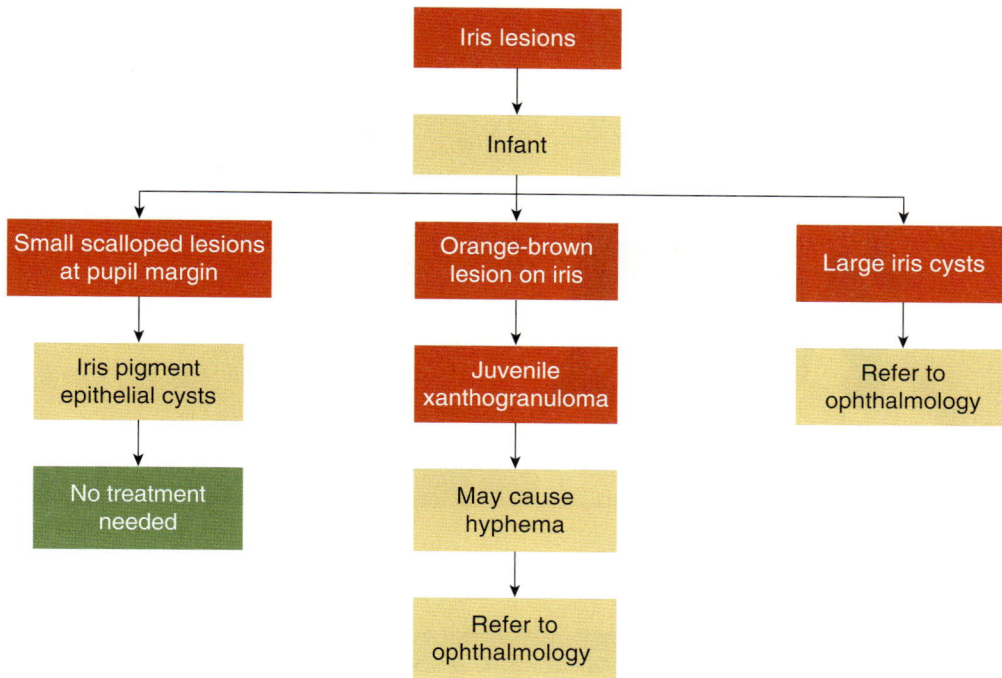

FIGURE 17–5 ■ Algorithm for evaluation and management of an infant with iris lesions.

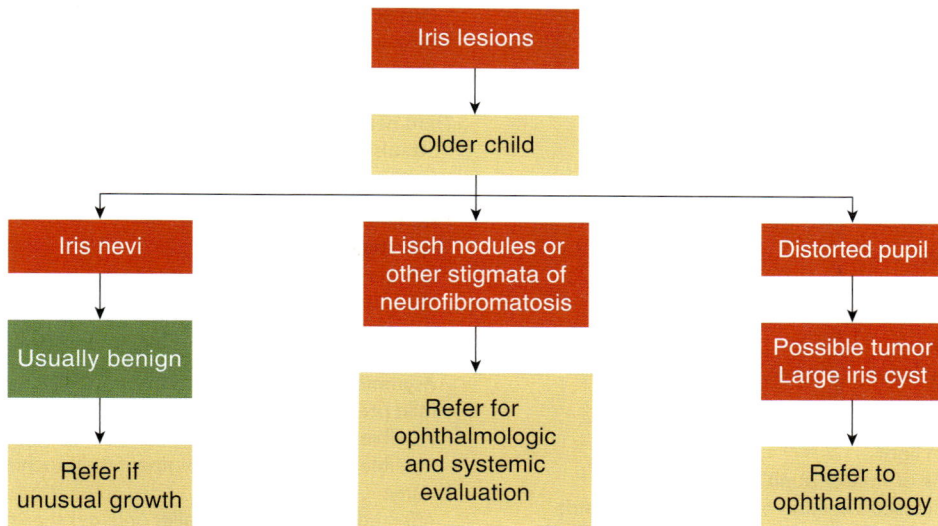

```
                        ┌─────────────────┐
                        │   Iris lesions  │
                        └─────────────────┘
                                 │
                                 ▼
                        ┌─────────────────┐
                        │   Older child   │
                        └─────────────────┘
                                 │
        ┌────────────────────────┼────────────────────────┐
        ▼                        ▼                         ▼
┌─────────────────┐    ┌─────────────────┐    ┌─────────────────┐
│    Iris nevi    │    │ Lisch nodules or│    │ Distorted pupil │
│                 │    │ other stigmata  │    │                 │
│                 │    │ of neurofibro-  │    │                 │
│                 │    │    matosis      │    │                 │
└─────────────────┘    └─────────────────┘    └─────────────────┘
        │                        │                         │
        ▼                        ▼                         ▼
┌─────────────────┐    ┌─────────────────┐    ┌─────────────────┐
│  Usually benign │    │    Refer for    │    │ Possible tumor  │
│                 │    │  ophthalmologic │    │ Large iris cyst │
└─────────────────┘    │   and systemic  │    └─────────────────┘
        │              │    evaluation   │             │
        ▼              └─────────────────┘             ▼
┌─────────────────┐                          ┌─────────────────┐
│    Refer if     │                          │    Refer to     │
│ unusual growth  │                          │  ophthalmology  │
└─────────────────┘                          └─────────────────┘
```

FIGURE 17–6 ■ Algorithm for evaluation and management of an older child with iris lesions.

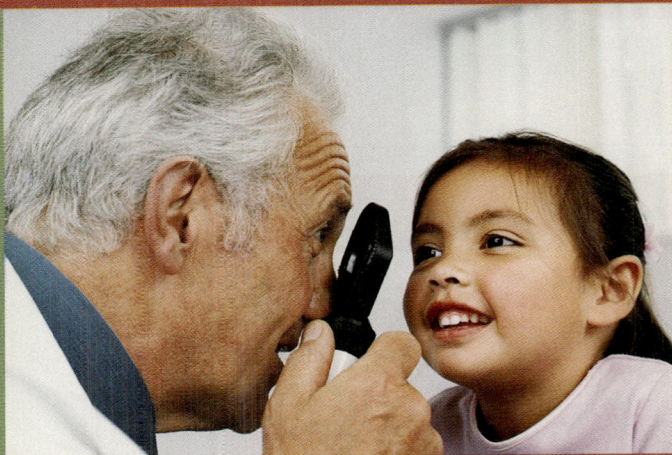

CHAPTER 18

Anisocoria

The Problem
"One of my child's pupils is larger than the other."

Common Causes
Physiological anisocoria
Horner syndrome
Iritis
Pharmacological

Other Causes
Third nerve palsy
Trauma
Congenital iris anomalies

KEY FINDINGS

History
Physiological anisocoria
  Mild asymmetry
  Variable (pupils sometimes equal)
Horner syndrome
  Pupils always unequal
  Worse in dim light
  Ptosis on side of smaller pupil
  Possible decreased sweating of face on affected side
  Unequal pupil color in congenital or early acquired cases
  Associated with some systemic disorders
    Neuroblastoma
    Thoracic or cervical surgery
    Birth trauma with cervical injury

Trauma
  History of direct ocular injury
Iritis
  History of juvenile idiopathic arthritis
  Ocular pain, redness
Pharmacological
  Exposure to topical medications or plants that
    affect pupil
Third nerve palsy
  Strabismus, ptosis
  Systemic diseases associated with third nerve palsy

Examination
Physiological anisocoria
  Difference between pupils less than 1.0 mm
  Variable, sometimes equal
  Greater in dim light
Horner syndrome
  Asymmetry greater in dim light
  Mild ptosis on affected side
  Possible unequal sweating on affected side
  Possible difference in iris pigment (heterochromia)
Trauma
  Affected pupil may be smaller or larger than normal pupil
  Other signs of ocular trauma
Iritis
  Pupil nonreactive, possibly irregular
  Possible cataract

WHAT SHOULD YOU DO?

Mild (<0.5 mm) anisocoria in young children is usually normal, particularly if it is variable. Anisocoria associated with other disorders, particularly Horner syndrome and third nerve palsy, is not an isolated finding. If a patient has ptosis along with anisocoria, referral to a pediatric ophthalmologist is indicated for evaluation of possible Horner syndrome or third nerve palsy. If the pupil does not react at all, referral is also indicated.

What Shouldn't Be Missed

Horner syndrome, particularly in older children, may result from serious diseases such as neuroblastoma. These patients require evaluation to look for these problems. Children with *iritis secondary to juvenile idiopathic arthritis (JIA)* may have no symptoms of ocular discomfort despite severe inflammation. In some of these patients, abnormal pupils due to scarring of the iris may be the first abnormality noted.

COMMON CAUSES

1. *Physiological anisocoria.* Mildly asymmetric pupils may occur in otherwise normal infants. This may be familial. The anisocoria is more noticeable in dim light. The hallmark of physiological anisocoria is variability, with the pupils sometimes appearing equal. Physiological anisocoria does not cause any problems with development of vision.
2. *Horner syndrome.* Horner syndrome occurs due to interruption of the oculosympathetic chain that begins in the hypothalamus, travels through the spinal cord to the thorax, and ascends along the internal carotid artery to the orbit. Lesions anywhere along this pathway may cause Horner syndrome. The syndrome is characterized by anisocoria (pupil smaller on the affected side), mild ptosis, and anhidrosis (decreased sweating on the affected side of the face) (Figure 18–1). It typically does not cause vision problems. It is important because of its association with other systemic conditions.
3. *Iritis.* Most patients with iritis (intraocular inflammation) have marked eye discomfort and seek medical attention because of this complaint. For unknown reasons, children with iritis associated with JIA usually do not experience significant eye pain. Because of this, even severe inflammation may go

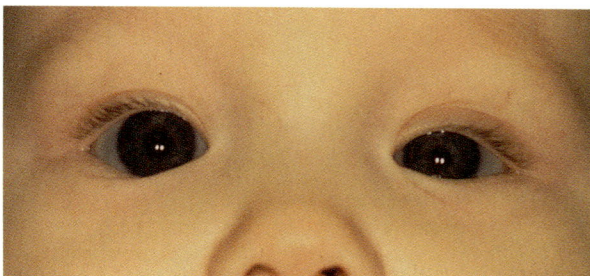

FIGURE 18–2 ■ Scarring of iris to anterior lens capsule in a patient with iritis.

unnoticed until substantial eye damage is present. Children with JIA sometimes present with nonreactive pupils due to scarring of the iris to the lens capsule (Figure 18–2).
4. *Pharmacological.* Several eye drops or exposure to certain plants may affect the pupil. This diagnosis can usually be established with a careful history, examination, and confirmatory drop testing (Table 18–1).
5. *Trauma.* Direct ocular injuries may result in damage to the muscles in the iris that control pupil size (Figure 18–3). In these patients, there is usually a recognized history of trauma.
6. *Third cranial nerve palsy.* Patients with third cranial nerve palsies usually have an enlarged pupil on the affected side, along with marked strabismus and ptosis. Congenital third nerve palsies

Table 18–1.

Pharmacological Causes of Anisocoria (Unilateral Topical Medication or Exposure)

- Affected pupil larger
  □ Atropine
  □ Scopolamine
  □ Cyclopentolate
  □ Tropicamide
  □ Phenylephrine
- Affected pupil smaller
  □ Pilocarpine
- Plant exposure (due to belladonna alkaloids—affected pupil larger)
  □ Jimsonweed
  □ Moonflower
  □ Black henbane
  □ Deadly nightshade

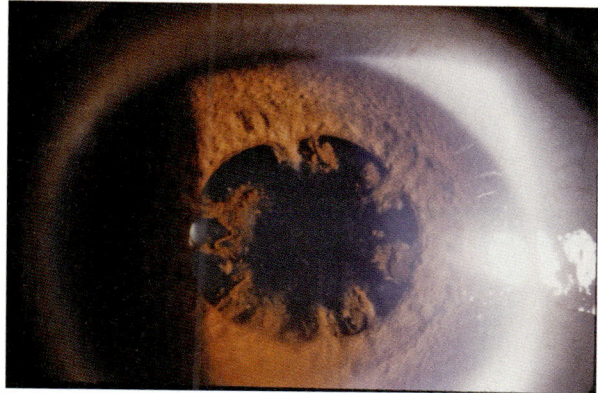

FIGURE 18–1 ■ Horner syndrome in a patient with neuroblastoma in the left lung apex. Note the smaller pupil and ptosis on the left.

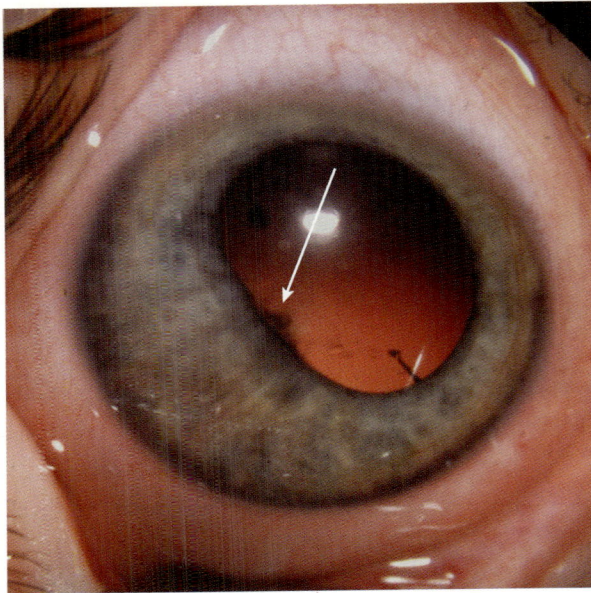

FIGURE 18–3 ■ Asymmetric pupil following trauma, with scarring of iris to anterior lens capsule (arrow).

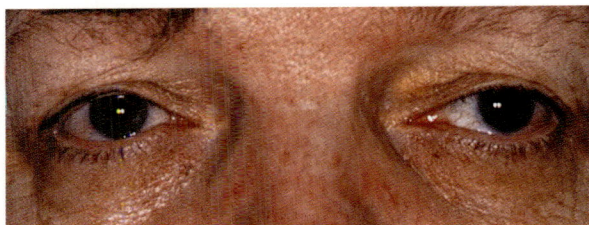

Table 18–2.

Anisocoria With Affected Pupil Smaller

- Horner syndrome
- Physiological
- Trauma
- Inflammation
- Congenital third cranial nerve palsy (uncommon)

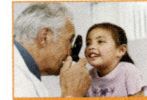

Table 18–3.

Anisocoria With Affected Pupil Larger

- Third cranial nerve palsy
- Pharmacological
- Trauma
- Inflammation
- Adie tonic pupil

sometimes present with a smaller pupil on the affected side. Partial third cranial nerve palsies present with variable ptosis and eye movement abnormalities, in which case the anisocoria is helpful in establishing a diagnosis (Figure 18–4).

APPROACH TO THE PATIENT

The presence of unequal pupils in children is concerning, primarily because this finding may result from serious underlying disorders. Most patients will be referred to an ophthalmologist. An appropriate evaluation can determine whether an underlying problem may be present and what additional investigations are warranted.

When the pupils are unequal, it is important to determine which pupil is abnormal. The iris sphincter muscles, which cause the pupil to become smaller, are under parasympathetic control. The iris dilator muscles, which cause the pupil to become larger, are under sympathetic control. If the abnormal pupil is smaller,

the anisocoria is usually worse in dim light, indicating a defect in dilation of the affected pupil (a sympathetic abnormality) (Table 18–2). If the affected pupil is larger, the anisocoria is usually worse in bright light, indicating an abnormality of constriction (a parasympathetic problem) (Table 18–3). If the pupil does not react at all, this usually indicates trauma, inflammation with scarring, or a pharmacological effect (Table 18–4).

History

Anisocoria may be brought to your attention by the patient's parents, or it may be noticed during a well-child evaluation. The history should include general questions about the child's health and development, and a neurological review of systems should be obtained. A history of arthritis increases the likelihood that the child may have iritis with secondary iris damage.

General questions about the anisocoria should include when it was first noted, which pupil is bigger (or

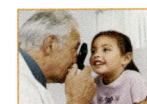

FIGURE 18–4 ■ Partial left third cranial nerve palsy. Note large left exotropia and slight ptosis. The left pupil is larger than the right.

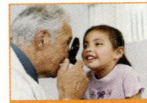

Table 18–4.

Pupil With No Reaction

- Trauma
- Pharmacological
- Inflammation
- Complete third cranial nerve palsy

Table 18–5.

Horner Syndrome Versus Third Nerve Palsy

	Anisocoria	Ptosis	Strabismus	Anhidrosis (decreased sweating on affected side of face)	Heterochromia (unequal pupil color)
Horner syndrome	Pupil smaller on affected side	Mild	No	Sometimes	Congenital—sometimes Acquired—no
Third cranial nerve palsy	Pupil larger on affected side (sometimes smaller in congenital palsies)	Severe	Marked (eye out and down)	No	No

smaller), whether the anisocoria is constant or variable, whether it is more noticeable in dim or bright light, and whether there has been any ocular trauma or exposure to medications or plants that could affect the pupils. More specific questions will be indicated based on the diagnoses being considered.

If Horner syndrome is suspected, questions should be asked about the child's birth. Difficult deliveries may cause Horner syndrome due to damage to the cervical portion of the oculosympathetic chain (although most infants with Horner syndrome do not have such a history and the etiology of the problem is not known). Horner syndrome may also be caused by a number of disorders along the neural pathway, including lesions in the brain, chest, and neck. Neuroblastoma is a common cause of acquired Horner syndrome in children.

Anisocoria due to third nerve palsy is accompanied by ptosis and strabismus. This is usually readily distinguished from Horner syndrome (Table 18–5).

Examination

A general ocular examination should be included in the evaluation of children with anisocoria, including measurement of visual acuity using appropriate methods for age. The pupil reaction to light should be checked to be sure the iris constricts concentrically. The pupil size should be measured in dim light and bright light. Some unusual congenital iris abnormalities may present with abnormal pupils, including colobomas (Figure 18–5A), large iris nevi, heterochromia (unequal pupil color), congenital iris ectropion (Figure 18–5B), and persistent pupillary membranes (Figure 18–5C).

Children with physiological anisocoria have normal irises, the asymmetry is mild (usually <0.5 mm), and the anisocoria is more noticeable in dim light. The remainder of the examination is normal. The pupil asymmetry in Horner syndrome is also more noticeable in dim light. In children with congenital or

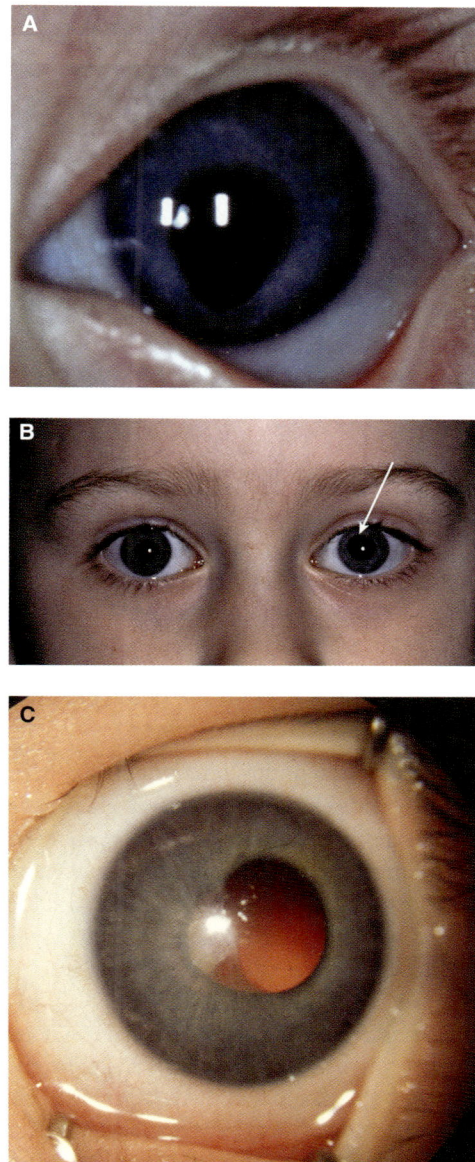

FIGURE 18–5 ■ Congenital iris anomalies causing abnormal pupil appearance. (A) Iris coloboma. (B) Congenital iris ectropion (ectropion uveae) (arrow). (C) Persistent pupillary membrane.

early-acquired Horner syndrome, the irises may have different colors.

If there is no pupillary reaction, the cause is likely pharmacological, trauma, or scarring of the iris due to iritis. Patients with complete third cranial nerve palsy also may have no pupil reaction. If the etiology is trauma, the child should be examined for other ocular and periocular injuries. If iritis is suspected, the child may also have a cataract. Because JIA is a common cause of iritis in children, an examination of the joints should be performed

Additional ocular examination should include evaluation for ptosis and strabismus. The eyelid height, levator muscle function, and extraocular movements should be assessed. The presence of ptosis indicates that Horner syndrome or a third cranial nerve palsy is likely present. The ptosis in Horner syndrome is mild (1 to 2 mm), whereas marked ptosis is typical with third nerve palsies. Strabismus (with the eye out and down) also occurs in third nerve palsies (Figure 18–4 and Table 18–5).

PLAN

In an infant with slight, variable anisocoria and otherwise normal ocular and systemic evaluation, no further evaluation is necessary. The evaluation of other patients with anisocoria is based on the determination of which pupil is abnormal (Figures 18–6, 18–7, and 18–8). If the pupil does not constrict at all, referral to an ophthalmologist is indicated. If anisocoria is accompanied by ptosis, the patient should be referred for evaluation of possible Horner syndrome or third cranial nerve palsy. If a diagnosis of acquired Horner syndrome is confirmed, an extensive evaluation is indicated to look for potential causes.

WHAT SHOULDN'T BE MISSED

Horner syndrome is one of the most common etiologies of nonphysiological anisocoria in children. If present from birth, it is usually benign, but urine vanillylmandelic acid may be measured to screen for neuroblastoma. Acquired Horner syndrome raises a significant concern for a serious underlying cause. Nonreactive pupils suggest the possibility of trauma or intraocular inflammation, which also requires prompt ophthalmic evaluation.

When to Refer

- Anisocoria accompanied by ptosis and/or strabismus
- Anisocoria greater than 1 mm
- History of ocular trauma
- Nonreactive pupil (unless clear history of exposure to medication to explain the finding)

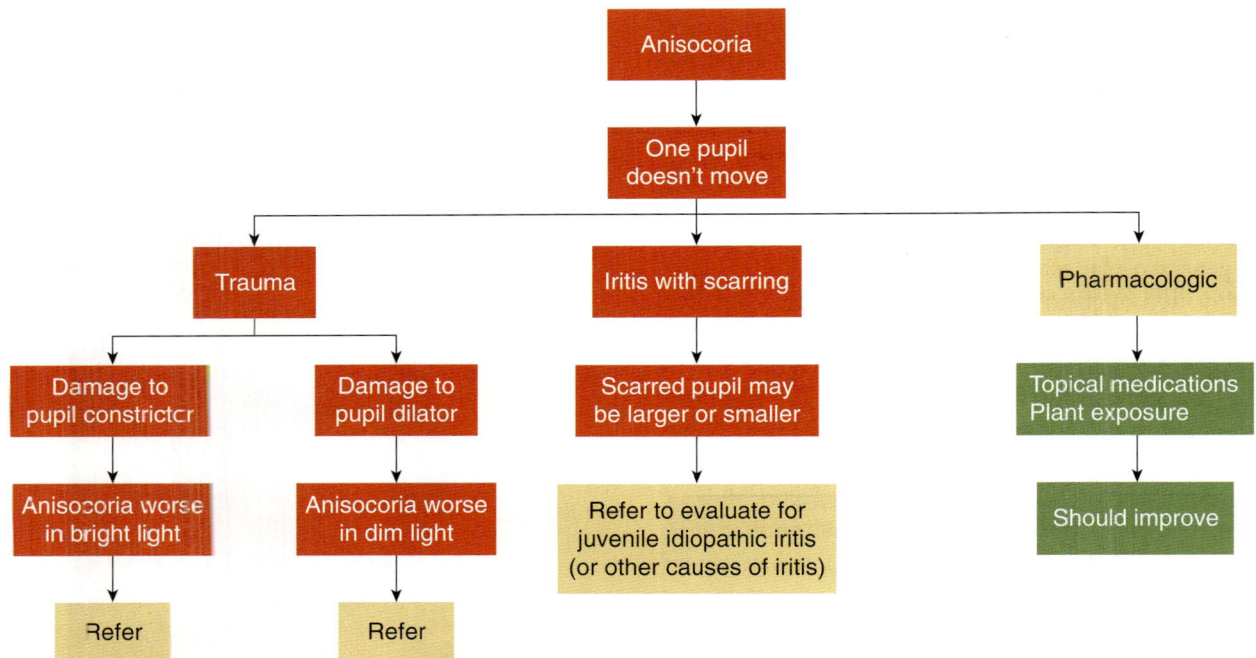

FIGURE 18–6 ■ Algorithm for evaluation and management of a child with anisocoria in which one pupil does not react.

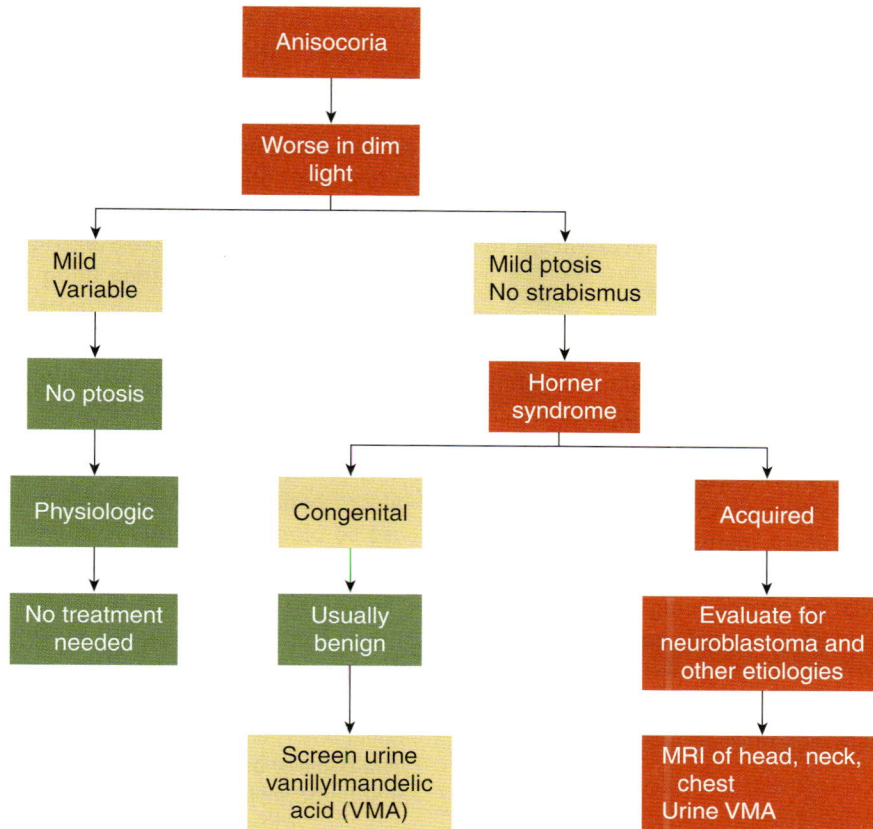

FIGURE 18–7 ■ Algorithm for evaluation and management of a child with anisocoria that is greater in dim light.

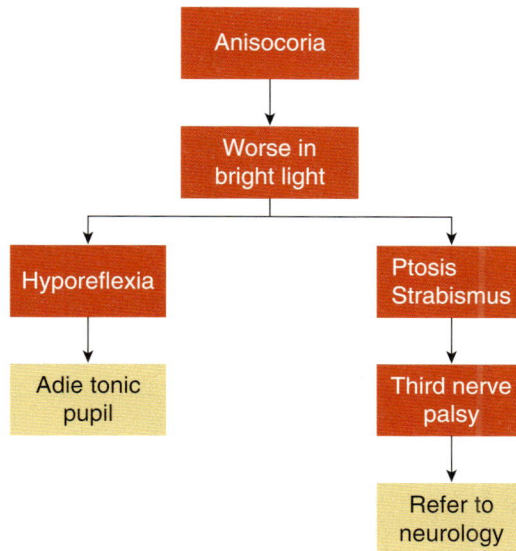

FIGURE 18–8 ■ Algorithm for evaluation and management of a child with anisocoria that is greater in bright light.

CHAPTER 19

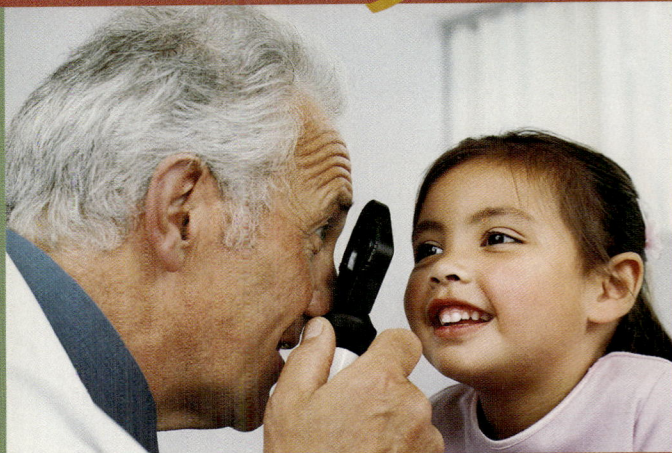

Abnormal Red Reflex

The Problem
"My child's eye reflex looks white."

Common Causes
Cataract
Retinoblastoma
Pseudoleukocoria

Other Causes
Retinal abnormalities
  Detachment
    Coat's disease
    Retinopathy of prematurity
  Retinal coloboma

KEY FINDINGS

History
General
  When first noticed?
  Getting worse?
  Does the eye wander?
  Does the child appear to see?
Cataract
  Family history of childhood cataracts
  Other systemic/developmental problems
Retinoblastoma
  Family history of retinoblastoma
Pseudoleukocoria
  Only noticed in photographs when taken
    from the side
Retinal disorder
  Premature birth
  Family history of retinal disease

Examination
General
  Assessment of red reflex with direct
    ophthalmoscope
  Vision
  Strabismus
Cataract
  Clouding of lens
Retinoblastoma
  White mass posterior to lens
Retinal detachment
  Grey mass posterior to lens
Pseudoleukocoria
  Red reflex appears normal when viewed from
    straight ahead
  Abnormal when viewed from side

WHAT SHOULD YOU DO?

Almost all patients whose parents report an abnormal red reflex should be referred to a pediatric ophthalmologist due to the potential serious implications of the possible diagnoses. Similarly, if the red reflex cannot be adequately visualized during a well-child examination, referral is indicated.

What Shouldn't Be Missed

Retinoblastoma is highly curable if it is identified while confined to the eye, but is potentially lethal if it spreads. Therefore, early diagnosis is very important.

The visual prognosis for infantile cataracts is directly related to the age at which they are detected and treated. Unilateral congenital cataracts should be removed by 6 weeks of age to maximize the potential for vision.

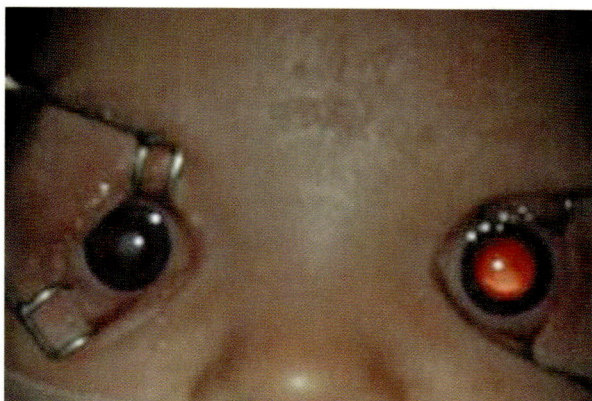

FIGURE 19–1 ■ Abnormal red reflex, right eye, secondary to infantile cataract.

FIGURE 19–2 ■ Retinoblastoma, left eye. (A) Abnormal red reflex. (B) Magnified view shows vascularized elevated white retinal mass. The lens is clear.

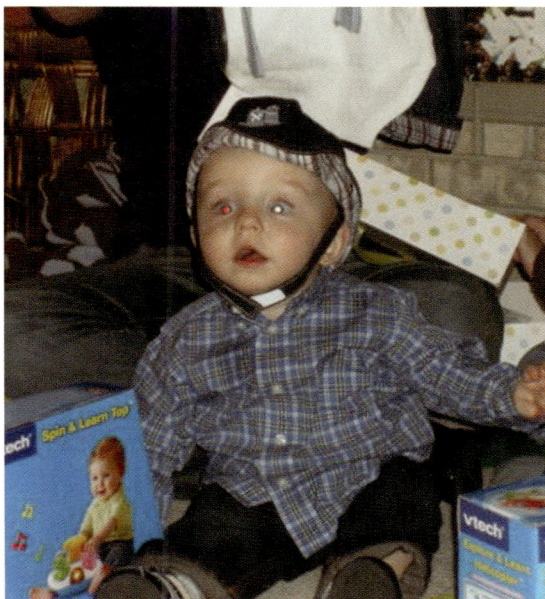

COMMON CAUSES

1. *Cataracts.* Cataracts in infants are most commonly identified by an abnormal red reflex (Figure 19–1). Due to the high risk of amblyopia in unilateral cataracts, prompt referral to a pediatric ophthalmologist is indicated. Bilateral cataracts may occur in association with several syndromes or diseases, and these children require evaluation for these systemic disorders (see Chapter 30).

2. *Retinoblastoma.* Retinoblastoma is rare, but it is the most common primary intraocular tumor in children. It most frequently presents due to an abnormal red reflex (Figure 19–2A and B). It is one of the few life-threatening disorders encountered in pediatric ophthalmology. Intraocular retinoblastoma is very treatable, but the mortality for metastatic disease is high. Identification of tumors before systemic spread is critical. Most children with large unilateral tumors will require enucleation (surgical removal of the eye), but the eye and vision may sometimes be preserved if the tumors are identified when they are small.

3. *Pseudoleukocoria.* The optic nerve head at the back of the eye is white. If a light is shined into the eye from an oblique angle temporally, the reflection from the optic nerve head may fill the pupillary opening, producing pseudoleukocoria (Figure 19–3). This usually requires evaluation by a pediatric ophthalmologist to verify.

4. *Retinal disorders.* Retinal disorders that cause detachments are rare in children. They most commonly occur in infants with retinopathy of prematurity and may also occur following

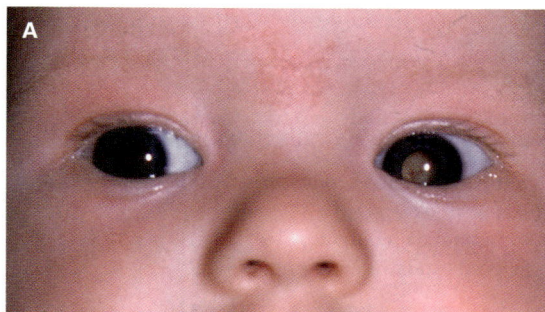

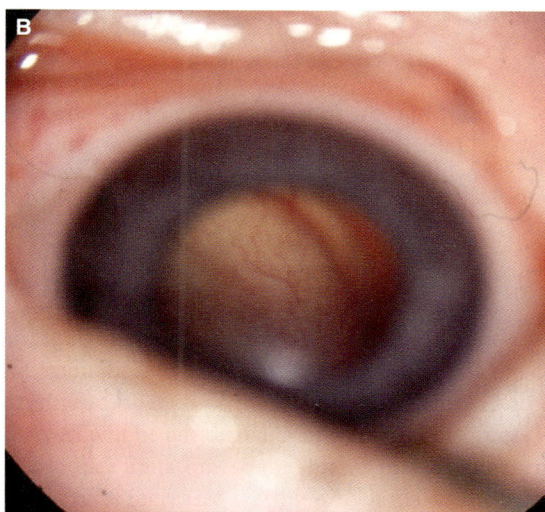

FIGURE 19–3 ■ Pseudoleukocoria, left eye. The light reflex in the left eye appears white due to a reflection from the optic nerve head (which is white). Note that the photograph is taken from the patient's left side.

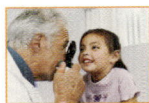

Table 19–1.

Causes of Retinal Detachment in Children

- Retinopathy of prematurity
- Systemic diseases
  - Incontinentia pigmenti
  - Familial exudative vitreoretinopathy
- Trauma
- Toxocara
- Coat's disease

trauma or due to rare familial disorders (Table 19–1). Large retinal colobomas may also produce leukocoria (Figure 19–4A and B). Toxocara infections may cause both retinal detachments and cataracts. They usually present as inflammatory white masses in the peripheral retina (Figure 19–5).

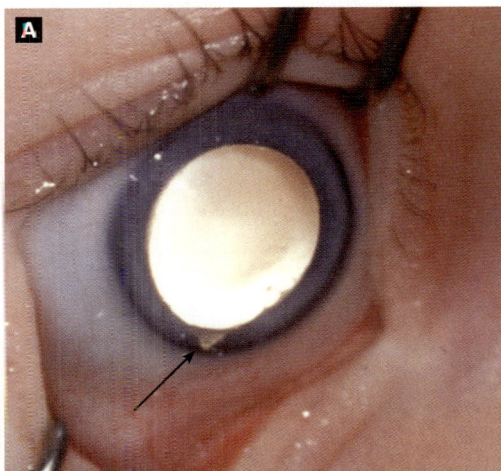

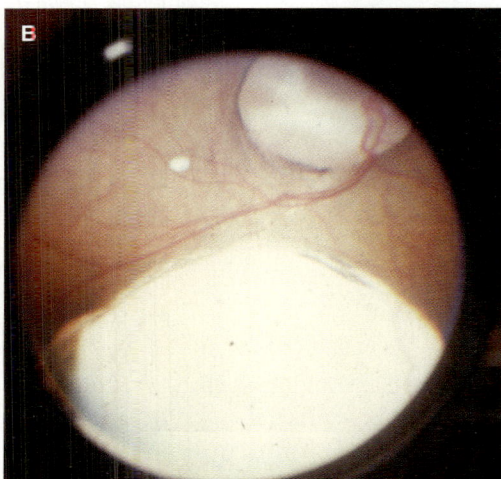

FIGURE 19–4 ■ Retinal coloboma. (A) Leukocoria secondary to reflection from abnormal retina. Note the small iris coloboma (arrow). (B) Fundus examination shows large inferior retinal coloboma.

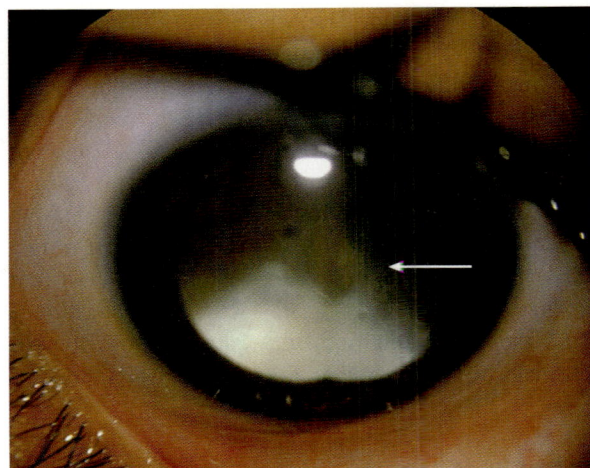

FIGURE 19–5 ■ Toxocara infection of the retina. These usually present as inflammatory white masses in the peripheral retina. Note the traction bands extending from the surface of the lesion (arrow).

APPROACH TO THE PATIENT

An abnormal red reflex is often the first abnormality noted in patients with potentially life- and vision-threatening disorders. Many of these occur in infants and young children, who are unable to vocalize complaints. *It is important to realize that in young children, even if one eye has extremely poor vision, as long as the other eye sees normally, the child will function well visually. Therefore, the absence of any complaints about the child's vision in no way rules out the possibility of unilateral eye problems.* Because of this, examination of the red reflex should be part of every routine well-child check.

History

Parents may come in to the pediatrician having noted an abnormal red reflex, or it may be noted during a routine examination. In either setting, one should ask how well the child appears to see. If the family has noticed an abnormal red reflex, the age when it was first noted should be determined. If only one eye is affected, the child will usually appear to see normally. If a child has a bilateral disorder, abnormal visual behavior will often be the first symptom noted by parents. If a child has decreased vision in one eye for any reason, strabismus often develops. This may be either esotropia or exotropia, and is often intermittent.

Questions about the child's general health may raise the suspicion of syndromes that may be associated with cataracts. Premature birth may lead to retinopathy of prematurity, which may cause retinal detachments. Retinoblastoma, cataracts, and many retinal disorders may be inherited, and therefore obtaining a family history is important.

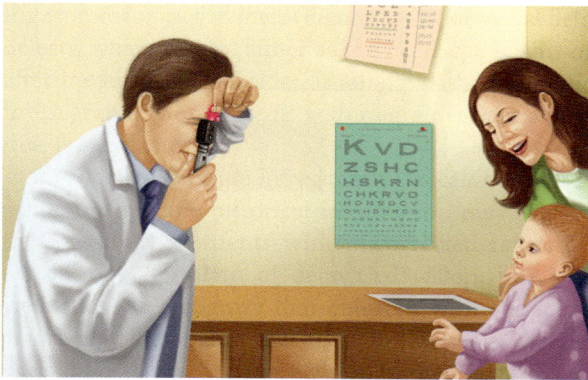

FIGURE 19–6 ■ Red reflex examination. This is most easily performed by using the direct ophthalmoscope from 2 to 3 feet away from the patient in a dim room. The examiner focuses on the child's face with the ophthalmoscope, and the red reflex can be compared between the two eyes.

Examination

The child's vision and examination of the anterior segment should be performed in the normal manner. *To best evaluate the red reflex, use the direct ophthalmoscope from 2 to 3 feet away from the patient in a dim room. Focus the ophthalmoscope on the patient's face. The red reflex can then be assessed and compared between the two eyes* (Figure 19–6). *The symmetry of the corneal light reflexes can also be noted at this time to screen for strabismus.* Pseudoleukocoria, retinoblastoma, and retinal colobomas usually cause a very white reflex, whereas retinal detachments are typically gray. The appearance of cataracts is highly variable. If a parent reports an abnormal red reflex, but it is not noted when shining the light into the patient's eyes from straight ahead, you should assess the red reflex as you move the direct ophthalmoscope from side to side. Tumors of the nasal retina, for instance, may not be noted until the light is shined into the eye from a lateral position (Figure 19–7A–D). This may be difficult to differentiate from pseudoleukocoria, which is also only noted when viewed from a lateral position.

PLAN

If a parent reports an abnormal red reflex or if you note this on examination, the child should be referred promptly to a pediatric ophthalmologist. This is particularly important for retinoblastoma, which may be lethal if it spreads beyond the eye. If an abnormal red reflex is found on a newborn screening, the patient should also be referred promptly. In a newborn, a cataract is the most likely etiology for leukocoria. If an infant has a unilateral cataract, surgical removal should be performed in the first 6 weeks of life to maximize the visual potential.

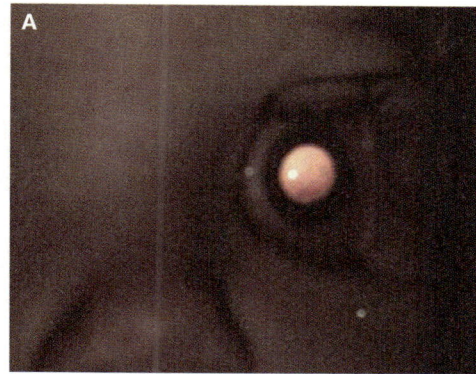

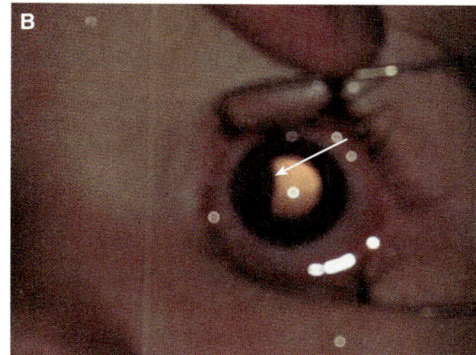

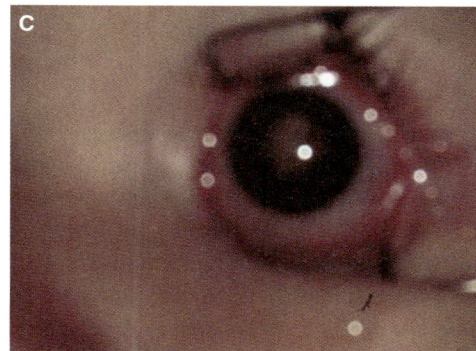

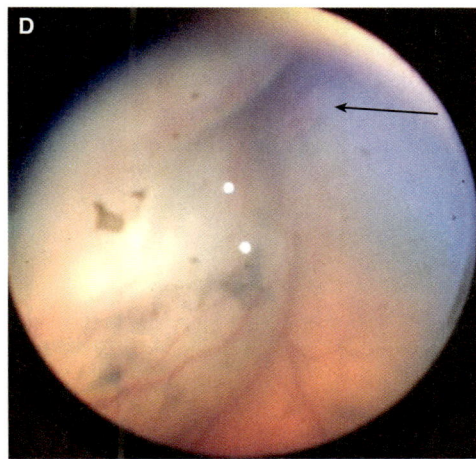

FIGURE 19–7 ■ Leukocoria due to nasal retinoblastoma, left eye. (A) Red reflex appears normal when viewed from straight ahead. (B) Crescent-shaped abnormality (arrow) begins to appear when light is moved to left. (C) Red reflex absent as light moved further to left. (D) Fundus examination reveals a large tumor filling the nasal retina. The optic nerve is marked by an arrow.

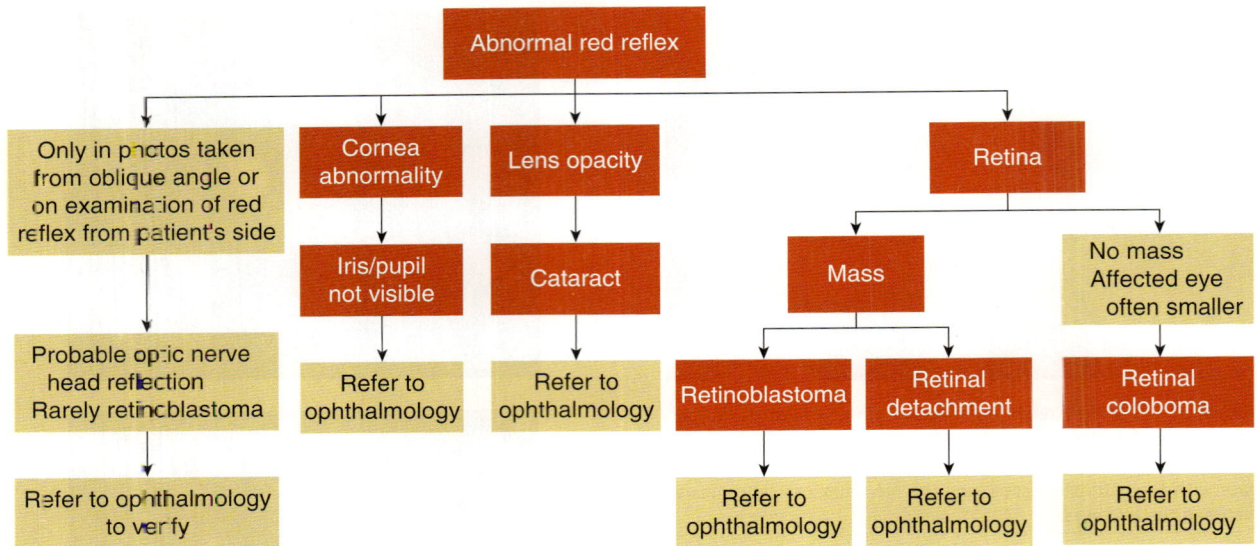

FIGURE 19–8 ■ Causes of an abnormal red reflex.

WHAT SHOULDN'T BE MISSED

Cataracts and retinoblastoma both often present with leukocoria. These are among the most treatable potentially vision- and life-threatening disorders in pediatric ophthalmology, and early referral is critical (Figure 19–8).

When to Refer

■ Any child with an abnormal red reflex should be referred to a pediatric ophthalmologist

CHAPTER 20

Retinal Hemorrhage

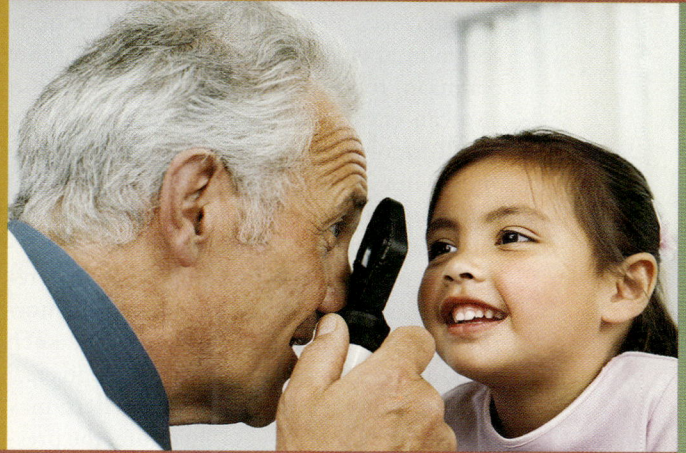

The Problem
Retinal hemorrhage

Common Causes
Normal birth
Child abuse

Other Causes
Major trauma
Systemic disease
  Glutaric aciduria type 1
  Bleeding disorder
  Sepsis
  Hypertension
  Neoplasm

KEY FINDINGS

History
Normal birth
  More common after vaginal delivery
  Frequent (even after uncomplicated delivery)
Child abuse
  History often not reliable
  Findings not consistent with given history
Major trauma
  Retinal hemorrhages uncommon
Systemic disease
  History corresponding to underlying disorder

Examination
Normal birth
  Range from few scattered to diffuse
    hemorrhages
Child abuse
  Widely variable, from no to massive retinal
    hemorrhage
  Retinoschisis cavity almost pathognomonic
    for shaking injury
Major trauma
  Usually only mild hemorrhage, even with
    severe injury
  Severe crush injuries very rarely cause
    retinoschisis
Systemic diseases
  Varies with underlying disorder

WHAT SHOULD YOU DO?

The presence of retinal hemorrhages is an exception to most of the other problems included in the symptoms section of this book. It is a sign, rather than a symptom, and therefore it is not an abnormality reported by parents or children. Pediatricians usually identify retinal hemorrhages because they are specifically looking for them due to associated problems. They are almost never noted during routine examinations due to their rarity and the difficulty of examining the retina in young children. Children with retinal hemorrhages should be referred to a pediatric ophthalmologist.

What Shouldn't Be Missed

The presence of diffuse retinal hemorrhages in a previously healthy infant or toddler should raise the strong suspicion of child abuse. If there is no other identifiable etiology, the patient will require an evaluation for occult systemic diseases and other evidence of child abuse.

COMMON CAUSES

1. *Normal birth.* Retinal hemorrhages are quite common after normal births. They are more common following vaginal deliveries, but also can occur after caesarean section. These usually resolve within the first few weeks of life and do not cause visual problems.

2. *Child abuse.* Retinal hemorrhages are an important finding in children who are victims of nonaccidental trauma. They are frequently associated with intracranial hemorrhages and other signs of trauma, such as bone fractures. They are not a universal finding, however, and other disorders may cause mild hemorrhages. Therefore, the presence of no or a few hemorrhages does not assist in the diagnosis of child abuse. The presence of diffuse multilayered hemorrhages (Figure 20–1) without another explanation is strong evidence for abuse, and the presence of perimacular folds and retinoschisis cavities is almost pathognomonic for abuse (Figure 20–2).

3. *Major trauma.* Even severe trauma rarely results in more than mild retinal hemorrhages. A rare exception is a severe crush head injury, which may mimic the finding of abuse.

4. *Systemic disease.* A number of systemic diseases may be associated with retinal hemorrhages (Table 20-1). The findings are variable and depend on the underlying disorder. These diseases include bleeding disorders, sepsis, hypertension, and hematological malignancies. Infectious diseases, such as congenital cytomegalovirus, may cause retinitis with retinal hemorrhage (Figure 20–3). Glutaric aciduria type 1, in particular, may cause retinal hemorrhages that are similar to those seen in abuse.

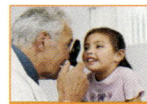

FIGURE 20–2 ■ Retinoschisis cavity following nonaccidental injury. The cavity is a clear, dome-shaped elevation over the posterior retina. A small, white perimacular fold is visible at the edge of the cavity (arrow). This finding is pathognomonic for nonaccidental injury (shaken baby) in the absence of a severe crush head injury.

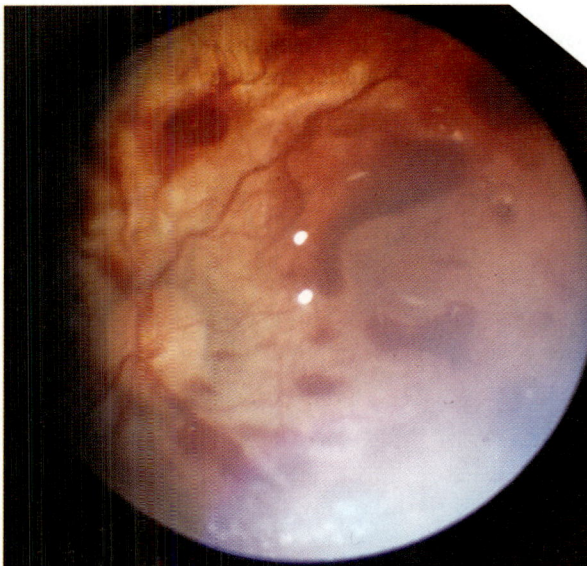

FIGURE 20–1 ■ Diffuse multilayered retinal hemorrhages in a patient with nonaccidental injury (child abuse).

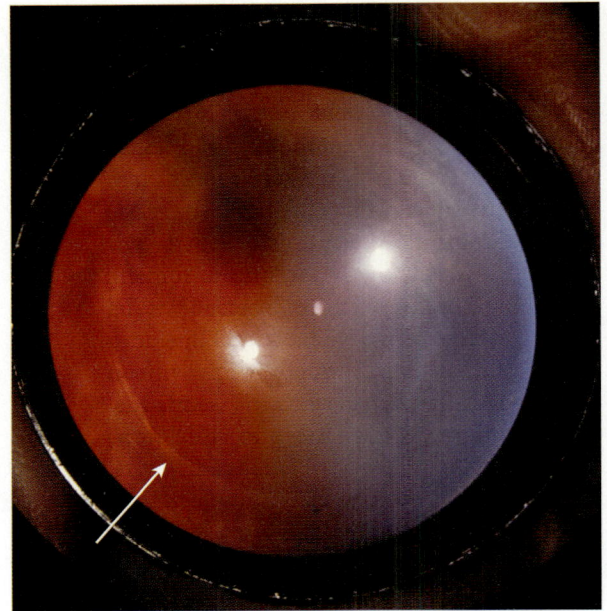

Table 20–1.

Causes of Retinal Hemorrhages in Children

- Normal childbirth
- Nonaccidental injury (child abuse)
- Severe intracranial trauma
- Massive intracranial hemorrhage (e.g., vascular malformation)
- Overwhelming sepsis
- Retinal infection (e.g., cytomegalovirus)
- Malignancy (e.g., leukemia)
- Bleeding diathesis
- Metabolic disease
  - Glutaric aciduria type 1
  - Osteogenesis imperfecta
- Extreme hypertension

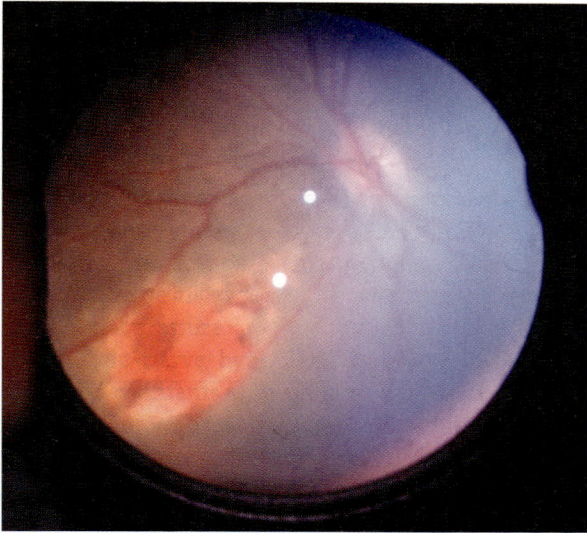

FIGURE 20–3 ■ Retinal hemorrhage secondary to congenital cytomegalovirus infection. The white appearance of the retina beneath the hemorrhage is due to retinal necrosis.

APPROACH TO THE PATIENT

The identification of retinal hemorrhages requires examination of the retina with an ophthalmoscope. Pediatricians use the direct ophthalmoscope for this examination. Direct ophthalmoscopy is often difficult in small children due to the small pupil, frequent eye movements, and limited field of view. Ophthalmologists use the indirect ophthalmoscope to evaluate the retina. This instrument provides a panoramic, 3-D view of the retina and can be performed through a small pupil even if the patient's eyes are moving.

History

Retinal hemorrhages will only rarely be noted during a routine pediatric examination due to their rarity and the difficulty of examining the retinas in young children. Most commonly, they will be identified because the patient has a specific problem that prompts retinal evaluation.

One of the most frequent and important causes of retinal hemorrhages in children is nonaccidental trauma. The presence of hemorrhages in patients suspected of shaking injuries may assist in the diagnosis, and severe ocular injuries may cause visual loss. The possibility of child abuse is usually raised when a child presents with injuries that are out of proportion to the history provided by the child's caretaker. An example is an obtunded child with an intracranial hemorrhage who is reported to have fallen a few feet from a couch onto a carpeted floor. Such children require a multidisciplinary evaluation to look for other evidence of abuse and rule out systemic diseases that could explain the findings. This includes intracranial and bone imaging, and evaluation for overwhelming infection, bleeding disorders, and hematological malignancies.

Examination

Examination of the retina in young children is difficult without indirect ophthalmoscopy. An exception to this is a comatose child with nonreactive pupils, which may occur if a child has been abused, suffered other major trauma, or has a severe systemic disease.

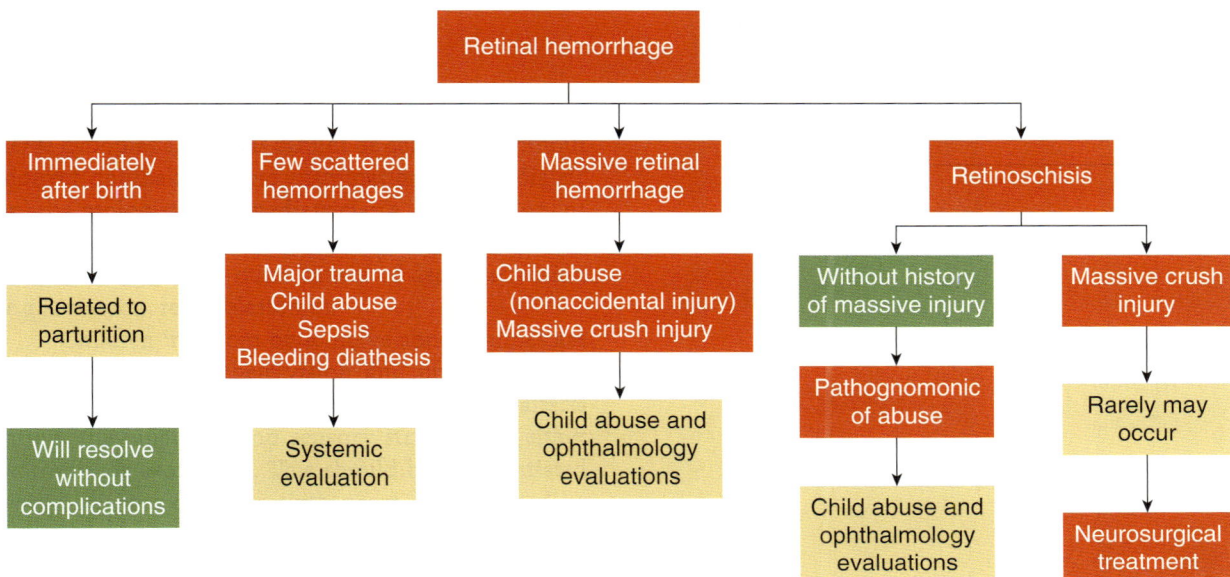

FIGURE 20–4 ■ Algorithm for evaluation of retinal hemorrhages in children.

PLAN

Children in whom retinal hemorrhages are identified, or who require examination to look for hemorrhages, should be referred to a pediatric ophthalmologist for indirect ophthalmoscopy. The presence and type of hemorrhages may be useful in establishing a diagnosis (Figure 20–1). Children with severe hemorrhages may be at risk for vision loss.

WHAT SHOULDN'T BE MISSED

Retinal examination is an important component of the evaluation of children who may have been abused. The presence of diffuse hemorrhages in the absence of another disorder that could explain them strongly suggests abuse. These children require a multidisciplinary evaluation and should not be returned to their homes until their safety can be assured.

When to Refer
■ Usually will not be noted during routine pediatric care
■ Outside of period immediately after birth, any patient with retinal hemorrhages should be referred for further evaluation

CHAPTER 21

Abnormal Optic Nerve

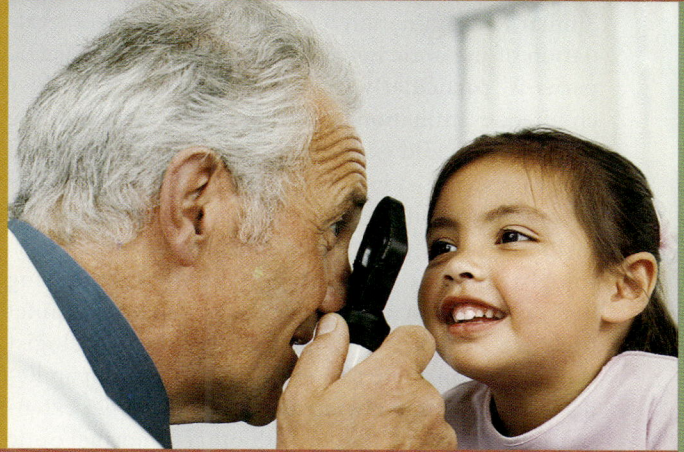

The Problem
The optic nerve is abnormal

Common Causes
Optic nerve hypoplasia
Papilledema
Optic nerve coloboma
Glaucoma

Other Causes
Pseudopapilledema
Myelinated nerve fibers
Albinism

KEY FINDINGS

History
Optic nerve hypoplasia
  If bilateral, often presents with poor vision and abnormal
    eye movements in infancy
  Unilateral hypoplasia may be associated with strabismus
    due to decreased vision
  If pituitary dysfunction, may have poor growth,
    developmental delay, and abnormal stress response
Papilledema
  Headache
  Double vision
  Transient visual obscuration (brief episodes of
    dimmed vision)
  Idiopathic intracranial hypertension
    Frequently associated with medication in children
      Corticosteroids, retinoic acid
    Also associated with obesity
Optic nerve coloboma
  Abnormal pupil appearance (if iris coloboma present)
  Poor vision or strabismus if fovea affected
  Associated systemic diseases
    CHARGE Association
Glaucoma
  May have family history
  Infants and young children
    Light sensitivity

Eye appears large, cornea cloudy
Older children
  Usually asymptomatic
Pseudopapilledema
  Optic disc drusen
  Trisomy 21
  Farsightedness
Myelinated nerve fibers
  Decreased vision due to myopia

Examination
Optic nerve hypoplasia
  Infant with poor vision, nystagmus
  Poor pupil responses
Papilledema
  Visual acuity usually normal (unless severe)
  Optic nerve elevated, swollen, hemorrhages,
    cotton wool spots
  Decreased outward movement of eye due to
    sixth nerve palsy
Optic nerve coloboma
  May have associated iris coloboma
  Variable involvement of optic nerve, retina
  Usually inferonasal quadrant
Glaucoma
  Infants and young children
    Corneal clouding, eye larger than normal
    Usually unable to visualize optic nerve
  Older children
    Enlarged cup:disc ratio
Pseudopapilledema
  Trisomy 21—abnormal vascular pattern
  Optic nerve drusen
    Irregular lumpy appearance
    White deposits within nerve
Myelinated nerve fibers
  White feathery appearance beginning at
    optic nerve
  Extend along course of retinal nerve fibers

WHAT SHOULD YOU DO?

Similar to examination for retinal hemorrhages, evaluation of the optic nerve is often difficult in pediatric patients, particularly infants and toddlers. In older children, examination of the nerve may be part of the routine well-child examination, or may be performed due to specific symptoms (such as headache). The presence of papilledema requires prompt evaluation, including neuroimaging and consultation with a neurologist. If the patient has an abnormal-appearing nerve, but no symptoms of increased intracranial pressure, referral to a pediatric ophthalmologist should be considered to evaluate for pseudopapilledema, which could obviate the need for further extensive testing. Most children with other abnormal optic nerve findings should be referred to a pediatric ophthalmologist.

What Shouldn't Be Missed

Optic nerve hypoplasia is a frequent cause of very poor vision and nystagmus in infants. Due to the difficulty of direct ophthalmoscopic evaluation of the optic nerves in infants with nystagmus, such patients require referral to a pediatric ophthalmologist. Optic nerve hypoplasia may be associated with pituitary abnormalities, and these patients may be unable to mount a normal stress response, potentially causing severe problems during even mild illnesses. This possibility should be kept in mind until the patient is evaluated by an endocrinologist.

Papilledema may occur in patients with idiopathic intracranial hypertension. In children, this is most commonly associated with medication use, such as corticosteroids or retinoic acid. Prompt evaluation is indicated to rule out intracranial tumors or other abnormalities and minimize the risk of vision loss associated with untreated papilledema.

COMMON CAUSES

1. *Optic nerve hypoplasia.* Optic nerve hypoplasia is a common cause of decreased vision in infants (Figure 21–1). This diagnosis usually cannot be made by the pediatrician due to the difficulty examining the optic nerves in infants with nystagmus. However, this potential diagnosis should be kept in mind while the evaluation is in progress, due to the risk of associated pituitary problems.
2. *Papilledema.* True papilledema usually results from increased intracranial pressure (Figure 21–2). This may occur due to space-occupying

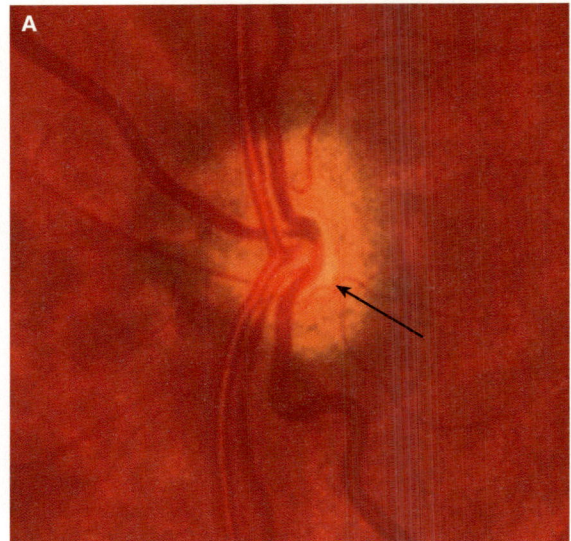

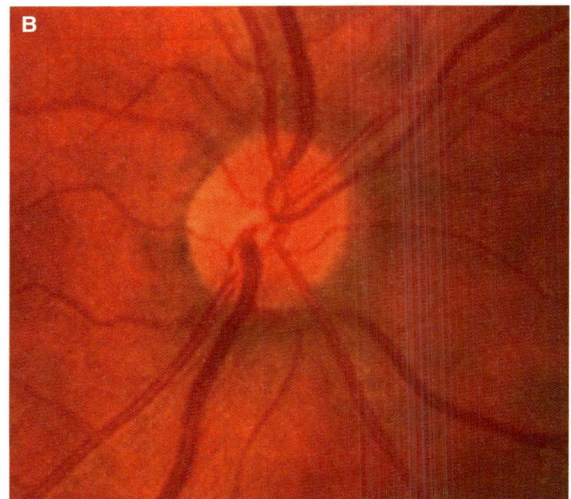

FIGURE 21–1 ■ Unilateral optic nerve hypoplasia. (A) The edge of the nerve is marked by an arrow. The surrounding depigmented area gives the "double ring sign." (B) The other optic nerve is normal.

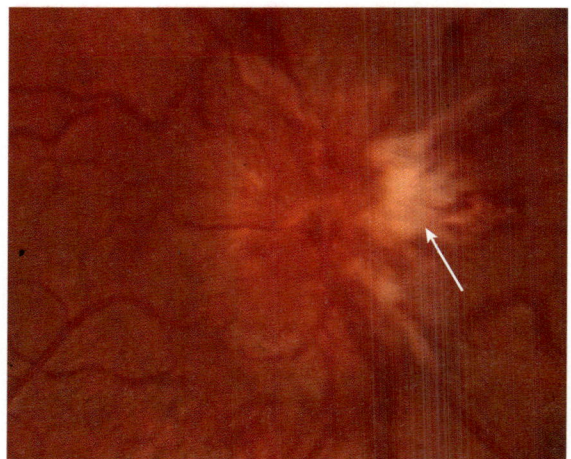

FIGURE 21–2 ■ Marked papilledema in a patient with idiopathic intracranial hypertension. Note obscuration of disc margin, cotton wool spots (arrow), and multiple splinter hemorrhages.

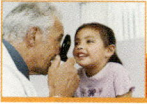

Table 21–1.

Causes of Papilledema

- Increased intracranial pressure
  - Intracranial mass lesion
  - Trauma
  - Idiopathic intracranial hypertension
- Orbital lesion
- Some optic neuritis

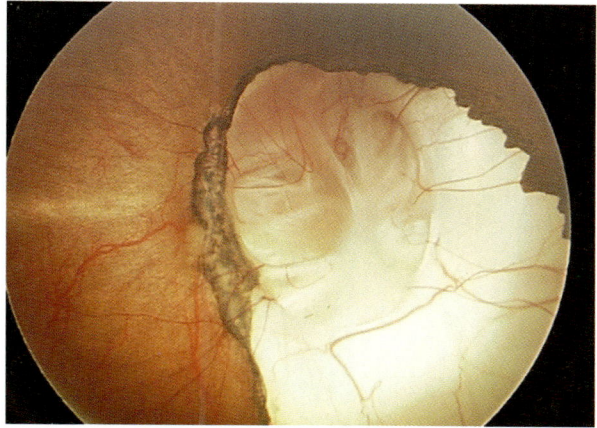

FIGURE 21–4 ■ Optic nerve coloboma in a patient with CHARGE association.

lesions, trauma, or idiopathic intracranial hypertension (pseudotumor cerebri) (Table 21–1). It may also arise due to tumors within the optic nerve (Figure 21–3A and B). The finding of papilledema warrants prompt evaluation.

3. *Optic nerve coloboma.* Optic nerve colobomas result from incomplete closure during the embryonic development of the eye (Figure 21–4). They are widely variable, both in appearance and in visual consequences.

4. *Glaucoma.* In infants and young children with glaucoma, the initial signs and symptoms include enlargement of the eye, corneal clouding, and light sensitivity. In older children and adults, the eye does not grow in response to increased intraocular pressure. The pressure causes damage to the optic nerve, producing an increase in the cup:disc ratio (Figure 21–5A and B). The vision loss affects the peripheral visual field first, with gradual constriction until the central vision is affected. Therefore, patients may have substantial loss of vision before the problem is detected. This is why glaucoma is sometimes called "the sneak thief of sight." This type of minimally symptomatic glaucomatous visual loss is much more common in adults (particularly the elderly) than in children.

5. *Pseudopapilledema.* The term pseudopapilledema describes patients who have an abnormality of the nerve with an appearance suggesting possible increased intracranial pressure (Table 21–2). Common causes include optic disc drusen (Figure 21–6) and Trisomy 21 (Figure 21–7). It is important to differentiate this abnormality from true papilledema, in order to avoid unnecessary testing.

6. *Myelinated nerve fibers.* This abnormality has a very distinctive appearance, with white, feathery opacities adjacent to the optic nerve (Figure 21–8). The myelinated nerve fibers themselves do not cause vision problems, but they are frequently associated with asymmetric myopia, which may cause amblyopia.

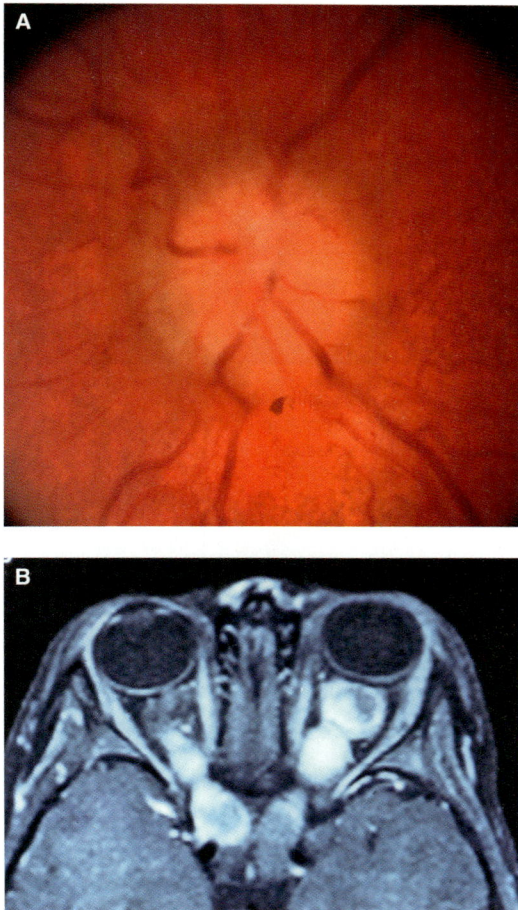

FIGURE 21–3 ■ Papilledema secondary to optic pathway glioma in a patient with neurofibromatosis. (A) Swollen optic nerve head with dilation of retinal vessels and splinter hemorrhages. (B) Magnetic resonance image showing bilateral large optic pathway gliomas.

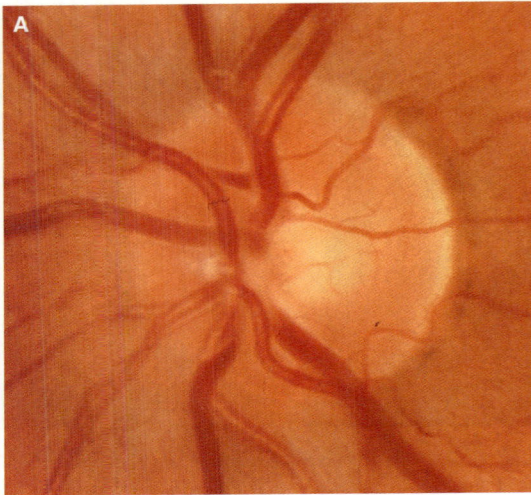

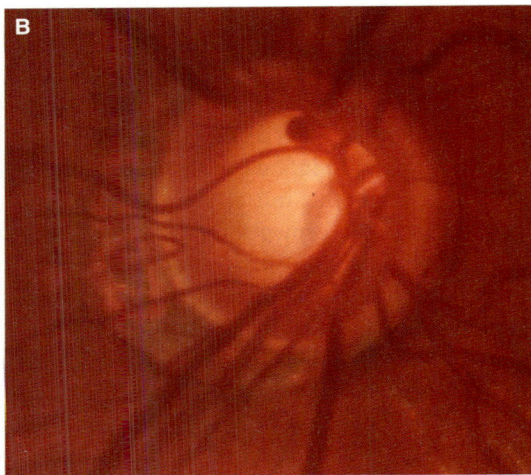

FIGURE 21–5 ■ Unilateral glaucoma. (A) Normal left optic nerve, with cup:disc ratio of approximately 0.3. (B) Right optic nerve with glaucomatous damage (cup:disc ratio of approximately 0.8).

APPROACH TO THE PATIENT

Unlike most of the other chapters in this section, the presence of an abnormal optic nerve is not something that patients or parents will report. However, optic nerve abnormalities may cause other problems that prompt evaluation of the nerve.

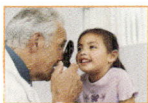

Table 21–2.

Causes of Pseudopapilledema

- Optic disc drusen
- Trisomy 21
- Marked farsightedness
- Myelinated nerve fibers

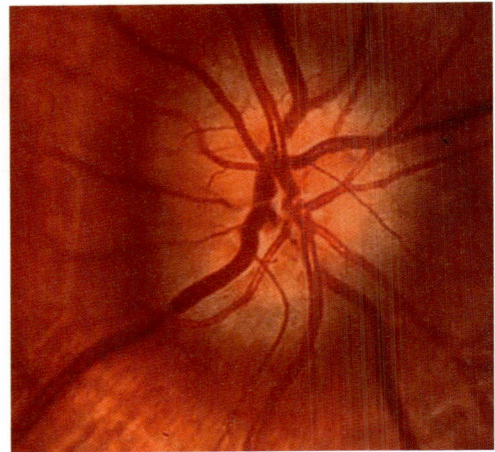

FIGURE 21–6 ■ Pseudopapilledema due to optic disc drusen. Note the abnormal branching pattern of the optic disc vessels, and that there is no obscuration of fine vessels as they cross over the nerve.

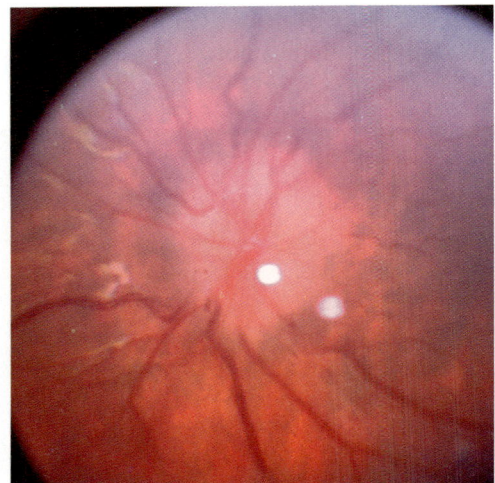

FIGURE 21–7 ■ Pseudopapilledema in a patient with Trisomy 21. Note the absence of an optic cup and the abnormal branching pattern of the optic nerve vessels.

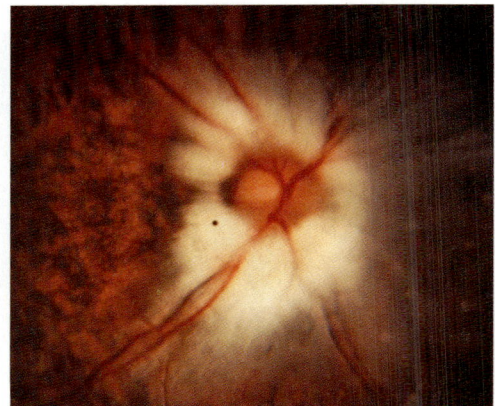

FIGURE 21–8 ■ Myelinated nerve fibers, right eye. Striking appearance of white, feathery-bordered opacity adjacent to the optic nerve. The optic nerve itself is normal.

History

The presence of optic nerve abnormalities may be detected during a regular well-child examination, or the optic nerve may be examined due to specific complaints (such as headache). If the child has no complaints, normal vision, and is incidentally found to have an abnormal optic nerve, then there is a good likelihood that this represents pseudopapilledema. However, specific questions should be asked regarding symptoms of increased intracranial pressure.

Optic nerve hypoplasia is in the differential diagnosis of infants with poor vision and nystagmus. Although it may be isolated, it is frequently a manifestation of septo-optic dysplasia. Affected children may have associated central nervous system and pituitary abnormalities, including developmental delay, seizures, and poor growth. An inability to mount a normal stress response due to adrenocorticotropic hormone deficiency may cause the child to have serious systemic problems precipitated by relatively minor illnesses.

If papilledema is suspected based on the child's complaints or is found on examination, specific questions should be asked. Headaches with nausea and vomiting may be caused by increased intracranial pressure. Horizontal diplopia may occur due to sixth cranial nerve palsy. A frequent symptom in patients with idiopathic intracranial hypertension is *transient visual obscurations*. These are brief (typically a few seconds) episodes in which the vision becomes dim or blacks out. Idiopathic intracranial hypertension in children is frequently due to medication, particularly retinoic acid and corticosteroids. If a patient with papilledema has been taking these medications, this diagnosis is very likely.

Examination

Infants with poor vision and nystagmus may have optic nerve hypoplasia, but this cannot be confirmed without indirect ophthalmoscopic examination by a pediatric ophthalmologist. The pediatrician's examination of such infants will be limited, but the red reflex should be evaluated to look for other causes of decreased vision (e.g., cataracts, retinoblastoma).

Children in whom optic nerve abnormalities are found should have their vision and pupil reactions checked. If a patient has a unilateral problem that affects vision, they may develop sensory strabismus (either esotropia or exotropia). This should be differentiated from esotropia due to a sixth nerve palsy caused by increased intracranial hypertension. The eye can move fully medially and laterally in sensory strabismus, whereas outward movement is limited in sixth cranial nerve palsy.

The visual acuity in patients with increased intracranial pressure is usually not affected early in the course of the disease, and therefore normal acuity does not rule out this diagnosis. Evaluation of the optic nerve usually reveals circumferential elevation of the optic nerve head, inability to visualize fine blood vessels as they cross over the surface of the nerve, retinal hemorrhages that are usually feathery and follow the course of the optic nerve fibers, and cotton wool spots.

Patients with pseudopapilledema have a "crowded" appearance of the nerve, and frequently have abnormal branching of the retinal blood vessels over the nerve. Optic disc drusen are a common form of pseudopapilledema in children (Figure 21–6). If they are superficial, white deposits may be visible within the nerve. Myelinated nerve fibers are white, arise just adjacent to the optic nerve, and follow an arcuate pathway along the course of the normal retinal nerve fiber layer (Figure 21–8).

PLAN

Infants with decreased vision and nystagmus should be referred to a pediatric ophthalmologist. The ophthalmological assessment will include evaluation of the optic nerves (Figures 21–9).

Children with true papilledema require prompt evaluation (Figures 21–10). Magnetic resonance imaging is performed initially to rule out a space-occupying lesion or sagittal sinus thrombosis. If the imaging is

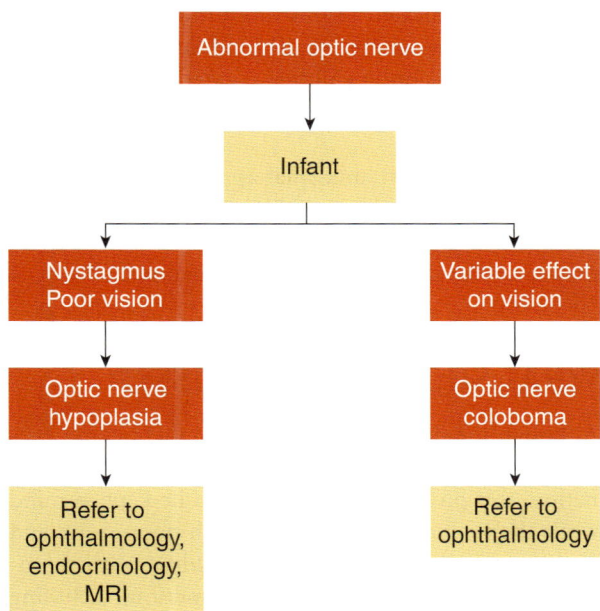

FIGURE 21–9 ■ Algorithm for evaluation and management of an infant with abnormal optic nerve(s).

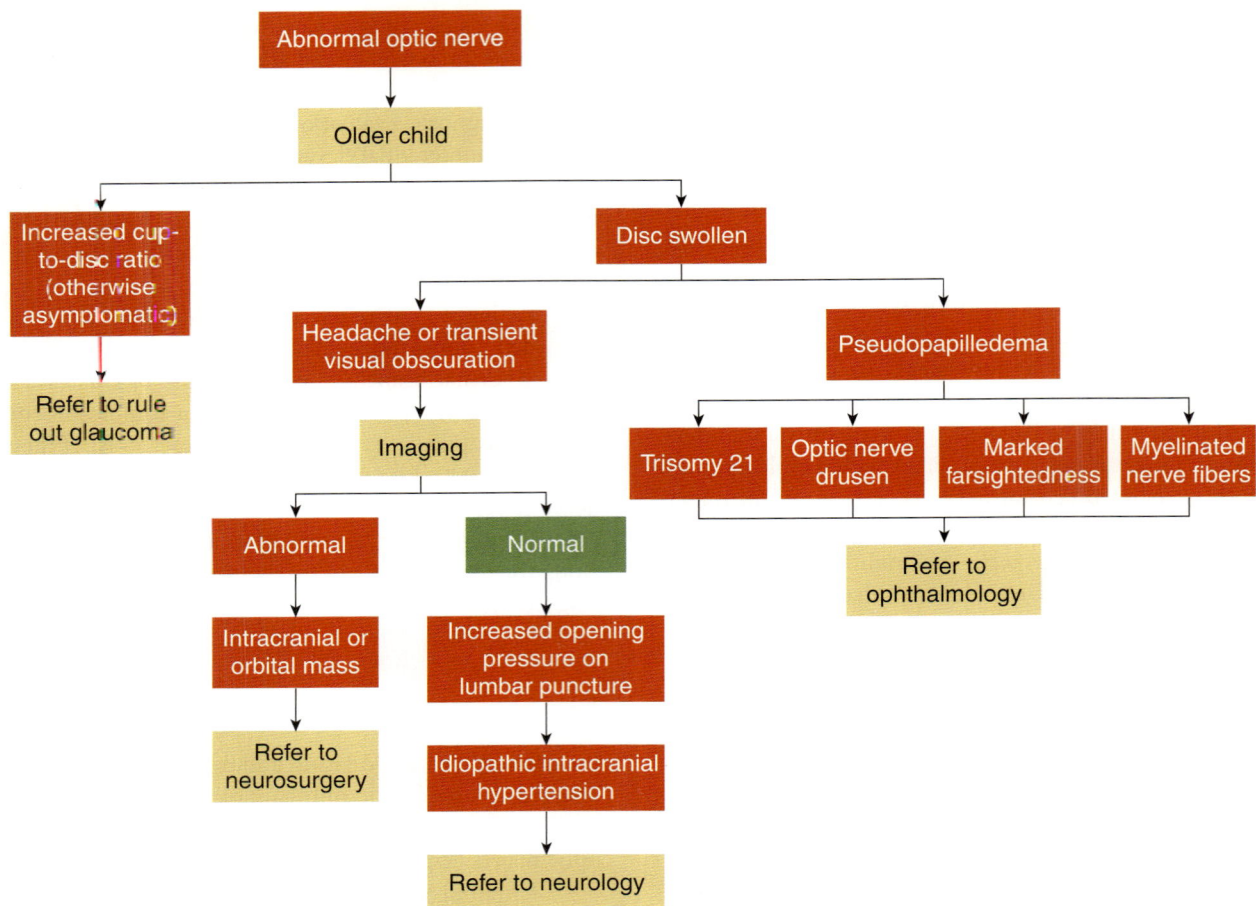

```
                    ┌─────────────────────┐
                    │ Abnormal optic nerve│
                    └─────────────────────┘
                               │
                        ┌─────────────┐
                        │ Older child │
                        └─────────────┘
```

FIGURE 21–10 ■ Algorithm for evaluation and management of an child with abnormal optic nerve(s).

normal, referral to a pediatric neurologist for lumbar puncture is indicated to measure intracranial pressure and evaluate the cerebrospinal fluid. Idiopathic intracranial hypertension in children is often due to medication, and discontinuation usually results in rapid improvement.

Children with abnormal-appearing optic nerves who are asymptomatic should be referred to a pediatric ophthalmologist. If pseuopapilledema is confirmed, this may spare the child unnecessary evaluations.

WHAT SHOULDN'T BE MISSED

Although the diagnosis of optic nerve hypoplasia cannot be made without a pediatric ophthalmology examination, this possible diagnosis should be kept in mind while the evaluation of an infant with poor vision and nystagmus is in progress. Some children with septo-optic dysplasia have pituitary dysfunction, including

adrenocorticotropic hormone deficiency. These children may be unable to mount a normal stress response and are at risk for decompensation during relatively minor illnesses.

Children with true papilledmea require prompt evaluation to establish a diagnosis and initiate treatment. Early intervention decreases the risk of permanent vision problems.

When to Refer

- Patients with papilledema should be referred promptly for imaging and neurological evaluation
- Patients with optic nerve hypoplasia will usually be referred due to decreased vision and nystagmus in infancy. The diagnosis cannot be established until the nerves are examined by an ophthalmologist.
- Patients with other optic nerve abnormalities found during routine well-child checks should be referred to a pediatric ophthalmologist.

Headache

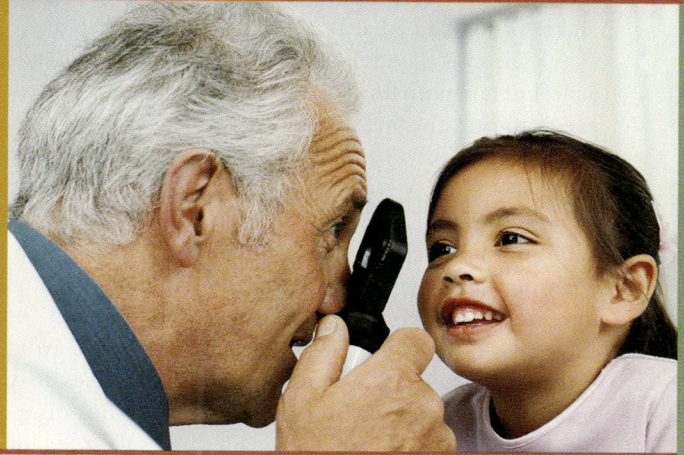

WHAT SHOULD YOU DO?

Headaches are a fairly frequent complaint in children, and most are not a serious problem. However, they may be an early symptom of serious disorders such as an intracranial tumor or idiopathic intracranial hyperten-sion. A careful history and examination are necessary to determine whether additional testing or referral to a pediatric ophthalmologist or neurologist is indicated. If the history is consistent with migraine or tension head-ache and the examination is otherwise normal, symp-tomatic treatment may be all that is necessary. If the history or examination suggests the possibility of increased intracranial pressure, then imaging studies and referral to a pediatric neurologist are indicated.

The eyes themselves are rarely the cause of headache, but an ophthalmological examination may be necessary to rule out this possibility.

What Shouldn't Be Missed

Migraine headaches are not uncommon in children. They may present with an initial complaint of abnormal visual phenomenon (prodrome). Recognition of migraines is important both for treatment and to avoid unnecessary testing. Less commonly, headaches may result from intracranial tumors or other serious disorders. The presence of papilledema indicates the need for prompt evaluation.

COMMON CAUSES

1. *Migraine headache.* Migraine headaches are more common in children than is often recognized. These may present with specific complaints of eye pain, which may be retro- or periorbital. Classic migraines are accompanied by prodromal syndromes, which are often visual, such as sparkling lights, jagged lines, or visual field defects (Figure 22–1). Most patients develop headaches in association with these phenomena, but the abnormal visual sensations sometimes occur without the headache (*acephalgic migraine*). The features of the headache, normal eye examination after the symptoms resolve, and the presence of a family history of migraines help in establishing a diagnosis.
2. *Tension headache.* Tension headaches also occur in children, but are less severe. Patients typically do not specifically complain of eye pain. The headaches tend to occur in specific situations, such as while at school.
3. *Eyestrain.* Eye problems rarely cause headaches, but an ophthalmological examination may be necessary if a diagnosis cannot be established. Patients with uncorrected refractive errors may squint chronically in an attempt to improve vision through a pinhole effect. Spectacle correction should resolve this problem. Occasionally, patients may have difficulty with accommodation (focusing of the lens at near) or convergence, which may cause complaints of eye fatigue or strain, particularly with reading.
4. *Increased intracranial pressure.* Headaches are a common symptom of increased intracranial pressure, which may occur for a variety of reasons. The visual acuity is usually normal unless the pressure is markedly elevated or prolonged to the point that optic nerve damage occurs. Etiologies include intracranial space-occupying lesions, hydrocephalus, and idiopathic intracranial hypertension (pseudotumor cerebri).

APPROACH TO THE PATIENT

Headaches are fairly common in children, and the pediatrician must decide which patients require only symptomatic care and which require further evaluation. Primary ocular problems only rarely cause headaches, but an ophthalmological evaluation may be indicated if a diagnosis cannot be established.

History

A careful history is very helpful in the evaluation of patients with headaches. Often a presumptive diagnosis can be identified based on the history alone. Occasional mild headaches that resolve without treatment usually do not require any further evaluation other than a screening examination (see below).

The history in migraine headaches can be variable, but certain features are common. The pain is usually fairly severe. If a child stops normal activities because of a headache, particularly while doing enjoyable activities, then migraine is the most likely diagnosis. The pain in migraine may occur in any location on the head, including the retro- or periorbital area, and the child may complain of specific eye pain. Migraines are frequently accompanied by nausea and vomiting, which can also occur in patients with increased intracranial pressure. The presence of prodromal visual symptoms, such as sparkling colored lights (scintillat-

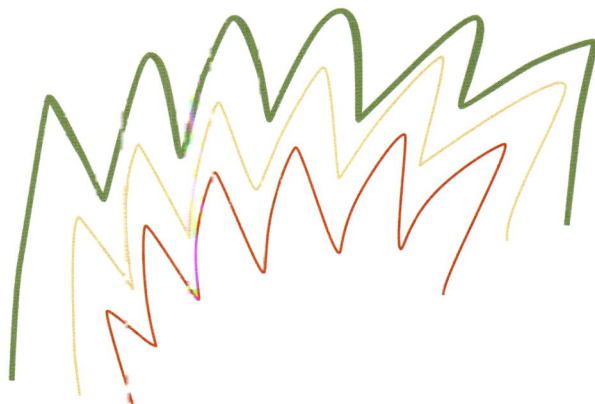

FIGURE 22–1 ■ Jagged lines. A form of visual prodrome that patients may describe in association with migraine headaches.

ing scotomas), jagged lines (Figure 22–1), or visual field defects, which resolve either as the headache begins or after the headache subsides, is almost pathognomonic for migraine. Most patients with migraines have a positive family history.

Eye problems are infrequently the cause of headaches, but specific historical information may suggest this possibility. Patients with uncorrected refractive errors may complain of decreased vision, but it is important to recognize that children with refractive errors may not realize that they do not see as well as others. Therefore, decreased vision is often first noticed by teachers or family members, when the child is unable to read something at a distance that others can. Difficulty with accommodation or convergence may cause complaints of eyestrain or eye fatigue, which is worse during reading.

Symptoms of increased intracranial pressure are initially often similar to those of headache, particularly migraine, but certain features help differentiate the two. The headaches with increased intracranial pressure tend to be chronic, rather than episodic. The presence of progressively worsening symptoms is very concerning for an enlarging intracranial lesion. Headaches due to increased intracranial pressure may awaken the child from sleep, which would be unusual with migraine. Patients with idiopathic intracranial hypertension may have symptoms of horizontal diplopia due to sixth nerve palsy and may also experience brief (few seconds) episodes of visual loss (*transient visual obscurations*). The visual field defects that may occur with migraines last longer (30–60 minutes) and resolve after the headache.

Examination

Patients who present for evaluation of headache should undergo a thorough neurological examination. The eye examination should include assessment of visual acuity, pupil reactions, confrontation visual fields, and ocular motility. The direct ophthalmoscope should be used to check for papilledema (Figure 22–2).

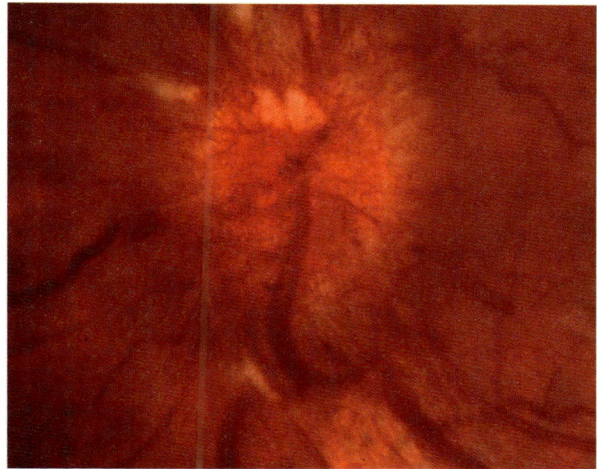

FIGURE 22–2 ■ Marked papilledema in a patient with idiopathic intracranial hypertension.

By the time patients with migraines are evaluated, the headaches have usually resolved and the examination is normal. If they happen to be seen during the headache, visual field defects or other visual abnormalities might be documented.

PLAN

A decision regarding management and further evaluation of headaches depends on consideration of all the factors above (Table 22–1). If papilledema is present, urgent referral for neuroimaging and pediatric neurological consultation is indicated. If the examination is normal, including the absence of papilledema, then the history may help determine an appropriate course of action. If the specific headache features are typical of migraine, and particularly if there is a positive family history, additional tests may not be necessary. If the history is less clear, neuroimaging may be considered. If the examination is normal except for decreased visual acuity, or if the patient has specific complaints of

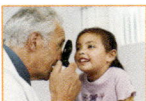

Table 22–1.

Features of different types of headaches

	Tension Headache	Migraine	Increased Intracranial Pressure
Severity	Mild to moderate	Moderate to severe	Moderate to severe
Stops activity	No	May	Yes
Vision changes	No	Possible prodromal scotoma	Transient visual obscuration
Papilledema	No	No	Yes

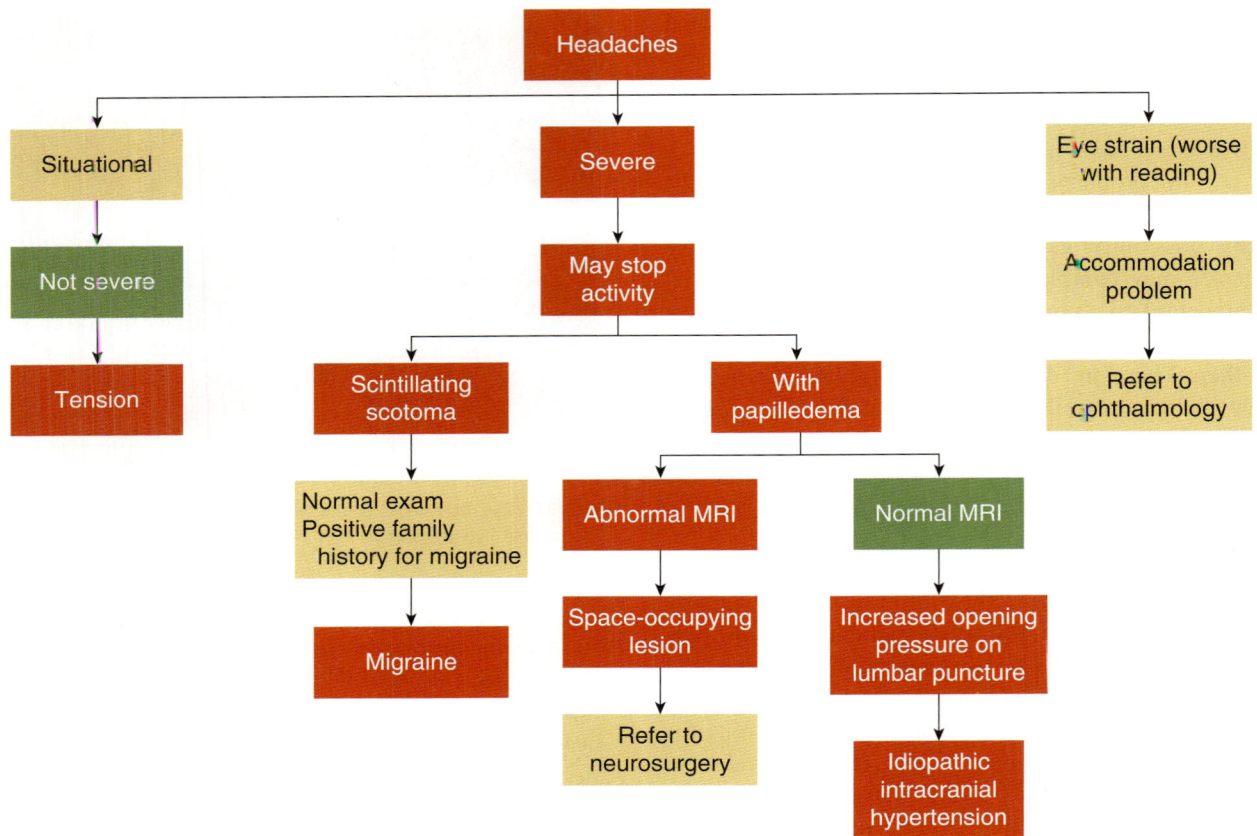

FIGURE 22–3 ■ Algorithm for evaluation of childhood headaches.

eyestrain that are worse with reading, referral to a pediatric ophthalmologist is warranted.

WHAT SHOULDN'T BE MISSED

Headaches are fairly common in children, and usually are not severe. However, very serious disorders, such as intracranial tumors, may present initially with headaches. The presence of papilledema on examination indicates the need for urgent evaluation (Figure 22–3).

When to Refer

- Any patient with a headache and papilledema should be referred promptly for neuroimaging and neurological consultation
- Patients with headache and other neurological abnormalities (e.g., cranial nerve palsy) should be referred promptly
- Patients with specific complaints of eyestrain, especially if worse when reading, should be referred to a pediatric ophthalmologist

CHAPTER 23

Learning Disorders

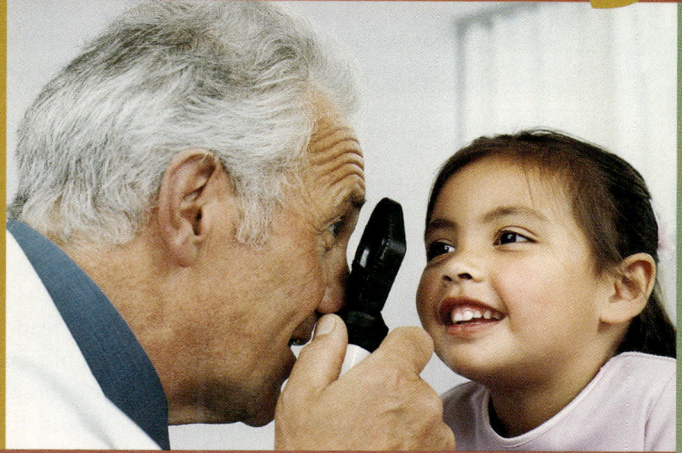

The Problem
"My child is having trouble at school."

Common Causes
Reading disorder (dyslexia)
Normal variation in rate of learning

Other Causes
Vision problem

KEY FINDINGS

History
Learning disorder
  Usually specific problem with reading
  Does well in other subjects (math, etc.)
  Understands things better when spoken, rather
    than written

Vision problem
  Blurred vision
  Double vision
  Convergence insufficiency

Examination
Learning disorder
  Normal eye examination
Vision problem
  Decreased visual acuity
  Strabismus
  Dry eyes

WHAT SHOULD YOU DO?

The majority of children with reading or other learning disorders do not have vision problems, but they should be evaluated by a pediatric ophthalmologist to rule out this possibility. Parents should be advised against optometric vision therapy because there is no evidence of benefit from this expensive and time-consuming treatment.

What Shouldn't Be Missed

Children with specific reading disorders, such as dyslexia, are usually of normal or above-normal intelligence. They have a specific problem processing written language. Early identification of such problems allows for the development of alternative teaching methods that can maximize the students' education.

COMMON CAUSES

1. *Dyslexia.* Children with dyslexia and other reading problems have specific difficulty processing written information. The disorder does not result from eye or ocular tracking problems, but rather from abnormalities in the portions of the cerebral cortex that process written information. Treatment programs based on "vision therapy" are of no benefit in treating this disorder.[1, 2]

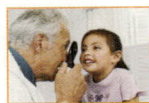

Table 23–1.

Eye Problems That May Cause Reading Difficulty

- Uncorrected refractive error
- Diplopia
- Convergence insufficiency
- Dry eye

Table 23–2.

Symptoms of Learning Disorder

- Trouble reading
- School performance better in nonreading activities (e.g., math)
- Understand spoken material better than written

2. *Vision problems.* Very few children with reading problems have primary ocular problems. However, they should be screened for these. Occasionally such children will be found to need glasses or have some form of strabismus or other vision abnormality that impedes reading (Table 23–1).
3. *Normal variation in rate of learning.* Normal children learn different tasks at different rates. The speed and ease at which children learn to read is quite variable, particularly during kindergarten and first grade. Patients are sometimes referred at this young age for evaluation of possible reading problems. Many of these patients are normal (both visually and cognitively), and will attain normal reading levels as they age.

APPROACH TO THE PATIENT

It is important to recognize reading disorders for several reasons. First, affected children often will benefit from alternative educational approaches, such as the use of books on tape rather than written information. Second, the families of such children may seek alternative treatments, such as optometric vision therapy. These evaluations typically result in recommendations for costly and time-consuming treatments, for which there is no scientific evidence of benefit.

History

Children with reading disorders are most commonly identified in early grade school. They are usually otherwise healthy. With specific questioning, the nature of the problem can often be identified (Table 23–2). Specifically, affected children have difficulty processing written information, and therefore often do better in subjects that do not require much reading, such as math. They understand things more readily when the material is spoken, rather than written. Educational testing may show normal or above-normal aptitude in other areas, but specific deficits in reading.

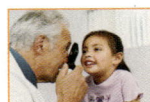

Dry eyes are not common in children, but they may produce difficulty with vision due to disruption of the tear film, which is important for focusing. Children with dry eyes may complain of frequent eye irritation or redness. When specifically questioned, they usually state their vision is initially clear, but becomes blurry with continued visual tasks, such as reading. This is because the normal blinking rate decreases with concentration. As the tear film evaporates, the images become blurred. If the patient blinks forcefully, the vision improves.

Some children with reading disorders may complain of problems with their vision, such as "I have trouble seeing the words." Most of these children have normal eye examinations. These complaints are the child's way of communicating that they are having trouble processing the words.

Examination

On examination, most children with reading disorders have normal visual acuity. They should be screened for strabismus and other ocular problems. This examination is usually normal.

PLAN

Children with reading problems should be evaluated by a pediatric ophthalmologist to rule out refractive errors, strabismus, dry eyes, or other vision problems (Figure 23–1). Most children will have normal examinations. Reading disorders are usually best addressed through the child's school, with employment of remedial or alternative learning strategies.

WHAT SHOULDN'T BE MISSED

Some well-meaning educators, family friends, or other therapists may recommend that children with reading problems seek out alternative treatments, such as optometric vision therapy. Such evaluations almost uniformly result in a recommendation for a costly course of vision therapy. Scientific reviews of such treatment show no evidence of benefit.

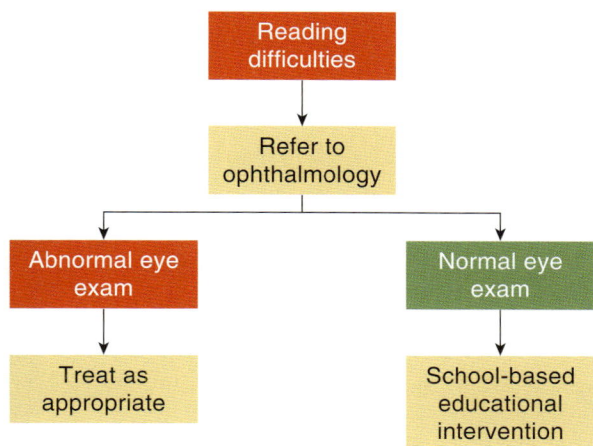

FIGURE 23–1 ■ Algorithm for evaluation and management of learning disorders.

REFERENCES

1. American Academy of Pediatrics, Section on Ophthalmology, Council on Children with Disabilities; American Academy of Ophthalmology; American Association for Pediatric Ophthalmology and Strabismus; American Association of Certified Orthoptists. Joint statement—Learning disabilities, dyslexia, and vision. *Pediatrics.* 2009;124:837–844.
2. Barrett BT. A critical evaluation of the evidence supporting the practice of behavioural vision therapy. *Ophthalmic Physiol Opt.* 2009;29:4–25.

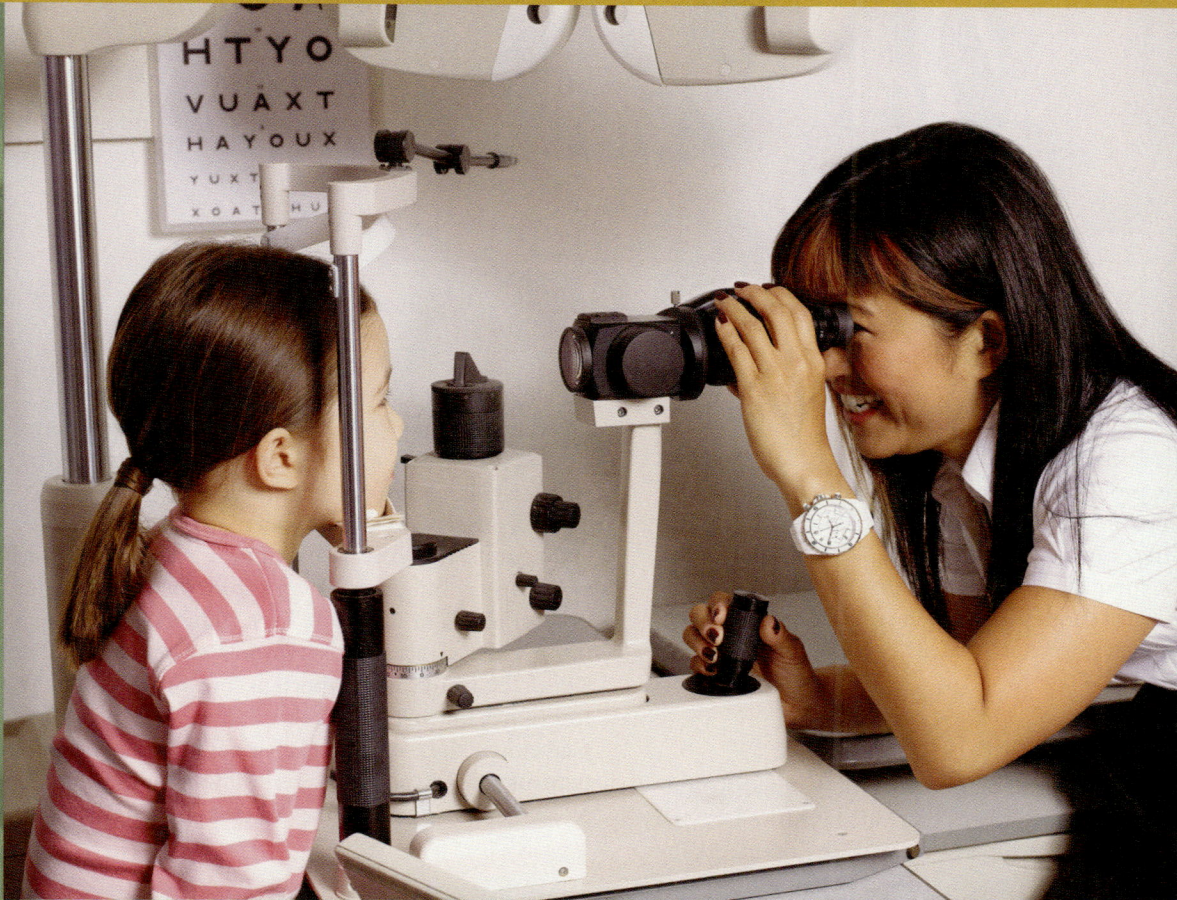

Diseases

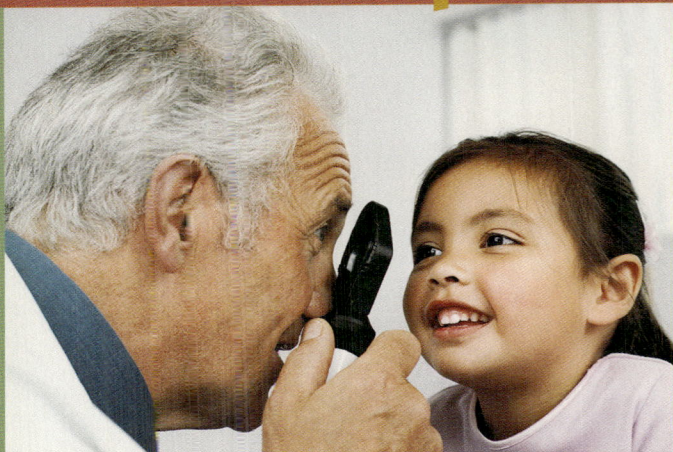

CHAPTER 24

Disorders of the Lacrimal System

DEFINITIONS AND EPIDEMIOLOGY

Disorders of the lacrimal system are among the most common problems encountered in pediatric ophthalmology. Approximately 6% of infants are born with nasolacrimal duct obstruction (NLDO). Many of these will improve spontaneously, but because NLDO is so common, lacrimal surgery is one of the most frequent surgical procedures performed by pediatric ophthalmologists.

ANATOMY AND PHYSIOLOGY

The lacrimal system functions by producing, distributing, and eliminating tears. Tears are produced by the lacrimal gland in the superolateral orbit, flow across the eye into the lacrimal puncta, travel through the lacrimal canaliculi to the lacrimal sac, then into the nares via the nasolacrimal duct (NLD) (Figure 24–1). The contraction of the eyelid muscles creates a pumping effect, which facilitates the normal drainage of tears.

A proper tear layer is vital to ocular health for several reasons. First, the natural flow of tears continuously rinses debris and other irritants from the eyes. Second, a normal tear film is required for comfort. Patients with dry eyes have recurrent symptoms of ocular irritation. Third, the tear film is important for normal vision. The tear film is the first surface that light rays come into contact with on the eyes. A regular smooth surface is required to focus these light rays properly. If the tear film is unstable, patients experience intermittent blurred vision.

Embryology

The lacrimal drainage system begins as a nest of ectodermal cells at the site of the future lacrimal sac. Cords of cells extend from this site to the eyelids and into the nares. Canalization of this tissue results in the formation of the lacrimal sac, canaliculi, and NLD. This canalization begins at the lacrimal sac and extends distally. The last portion to canalize is the opening of the NLD into the nares.

PATHOGENESIS

NLDO is by far the most common lacrimal problem encountered in children, occurring in approximately 6% of infants. It results from incomplete canalization of the NLD during embryological development. Because the opening of the duct into the nares is normally the last portion to canalize, this is the most common site of obstruction (Figure 24–2).

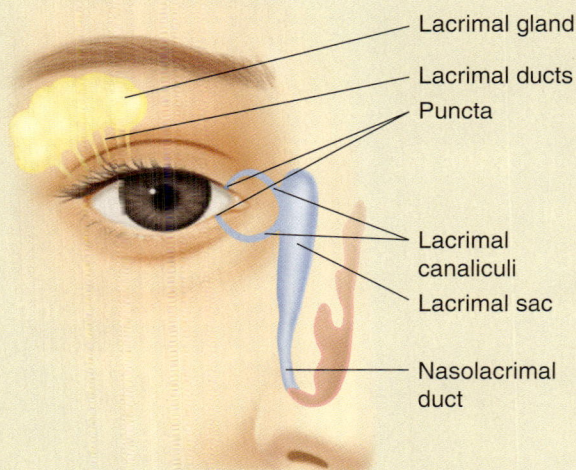

Lacrimal gland
Lacrimal ducts
Puncta
Lacrimal canaliculi
Lacrimal sac
Nasolacrimal duct

FIGURE 24–1 ■ Drawing of lacrimal system.

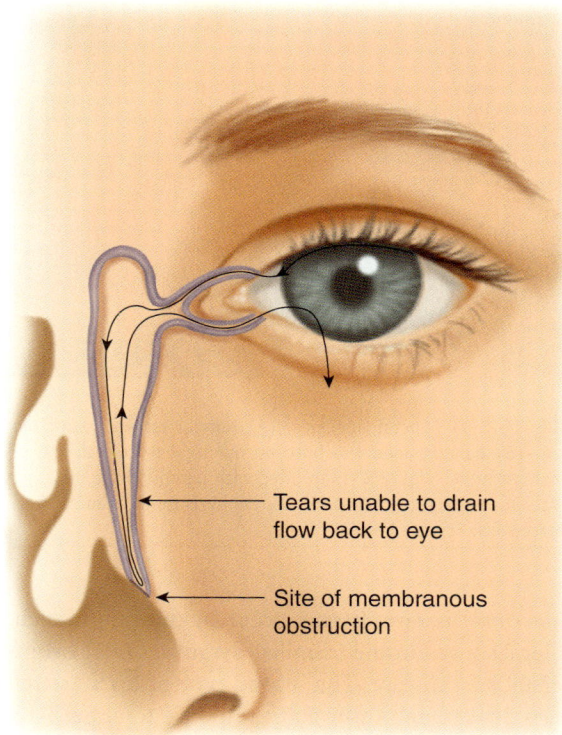

FIGURE 24-2 ■ Nasolacrimal duct obstruction. The tears drain into the nasolacrimal duct, where they encounter a membrane at the site of obstruction, causing the tears to flow back to the eyelid and onto the cheek. (Modified and reprinted with permission from Lueder GT. Balloon catheter dilation for treatment of older children with nasolacrimal duct obstruction. *Arch Ophthalmol.* 2002;120:1685–1688. Figure 1. Copyright American Medical Association. All Rights Reserved.)

The blocked flow of tears produces 2 clinical problems. The first is overflow tearing (*epiphora*). Because the tears cannot drain into the nares, they back up through the lacrimal sac and canaliculi, resulting in an increased tear lake in the eyes. This is easily conceptualized as a simple plumbing problem, with the lacrimal duct obstruction analogous to a clogged pipe. In this analogy, the resistance to flow of fluid results in collection of liquid in the sink (the normal tear layer on the eyelids), and eventually the sink overflows (epiphora).

The second clinical problem associated with NLDO is recurrent lacrimal infection. Normal flora bacteria are present in the tear film. These usually do not cause problems because they are continuously flushed from the eyes through the tear sac into the nares. However, if the tear drainage is blocked, the bacteria can accumulate in the lacrimal sac. This moist, warm environment is ideally suited to bacterial growth, and therefore recurrent infection (*dacryocystitis*) commonly results. The dacryocystitis that occurs in association with typical infantile NLDO is usually chronic, intermittent, and low-grade. Much less commonly, acute

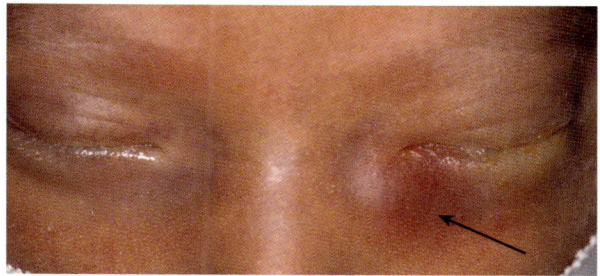

FIGURE 24-3 ■ Infected mucocele. Erythema and edema overlying left lacrimal sac (arrow).

dacryocystitis occurs. This presents with swelling and erythema overlying the lacrimal sac.

Approximately 1% to 2% of children with NLDO will present with a *mucocele* (amniotocele, dacryocele, dacryocystocele). This usually is present at birth, with a distended mass overlying the lacrimal sac. Mucoceles are initially blue-tinged, but may become erythematous and inflamed if they become infected (Figure 24–3). Mucoceles are almost always associated with an NLD cyst beneath the inferior turbinate (Figure 24–4). If the cyst is large, it may cause problems with airway obstruction.

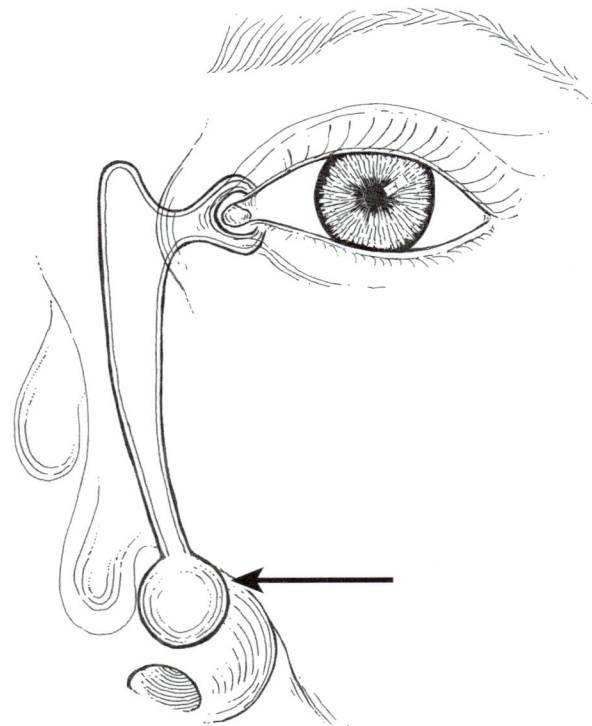

FIGURE 24-4 ■ Nasolacrimal duct cyst (arrow). These are almost always present in infants with mucoceles. (Reprinted with permission from Lueder GT. Endoscopic treatment of distal nasolacrimal duct abnormalities in children with complicated nasolacrimal obstruction. *JAAPOS.* 2004:8(2);128-132. Copyright Elsevier.)

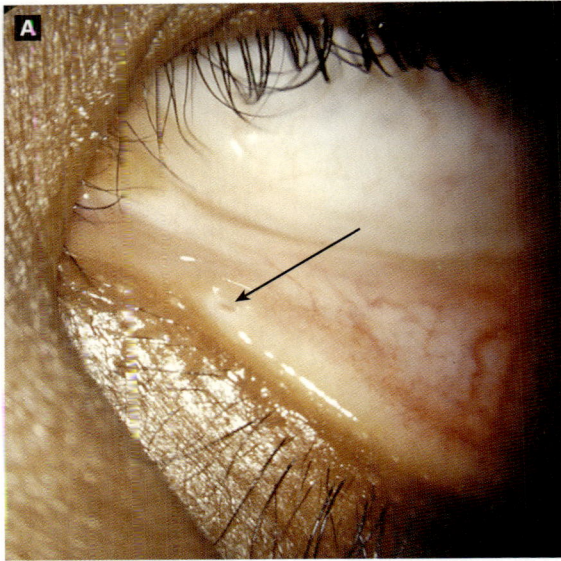

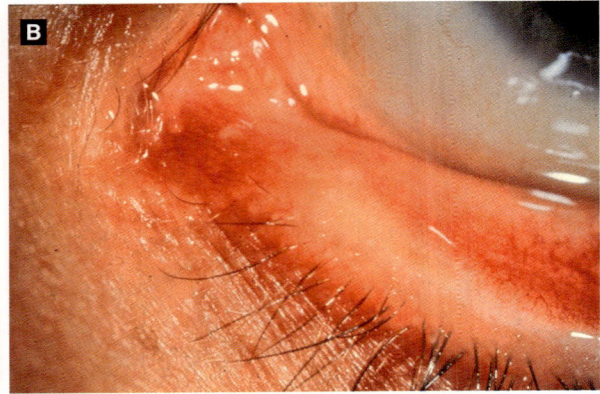

FIGURE 24–5 ■ Punctal agenesis. (A) Normal lacrimal punctum (arrow). (B) Punctal agenesis. Note no opening at normal site of lacrimal punctum. (Figure B is reprinted with permission from *Semin Ophthalmol.* 1997;12(2):109-116. Copyright Informa Medical and Pharmaceutical Science.)

Rare embryological abnormalities of the lacrimal system include *punctal or canalicular agenesis*, and *lacrimal sac fistulae*. Punctal and canalicular agenesis results from incomplete canalization of these structures (Figure 24–5). Because the tears have nowhere to drain, these children present with epiphora. Lacrimal sac fistulae result from aberrant cords of tissue that extend from the lacrimal sac to the skin, typically between the eye and the nares. If the fistulae are patent, tears may flow through them, producing epiphora (Figure 24–6). *Crocodile tears* are an unusual disorder in which aberrant innervation of the lacrimal gland causes tearing to occur during chewing or swallowing (Figure 24–7).

Dry eyes result from abnormal tear production. This is a relatively uncommon problem in children. There are 2 types of tears. The first are basal tears, which are important for maintaining ocular health and clear vision. Absence or reduction of basal tear production

(*alacrima*) is rare. It may occur in conditions such as Riley-Day syndrome (familial dysautonomia) or graft-versus-host disease. The second type of tears are reflex tears, which are produced in response to either irritation or emotional stimuli. These tears are produced when someone is crying. Some infants do not produce reflex tears. This does not cause vision problems because the basal tears function normally.

Patients with poor tear films have poor vision due to disruption of light focusing. A useful analogy to help understand this is looking into a puddle on a sidewalk after a rain. Initially, if the puddle is intact, one can see a clear image, similar to a mirror. As the puddle evaporates, it gradually breaks up into smaller parts, and the image becomes irregular. When patients with

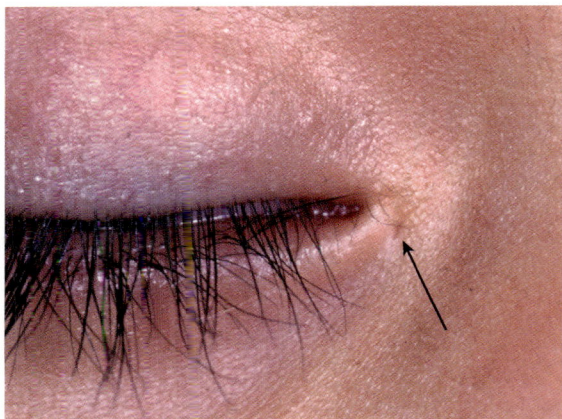

FIGURE 24–6 ■ Lacrimal fistula (arrow). (Reprinted with permission from *Semin Ophthalmol.* 1997;12(2):109-116, Copyright Informa Medical and Pharmaceutical Science.)

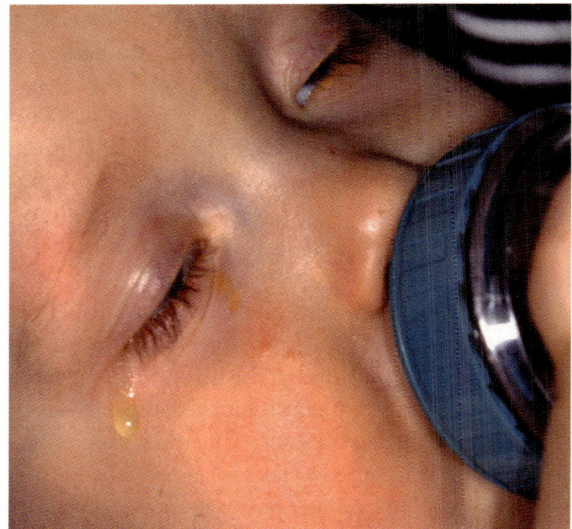

FIGURE 24–7 ■ Crocodile tears, produced when infant sucks from bottle.

dry eyes blink, their tear film is intact immediately after the blink, and they see clearly. As the tears evaporate, the image becomes blurry, and patients need to blink repeatedly to keep things clear.

CLINICAL PRESENTATION

Presentation of Lacrimal Disorders

NLDO usually appears in the first few weeks of life with variable symptoms of overflow tearing, recurrent periocular mucopurulent discharge, or both (Figure 24–8). If there is significant overflow of tears onto the eyelids, erythema and irritation of the eyelid skin may also be present. Of note, the infants themselves typically do not seem particularly bothered by their condition.

Infants with *mucoceles* present at or shortly after birth with blue-tinged, distended masses overlying the lacrimal sac. If they become infected, the swelling may increase and the area becomes erythematous (Figure 24–3). Purulent discharge may be expressed with gentle pressure over the sac (Figure 24–9). If the mucoceles are large, they can interfere with the airway. Problems range from difficulty during feeding (because the patients' mouths are obstructed by feeding and they cannot breathe normally due to obstruction of nasal airflow) to frank respiratory distress.

Acute dacryocystitis in older children presents with swelling and erythema overlying the lacrimal sac. Purulent discharge is often present. Unlike the more common low-grade dacryocystitis associated with typical infantile NLDO, acute dacryocystitis in older children

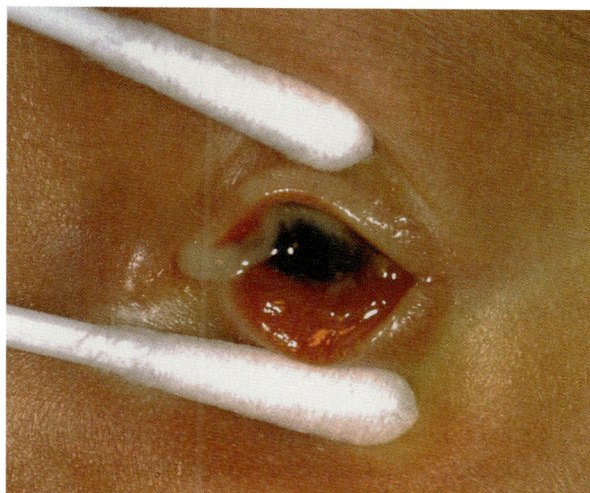

FIGURE 24–9 ■ Infected mucocele. Purulent reflux with pressure over lacrimal sac.

may present with systemic symptoms, including fever. This disorder may be associated with diverticula of the lacrimal sac, which are prone to infection due to stasis of flow within the diverticula.

Patients with *punctal or canalicular atresia* present with symptoms of overflow tearing only, because the tears cannot gain entrance into the lacrimal outflow system. They do not develop infections because bacteria are unable to reach the lacrimal sac. Therefore, if an infant presents with excess tearing only, punctal and canalicular atresia needs to be considered as possible diagnoses. However, because typical NLDO is much more common, and may present with variable symptoms (sometimes epiphora only, sometimes infection without epiphora, most frequently with both), a child with only epiphora is more likely to have NLDO than punctal or canalicular agenesis.

Patients with *lacrimal sac fistulae* typically present with epiphora. The opening of the fistula is usually very small, and often is not visible to the family (Figure 24–6). Sometimes they will notice specifically that the tears arise from the site of the fistula opening on the skin between the eye and the nose, but usually they simply only note excess tears. Patients with fistulae usually do not have symptoms of infection.

Presentation of Dry Eyes

Patients with decreased tear production present in different manners, depending on the type of tear deficiency they have. Absence of reflex tearing is much more common than absent basal tearing. Children with *absent reflex tears* usually present because the parents note that their babies do not appear to cry when they are upset. The children make the same noises and facial grimacing that a crying child makes, but no tears are produced.

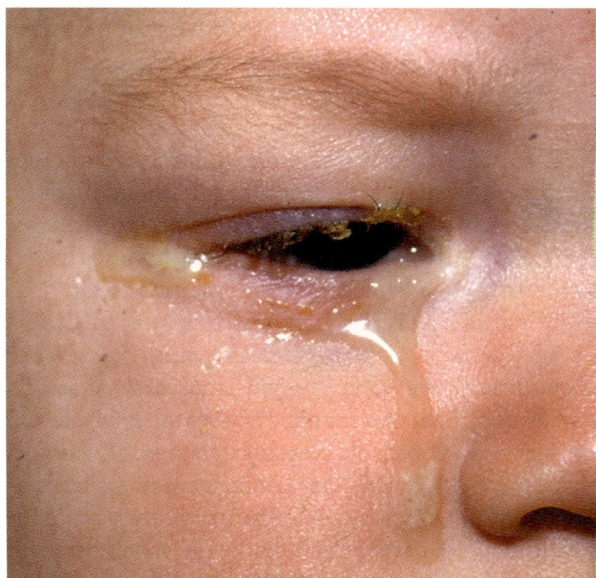

FIGURE 24–8 ■ Epiphora (overflow tearing) and mucoid discharge secondary to lacrimal obstruction and infection.

However, these children have no symptoms of ocular irritation and their examinations are otherwise normal.

Patients with *decreased basal tears* present with symptoms of chronic ocular irritation, light sensitivity, and blurred vision. Paradoxically, they may also have intermittent excess tearing. This is because they have a chronic low level of basal tears. They develop ocular irritation, which produces a bolus of reflex tears, which may cause epiphora. Once the reflex tears evaporate, the eyes again become irritated, and the cycle repeats itself.

TREATMENT

Treatment of Lacrimal Disorders

NLDO is initially treated conservatively, because most patients spontaneously improve during the first 6 to 12 months of life. Lacrimal massage may be recommended. Massage is performed by gently pressing on the lacrimal sac between the eye and the nose. The purpose is to increase pressure in the lacrimal sac, which is transmitted through the lacrimal duct to the site of obstruction. It is difficult to prove whether massage has any real effect on outcomes, due to the natural history of spontaneous improvement in most cases. However, some studies suggest that it is useful. In practical terms, it is worth performing as long as the infant is not particularly bothered by the procedure. If recommended, it is important to demonstrate the proper technique to the parents. Gentle pressure at the medial eyelid will compress the sac (Figure 24–10). Parents may see reflux of tears and discharge from the lacrimal puncta if they are massaging in the correct location.

If patients with NLDO have significant discharge and drainage, topical antibiotics may be prescribed. Most antibiotics will temporarily improve the symptoms, but it is important that the parents understand that they will not cure the obstruction itself. Once the antibiotics are discontinued, the symptoms will typically recur unless the underlying obstruction has resolved. Antibiotics are usually not used if only mild crusting is present, but may be used as needed for exacerbations.

WHAT THE OPHTHALMOLOGIST WILL DO

Typical Nasolacrimal Obstruction

If patients with NLDO do not improve, referral to a pediatric ophthalmologist is indicated. Nasolacrimal probing is performed by passing metal probes through the lacrimal puncta and canaliculi, into the lacrimal sac, then through the lacrimal duct into the nares (Figure 24–11A and B). In patients with typical NLDO,

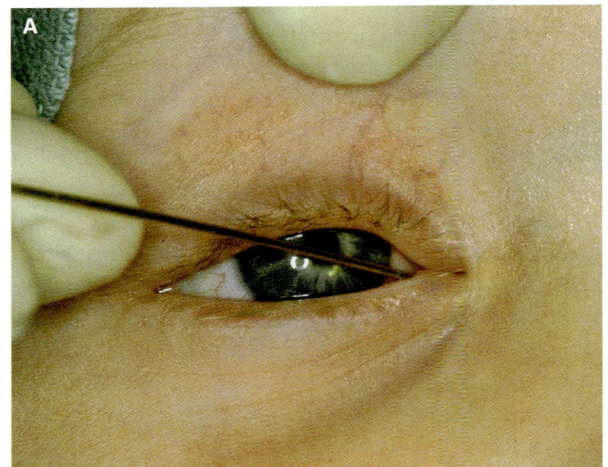

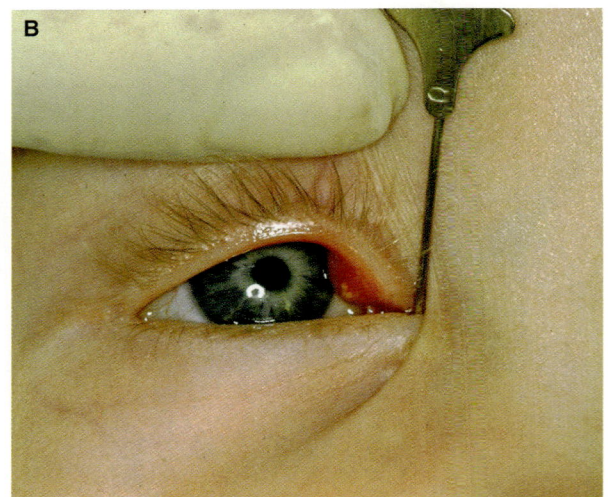

FIGURE 24–11 ■ NLD probing. (A) Probe is inserted into lacrimal puncta and passed through the canaliculus to the lacrimal sac. (B) Probe is then rotated and passed vertically through the NLD.

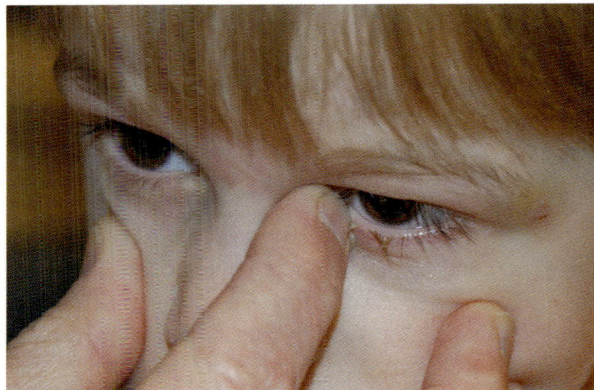

FIGURE 24–10 ■ Lacrimal massage. Gentle pressure is placed over the left lacrimal sac, between the eye and the nose.

a popping sensation is palpable as the probe passes through the obstruction in the distal duct.

There are 2 approaches to surgical treatment of NLDO. Some ophthalmologists perform nasolacrimal probing in awake children in the office at a young age. The advantage of this approach is that the problem is solved earlier and general anesthesia is not required. The disadvantage is the discomfort of the procedure, and the treatment of infants who might have spontaneously improved with additional time. The alternative approach is to wait until infants are older (usually 9 to 12 months of age), then perform the procedure in the operating room. The disadvantages of this approach are the need for anesthesia and the increased cost. The advantages are decreased discomfort, the avoidance of treating children who spontaneously improve, and the ability to perform additional procedures (such as stent placement) if atypical findings are discovered during surgery. Both of these approaches are acceptable.

If symptoms persist after the initial probing, repeat probing with additional procedures such as stent placement or balloon catheter dilation of the stenotic NLD may be indicated.[1] The latter procedure is performed by passing a balloon catheter into the distal duct. The balloon is inflated, which creates a dilation of the obstructed area (Figure 24–12). If these procedures do not work, dacryocystorhinostomy (DCR) is usually performed. In this procedure, a new opening is created between the lacrimal sac and nasal cavity to allow an alternative path for tear drainage. In older children with acute dacryocystitis, DCR is more often necessary to relieve symptoms.

NLDO is a common ocular complication of Trisomy 21. These children may have typical NLDO, but also have a higher incidence of associated lacrimal abnormalities. The success rate of NLD probing is decreased in the patients with Trisomy 21, and additional procedures are more often necessary to alleviate the symptoms.[2]

Mucoceles

Infants with mucoceles require more aggressive treatment. If the mucoceles become infected, a frank abscess may develop in the distended lacrimal sac. Because neonates are relatively immunocompromised, they are at increased risk for systemic spread of infection. Larger mucoceles may cause airway obstruction due to NLD cysts in the nares, in which case urgent treatment with lacrimal probing and endsocopic removal of the cyst is indicated.

If an uninfected mucocele is present at birth, conservative treatment with topical antibiotics and massage is recommended. If the mucocele becomes acutely infected, or does not improve with conservative treatment, surgical treatment is indicated. Some ophthalmologists treat these patients with bedside probing in the hospital. Because these patients almost always have NLD cysts, others prefer to treat with nasolacrimal probing and nasal endoscopy to remove the cysts (Figure 24–13).[3] Systemic antibiotics (parenteral or oral) should be used if the mucoceles are infected, due to the risk of sepsis.

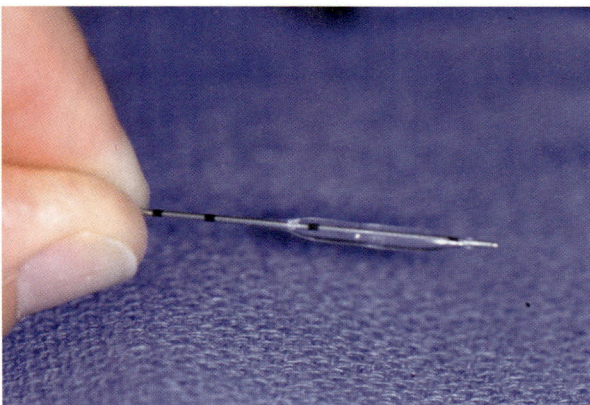

FIGURE 24–12 ■ Balloon catheter (Atrion Medical Products, Birmingham, Alabama). The catheter is placed into the distal NLD and inflated, providing increased dilation of the stenotic duct.

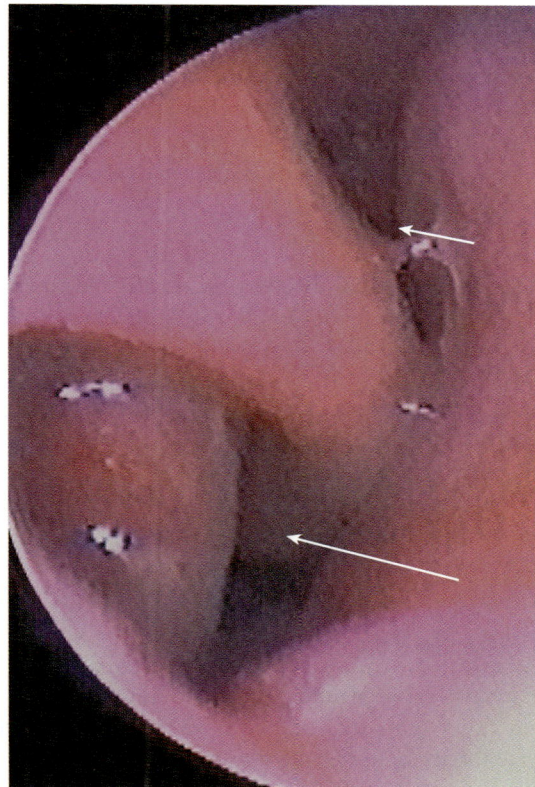

FIGURE 24–13 ■ Endoscopic view of NLD cyst (long arrow) beneath inferior nasal turbinate (short arrow). (Reprinted with permission from SLACK Incorporated, Lueder GT. Neonatal dacryocystitis associated with NLD cysts. *J Pediatr Ophthalmol Strabismus*. 1995;32(2): 102–106.)

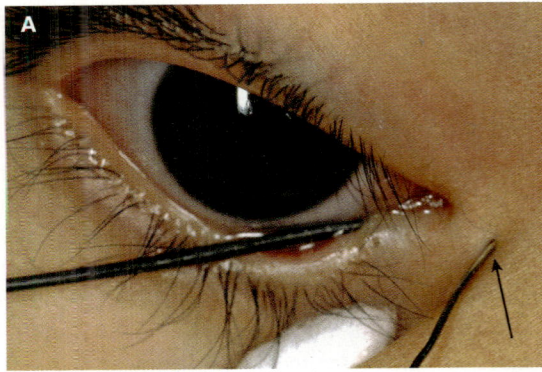

FIGURE 24–14 Lacrimal fistula surgery. (A) One probe is placed in the normal lacrimal canaliculus. The other probe (arrow) is passed through the fistula. (B) The fistula tract (arrow) is dissected and excised. (Figure B is reprinted with permission from *Semin Ophthalmol*. 1997;12(2):109–116. Copyright Informa Medical and Pharmaceutical Science.)

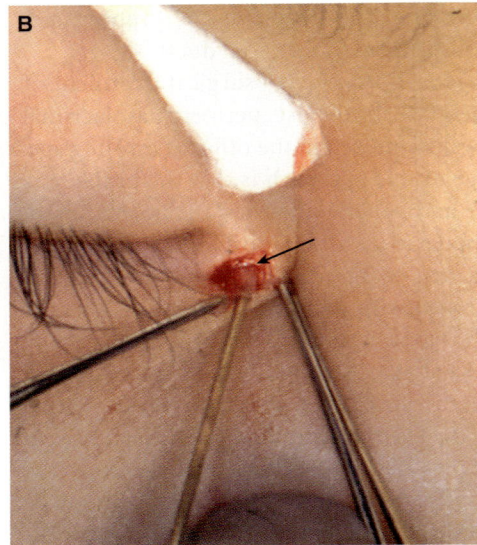

Punctal/Canalicular Atresia

The treatment of children with punctal or canalicular atresia is either simple or difficult. If the puncta are blocked by a membrane, simple dilation and probing will cure the problem. If the canaliculi are atretic, initial treatment usually consists of exploration of the eyelid to see whether any normal tissue can be identified and probed. If the entire canaliculus is absent, treatment is difficult. Placement of a Jones tube is usually recommended. This is a glass funnel that is inserted at the medial canthus and which extends into the lacrimal sac. These are prone to complications, and often are not placed until the teenage years.

Lacrimal Fistulae

Patients with lacrimal fistulae may require treatment if they have symptomatic epiphora or infection. Treatment consists of surgical removal of the fistula (Figure 24–14A and B). Probing and stent placement may be performed concurrently to decrease the risk of scar tissue formation that could block the normal duct.

TREATMENT OF TEAR FILM DISORDERS

Absent Reflex Tearing

Patients with absent reflex tearing do not require treatment, other than reassurance to the parents that the children will not suffer any vision problems related to this problem.

Absent Basal Tears (Alacrima)

Patients with absent basal tearing are prone to significant symptoms and potentially severe complications, such as corneal infection and scarring. Symptomatic treatment includes the use of lubricating eyedrops, although this may be difficult because children are often averse to using drops. Moisture chamber glasses can be made that decrease the evaporation of tears. Surgical occlusion of the lacrimal puncta with either plugs or cautery allows the tears that are produced to remain in the eye for longer periods, and often is quite helpful. These children require regular ophthalmic examinations to monitor for complications.

LACRIMAL TRAUMA

Trauma to the lacrimal system almost always occurs in conjunction with eyelid lacerations. Medial lower eyelid lacerations may extend through the lacrimal canaliculi, disrupting the connection between the lacrimal puncta and lacrimal sac (Figure 24–15).

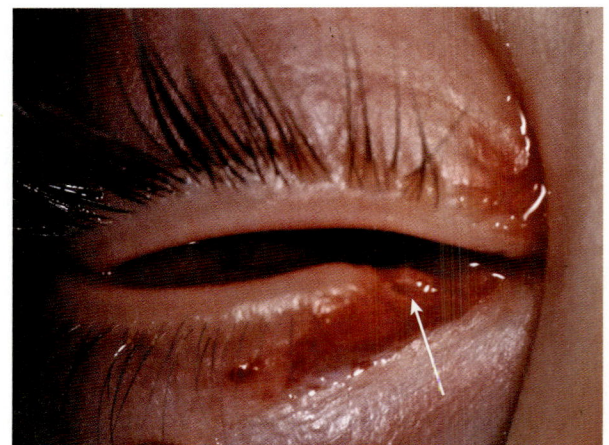

FIGURE 24–15 ■ Canalicular laceration. The distal cut end of the canaliculus is visible (arrow).

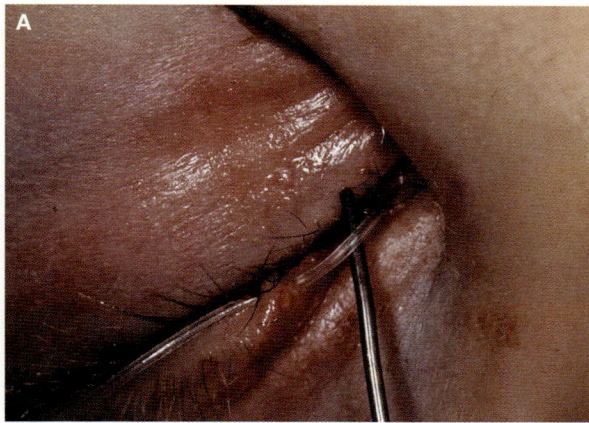

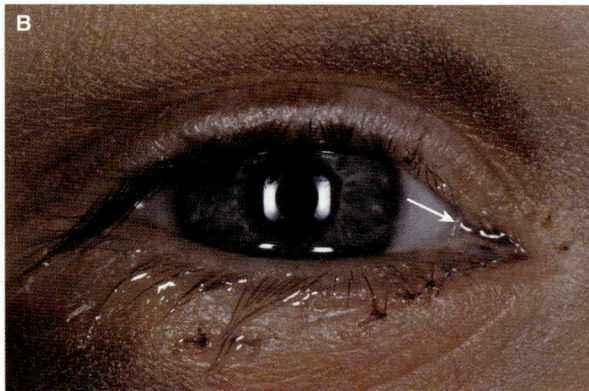

FIGURE 24–16 ■ Canalicular laceration repair. (A) A lacrimal stent has been placed between the cut ends of the lacrimal canaliculus. (B) One week after surgery the lower eyelid is in good position. There is some residual tearing and mucoid discharge due to edema and the presence of the stent (arrow). The patient's tear drainage returned to normal after the wound healed and the stent was removed.

A common cause of this in children is dog bites, in which one of the animal's jaws causes traction on the lower eyelid and tearing of the lacrimal canaliculus. These injuries may be hard to recognize. Careful inspection is indicated in any patient with a medial lower eyelid laceration to search for canalicular lacerations. Surgical repair is performed by reuniting the cut ends of the lacerated canaliculus (Figure 24–16). Stents are placed to maintain the patency of the canaliculus during the healing process.

REFERENCES

1. Becker B, Berry FD, Koller H. Balloon catheter dilatation for treatment of congenital nasolacrimal duct obstruction. *Am J Ophthalmol.* 1996;121:304–309.
2. Coats DK, McCreery KMB, Plager DA, Bohra L, Kim DS, Paysse EA. Nasolacrimal outflow drainage anomalies in Down's syndrome. *Ophthalmology.* 2003;110:1437–1441.
3. Lueder GT. Endoscopic treatment of intranasal abnormalities associated with nasolacrimal duct obstruction. *JAAPOS.* 2004;8:128–132.

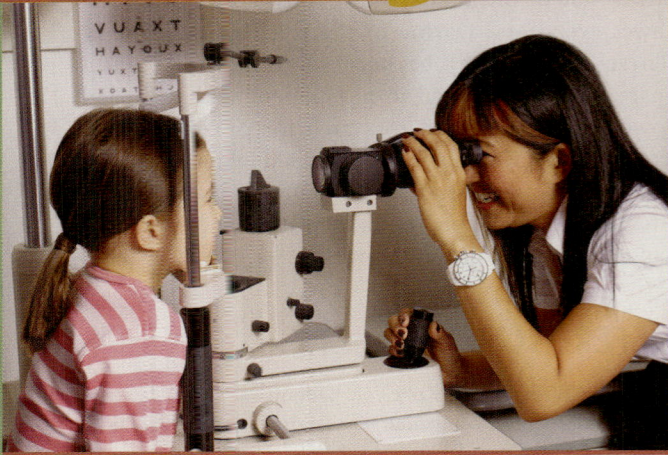

CHAPTER 25

Disorders of the Eyelids

DEFINITIONS AND EPIDEMIOLOGY

The most common eyelid abnormality in children is *ptosis* (blepharoptosis), which causes drooping of the eyelid. The upper eyelid normally rests just below the junction of the cornea and sclera (the limbus) superiorly. *Eyelid retraction* is the opposite of ptosis—the upper eyelid rests too high on the globe, such that the sclera above the iris is visible. *Lagophthalmos* is present if the eyelids do not close completely.

The eyelashes are normally directed away from the eye. *Entropion* is present if the eyelid and lashes are directed inward. *Ectropion* is present if the eyelashes are turned outward and the eyelid does not rest directly against the eyeball. *Distichiasis* is a condition in which patients have an extra row of abnormal eyelashes on the posterior eyelid margin.

Abnormalities of the eyelid structures occur in association with many craniofacial abnormalities. Examples of these include *hypotelorism*, in which the orbits and eyelids are closer together than normal; *hypertelorism*, in which these structures are farther apart than normal; and *telecanthus*, in which the distance between the inner eyelid margins (medial canthi) is abnormally wide. These abnormalities do not usually cause vision problems, but analysis of the different relationships of the eyelid structures may be useful in identifying specific syndromes. *Epicanthal folds*, extra medial eyelid tissue, are fairly common in infants. They are the most common cause of pseudostrabismus, the appearance of eye crossing despite normal ocular alignment.

ANATOMY AND EMBRYOLOGY

The upper eyelid is lifted by the *levator palpebrae superiorus muscle*, which originates in the posterior orbit. It travels forward and divides into an anterior portion, the *levator aponeurosis*, and a posterior portion, *Müller's muscle*. Both of these insert onto to the *tarsal plate (tarsus)*, the firm connective tissue that gives substance to the eyelid (Figure 25–1). The levator aponeurosis has attachments to the skin, which create the superior eyelid fold. The levator muscle is innervated by the third cranial nerve. Müller's muscle is sympathetically innervated.

The eyelids close by contraction of the *orbicularis oculi muscle*, which is arranged in a circular configuration around the upper and lower eyelids. It is innervated by the seventh cranial nerve.

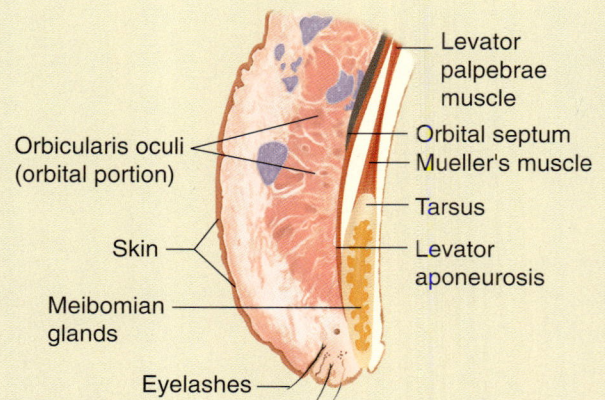

FIGURE 25–1 ■ Cross-sectional view of upper eyelid anatomy.

Embryology

The eyelids initially form from ectoderm at 4 to 5 weeks gestation. The upper and lower eyelids move toward each other and fuse at 10 weeks. Mesodermal tissue enters the lid and forms the musculature of the eyelid. During the fifth month of gestation the eyelids separate.

DISORDERS OF EYELID FUNCTION

Ptosis

Ptosis is caused by dysfunction of the levator muscle. In children it may be congenital or acquired. Most commonly it is congenital, secondary to underdevelopment of the muscle. Ptosis may be bilateral or unilateral, and may be idiopathic, familial, or associated with other syndromes (e.g., Turner syndrome). Congenital ptosis is commonly an isolated finding in otherwise normal children. Acquired ptosis may develop secondary to third cranial nerve palsy or eyelid or orbital lesions. *Myasthenia gravis* and *chronic progressive external ophthalmolplegia* may also cause ptosis, as can many other disorders (Table 25–1).

Evaluation

Ptosis can be generally categorized as mild, moderate, or severe. Mild ptosis is more easily noticed if unilateral, in which case one eyelid is slightly lower than the other. This does not produce visual problems and no treatment is necessary. In patients with severe ptosis, the eyelid partially or completely blocks the pupil, and

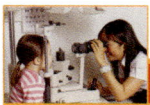

Table 25–1.

Partial List of Causes of Ptosis

- Idiopathic infantile ptosis
- Familial
  □ Blepharophimosis
  □ Congenital fibrosis of the extraocular muscles
  □ Chronic progressive external ophthalmoplegia
    – Kearns-Sayre syndrome
- Trauma
- Associated with syndromes
  □ Turner syndrome
  □ Cornelia de Lange syndrome
  □ Fetal alcohol syndrome
  □ Multiple others
- Myasthenia gravis
- Third cranial nerve palsy
- Horner syndrome
- Marcus-Gunn jaw winking
- Orbital disease
- Eyelid disease

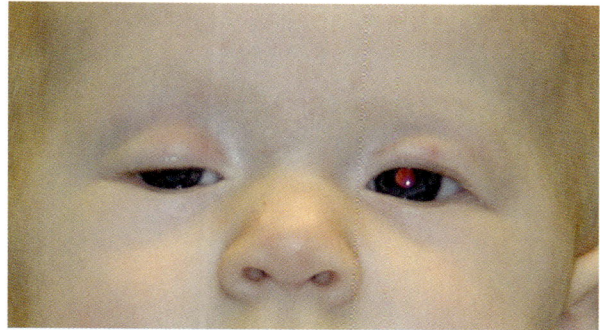

FIGURE 25–2 ■ Marked congenital ptosis with pupil covering right pupil. Note absence of right upper eyelid crease.

therefore interferes with vision (Figure 25–2). Infants with severe ptosis require early surgical correction to prevent amblyopia. In children with moderate ptosis the eyelid partially blocks the pupil. Ptosis may cause amblyopia either directly by blocking vision or indirectly by inducing astigmatism by the weight of the eyelid on the cornea.[1] Children with moderate-to-severe ptosis often have a prominent brow lift with arched eyelids, which they adopt to help elevate the eyelid by using the frontalis muscles (Figure 25–3). They also frequently develop a chin-up head posture to see below the drooping eyelid (Figure 25–4).

Evaluation of ptosis requires assessment of the degree of the levator muscle function. This is done by noting the amount of elevation of the eyelid between downgaze and upgaze. In normal patients the eyelid excursion measures approximately 15 mm. In moderate ptosis (with some residual function of the levator muscle), patients usually have 5 to 10 mm of movement. In severe ptosis, movement is 4 mm or less (Figure 25–5A and B). In many cases of childhood ptosis, the levator muscle is stiff in addition to being weak. This may cause the eyelid to not fully close, and the distance between

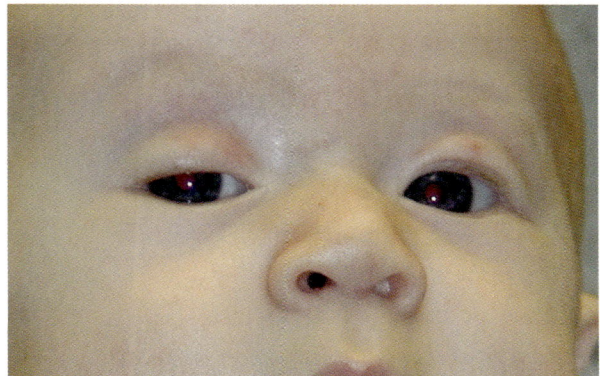

FIGURE 25–3 ■ Compensatory right brow lift to elevate eyelid above pupil.

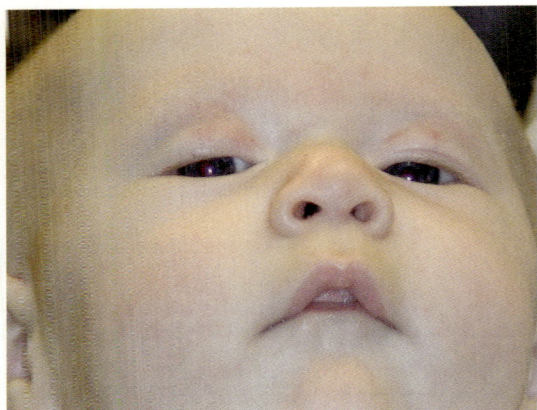

FIGURE 25–4 ■ Compensatory chin-up head posture to allow viewing beneath eyelid.

the upper and lower eyelids may actually increase in downgaze (Figure 25–5C). The normal eyelid crease forms by fibers of the levator muscle extending to the eyelid skin. Because the levator muscle is weak in

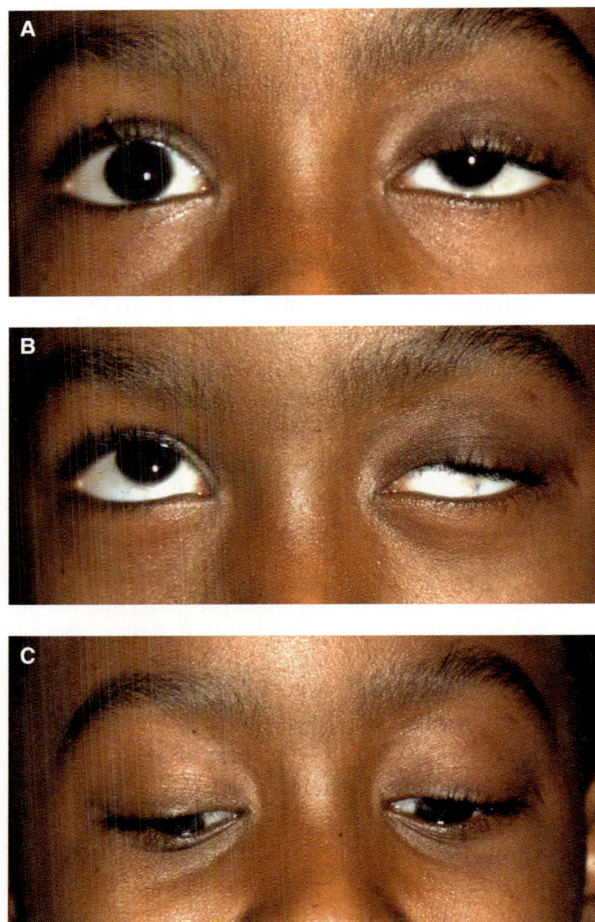

FIGURE 25–5 ■ (A) Ptosis partially covering left pupil. (B) Minimal movement of left upper eyelid in upgaze. (C) Stiffness of left upper eyelid limits movement in downgaze, creating an increased distance between the upper and lower eyelid compared to normal right eye.

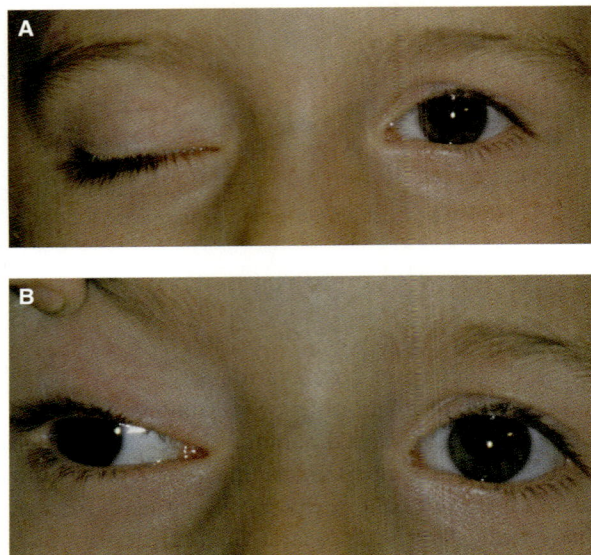

FIGURE 25–6 ■ (A) Complete ptosis, right eye secondary to third cranial nerve palsy. (B) When eyelid is manually elevated, the eye is noted to be down and out, and right pupil is larger than left.

patients with ptosis, they often have decreased eyelid skin creases (Figure 25–2).

If ptosis is not an isolated abnormality, most patients will have other findings that suggest a diagnosis. *Third cranial nerve palsies* typically also involve the pupil (which is dilated, except in some congenital cases in which the affected pupil is smaller than the other) and extraocular muscles (with the eye out and down) (Figures 25–6A and B). *Orbital or eyelid lesions* may produce proptosis with visible thickening or masses within the eyelid. Contiguous *sinus infections* may cause ptosis due to inflammation and edema (Figure 25–7A and B). Patients with *ocular myasthenia gravis* usually have variable strabismus and ptosis (Figure 25–8). These are usually most noticeable when the patient is fatigued. Examination may reveal a *Cogan lid twitch*, in which the eyelid briefly elevates more than normal when the patient's gaze is quickly directed from down to up.

Patients with *chronic progressive external ophthalmoplegia* (CPEO) typically have progressive ptosis and restrictive strabismus, most commonly involving the inferior rectus muscles. A form of this disorder associated with mitochondrial abnormalities is *Kearns-Sayre syndrome*, which includes CPEO, pigmentary retinopathy (Figure 25–9A and B), and cardiac conduction defects.

Treatment

The treatment of ptosis depends on the patient's age and the severity of the eyelid droop. Mild ptosis usually does not require any treatment. Children with severe ptosis that occludes the eyes are at high risk for amblyopia,

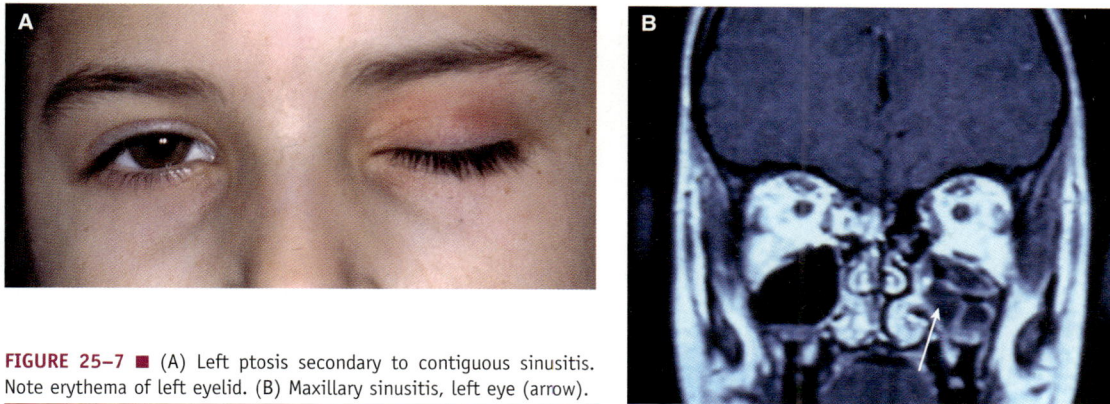

FIGURE 25–7 ■ (A) Left ptosis secondary to contiguous sinusitis. Note erythema of left eyelid. (B) Maxillary sinusitis, left eye (arrow).

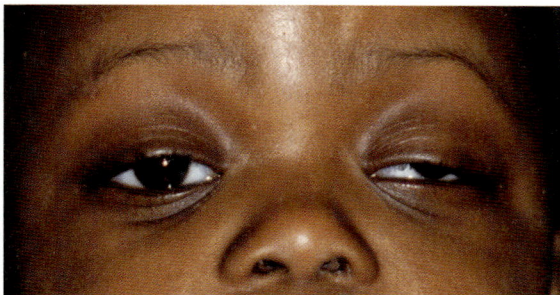

FIGURE 25–8 ■ Ptosis and strabismus in a patient with myasthenia gravis.

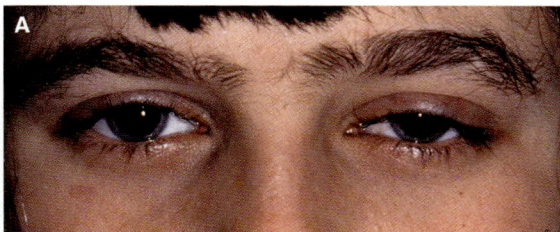

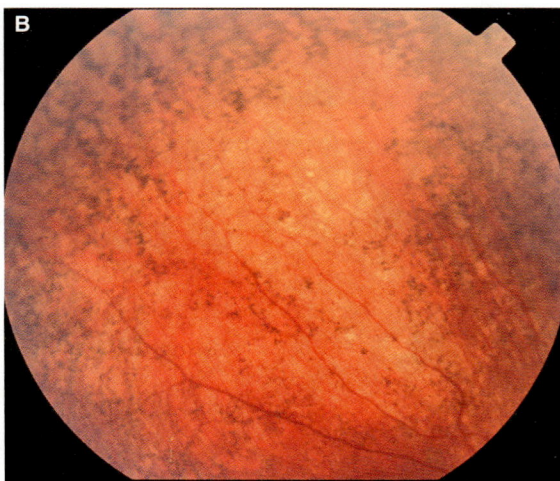

FIGURE 25–9 ■ Kearns-Sayre syndrome. (A) Bilateral ptosis, left greater than right. (B) Pigmentary retinopathy.

particularly if the ptosis is unilateral (similar to the risk of amblyopia in unilateral congenital cataracts). If the ptosis is moderate and the vision is developing normally, treatment is often delayed until approximately 4 to 5 years of age.

Surgery is required to correct ptosis. The type of surgery depends on the degree of function of the patient's levator muscle. In severe cases of congenital ptosis the levator usually has almost no function. These patients typically lift their brow to recruit the frontalis muscle to assist in elevating the lid (Figure 25–3). Surgical correction of severe ptosis takes advantage of this by attaching the eyelid directly to the frontalis muscle with strips of donor or autologous fascia or synthetic material (Figure 25–10). After surgery, when the patient elevates the brow, the force is transmitted directly to the eyelid (Figure 25–11). Even with a good surgical outcome, the eyelid height will vary depending on how alert the patient is. The most common complication of frontalis suspension surgery is corneal exposure due to incomplete eyelid closure. Exposure of the implant material or recurrent granuloma formation may also occur, sometimes requiring removal of the material (Figure 25–12). Over time the drooping of the eyelid may recur, necessitating repeat surgery.

Patients with moderate ptosis have some residual function of the levator muscle. Surgery in these patients consists of tightening the muscle (levator muscle resection) (Figure 25–10), normally performed through an incision in the eyelid crease to minimize scarring. This surgery generally results in a more normal appearance of the eyelid than does frontalis suspension surgery, and there are fewer complications.

OTHER FORMS OF PTOSIS

Pseudoptosis. Patients may sometimes appear to have mild ptosis due to overhanging of the brow skin. This can be distinguished by elevating the brow tissue and

Levator
aponeurosis

Tarsus

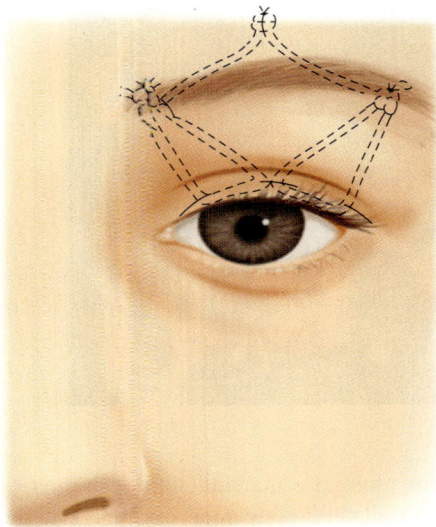

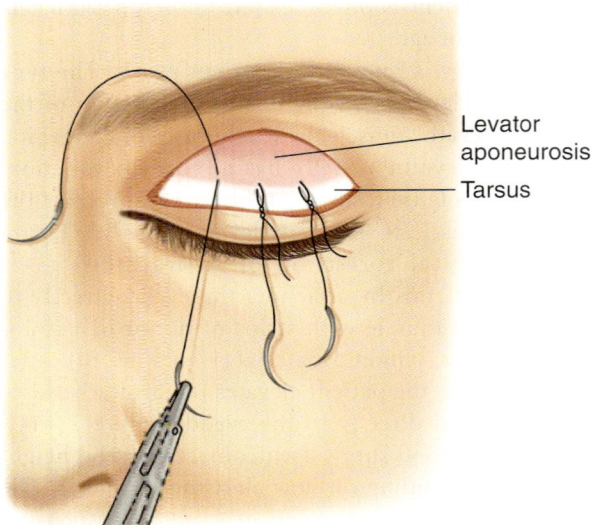

FIGURE 25–10 ■ Ptosis surgery. (Top) Frontalis sling. The eyelid is attached to the frontalis muscle using either fascia lata or synthetic material. (Bottom) Levator muscle resection. A portion of the levator muscle is removed, and the shortened muscle is reattached to the tarsus.

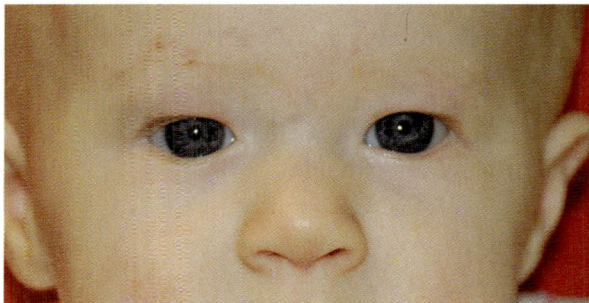

FIGURE 25–12 ■ Postoperative exposure of ptosis sling material (arrow) at site of brow incision.

examining the eyelid and levator muscle function, which are found to be normal (Figure 25–13A and B).

Patients may also appear to have ptosis due to other ocular conditions:

■ Patients with increased light sensitivity (due to a corneal problem, for example) may voluntary keep their eyelid closed to decrease their symptoms.
■ Patients with vertical strabismus may appear to have ptosis on the side with the lower eye because the eyelid normally moves in conjunction with the eye.
■ Patients with intermittent exotropia may close the eye when exotropia is manifest.

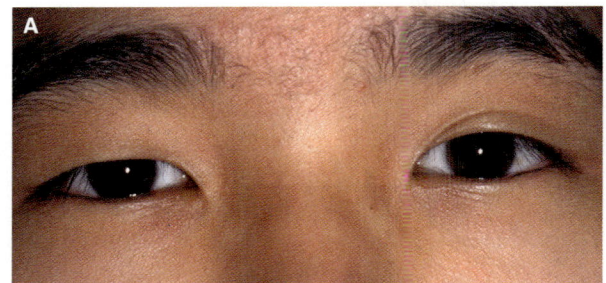

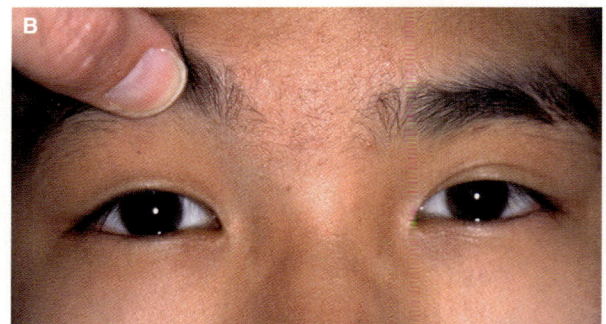

FIGURE 25–11 ■ Postoperative appearance of patient in Figure 25–2 after ptosis sling procedure, right eye.

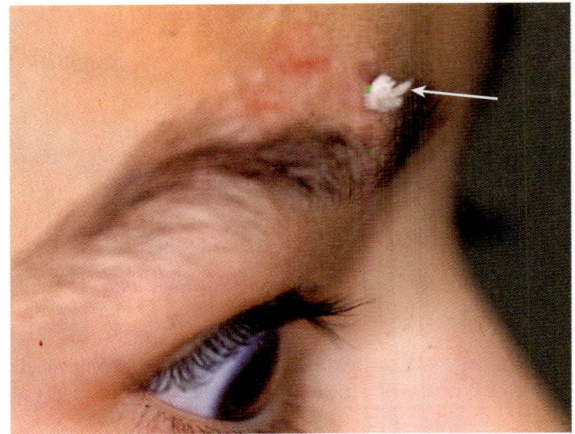

FIGURE 25–13 ■ (A) Pseudoptosis, right eye, due to overhanging eyelid skin. (B) When skin is manually elevated, the eyelid heights are seen to be symmetric.

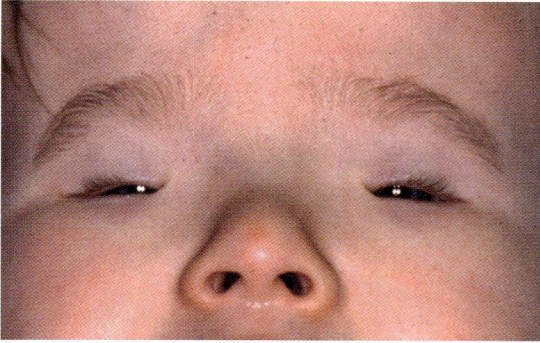

FIGURE 25–14 ■ Blepharophimosis syndrome. Note marked bilateral ptosis, narrow interpalpebral fissures (horizontal opening of the eyelids), and epicanthus inversus (epicanthal fold more prominent on lower eyelids).

Blepharophimosis syndrome is an autosomal dominant disorder characterized by ptosis, epicanthus inversus (an epicanthal fold that is most prominent on the lower eyelid), and short vertical and horizontal eyelid fissures (blepharophimosis) (Figure 25–14). The ptosis frequently requires a sling procedure in infancy to prevent amblyopia. Surgery to reduce the prominent epicanthal folds is often performed.

Marcus-Gunn jaw winking is an unusual form of ptosis related to miswiring between the fifth and seventh cranial nerves. When affected children chew or move their jaw, there is a synchronous elevation and lowering of the eyelid (Figure 25–15A and B). Treatment of patients with Marcus-Gunn jaw winking ptosis pres-

ents a unique challenge, due to the variability of eyelid height. Surgery to elevate the eyelid may result in an exaggerated eyelid retraction when the jaw moves. Some surgeons recommend extirpation of the levator muscle combined with a frontalis suspension procedure to avoid this problem. Parents are often not enthusiastic about this option, and may choose a partial levator resection, with the goal of elevating the eyelid somewhat, while attempting to minimize the retraction.

EYELID RETRACTION

True eyelid retraction is uncommon (Table 25–2). The appearance of eyelid retraction is usually secondary to some other problem. The most common of these is

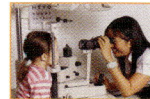

Table 25–2.

Causes of Eyelid Retraction

- Ptosis in opposite eye
- Orbital mass (proptosis)
  - Tumor
  - Thyroid ophthalmopathy
- Marcus-Gunn jaw winking
- Surgical overcorrection
- Eyeball enlargement
  - High myopia (with enlarged eye)
  - Infantile glaucoma with buphthalmos

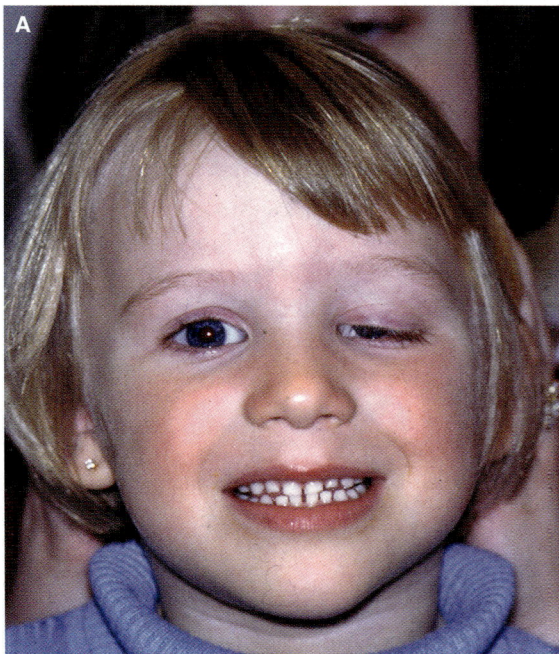

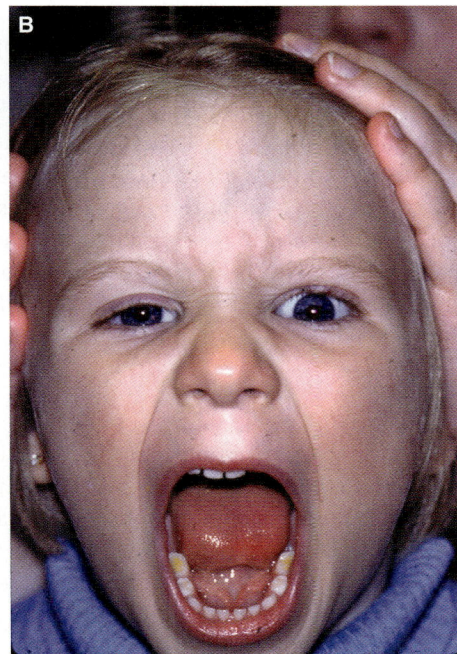

FIGURE 25–15 ■ Marcus-Gunn jaw winking ptosis. (A) Ptosis, left upper eyelid. (B) Elevation of left upper eyelid due to synkinesis with jaw opening.

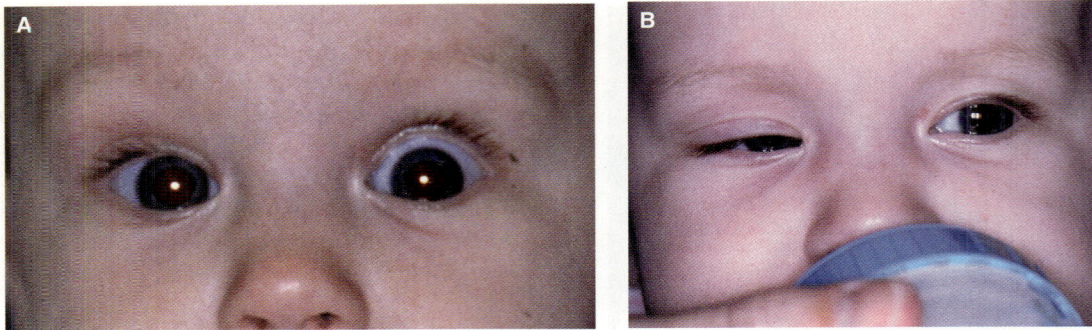

FIGURE 25–16 ■ (A) Retraction of left upper eyelid, present when infant is awake and alert. (B) Ptosis of right upper eyelid, noted as patient becomes sleepy while taking bottle. The eyelid retraction results from excess innervation to the left upper eyelid, which occurs when the infant attempts to lift the ptotic right upper eyelid.

proptosis, in which the eye bulges forward due to an orbital abnormality, such as a tumor or thyroid-related enlargement of the extraocular muscles. As the eye moves forward, the lid is pushed upward, creating the appearance of retraction.

Lid retraction may also occur due to mild or moderate ptosis of the opposite eye. This is because innervation to the eyelids is distributed equally to both eyes. If one eye has ptosis and the patient supplies extra innervation to this weaker eyelid to elevate it, the same excess innervation is sent to the normal eye, creating overelevation of the unaffected eyelid (Figure 25–16A and B).

Eyelid retraction may also occur due to surgical overcorrection of ptosis.

Presentation

Even mild eyelid retraction is often easily recognized due to visibility of the white sclera above the pupil. If the eyelid retraction is due to proptosis, this should also be detectable on examination. Patients with marked proptosis may have accompanying limitation of extraocular movements and corneal irritation due to exposure. If the eyelid retraction is a secondary effect of ptosis in the opposite eye, the ptosis may be visible if the ptotic eye is covered (but observed behind the occlusion) or if the patient is examined when they are sleepy (e.g., after an infant feeds) (Figure 25–16A and B).

Treatment

The treatment of eyelid retraction depends on its etiology. Surgical overcorrection of ptosis is fairly common in the immediate postoperative period, and usually improves with time. If it does not, surgery to lower the eyelid may be necessary. If the eyelid retraction is due to ptosis of the opposite eye, surgical correction of the ptotic eyelid may be indicated. If the eyelid retraction is due to proptosis of the eyeball, treatment is directed toward the underlying orbital disorder.

LAGOPHTHALMOS

Closure of the eyelid is produced by the orbicularis muscle, which is innervated by the seventh cranial nerve. Lagophthalmos (incomplete eyelid closure) most commonly occurs in association with facial nerve palsy. It may also develop in neuromuscular diseases, as a consequence of proptosis, or in patients whose eyelids are stiffer than normal, which could occur with an infiltrative process. Transient mild lagophthalmos somtimes occurs in normal newborns. Paradoxically, some patients with severe ptosis may have stiff levator muscles that prevent full eyelid closure, resulting in both ptosis and lagophthalmos (Table 25–3).

Presentation

Mild incomplete eyelid closure is common in infancy. This usually does not produce any ocular problems and resolves spontaneously. Acquired lagophthalmos is most commonly due to seventh cranial nerve palsy (Figure 25–17). *Bell's palsy* is an idiopathic form of this disorder. Affected children may develop excess tearing and photophobia due to corneal exposure (*exposure keratitis*), and are at risk for corneal infection and ulceration in severe cases (Figure 25–18).

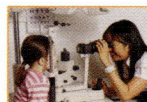

Table 25–3.

Causes of Lagophthalmos (Incomplete Eyelid Closure)

- Seventh cranial nerve palsy
  □ Bell's palsy
- Severe congenital ptosis with stiff eyelid levator muscles
- Normal newborns during sleep
- Neuromuscular diseases
- Any of the conditions in Table 25–2

Treatment

The treatment of lagophthalmos is directed toward protection of the cornea from damage due to incomplete closing of the eyelids. In severe cases this can lead to corneal infection or scarring, potentially affecting vision (Figure 25–18). In conditions that are expected to improve (Bell's palsy, for example), protection of the cornea during the recovery phase is indicated. Depending on the degree of irritation, lubrication with artificial tears or ophthalmic lubricating ointment may suffice. More severe cases may require closing of the eyelid during sleep with tape, or special moisture-chamber glasses that form a seal around the eye to help maintain moisture. Surgical options for more severe cases include either a temporary or permanent lateral tarsorraphy (sewing together of the outer portions of the eyelids to decrease exposure) (Figure 25–17B), or implantation of a gold or platinum

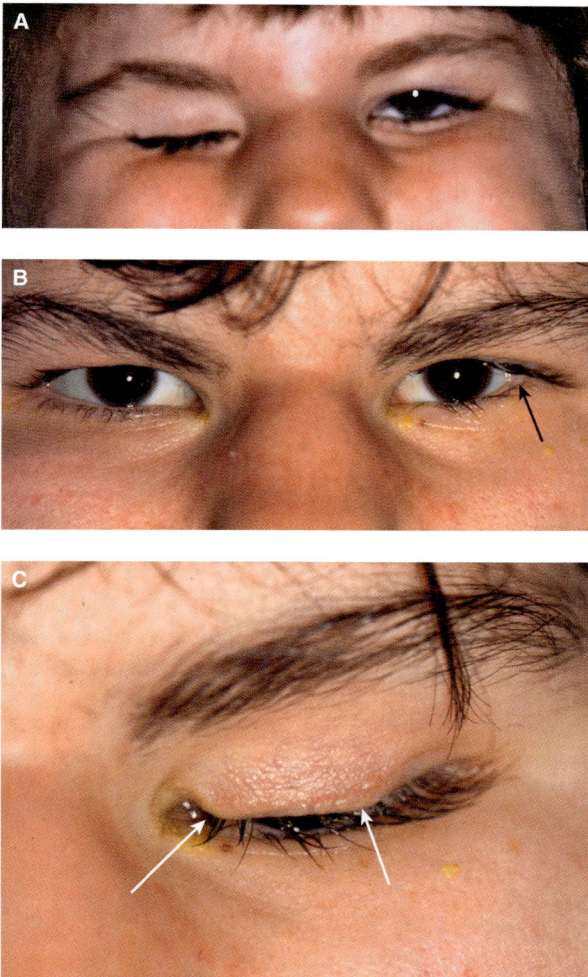

FIGURE 25–18 ■ Severe corneal exposure keratopathy due to lagophthalmos with inability to protect cornea.

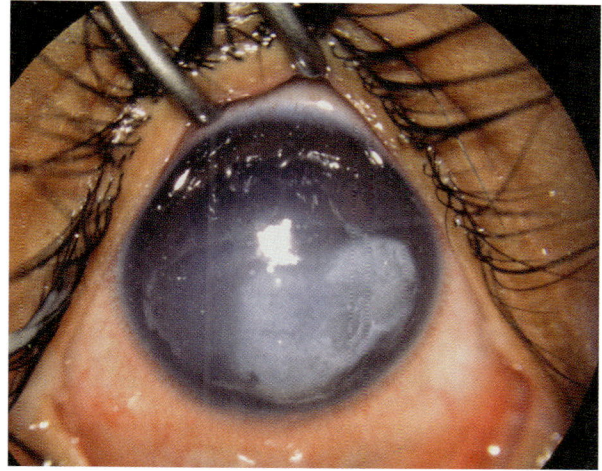

FIGURE 25–17 ■ (A) Lagophthalmos, left eye, secondary to seventh cranial nerve palsy. (B) Appearance after lateral tarsorrhaphy (surgical joining of lateral upper and lower eyelids—arrow). (C) Platinum weight in upper eyelid (edges of weight marked by arrows), allowing almost complete closure of eyelid.

weight in the upper eyelid to improve closure (due to the weight of the implant) (Figure 25–17C).[2]

DISORDERS OF EYELID POSITION

Entropion

Entropion refers to an inward turning of the eyelid. In children, it most frequently occurs due to *epiblepharon*, an extra fold of skin on the lower eyelid that causes the eyelashes to turn inward (Figure 25–19A). This may result in corneal irritation.

Presentation

Entropion secondary to epiblepharon is often asymptomatic in young children. If the misdirected eyelashes cause corneal irritation, the children may have symptoms of photophobia and excess tearing, sometimes with a mucoid ocular discharge. These symptoms are similar to those of typical nasolacrimal duct obstruction, and examination of the eyelid margins is needed to distinguish these disorders.

Treatment

If patients have persistent corneal irritation due to epiblepharon, surgical treatment to evert the eyelids is highly effective (Figure 25–19B).[3]

OTHER CONGENITAL EYELID ABNORMALITIES

Congenital structural anomalies of the eyelids are rare. The most severe is *cyrptophalmos*, in which the eyelids are fused together, and the underlying eye is markedly abnormal. Eyelid *colobomas* are notches or larger defects

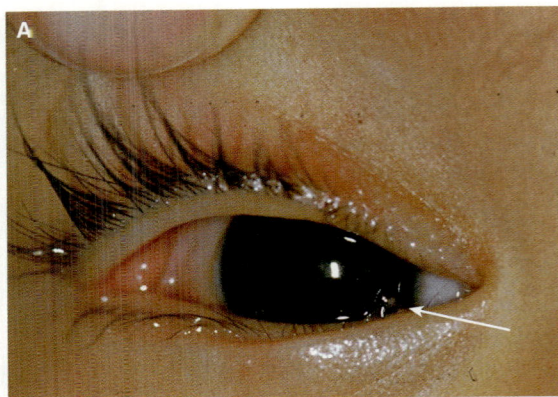

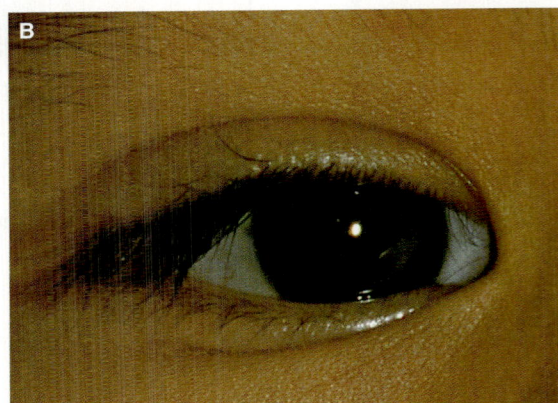

FIGURE 25–19 ■ (A) Epiblepharon, right eye. Extra fold of skin on medial right lower eyelid causes lashes to rub against the cornea (arrow), causing increased tearing and mucoid discharge. (B) Same patient 4 years after surgical treatment to normalize the eyelid position.

of the eyelids themselves (Figure 25–20). These are most commonly associated with *Goldenhar syndrome.* Large colobomas may require surgical treatment to prevent exposure damage to the eye. *Ankyloblepharon* describes partial incomplete separation of the eyelids, usually with small strands of residual tissue between the upper

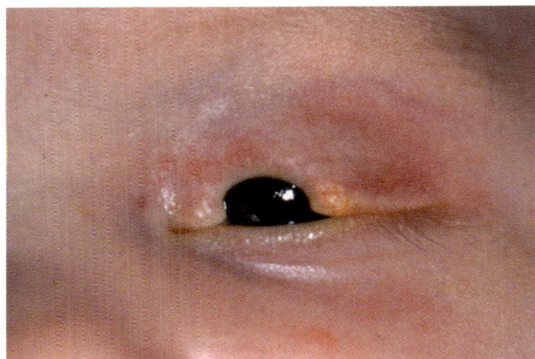

FIGURE 25–20 ■ Congenital left upper eyelid coloboma.

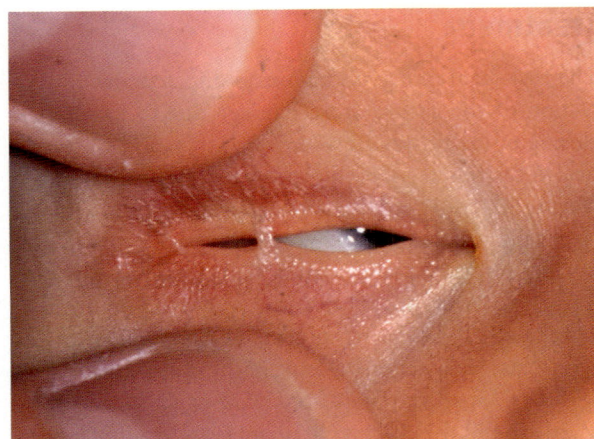

FIGURE 25–21 ■ Ankyloblepharon. Small strands of tissue cause adhesion between right upper and lower eyelid.

and lower eyelid that prevents full separation of these structures (Figure 25–21). Surgical separation of the bands restores the eyelids to normal.

EYELID EDEMA

Eyelid changes are frequently early signs of systemic conditions that cause edema. This occurs because the tissue of the eyelids is fairly loose and it is easy for fluid to accumulate in this area. The eyelid swelling is usually most noticeable on awakening because of dependent edema associated with sleeping position. This is usually a nonspecific finding, but it should prompt a search for underlying causes of edema (Figure 25–22).

DISORDERS OF THE EYELASHES

Distichiasis

In distichiasis, patients are born with a row of abnormal eyelashes that arise from the meibomian gland orifices on the posterior margin of the eyelid (Figure 25–23).

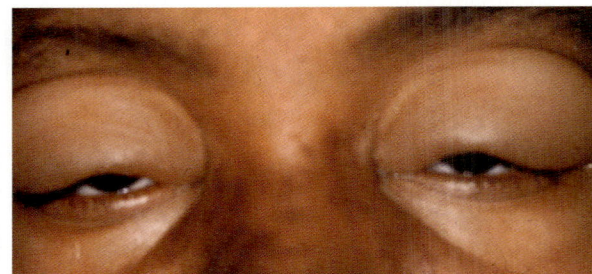

FIGURE 25–22 ■ Marked bilateral eyelid edema as the first manifestation of systemic lupus erythematosis.

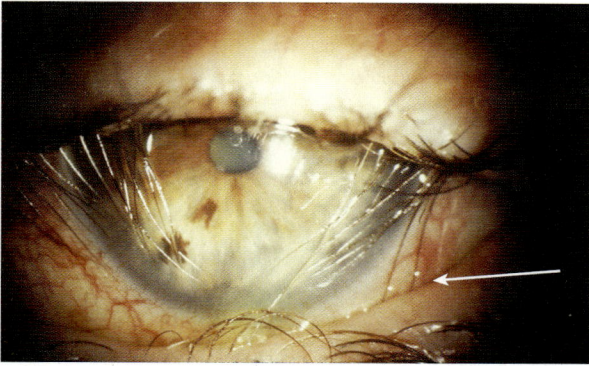

FIGURE 25–23 ■ Distichiasis. Note abnormal row of eyelashes (arrow) that arise posterior to the normal row of eyelashes.

Superficially the appearance is similar to epiblepharon, with misdirection of eyelashes against the eyeball. However, in distichiasis there are 2 rows of lashes, and the eyelid itself is in normal position. The lashes in distichiasis are relatively soft and are often well-tolerated. In some patients they cause chronic ocular irritation by rubbing on the cornea, with symptoms similar to epiblepharon. Surgical treatment requires removal of the lashes, usually with electrolysis or cryotherapy. The eyelid may be surgically separated during this procedure to preserve the normal eyelashes.

Trichotillomania

Trichotillomania is a disorder in which patients repeatedly pull out their hair. This behavior is sometimes limited to the eyelashes. It is a form of obsessive-compulsive disorder. Patients are aware of the behavior, but are unable to control it. They often disguise it from family members (for instance, only doing it when they are alone in their bedrooms), and they may deny that they do it. The examination findings in trichotillomania are characteristic: the lashes are missing in segmental areas, rather than diffusely, and the hair shafts are broken at irregular lengths (Figure 25–24A and B). The eyelids themselves show no signs of inflammation or other problems. Treatment is usually directed at the underlying behavior, sometimes with the assistance of mental health professionals.[4]

OTHER EYELID LESIONS

Chalazia (Hordeola, Sty)

Chalazia and hordeola are the most common eyelid lesions in children. They result from plugging of the sebaceous glands within the eyelid. The lesions initially incite an inflammatory lipogranulomatous reaction, creating an erythematous nodule of either the upper or lower eyelid

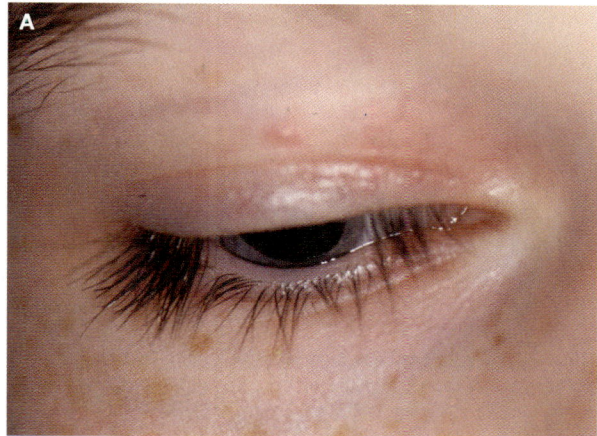

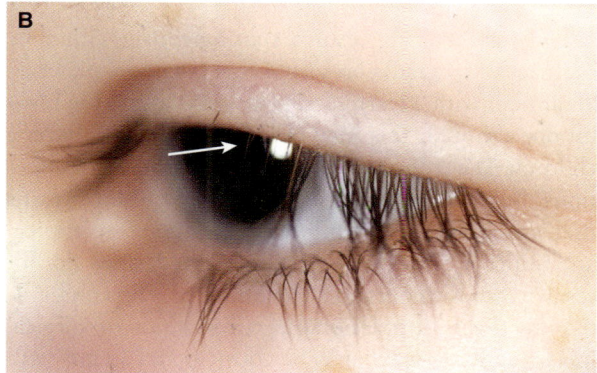

FIGURE 25–24 ■ Trichotillomania. (A) Note segmental loss of eyelashes in center portion of upper eyelid. (B) Eyelashes broken at different lengths (arrow).

(Figure 25–25). In some patients the sty itself may not be visualized discretely. The eyelid may be erythematous and edematous, with an appearance similar to preseptal cellulitis (Figure 25–26). If a sty does not spontaneously drain or resolve, it may turn into a chronic nodule of the eyelid. Some patients develop a *pyogenic granuloma* of the tarsal conjunctiva adjacent to the lesion, which appears as a fleshy, pink, pedunculated mass (Figure 25–27).

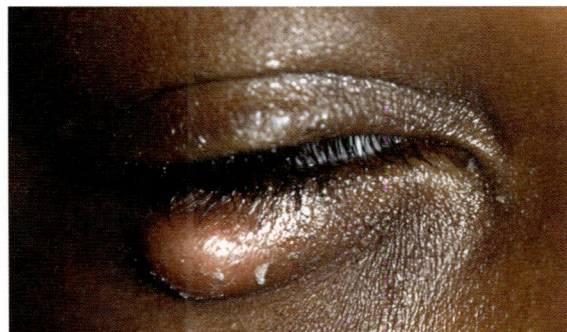

FIGURE 25–25 ■ Chalazion, right lower eyelid.

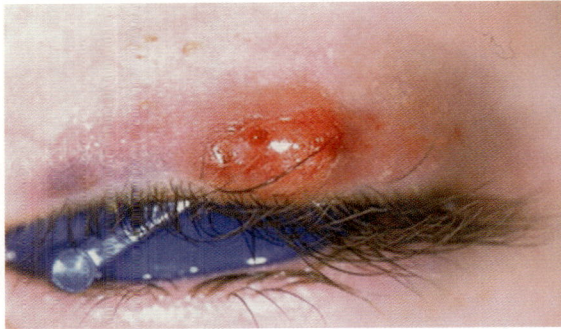

FIGURE 25–26 ■ Erythema and edema of right upper eyelid secondary to chalazion (the blue object is a globe protector, placed during surgical drainage of the chalazion).

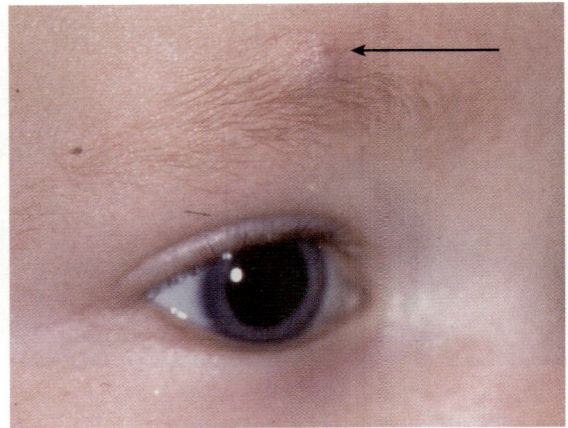

FIGURE 25–28 ■ Pilomatrixoma right upper eyebrow (arrow).

Most chalazia resolve spontaneously, either by drainage or by gradual resorption of the lipoid material. Treatment with a warm compress may hasten the resolution, although this may be difficult to do in young children. The styes themselves are not the result of infections, but staphylococcal bacteria may produce toxins that exacerbate the condition, and therefore topical antibiotics are sometimes useful. If the lesions do not resolve over the course of 1 to 2 months with conservative treatment, intralesional corticosteroids or surgical incision and drainage may be considered. Patients with recurrent chalazia often have underlying blepharitis, which may benefit from oral antibiotics or regular eyelid scrubs with baby shampoo.

Pilomatrixoma (Calcifying Epithelioma of Malherbe)

Pilomatrixomas are benign tumors that arise from hair gland follicles. They present as firm subcutaneous nodules. Periocular lesions may occur in the eyebrow or on the eyelid tissue (Figure 25–28). They may have a whitish yellow or purplish appearance. Subcutaneous calcium may be visible. Surgical excision may be indicated to establish a diagnosis, and is curative (Figure 25–29).

Papilloma

Papillomas are benign epithelial hyperplasias that may develop on the eyelid or conjunctiva. These lesions usually have a keratinized appearance, similar to cauliflower (Figure 25–30). Some papillomas are caused by papillomaviruses (verucca vulgaris). Excision of the lesion at the base is usually curative, although lesions caused by papillomavirus may recur.

Tinea

Periocular fungal infections may occur in a pattern that is typical of ringworm, in which case it may be easily

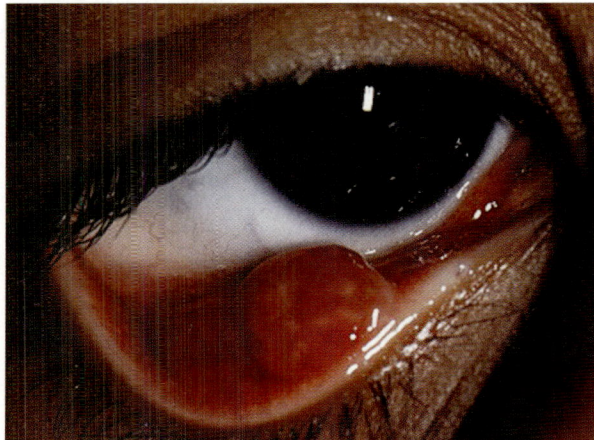

FIGURE 25–27 ■ Pyogenic granuloma associated with chalazion on tarsal conjunctiva surface of right lower eyelid.

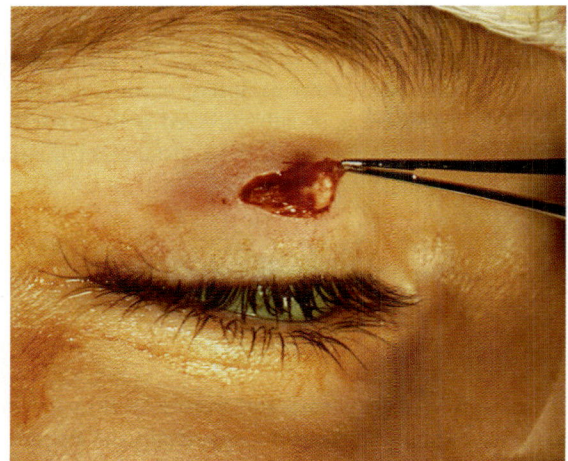

FIGURE 25–29 ■ Surgical removal of pilomatrixoma. Note white, chunky appearance of lesion.

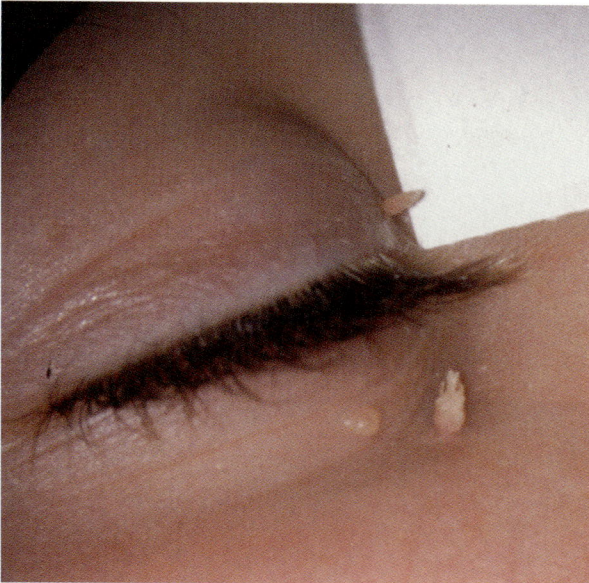

FIGURE 25–30 ■ Multiple eyelid papillomas.

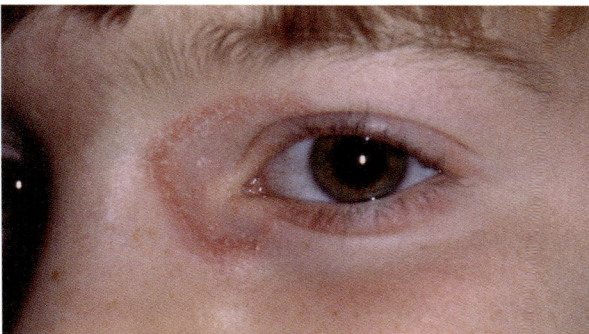

FIGURE 25–32 ■ Right upper eyelid choristoma.

recognized (Figure 25–31). However, dermatophytic infections may cause nonspecific erythema and inflammation that is misdiagnosed as preseptal cellulitis. The presence of scaling, loss of eyelashes, and worsening with topical corticosteroids should raise suspicion for tinea infection. The diagnosis may be confirmed with KOH scrapings. Treatment with oral griseofulvin is usually effective.

Choristomas

Choristomas are lesions composed of normal tissue in an abnormal location. Common ocular examples of choristomas include orbital dermoid cysts and corneal dermoids. Less commonly, choristomas may be present on the eyelids at birth (Figure 25–32). Surgical excision is usually curative.

Capillary Hemangioma

Capillary hemangiomas may occur on the eyelids or within the orbit. They are discussed in Chapter 26.

Juvenile Xanthogranuloma

Juvenile xanthogranuloma (JXG) is a benign, self-limited disorder of children that usually occurs in infants and young children. Most cases involve only the skin, characterized by sharply demarcated yellow nodules that vary in size from a few millimeters to several centimeters. The lesions normally involute spontaneously. The most common ocular manifestations of JXG involve the eyelid, iris, and ciliary body. Eyelid lesions are usually single and often represent the only manifestation of the disease (Figure 25–33). Excisional biopsy is both diagnostic and curative. If other lesions are present and the diagnosis is not in question, observation of eyelid

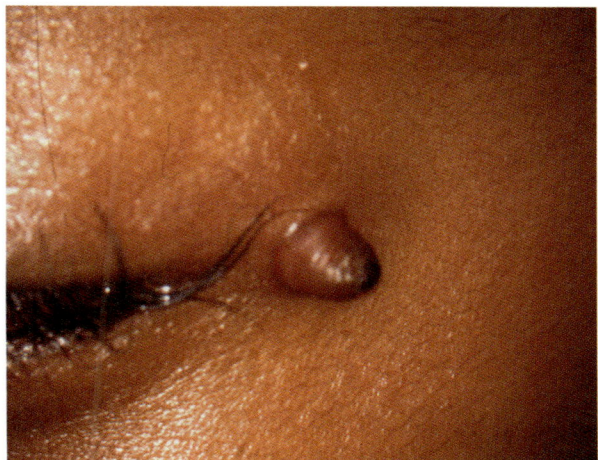

FIGURE 25–31 ■ Tinea infection of eyelids, with classic ringworm appearance.

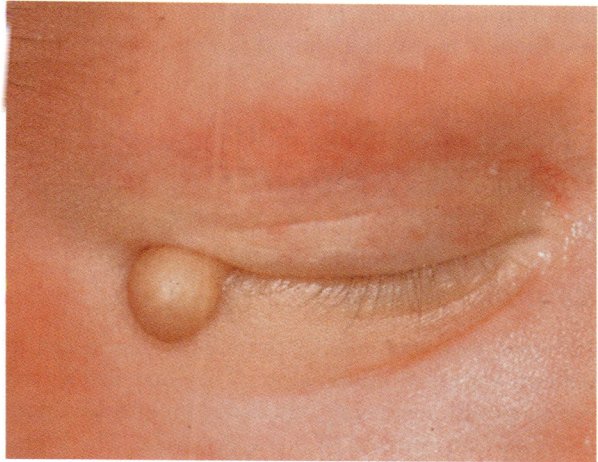

FIGURE 25–33 ■ Eyelid juvenile xanthogranuloma.

lesions usually results in spontaneous regression. Iris involvement in JXG is discussed further in Chapter 29.

EYELID AND EYELASH DISORDERS ASSOCIATED WITH SYSTEMIC DISEASES

Neurofibromatosis

Plexiform neurofibromas of the eyelids may occur in patients with neurofibromatosis. They may involve the eyelid, usually producing a gradually progressive thickening and enlargement of the upper eyelid. The lateral portion is usually more affected, which produces an S-shaped deformity of the eyelid (Figure 25–34).

Poliosis

Poliosis results from decreased or absent melanin within the hair. Eyelash poliosis may be segmental or diffuse (Figure 25–35A and B). Poliosis of the scalp hair may occur in *Waardenburg* syndrome. This is an autosomal dominant disorder caused by a mutation of the *PAX3* gene. In addition to a white forelock on the scalp, associated abnormalities include lateral displacement of the medial canthi, iris heterochromia, abnormal retinal pigment epithelium, and hearing loss. Other diseases in which eyelash poliosis may occur include inflammatory disorders, such as blepharitis, Vogt-Koyanagi-Harada syndrome, and vitiligo.

Alopecia

Alopecia is an autoimmune disorder characterized by loss of hair without scarring. In alopecia areata the loss of hair is irregular and most commonly involves the scalp. The eyelashes may also be affected. Alopecia totalis affects the entire scalp, and alopecia universalis affects the entire body. Latanaprost is a prostaglandin analogue used in the treatment of glaucoma. It increases pigment

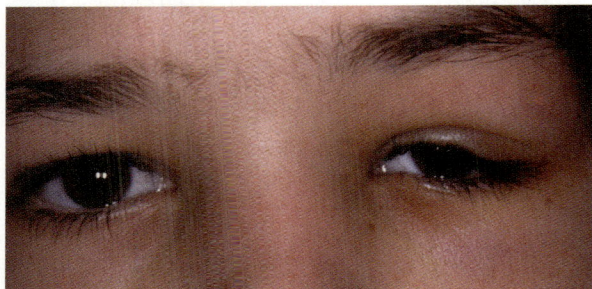

FIGURE 25–35 ■ Eyelash poliosis. (A) Segmental loss of pigment in medial upper eyelashes in a patient with vitiligo. (B) Diffuse bilateral eyelash poliosis.

within the iris and increases eyelash growth (hypertrichosis), and is being investigated as a treatment for patients with eyelash loss due to alopecia (NIH Study NCT00187577, clinicaltrials.gov).

Ichthyosis

The ichthyoses are a group of inherited skin disorders characterized by scaling and dryness of the skin. The clinical findings are a result of an increased rate of formation of the stratum corneum as well as a decreased rate of desquamation. Ichthyosis vulgaris is a very common disorder and it is generally mild. A particularly severe form of neonatal ichthyosis is the harlequin fetus, which is classified separately from the other ichthyoses. The most common ocular manifestations of the ichthyoses include corneal opacities and eyelid thickening and ectropion (Figure 25–36). Patients with significant ectropion require lubrication to protect the eyes. The ectropion may spontaneously improve. Surgery may be necessary if the ectropion persists.

Epidermolysis Bullosa

Epidermolysis bullosa (EB) is a group of disorders characterized by recurrent blistering of the skin. The severity of the disease depends on which layer of the skin is affected. The junctional and dystrophic forms of EB, in which cleavage abnormalities develop within the basal layer of the epidermis and superficial dermis, respectively,

FIGURE 25–34 ■ Eyelid plexiform neurofibroma causing S-shaped deformity of left upper eyelid in a patient with neurofibromatosis.

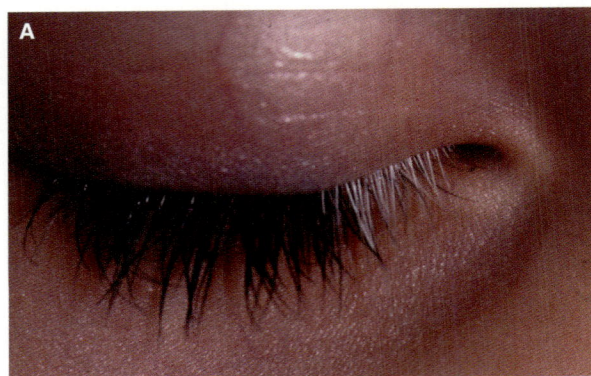

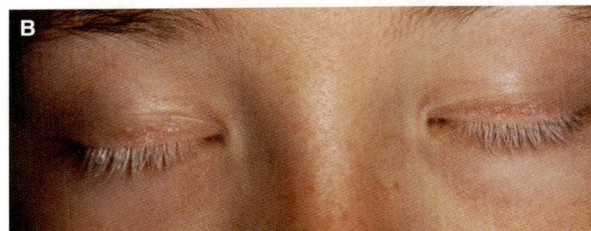

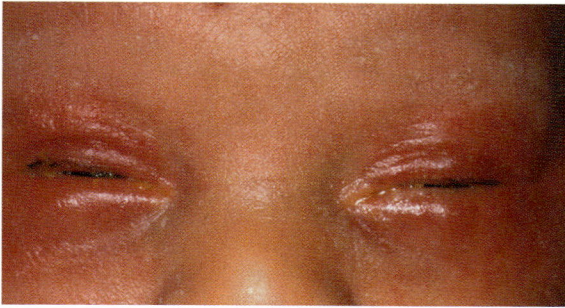

FIGURE 25–36 ■ Eyelid thickening and ectropion (outward turning) of lower eyelid in a patient with ichthyosis.

are often associated with ocular complications. These include corneal erosions and scarring, blepharitis, scarring of the eyelids, and lacrimal obstruction (Figure 25–37A and B). Ophthalmic treatment includes ocular lubrication and may require corneal or eyelid surgery.

EYELID TRAUMA

Direct blunt injuries to the eyes, such as from a fist or a ball, may cause swelling and ecchymosis of the eyelids. Such injuries usually resolve without sequela. When

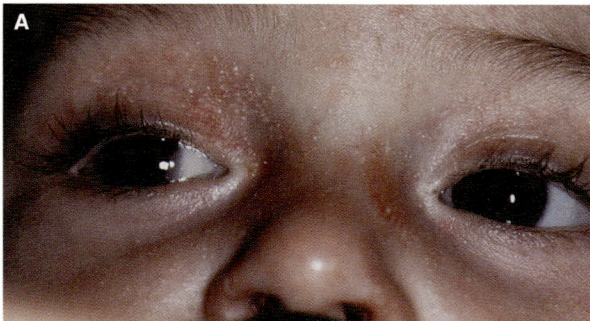

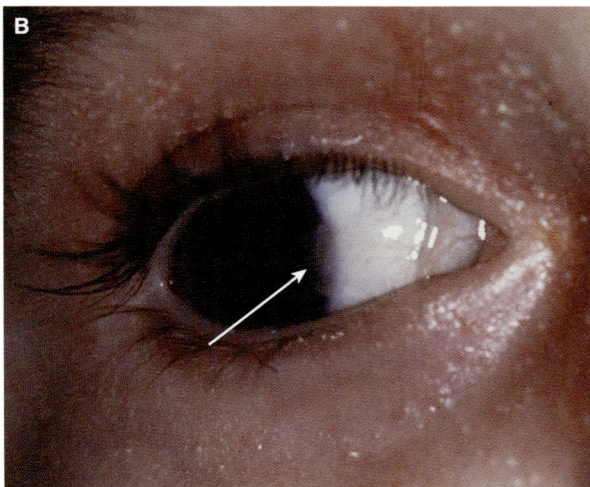

FIGURE 25–37 ■ Epidermolysis bullosa. (A) Periocular skin changes. (B) Peripheral corneal opacity (arrow).

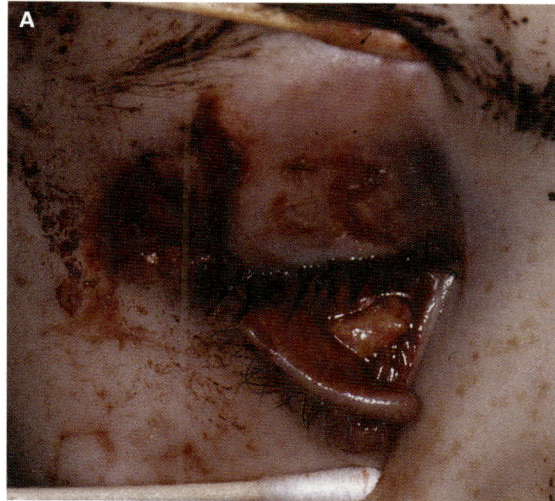

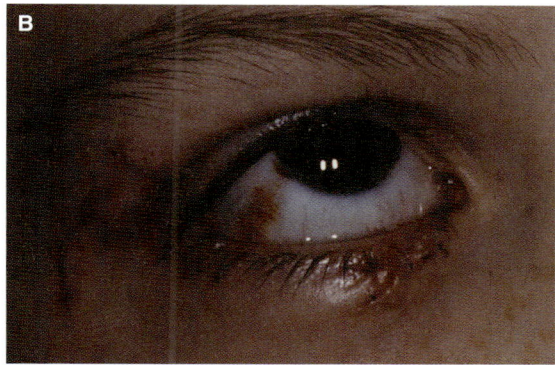

FIGURE 25–38 ■ (A) Severe eyelid laceration involving upper and lower eyelids. (B) Two weeks following surgical repair.

patients present with this type of trauma, it is important to search for associated injuries, such as orbital fractures, ocular lacerations, or hyphemas.

Lacerations of the eyelids require careful surgical repair. It is important to restore the normal shape of the eyelid and its apposition to the eyeball (Figure 25–38A and B). If this is not done, the patient may develop ocular irritation due to the eyelid rubbing against the eyeball, or abnormal tearing due to laxity of the eyelid.

Cyanoacrylate

Children occasionally will rub their eyes after using cyanoacrylate (Super-glue), causing the eyelashes to stick together (Figure 25–39). This is not painful unless an uneven surface is present on the inner eyelid. Conservative treatment with warm compresses and ocular lubricants may be used if the patient does not have eye pain. The eyelids usually spontaneously separate within 1 to 2 weeks. If pain is present, the eyelids may need to be separated to examine the eye.

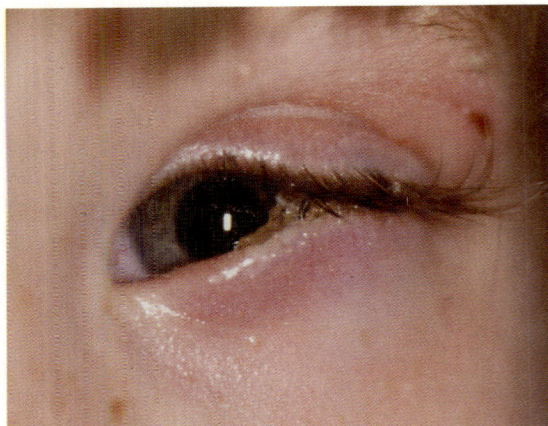

FIGURE 25-39 ■ Lateral eyelids stuck together by cyanoacrylate adhesive.

REFERENCES

1. Anderson RL, Baumgartner SA. Amblyopia in ptosis. *Arch Ophthalmol*. 1980;98:1068–1069.
2. Seiff SR, Boerner M, Carter SR. Treatment of facial palsies with external eyelid weights. *Am J Ophthalmol*. 1995; 120:652–657.
3. Jeong S, Park HJ, Park YG. Surgical correction of congenital epiblepharon: low eyelid crease reforming technique. *J Pediatr Ophthalmol Strabismus*. 2001;38:356–358.
4. Mawn LA, Jordan DR. Trichotillomania. *Ophthalmology*. 1997;104:2175–2178.

CHAPTER 26

Disorders of the Orbit

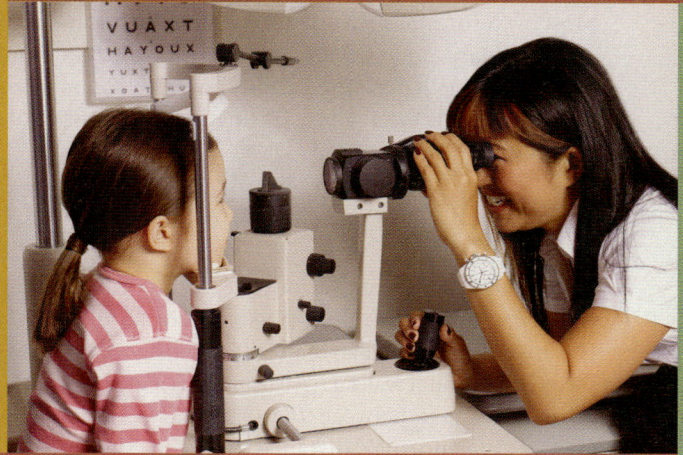

ANATOMY AND EMBRYOLOGY

The orbit is the space in the skull in which the eye and extraocular muscles are located. It is cone-shaped, widest anteriorly and tapering to the orbital apex, through which the optic nerve passes. The orbits are demarcated by the bones of the skull (Figure 26–1). The roof consists of a portion of the frontal bone and the lesser wing of the sphenoid bone. The frontal lobes of the brain lie above this area. The medial orbital wall is composed of the lacrimal bone and portions of the ethmoid, maxilla, and sphenoid bones. The ethmoid sinuses are adjacent to this wall. The floor of the orbit is composed of the maxilla and a portion of the zygomatic bone. It lies above the maxillary sinus. The lateral wall is formed by the zygomatic bone and the greater wing of the sphenoid.

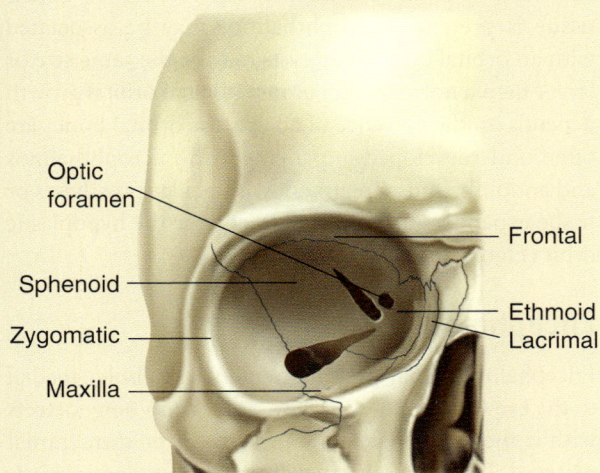

Openings in the orbit allow for passage of other structures (Figure 26–2). The optic nerve, ophthalmic artery, and sympathetic fibers pass through the optic foramen posteriorly at the apex of the orbit. Cranial nerves III, IV, and VI, and portions of cranial nerve V travel through the superior orbital fissure. The infraorbital nerve (a branch of cranial nerve V) is transmitted through the infraorbital fissure.

All of the extraocular muscles except the inferior oblique muscle arise at the annulus of Zinn at the apex of the orbit and extend anteriorly to insert on the globe. A layer of connective tissue joins these muscles to form a cone-shaped space. Orbital disorders may be classified as *intraconal* (within this group of muscles) or *extraconal* (outside of the muscle cone but still within the orbit). The orbital septum lies beneath the orbicularis muscle, and separates the orbit into the *preseptal* and *postseptal* spaces. The lacrimal gland is located in the lacrimal fossa in the superolateral portion of the orbit.

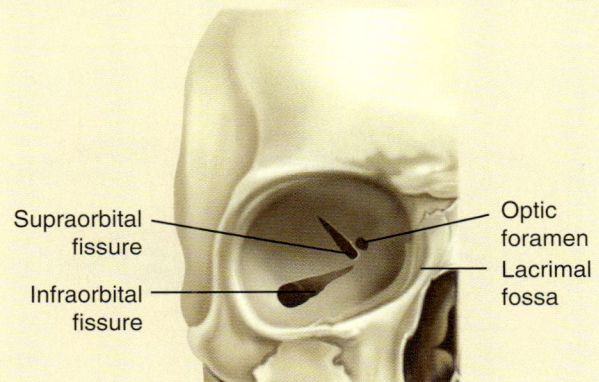

FIGURE 26–1 ■ The orbit is delineated by the cranial bones that surround it.

FIGURE 26–2 ■ The posterior orbital openings, through which the optic nerve, blood vessels, and nerves pass (see text).

Embryology

Most of the orbital structures arise from the frontonasal and maxillary processes of neural crest cells that surround the optic cups. The various bones that comprise the orbital walls usually fuse during the sixth month of gestation.

DEFINITIONS

Measurements between various eyelid and ocular structures may be used to describe some orbital disorders. *Hypotelorism* is a smaller-than-normal distance between the medial orbital walls. *Hypertelorism* is a greater-than-normal distance between the orbits. *Telecanthus* is a greater-than-normal distance between the medial canthi. In telecanthus, the orbits themselves are often normal (Figure 26–3).

Orbital disorders are uncommon in children. The most frequent abnormalities are discussed in this chapter. There are a large number of rare entities that can affect the orbit, which are beyond the scope of this text.

PATHOGENESIS

Orbital disorders may arise from a variety of conditions, including congenital anomalies, trauma, infections, tumors, vascular and lymphatic malformations, and inflammatory conditions. Because the orbit is demarcated by bony structures, space-occupying lesions can create problems either by causing forward displacement of the eyeball (*proptosis*) or by compression of vital structures, most importantly the optic nerve.

CLINICAL PRESENTATION

Orbital problems are most commonly identified by proptosis, in which the globe is displaced anteriorly and appears to bulge from the socket. As the eyeball moves

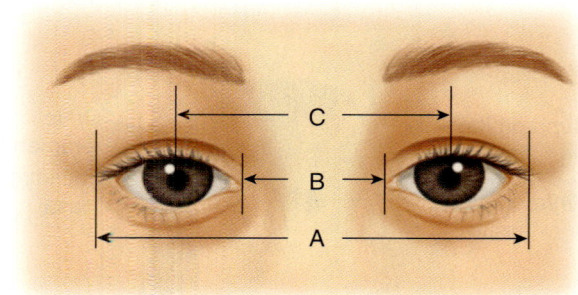

FIGURE 26–3 ■ Orbital measurements. (A) Outer canthal distance. (B) Inner canthal distance. (C) Interpupillary distance.

forward, the eyelids are displaced, which can give the clinical appearance of eyelid retraction, in which the sclera is visible between the upper and lower eyelid and the cornea. In some patients the asymmetric appearance of the eyes may be mistakenly interpreted as ptosis of the normal eye. In some conditions, particularly traumatic fractures, the eye may be displaced posteriorly (enophthalmos) and appear sunken-in. In inflammatory and infectious processes, the periocular area may become erythematous and edematous. The presence of pain is variable, and this symptom may be helpful in establishing a diagnosis.

If proptosis progresses, patients develop signs and symptoms of corneal exposure due to incomplete coverage of the eye by the stretched eyelids. These symptoms include ocular redness, light sensitivity, and foreign body sensation. If the extraocular muscles are involved, patients develop strabismus and diplopia. If the optic nerve is compressed, vision may decrease.

CONGENITAL ANOMALIES

Craniofacial Malformations

Many craniofacial malformations have associated orbital findings. In most, the orbit is shallow and the eye appears protuberant. Disorders secondary to *craniosynostosis* include *Crouzon, Apert, Pfeiffer, and Saethre-Chotzen syndromes*. The most common ocular problems associated with craniosynostosis syndromes are corneal exposure and strabismus (Figure 26–4A and B). Compression of the optic nerve may also occur.

Anophthalmos and Microphthalmos

In these disorders the eye is underdeveloped (microphthalmos) or absent (anophthalmos). True anophthalmos is very rare. In most cases at least some vestige of ocular tissue is present. Microphthalmos may be associated with an orbital cyst. These cysts may be the same size or larger than a normal eye. Because normal orbital growth depends on the presence of an eye, the orbital bones are often underdeveloped in patients with microphthalmos and anophthalmos. Treatment with ocular prostheses or tissue expanders may be used to enlarge the hypoplastic orbit (Figure 26–5).[1]

Encephalocele

Encephaloceles may present in infancy as a bulge medial to the eye (Figure 26–6). These result from bony defects within the skull that allow protrusion of intracranial material. They may superficially appear similar to infantile mucoceles. Encephaloceles can be distinguished from mucoceles by their location above the medial

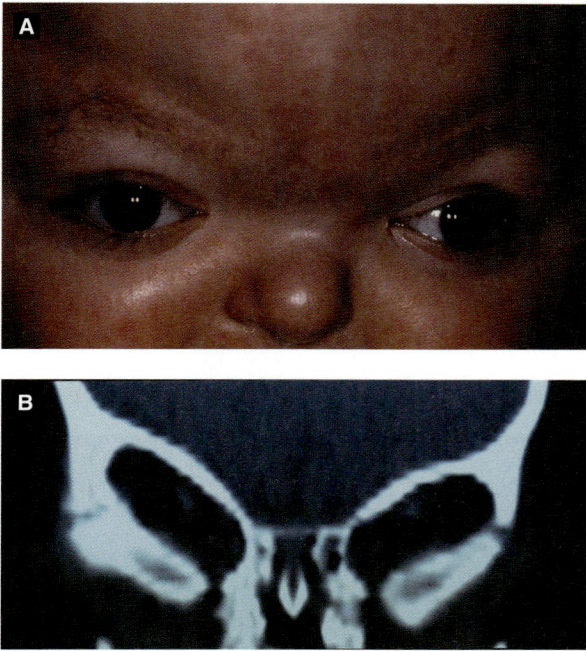

FIGURE 26–4 ■ Apert syndrome. (A) Note hypertelorism, mild proptosis, and strabismus (left exotropia). (B) Computed tomography showing markedly abnormal shape of orbits.

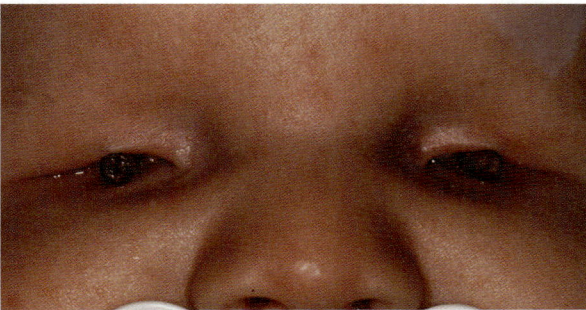

FIGURE 26–5 ■ Bilateral severe microphthalmos. Conformers are in place to increase growth of the orbit.

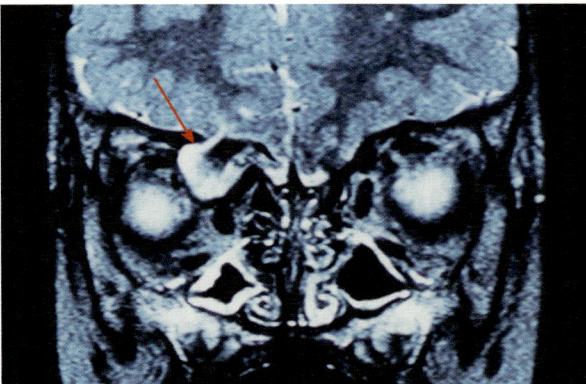

FIGURE 26–6 ■ Magnetic resonance image of right superior orbital encephalocele (arrow).

canthus, noninflamed appearance, and frequent presence of visible pulsations within the lesion (due to transmission of intracranial pressure).

TRAUMA

Blunt Orbital Trauma

Blunt trauma to the eye may cause fractures of the orbital bones. Major trauma, such as a motor vehicle accident, can cause multiple fractures. The most common injuries result from direct trauma to the ocular area. The bony rims of the orbit extend beyond the eyeball itself, and therefore the globe is relatively protected from blunt injuries with large objects. Smaller objects, such as fists or small balls, may impact the globe directly. Transmission of the force from such an impact, or by direct trauma to the inferior orbital rim, may cause a *blowout fracture*, in which the floor of the orbit is fractured. This may cause herniation of the extraocular muscles or the globe through the fracture.

Presentation of blunt orbital trauma

Patients with orbital trauma usually present with periocular edema and ecchymosis. Specific clinical signs of blowout fracture include enophthalmos (the eye appears sunken in the orbit) and strabismus. Strabismus most commonly results from restriction of the inferior rectus muscle, which limits elevation of the eye (Figure 26–7A and B).

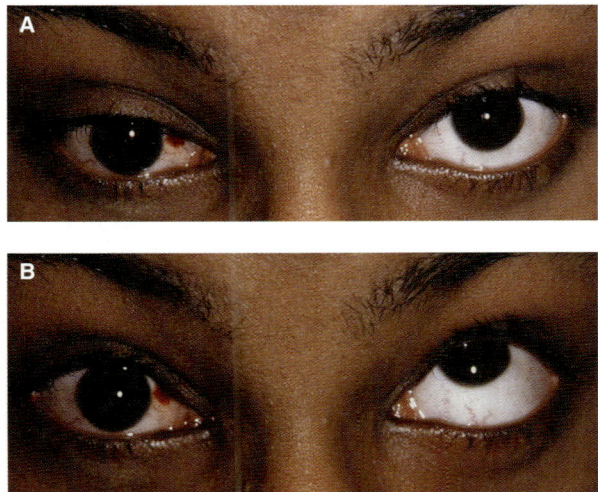

FIGURE 26–7 ■ Ocular motility in orbital blowout fracture, right eye. (A) The right eye is lower than the left eye when looking straight ahead. Note conjunctival injection and subconjunctival hemorrhage on right. (B) Right eye cannot elevate in attempted upgaze (left eye is elevating normally).

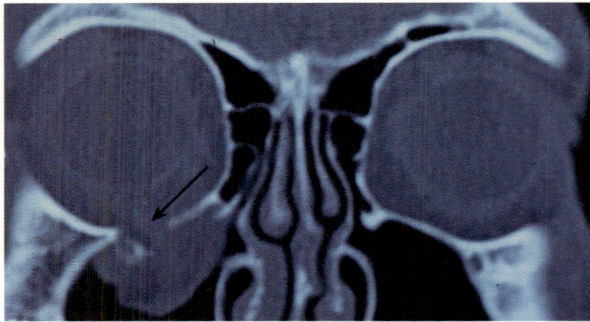

FIGURE 26-8 ■ Computed tomography, right orbital blowout fracture. There is a fracture of the right orbital floor (arrow), with intraorbital contents extending into the maxillary sinus.

Extraocular muscles that have limited movement can be assessed with *forced ductions*, in which the eye is grasped with forceps (after instillation of a topical anesthetic) and moved by the examiner. An inability to move the eye suggests entrapment. In the early posttraumatic period, however, edema of the muscle may also cause some limitation of forced ductions. If the eye moves freely with forced ductions, but does not function normally, then the movement abnormality is likely due to damage to the nerve that supplies the muscle. A diagnosis of entrapment can be confirmed by imaging studies, most commonly computed tomography (Figure 26–8). Children with orbital trauma should be examined for associated ocular injuries.

Treatment of blunt orbital trauma

Treatment of small, nondisplaced fractures is usually not necessary. Surgical repair is indicated if there is radiographic evidence of entrapment and significant enophthalmos or strabismus. In most cases surgery is delayed 1 to 2 weeks to allow edema to decrease and to determine whether the strabismus improves (which can occur due to reduction of muscle edema or hemorrhage).

An important exception requiring early treatment in children is the *white-eyed blowout fracture*, in which the inferior rectus muscle becomes entrapped in the orbital floor fracture. These patients have only mild periocular signs of trauma. They are unable to elevate their eyes. They often experience nausea or bradycardia when they attempt to do so, due to the oculocardiac reflex. Urgent repair is indicated in patients with white-eyed blowout fractures due to the risk of muscle necrosis.[2]

Orbital Hemorrhage

Trauma to the orbit may cause retro-orbital hemorrhage. If the hemorrhage is large enough, patients may

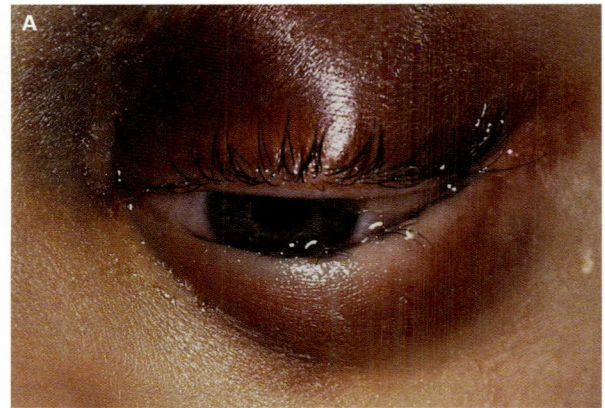

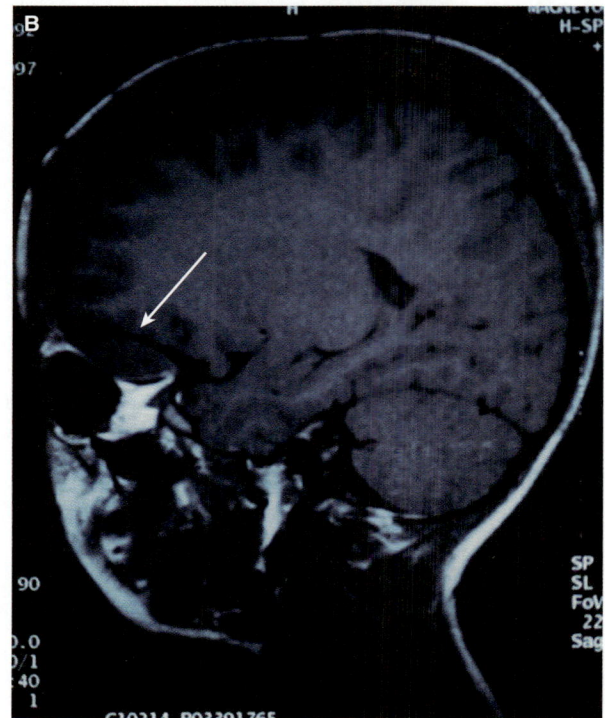

FIGURE 26-9 ■ Orbital hemorrhage following mild blunt trauma in a patient with factor IX deficiency. (A) Proptosis and marked periocular ecchymosis. (B) Magnetic resonance imaging shows superior subperiosteal (arrow) and subdural hemorrhage. (Figures A and B are reprinted with permission from Guirgis MF, Segal WA, Lueder GT. Subperiosteal orbital hemorrhage as initial manifestation of Christmas disease [factor IX deficiency]. *Am J Ophthalmol.* 2002;133(4): 584–585. Copyright Elsevier.)

present with proptosis and periocular ecchymosis (Figure 26–9A). In severe cases limited extraocular movements and decreased vision may also be present. The diagnosis is confirmed by the history and imaging findings (Figure 26–9B). Small hemorrhages may resolve spontaneously. Larger hemorrhages that cause significant proptosis, diplopia, or impair vision require surgical drainage. Rarely, orbital hemorrhage following relatively minor trauma may be the initial manifestation of a bleeding disorder (Figure 26–9).

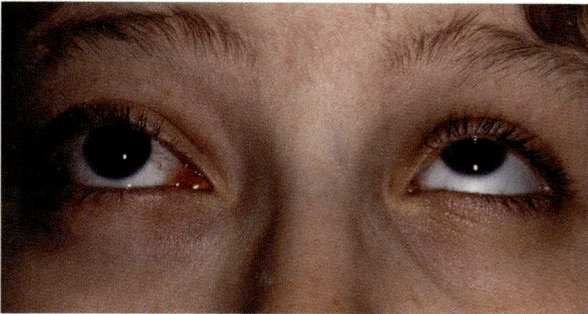

FIGURE 26-10 ■ Right proptosis and limited elevation secondary to orbital rhabdomyosarcoma. The left eye is elevating normally. Note stretched appearance of right lower eyelid.

ORBITAL MALIGNANCIES

Rhabdomyosarcoma

Rhabdomyosarcoma (RMS) is the most common primary orbital tumor in childhood. The orbit is the primary tumor location in approximately 10% of patients. RMS arises from mesenchymal cells. It may develop at any age, but is most common between 5 and 10 years. The classic presentation is rapid painless proptosis (Figure 26–10). Edema and palpable masses are sometimes present. Lesions may be visible on the conjunctiva (Figure 26–11). Imaging studies are performed to evaluate the extent of the lesion (Figure 26–12).

The diagnosis of RMS is confirmed by biopsy. The prognosis is dependent on the extent of the disease and the histopathological type. Embryonal tumors are the

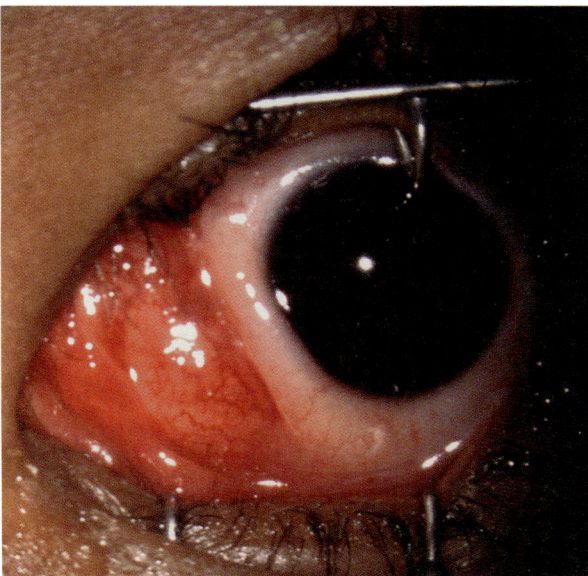

FIGURE 26-12 ■ Magnetic resonance image of right inferior orbital rhabdomyosarcoma (arrow) (same patient as Figure 26–10).

most common type of orbital RMS in children. Their prognosis is good. The alveolar type is less common and has the worst prognosis. The pleomorphic type is the least common and has the best prognosis. Treatment usually consists of chemotherapy and radiation.

Metastatic Orbital Tumors

The orbit is a site of metastases for many neoplasms. The most common metastatic orbital tumor in children is *neuroblastoma*. Orbital involvement occurs in approximately 20% of children with this tumor. The primary tumor in young children usually arises in the adrenal glands or in the sympathetic ganglion. In addition to proptosis, the presence of periocular ecchymosis is highly suggestive of neuroblastoma (Figure 26–13). Other ocular manifestations of neuroblastoma include

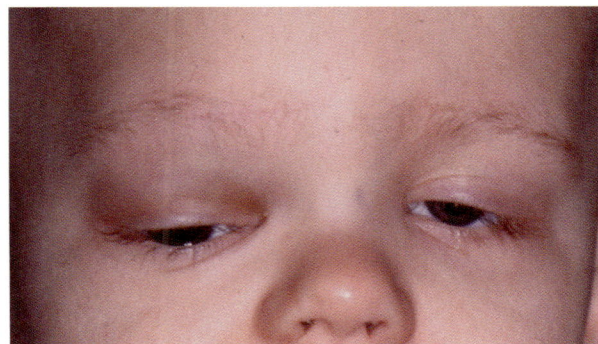

FIGURE 26-11 ■ Orbital rhabdomyosarcoma extending onto conjunctival surface.

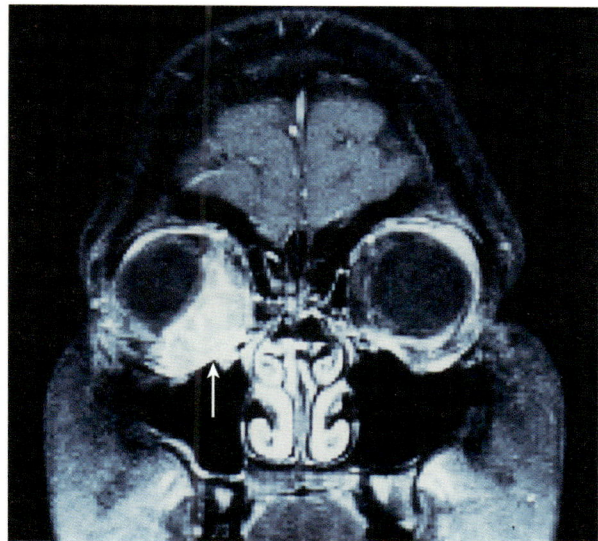

FIGURE 26-13 ■ Right upper eyelid ecchymosis and downward displacement of right eye secondary to metastatic neuroblastoma in right orbit.

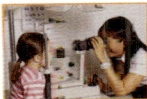

Table 26–1.

Orbital Tumors in Children

- Rhabdomyosarcoma
- Neuroblastoma
- Leukemia
- Lymphoma
- Langerhans cell histiocytosis
- Eosinophilic granuloma
- Osteogenic sarcoma
- Fibrous histiocytoma
- Ewing sarcoma

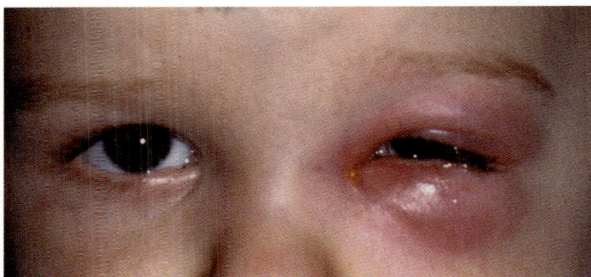

FIGURE 26–15 ■ Preseptal cellulitis that progressed to an eyelid abscess despite treatment with antibiotics. Culture of material obtained during surgical drainage revealed methicillin-resistant *Staphylococcus aureus*.

Horner syndrome and *opsoclonus*. Opsoclonus is an unusual motility abnormality characterized by irregular, rapid, multidirectional eye movements. The diagnosis of neuroblastoma is established by biopsy. The tumor is difficult to treat, with a poor prognosis despite radiation and chemotherapy.

Many other tumors may occur in the orbit, including leukemia and Langerhans cell histiocytosis (Table 26–1).

INFECTIONS

Preseptal Cellulitis

Periorbital infections are separated into those that are limited to the structures anterior to the orbital septum (preseptal cellulitis) and those that affect structures posterior to the septum (orbital cellulitis). Preseptal cellulitis is a fairly common infection of children. It is characterized by inflammation, erythema, and edema of the eyelids (Figure 26–14). The eyeball itself is not affected. Preseptal cellulitis most commonly arises from skin trauma (e.g., an abrasion or insect bite) or in association with upper respiratory or sinus infections. The most common pathogens are staphylococcal or streptococcal species.

Treatment of preseptal cellulitis

Outpatient treatment with a broad-spectrum antibiotic such as ampicillin-clavulanic acid or a cephalosporin is appropriate for mild cases. Patients with infections that progress despite oral antibiotics may require hospitalization for intravenous antibiotics. Infections due to methicillin-resistant staphylococci should be suspected if the infection does not respond to standard antibiotic treatment (Figure 26–15).

Orbital Cellulitis

Infections posterior to the orbital septum are a much more serious problem, with the potential for vision-threatening complications. Orbital cellulitis in children most commonly arises from contiguous spread of infection from infected sinuses. It may also occur following trauma. Clinically, the symptoms include those of preseptal cellulitis, but patients also show signs of orbital involvement (Figure 26–16). These include proptosis, limitation

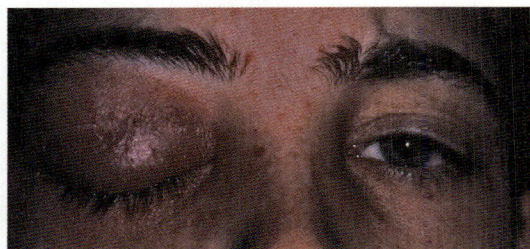

FIGURE 26–14 ■ Preseptal cellulitis. Marked erythema and edema of left periocular skin.

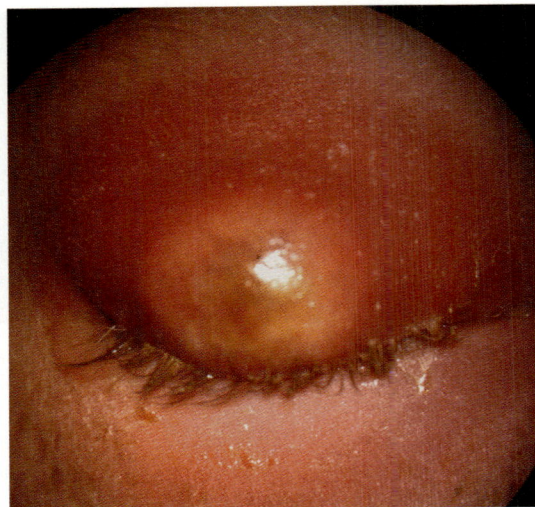

FIGURE 26–16 ■ Edema, erythema, and ptosis of right eyelid secondary to orbital cellulitis.

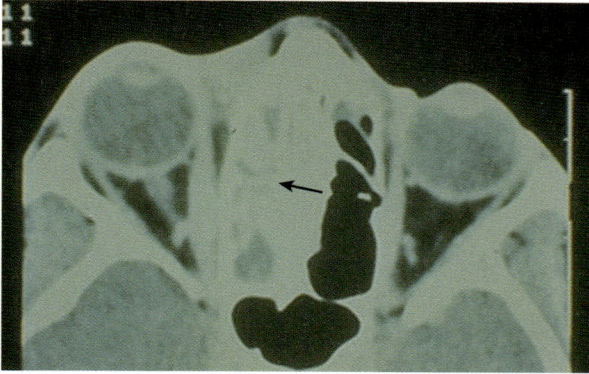

FIGURE 26–17 ■ Orbital computed tomography, orbital cellulitis. Note proptosis and marked opacification of adjacent right ethmoid sinuses (arrow).

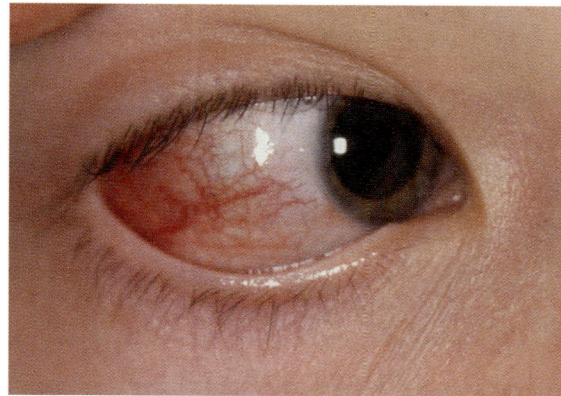

FIGURE 26–18 ■ Orbital myositis (pseudotumor). Note conjunctival erythema and edema overlying right lateral rectus muscle.

of extraocular movements, abnormal pupil responses, and decreased vision. Systemic symptoms, including fever and lethargy, are common. The most common pathogens are similar to those in preseptal cellulitis (streptococcal and staphylococcal species). Older children may have mixed infections, including anaerobes.

Treatment of orbital cellulitis

Prompt treatment with intravenous antibiotics is indicated to minimize the risk of sight-threatening complications. Imaging studies of the orbit are indicated. They frequently show contiguous sinus disease (Figure 26–17). A common finding in children with orbital cellulitis is a subperiosteal abscess. These abscess are unusual in that they may respond to medical treatment alone in some patients. Intravenous antibiotics should be the initial treatment in children younger than 9 years of age whose abscess are isolated to the medial or inferior periosteum and who have contiguous ethmoid sinusitis. Surgical drainage is indicated in older children and in younger children whose abscesses do not improve after 48 to 72 hours of intravenous antibiotic treatment.[3] Immediate drainage is necessary in patients whose vision is acutely threatened (due to optic nerve compression). Otolaryngological consultation is usually indicated to assist with the management of sinus disease.

INFLAMMATION

Orbital Pseudotumor (Idiopathic Orbital Inflammation; Myositis)

This is an idiopathic condition characterized by unilateral or bilateral inflammation of orbital tissue and extraocular muscles. It usually presents with the rapid onset of marked periocular pain, accompanied by proptosis and inflammation of the eye and eyelid tissue.

Systemic symptoms of lethargy and fever are common. The appearance is similar to that seen in orbital cellulitis or a rapidly growing orbital mass (such as tumor or bleeding within a lymphangioma). Focal erythema and inflammation overlying the extraocular muscle insertions are frequently seen (Figure 26–18). The presence of pain that is out of proportion to the physical findings is suggestive of orbital pseudotumor. Imaging studies may show thickening of the sclera and enlargement of the extraocular muscles, and are useful in ruling out orbital masses or abscesses. Acute thyroid eye disease (see below) may sometimes present in a similar fashion. An imaging finding that may help distinguish these entities is the extent of enlargement of the extraocular muscles. In patients with orbital pseudotumor this often extends to the eyeball itself due to involvement of the muscle tendon, whereas the thickening seen in thyroid disease is limited to the muscle itself (Figure 26–19A and B).

Treatment of orbital pseudotumor

Orbital pseudotumor characteristically responds very rapidly to oral corticosteroids, which is helpful in establishing a diagnosis. Most patients experience a marked reduction in symptoms within 12 to 24 hours. Biopsy is usually not necessary in patients who have typical clinical and radiographic findings and who demonstrate this rapid response. However, some tumors and other inflammatory conditions may also respond to corticosteroids, and biopsy may be necessary if the diagnosis is in doubt. Patients with orbital pseudotumor usually require prolonged treatment with corticosteroids, and relapses may occur when the medication is tapered.

Thyroid Eye Disease (Graves Disease)

Thyroid eye disease is much less common in children than in adults. It is characterized by autoimmune thickening of the extraocular muscles. Ocular symptoms include

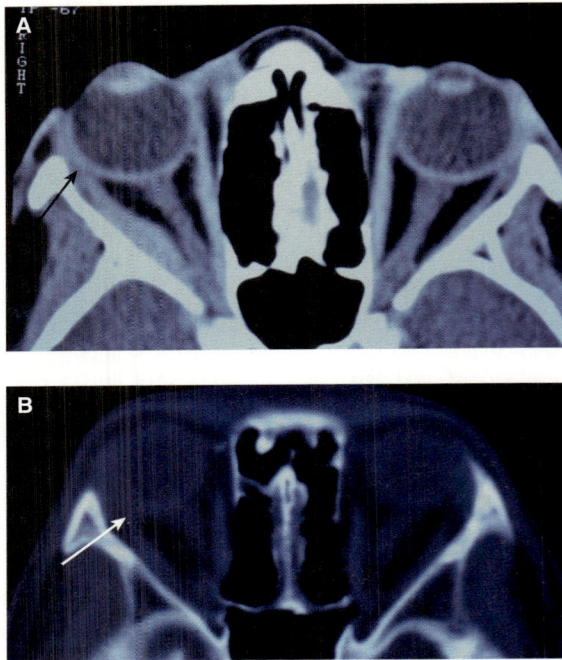

FIGURE 26–19 ■ Differentiating orbital pseudotumor and thyroid ophthalmolopathy (Graves disease) by imaging. (A) Orbital pseudotumor: thickening of right lateral rectus muscle extends through the tendon to insertion of muscle on globe (arrow). (B) Thyroid ophthalmopathy: thickening of muscle limited to the muscle itself and stops (arrow) before insertion of muscle on globe. Note also that the medial and lateral rectus muscles in both orbits are thickened in thyroid disease, compared with normal muscles other than the right lateral rectus muscle in orbital myositis.

proptosis, strabismus, eyelid retraction, corneal exposure, and compression of the optic nerve. The ocular symptoms do not necessarily correlate with the systemic disease, and ocular symptoms may progress despite successful systemic treatment. In severe cases, orbital decompression may be indicated. In this procedure portions of the bony orbital wall are removed to decrease congestion within the orbit.

VASCULAR AND LYMPHATIC MALFORMATIONS

Capillary Hemangioma

Capillary hemangiomas are benign proliferations of capillaries that develop in the neonatal period. The most common ocular problem associated with hemangiomas is periocular involvement of either the eyelids or orbit. Lesions that develop on the eyelids usually appear within the first 1 to 2 weeks of life, gradually enlarge over the next few months (Figure 26–20), stop growing, then gradually regress during the first 4 to 5 years of life. Hemangiomas that develop primarily in the orbit usually do not become clinically evident until 1 to 2 months of age, because they must grow large enough to produce

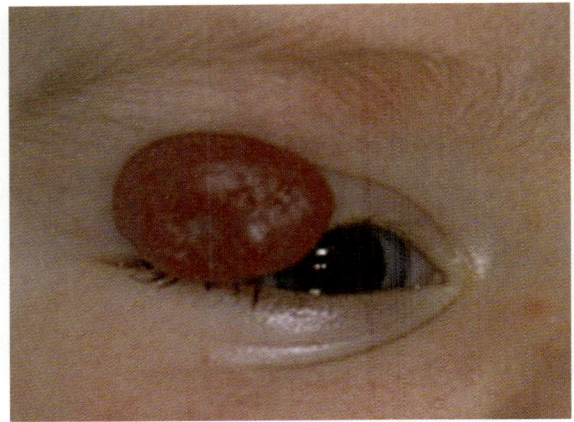

FIGURE 26–20 ■ Hemangioma, right upper eyelid, causing amblyopia both by obstructing vision and inducing astigmatism.

visible abnormalities. They commonly present with proptosis or a subcutaneous mass (Figure 26–21A and B).

Although capillary hemangiomas are histologically benign, they have the potential to affect vision. The infant's eye is particularly susceptible to amblyopia due to unilateral visual problems, which may occur in hemangiomas either due to direct obstruction of vision, or more subtly by inducing astigmatism by pressure on the globe (Figure 26–20). The diagnosis of superficial capillary hemangiomas is usually readily made by their vascular appearance. In deeper lesions, the vascular

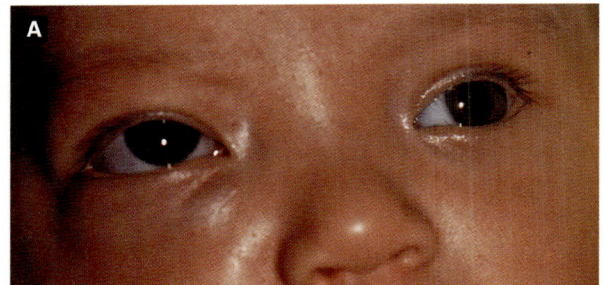

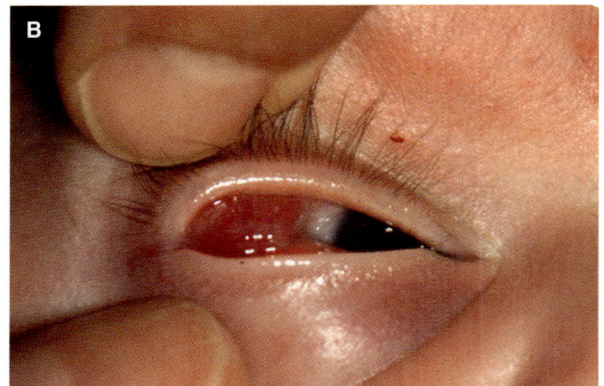

FIGURE 26–21 ■ Right orbital capillary hemangioma. (A) Right proptosis, upward displacement of globe, and discoloration of lower eyelid. (B) Vascular lesion visible in right lateral conjunctiva.

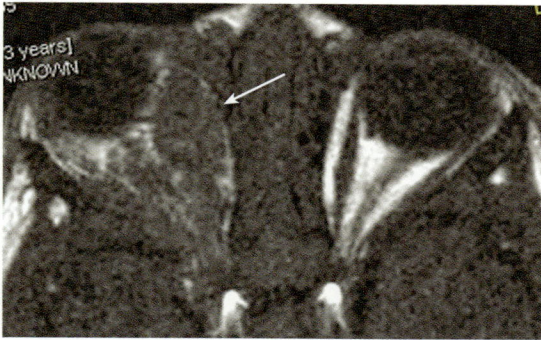

FIGURE 26–22 ■ Hemangioma. Magnetic resonance image showing large lesion in right medial orbit (arrow).

characteristics may not be readily apparent. Because of this, orbital lesions may require imaging studies or biopsy for confirmation (Figure 26–22).

Treatment of periocular hemangiomas

If periocular hemangiomas do not cause vision problems, treatment is usually not necessary because most hemangiomas will ultimately regress spontaneously. If the lesions are amblyogenic, treatment is indicated. In the past, this usually consisted of topical, oral, or local injections of corticosteroids (Figure 26–23). Surgical treatment of superficial lesions can also be effective (Figure 26–24A and B). The recent introduction of systemic propranolol has proven remarkably effective in the management of this disorder.[4]

Lymphangioma

Lymphangiomas are abnormal lymphatic structures that develop in the orbit. They are present at birth and may cause neonatal proptosis. More commonly they do not become clinically evident until later in childhood. Forward extension of the lymphatic structures may present as cystic-appearing lesions on the conjunctiva (Figure 26–25). Lymphangiomas may enlarge

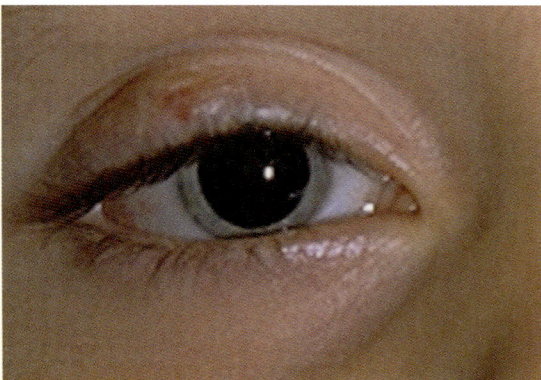

FIGURE 26–24 ■ Hemangioma, left upper eyelid. (A) Preoperative appearance. (B) Three months following surgical excision.

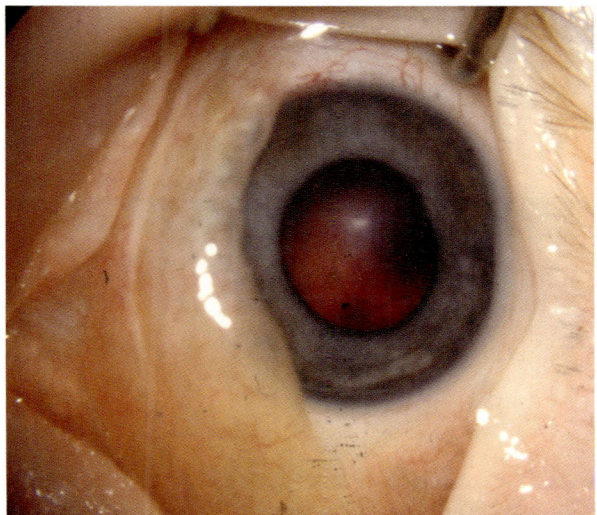

FIGURE 26–23 ■ Hemangioma, same patient as Figure 26–20, 5 years after corticosteroid injection.

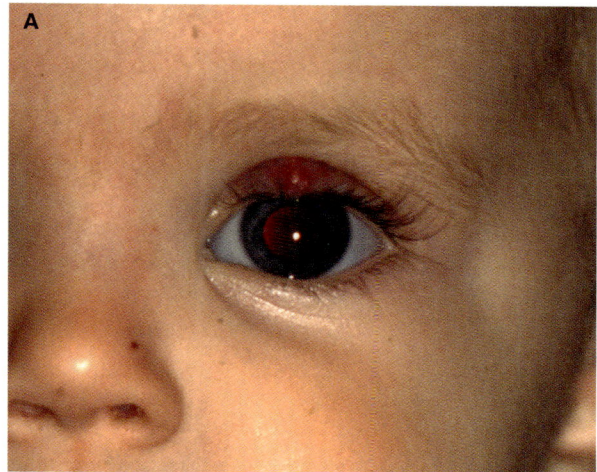

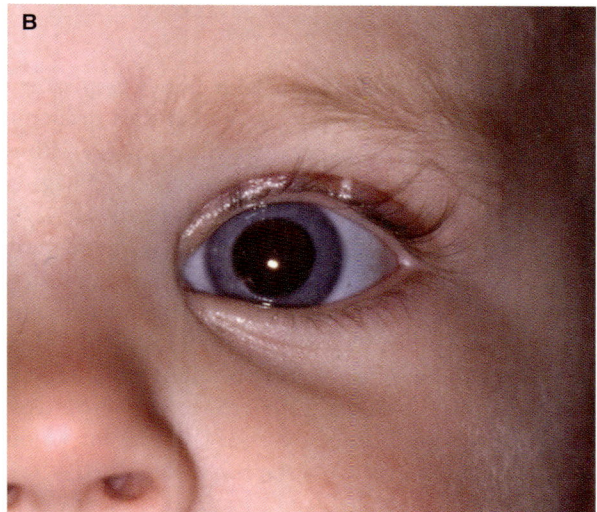

FIGURE 26–25 ■ Orbital lymphangioma extending onto medial conjunctiva.

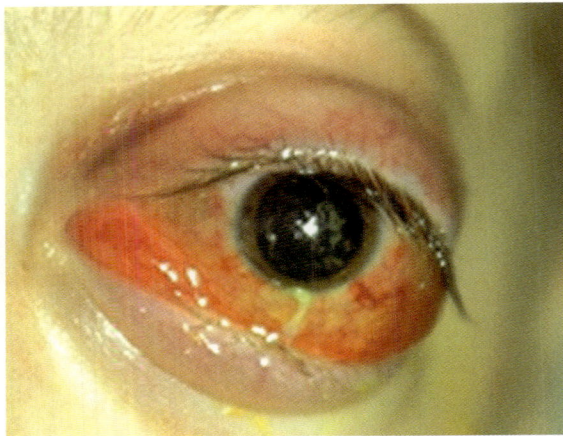

FIGURE 26–26 ■ Marked proptosis due to hemorrhage within orbital lymphangioma.

FIGURE 26–28 ■ Orbital varix, left eye. (A) Mild proptosis, left eye (note asymmetry of upper eyelids). (B) Increased proptosis visible during Valsalva maneuver.

intermittently in association with upper respiratory infections. Orbital lesions may present in a dramatic fashion with rapid proptosis due to hemorrhage within the lesion (chocolate cyst) (Figure 26–26). Imaging studies reveal a cystic orbital lesion (Figure 26–27). Fluid levels are sometimes present due to the hemorrhage. In most instances surgery on lymphangiomas is not recommended because the lesions insinuate themselves within other vital structures within the orbit. This creates a high risk of complications with surgical resection. With marked hemorrhage and proptosis, surgical drainage may be necessary to prevent vision loss, or to obtain tissue to establish a diagnosis.

Orbital Varix

Orbital varices are uncommon venous malformations that enlarge with Valsalva maneuvers, producing intermittent proptosis (Figure 26–28A and B). The diagnosis is established by a characteristic history, clinical findings, and imaging. Small areas of calcification (phleboliths) are a common radiographic finding. Similar to lymphangiomas, treatment is complicated by the inter-

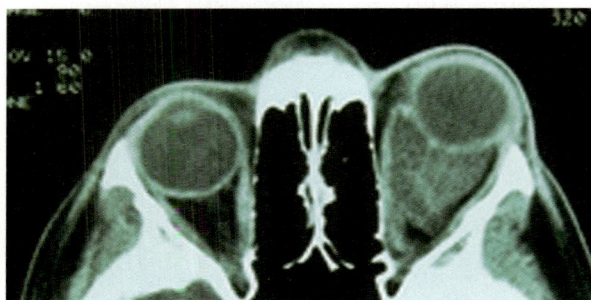

twining of the varix with normal tissues. In severe cases in which vision is threatened, embolization with or without surgical resection may be indicated.

OTHER ORBITAL LESIONS

Orbital Dermoid

Orbital dermoids are one of the most common orbital lesions in childhood. They develop due to sequestration of tissue within cranial sutures during embryonic development. Histologically, they are choristomatous cysts that have keratinized epithelial linings and dermal elements such as hair, sweat glands, and sebaceous glands. Clinically, they are smooth, whitish-yellow lesions that may have hair on the surface. They most commonly develop in the superolateral orbit and present clinically as slightly mobile cystic lesions in this location (Figure 26–29). They may also develop superonasally in

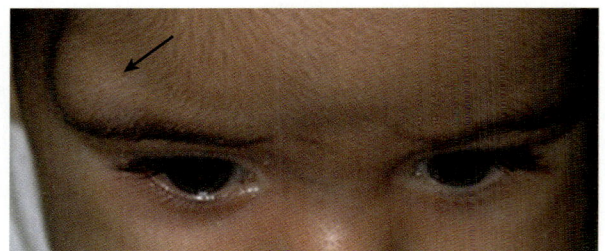

FIGURE 26–27 ■ Orbital lymphangioma following hemorrhage. Computed tomography shows marked proptosis of left globe and cystic appearance of orbital lesion.

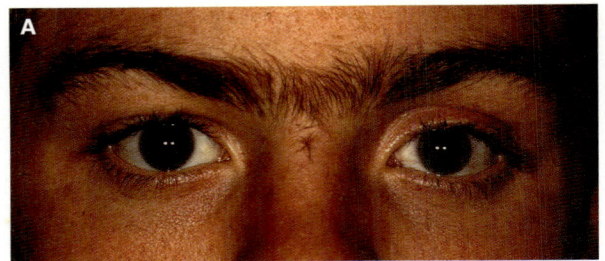

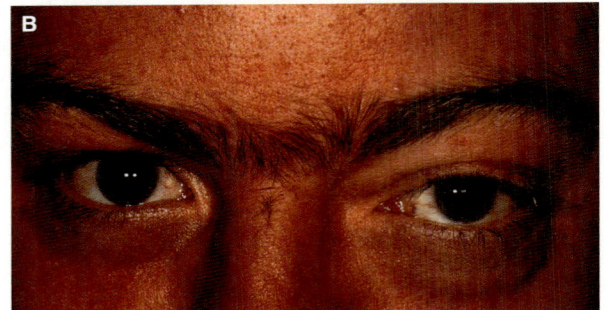

FIGURE 26–29 ■ Orbital dermoid cyst, right superolateral orbit (arrow).

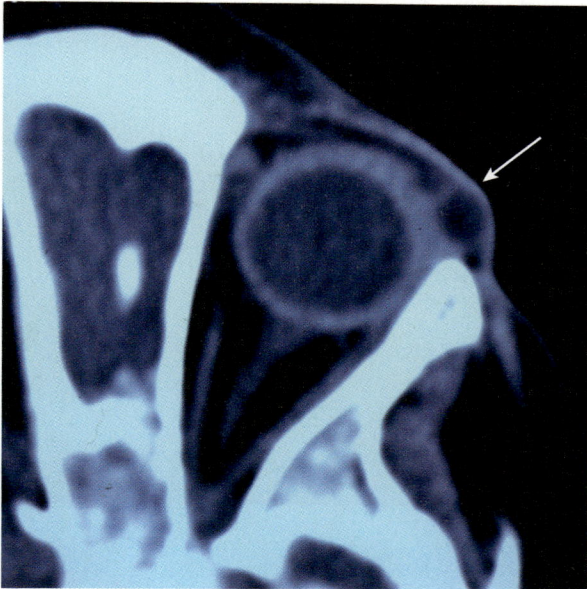

FIGURE 26–30 ■ Computed tomography, right orbital dermoid cyst (arrow).

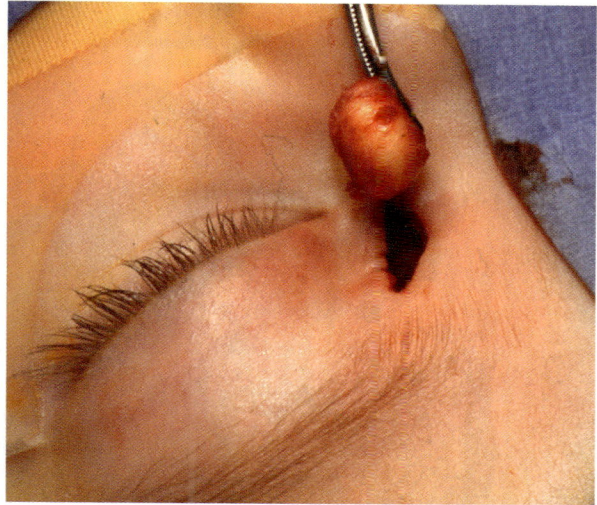

FIGURE 26–31 ■ Medial orbital dermoid cyst excision. Note yellow, smooth, cystic apperance of lesion.

the orbit, or rarely within the orbit itself, in which case they may present with proptosis. The material within the cyst may elicit an inflammatory response if traumatic rupture occurs. Imaging studies reveal a characteristic cystic appearance (Figure 26–30), but these are often not necessary if the clinical examination is typical. Surgical excision is usually recommended to remove the lesion before further growth, verify the diagnosis, and prevent potential complications due to traumatic rupture and inflammation (Figure 26–31).

Teratoma

Teratomas are rare orbital lesions that may present with marked proptosis in the neonatal period. Histologically they contain a mixture of ectodermal, endodermal, and mesodermal tissues. They are usually benign histologically, but surgical excision is normally required due to marked disfigurement. The visual prognosis is poor.

REFERENCES

1. Gossman MD, Mohay J, Roberts DM. Expansion of the human microphthalmic orbit. *Ophthalmology*. 1999;106: 2005–2009.
2. Burnstine MA. Clinical recommendations for repair of isolated orbital floor fractures: an evidence-based analysis. *Ophthalmology*. 2002;109:1207–1213.
3. Garcia GH, Harris GJ. Criteria for nonsurgical management of subperiosteal abscess of the orbit. *Ophthalmology*. 2000;107:1454–1458.
4. Léauté-Labrèze C, Dumas de la Roque E, Hubiche T, Boralevi F, Thambo JB, Taïeb A. Propranolol for severe hemangiomas of infancy. *N Engl J Med*. 2008;358: 2649–2651.

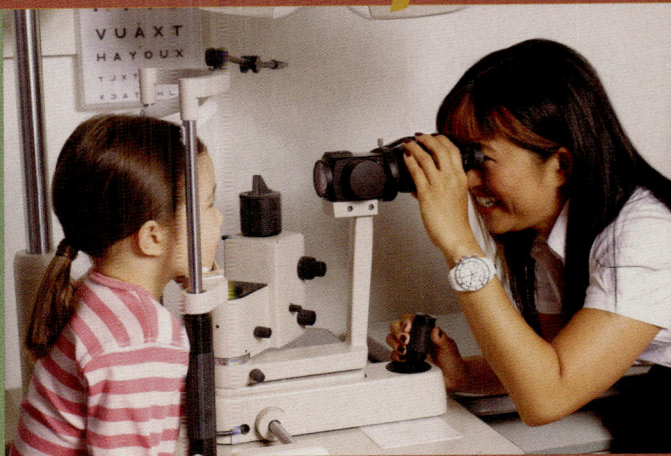

CHAPTER 27

Diseases of the Conjunctiva

DEFINITIONS AND EPIDEMIOLOGY

The conjunctiva is the clear layer of tissue that lines the inner eyelids (*tarsal or palpebral conjunctiva*) and the eyeball itself (*bulbar conjunctiva*). It extends from the eyelid margin to the edge of the cornea. Histologically, the conjunctiva is composed of an epithelial layer that contains goblet cells, a substantia propria layer that contains lymphatic vessels, and a lymphoid layer that is active in generating immune responses. The conjunctiva is normally clear, with a few visible blood vessels supplied by the anterior ciliary artery. The vessels become dilated when they are irritated (blood-shot eyes).

The conjunctiva is important in maintaining a normal tear film in the eye. The tears are composed of 3 layers (Figure 27–1). The bulk of the tear film is composed of the *liquid aqueous layer*, which is secreted by the lacrimal glands. The external surface of the tear film is composed of the *lipid layer*. This layer is formed by lipids secreted by the meibomian glands in the eyelids. The lipid layer maintains stability of the tear film and retards evaporation. The basal layer of the tear film is the *mucin layer*. This layer is secreted by the conjunctival goblet cells. Its primary function is to promote adhesion between the tear film and the eyeball and lubricate the eye. Abnormalities of any of these layers may cause dysfunction of the tears, with secondary ocular complications.

Inflammation of the conjunctiva due to allergies or infection (pink eye) is one of the most common ocular problems encountered by pediatricians.

PATHOGENESIS

The conjunctiva has a limited number of ways to respond to stimuli. The most common is dilation of the conjunctival blood vessels, which may occur as a reac-

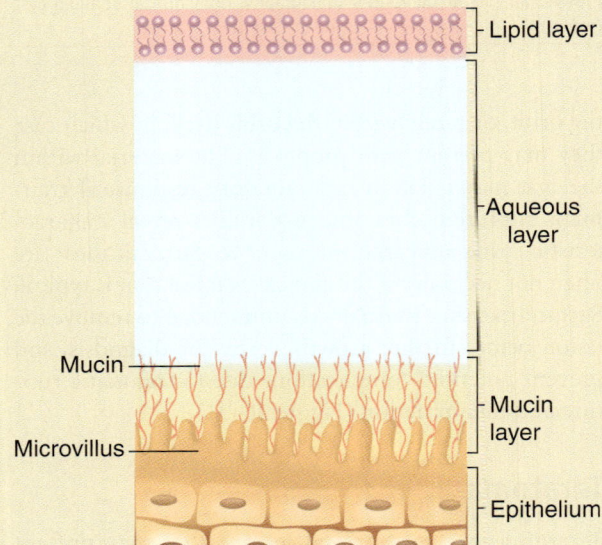

FIGURE 27–1 ■ Drawing of tear layers.

tion to external irritation (e.g., smoke), infection, trauma, or inflammation. These conditions may also cause edema of the conjunctiva, which produces a milky thickening of the conjunctival tissue (chemosis) (Figure 27–2). If the conjunctiva is diffusely damaged, the surfaces may scar. This can produce adhesion of the conjunctiva between the globe and the inner lining of the eyelid (symblepharon) (Figure 27–3). If a large area of the conjunctiva is injured, tear film dysfunction may develop due to loss of the mucin tear layer that is normally produced by the conjunctival goblet cells. In this condition the tear production is normal, but the tears do not function properly because they cannot adhere to the eye.

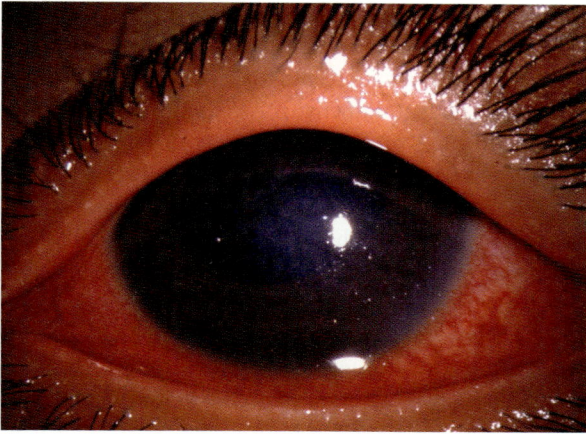

FIGURE 27–2 ■ Thickening (chemosis) and injection (engorged blood vessels) of conjunctiva following blunt trauma (air bag).

The tarsal conjunctiva has 2 common responses to inflammation. The first is *papillae*. This is a vascular reaction of the conjunctiva in which abnormal capillaries are surrounded by areas of inflammation. Because the conjunctiva is attached to the underlying tissue by fibrous septa, the follicles usually appear as multiple, small, elevated mounds with vessels in their centers (Figure 27–4A). These can vary from a fairly smooth, velvet-like appearance to multiple large nodules (*giant papillary conjunctivitis*) (Figure 27–4B).

The second type of conjunctival reaction is *follicles*. These are produced by clusters of lymphoid tissue within the conjunctiva, most readily visible on the inner surface of the lower eyelid. They may enlarge in response to certain infections or medication and are analogous to the swollen lymph glands in the neck that may develop in response to pharyngitis. They appear as pink, smooth, elevated nodules (Figure 27–5).

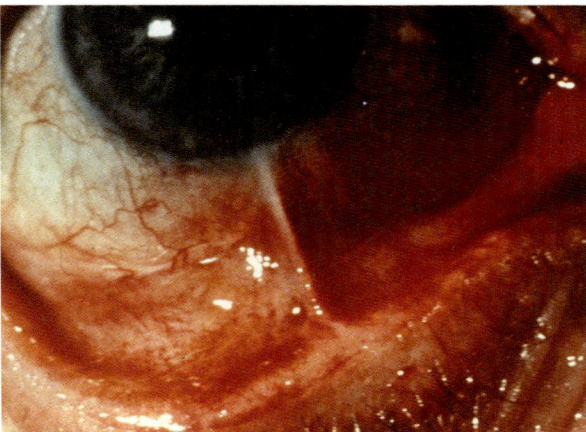

FIGURE 27–4 ■ Papillary responses of conjunctiva to inflammation. (A) Papillae are usually small nodules with vascular cores. (Photograph contributed by Anthony Lubniewski, MD.) (B) Giant papillary conjunctivitis of the upper tarsal conjunctiva, best seen with eversion of eyelid. Most commonly found in contact lens-related inflammation.

PRESENTATION

Most conjunctival disorders present with various degrees of conjunctival inflammation, edema, and dilation of the conjunctival blood vessels (commonly called *injection* of the blood vessels). The main etiologies are discussed below.

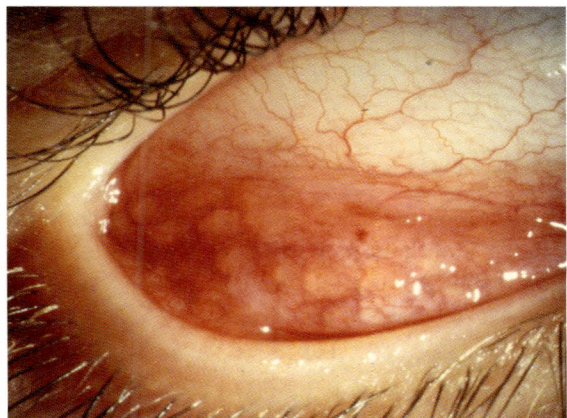

FIGURE 27–3 ■ Symblepharon (scar tissue) between tarsal (eyelid) and bulbar (eyeball) conjunctiva following a chemical injury.

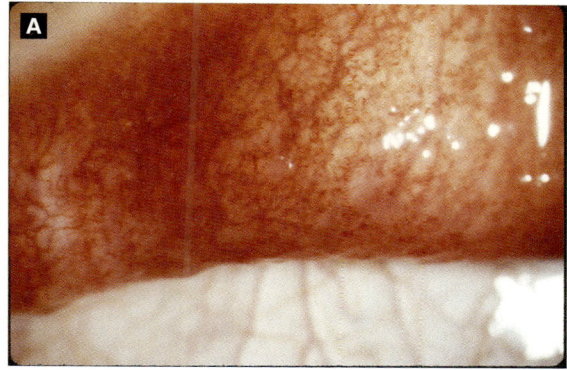

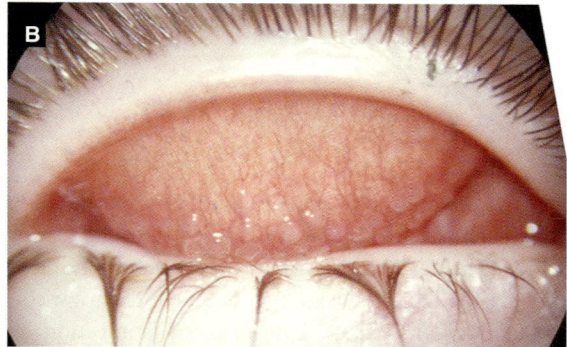

FIGURE 27–5 ■ Follicular conjunctival reaction. Larger smooth nodules without a central vessel, producing a lumpy appearance on the inner lining of the lower eyelid.

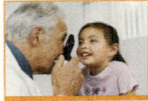

Table 27–1.

Differential Diagnosis of Follicular Conjunctivitis

- Adenovirus
- Herpes simplex virus
- Chlamydia (follicles not present in neonates)
- *Molluscum contagiosum*
- Topical medication
  - Atropine
  - Dipivefrin
  - Brimonidine
  - Topical antivirals
  - Phospholine iodide

Follicular Conjunctivitis

One type of conjunctivitis that has a fairly specific differential diagnosis is follicular conjunctivitis, which presents with a follicular reaction of the conjunctiva lining the lower eyelid (Table 27–1 and Figure 27–5). The most common etiology of follicular conjunctivitis is infection, and several organisms are associated with this particular response. The most common is adenovirus, which is a frequent cause of infectious conjunctivitis (pink eye). Herpes simplex virus (HSV), if it involves the eye, may cause follicular conjunctivitis, and this finding may be helpful in establishing a diagnosis. Chlamydial conjunctivitis also may cause a follicular reaction. However, neonates do not produce follicles, and therefore they are not present in ophthalmia neonatorum secondary to chlamydial disease. Chlamydia is a common sexually transmitted disease in adolescents, and the presence of follicular conjunctivitis in this setting should prompt testing for this pathogen. Patients with *Molluscum contagiosum* that involve the eyelids and periocular structures may develop a secondary follicular conjunctivitis. This resolves with treatment of the eyelid lesions. Finally, follicular conjunctivitis may occur as a side effect of topical ocular medications, such as dipivefrin, brimonidine, and atropine.

INFECTIONS

Infectious conjunctivitis is one of the most common pediatric ophthalmology disorders encountered by pediatricians. Viral etiologies are most frequent, followed by bacterial and chlamydial.

Viral Conjunctivitis

Clinically, viral conjunctivitis usually produces symptoms of ocular irritation and discharge. Examination reveals injection of the conjunctival blood vessels, chemosis, and a mucoid discharge. A follicular reaction of the tarsal conjunctiva is often present. Most patients with viral conjunctivitis have other manifestations of viral infection, most commonly upper respiratory infection.

Most viral conjunctivitis is caused by *adenoviruses*. Certain serotypes may produce specific types of reactions, such as pharyngoconjunctival fever, hemorrhagic conjunctivitis, or follicular conjunctivitis. *Epidemic keratoconjunctivitis (EKC)* is a highly contagious form of viral conjunctivitis associated with adenovirus types 8, 19, and 37. It presents with a follicular conjunctivitis and is often accompanied by preauricular lymphadenopathy. Unlike most forms of viral conjunctivitis, EKC usually is associated with multiple fine corneal epithelial and subepithelial opacities, which are not visible without a slit lamp. The diagnosis can be made clinically. Confirmatory office testing with rapid immunochromatography is available (RPS Adenodetector, Rapid Pathogen Screening, Inc., South Williamsport, PA). Patients with EKC should be kept out of school because of the highly contagious nature of the disease. Treatment is usually supportive. Topical corticosteroids may be used in patients with marked symptoms due to corneal changes. These are effective in improving symptoms, but may prolong recovery.

Herpes Virus

HSV and *herpes zoster virus* may cause conjunctivitis. Primary HSV (usually HSV1) is most likely to present with symptoms of conjunctivitis, usually accompanied by vesicles on the eyelid and a follicular reaction of the tarsal conjunctiva (Figure 27–6). Recurrent HSV more commonly involves the cornea. Topical treatment of isolated HSV conjunctival disease is usually not necessary. Acyclovir is usually used if the cornea is involved.

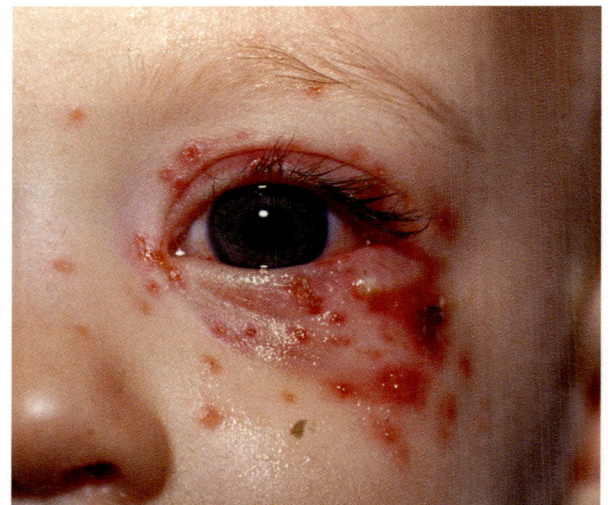

FIGURE 27–6 ■ Primary HSV affecting the periocular skin and conjunctiva. Note vesicular lesions on skin and erythema and thickening of inferior conjunctiva.

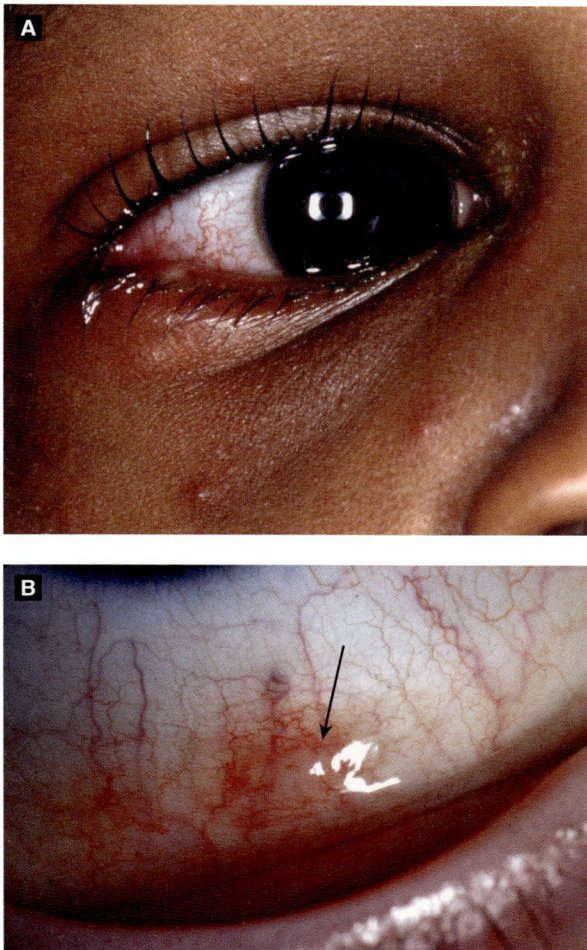

FIGURE 27–7 ■ Varicella conjunctivitis. (A) Note pox lesion on lower eyelid and adjacent conjunctival inflammation. (B) Varicella pox lesion (arrow) on bulbar conjunctiva.

Varicella may also cause conjunctivitis (Figure 27–7A), including small vesicles or ulcerations on the bulbar conjunctiva (Figure 27–7B). These almost always resolve without sequela, and treatment is not necessary, although topical antibiotics may be used to prevent secondary infection.

Bacterial Conjunctivitis

Bacterial conjunctivitis has symptoms that are similar to viral conjunctivitis, but it is usually associated with a mucopurulent ocular discharge. The most common organisms in children are *Streptococcus pneumoniae* and *Moraxella*. The use of vaccines has decreased the incidence of *Haemophilus* infections. The disorder is usually self-limited, but topical antibiotics are usually used to speed up the recovery. Many broad-spectrum antibiotics are available for treatment, including trimethoprim-polymixin B, aminoglycosides, and erythromycin. Newer medications, such as fourth-generation fluoro-

quinolones, are more rapidly effective, but are considerably more expensive than the alternatives. Cultures are typically not necessary unless the infection is severe or not improving with conventional therapy.

Neisseria gonorrhoea is a potentially severe form of bacterial conjunctivitis that may occur as a sexually transmitted disease in older children or acquired in neonates by exposure to an infected birth canal (ophthalmia neonatorum). This usually presents with hyperpurulent discharge and may progress rapidly to involve the cornea, potentially causing perforation. Erythromycin ointment is used in newborns as prophylaxis against *N gonorrhoea* and Chlamydia infections.

Neisseria meningiditis is another rare cause of bacterial conjunctivitis that presents with hyperpurulent discharge. *N meningiditis* has the potential for rapid systemic spread, leading to meningitis or septicemia. Affected patients require systemic treatment in addition to topical antibiotics, and individuals exposed to the patient require prophylactic treatment with rifampin to prevent disease.[1]

Chlamydial Conjunctivitis

Chlamydial conjunctivitis results from infection with *Chlamydia trachomatis*. It may occur as a form of ophthalmia neonatorum acquired through an infected birth canal (Figure 27–8), or as a sexually transmitted disease in older children. In older patients the conjunctivitis is usually accompanied by urethritis or cervicitis. Clinical symptoms include mild discharge. Corneal infiltrates are often present. The presence of a marked conjunctival follicular response is highly suggestive of chlamydial infections in adolescents.

Neonates with chlamydial infection acquired at birth usually present in the first week of life with conjunctival swelling and moderate discharge. Unlike older patients, the conjunctiva in neonates does not produce follicles, and therefore follicular changes are not seen in neonates with chlamydial conjunctivitis.

In both newborns and older patients, the diagnosis of Chlamydia may be established by culture, polymerase chain reaction, direct fluorescent antibody, or enzyme immunoassay tests. Erythromycin ointment is used prophylactically in newborns to prevent infection with

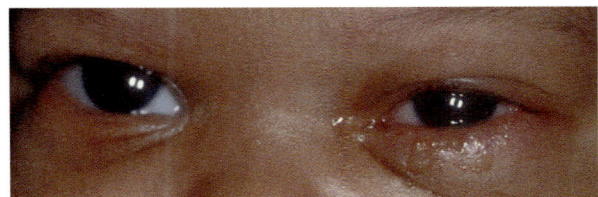

FIGURE 27–8 ■ Neonatal chlamydial conjunctivitis, left eye.

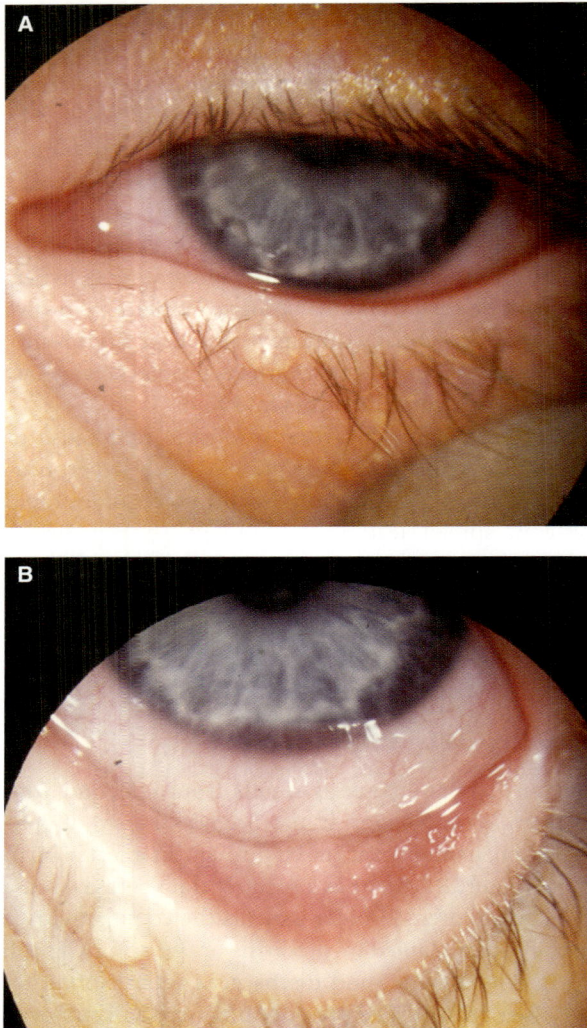

FIGURE 27–9 ■ *Molluscum contagiosum*. (A) Lower eyelid lesion. Note injection of conjunctiva and increased tear lake. (B) Follicular conjunctivitis secondary to *M contagiosum*.

N gonorrhoea and Chlamydia. If infants do become infected, systemic treatment with erythromycin is needed due to the risk of pneumonia. Older patients require systemic treatment and evaluation for other sexually transmitted diseases.

Molluscum contagiosum

M contagiosum results from a DNA pox virus that is spread by direct contact. It produces elevated smooth nodules with umbilicated centers (Figure 27–9A). The lesions may develop anywhere on the body. Lesions on or near the eyes may shed viral particles into the tear film, causing follicular conjunctivitis (Figure 27–9B). Several treatment options are available. Removal of the core with a small needle is usually effective. Recurrences may occur if not all of the lesions are treated.

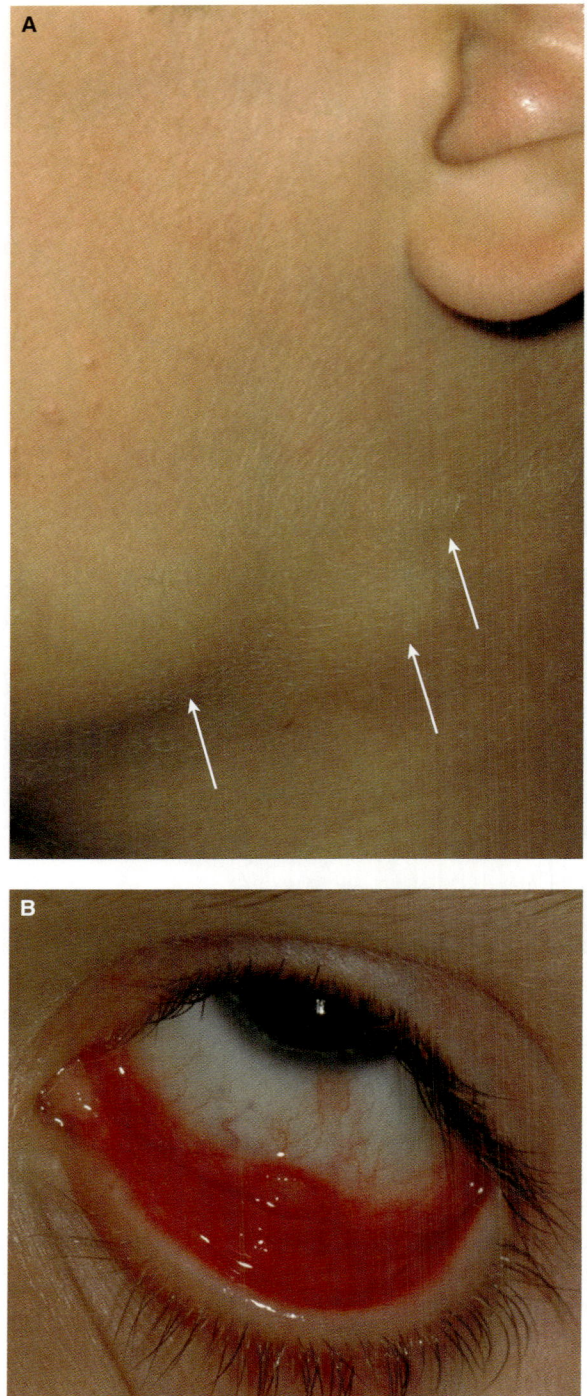

FIGURE 27–10 ■ Parinaud oculoglandular syndrome in a patient with tularemia. (A) Submandibular and cervical adenopathy (arrows). (B) Conjunctival granuloma.

Parinaud Oculoglandular Syndrome

Parinaud oculoglandular syndrome presents with a unilateral conjunctivitis accompanied by conjunctival granulomas and preauricular and submandibular lymph node enlargement (Figure 27–10A and B). The most common etiology is *Bartonella henselae*

(Cat-scratch disease). It may also be caused by many unusual infections, including tuberculosis, leprosy, tularemia, syphilis, sporotrichosis, and coccidioidomycosis. Treatment is directed at the underlying causative organism.

INFLAMMATION

Episcleritis

Episcleritis is an idiopathic disorder characterized by focal inflammation of the episcleral tissue. It presents with a wedge-shaped area of erythema and edema medial or lateral to the cornea (Figure 27–11A and B). Small nodules are sometimes present within the affected area (*nodular episcleritis*). Episcleritis is usually unilateral. Patients characteristically have no symptoms of discomfort or ocular irritation. Episcleritis is usually an isolated abnormality, but occasionally occurs in patients with autoimmune disease. It is typically self-limited, lasting 1 to 2 weeks. Treatment is not necessary because patients are asymptomatic and the disease resolves spontaneously.

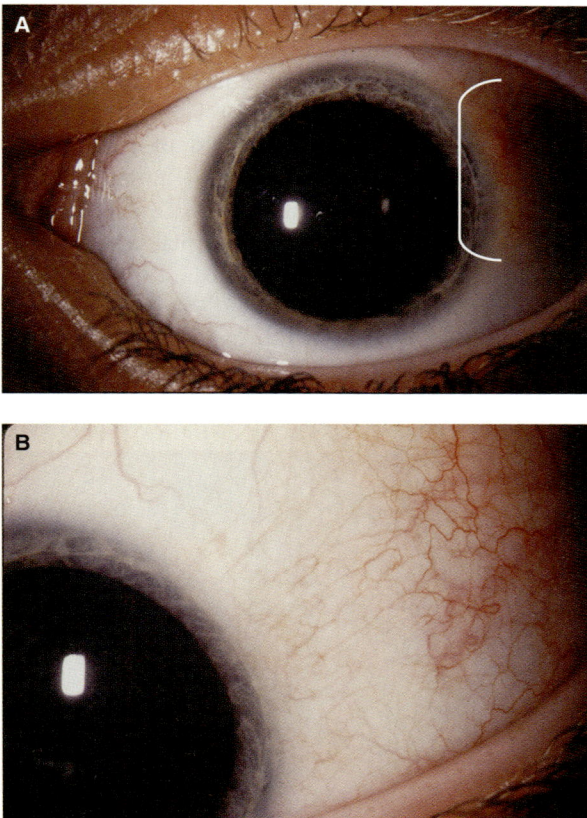

FIGURE 27–11 ■ (A) Focal area of episcleral inflammation temporally (marked). The remainder of the conjunctiva is white. (B) Magnified view of focal area of episcleritis.

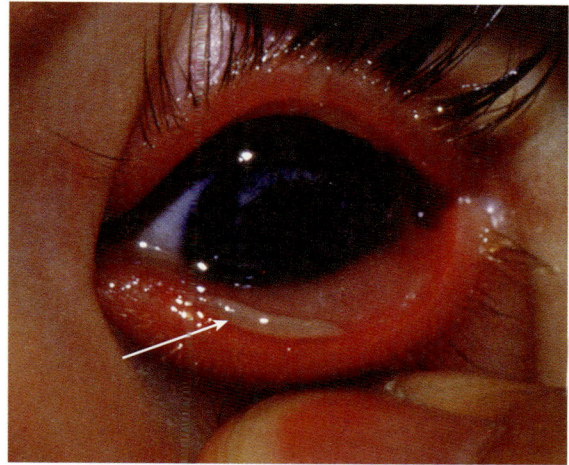

FIGURE 27–12 ■ Stevens-Johnson syndrome. Note pseudomembrane (arrow) with thickening and erythema of conjunctiva on inner lower eyelid.

Stevens-Johnson Syndrome (Erythema Multiforme)

Stevens-Johnson syndrome (SJS) is a systemic inflammatory disorder that affects the skin and mucous membranes, including the conjunctiva. Patients develop angiitis as a reaction to inciting agents, including infections, vaccines, and many medications. SJS is a potentially severe disorder, with a mortality of approximately 10%. Systemic manifestations include a prodromal flu-like illness, followed by the development of bullous skin and mucosal lesions.

Inflammation of the conjunctiva occurs in approximately half of patients with SJS. The conjunctiva is injected and vesicular lesions develop, often with mucoid discharge. Membranous or pseudomembranous conjunctivitis may develop (Figure 27–12), which may lead to scarring of the conjunctival surfaces (symblepharon). The acute phase may resolve without sequela, but patients are at risk for severe complications due to scarring, including eyelid malposition and tear film dysfunction.

Initial ophthalmic treatment of SJS includes frequent ocular lubrication and topical antibiotics to prevent secondary infection. Attempts to prevent symblepharon formation by lysis of adhesions or the use of amniotic membrane grafts is sometimes performed.[2] Careful ophthalmological monitoring is important for these patients.

External Beam Radiation

Radiation may be used to treat ocular and periocular tumors, such as retinoblastoma and orbital rhabdomyosarcoma. This may cause several ocular complications, including cataracts and radiation retinopathy. Acute changes at the time of radiation also include erythema and inflammation of the eyelids and conjunctiva (Figure 27–13A and B). This can be treated with

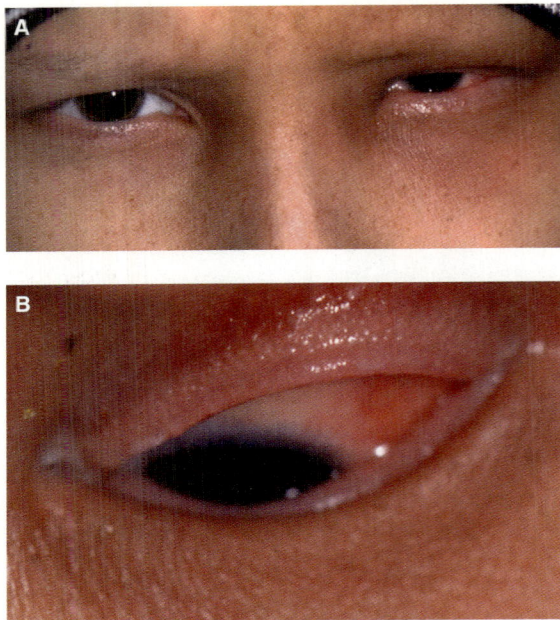

FIGURE 27–13 ■ Radiation conjunctivitis following external beam irradiation. (A) Note discoloration and thickening of left eyelids. (B) Note loss of eyelashes and conjunctival inflammation.

lubrication and topical medication, and usually improves with time. Chronic problems with dry eyes and ocular irritation may occur with higher doses of radiation.

Pyogenic Granuloma

Pyogenic granulomas are a form of conjunctival inflammation characterized by a fleshy, vascular appearance. Histologically, they are actually neither pyogenic nor granulomas. They may occur in response to trauma, such as following strabismus surgery. They most commonly occur on the tarsal conjunctiva (inner eyelid lining) in association with chronic chalazia (Figure 27–14). They often respond to topical corticosteroids.

SYSTEMIC DISEASES INVOLVING THE CONJUNCTIVA

Kawasaki Disease

Kawasaki disease (*mucocutaneous lymph node syndrome*) is a vasculitic disorder of unknown etiology that occurs in young children. Systemic signs and symptoms include fever, mucous membrane changes, edema or erythema of the hands and feet, a polymorphous rash, and lymphadenopathy. The most important potential complication is coronary artery disease.

Ocular involvement in Kawasaki disease consists of conjunctival injection, which typically does not extend to the edge of the cornea (the limbus). Mild anterior iritis is detectable in many patients on slit lamp

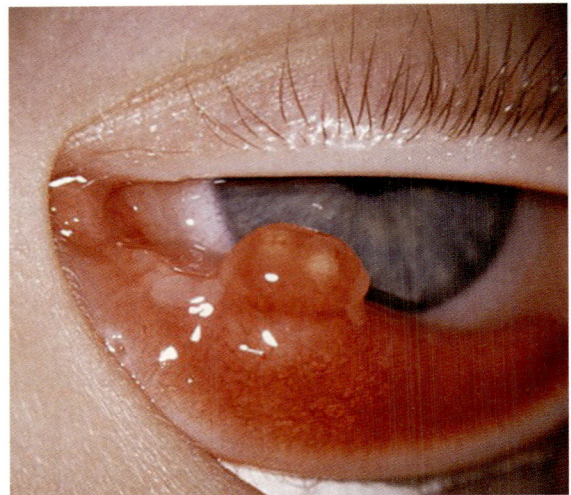

FIGURE 27–14 ■ Pyogenic granuloma of lower tarsal conjunctiva, formed in response to a chalazion. Note fleshy, vascular appearance of lesion.

examination early in the course of the disease.[3] This iritis is self-limiting, and topical corticosteroid treatment is not needed. Systemic treatment includes intravenous immunoglobulin and aspirin.

Ataxia-Telangiectasia

Ataxia-telangiectasia is a rare autosomal recessive phakomatosis caused by a defect of the ATM gene on chromosome 11. Systemic abnormalities include ataxia due to cerebellar dysfunction, and defective T-cell function with recurrent infections and increased risk of malignancies. Ocular changes include abnormal eye movements and conjunctival blood vessels. The abnormal eye movements are caused by inability to generate normal saccades, similar to that seen in ocular motor apraxia. The conjunctiva develops telangiectatic vessels by age 5 years in over 90% of patients (Figure 27–15). This specific finding may be helpful in identifying the diagnosis.

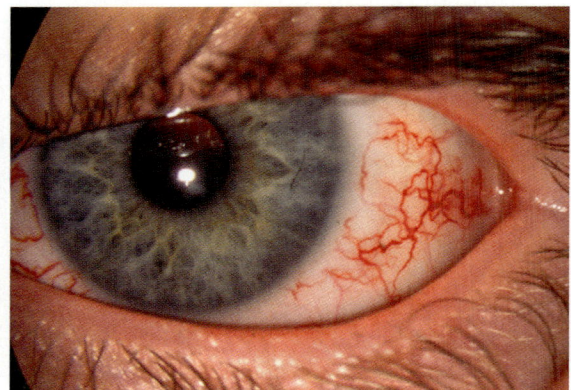

FIGURE 27–15 ■ Ataxia-telangiectasia. Note enlargement and tortuosity of conjunctival blood vessels.

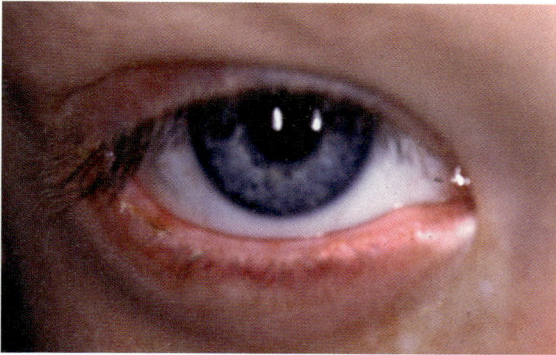

FIGURE 27–16 ■ GVHD. Note marked thickening and erythema of lower eyelid.

Graft-Versus-Host Disease

Graft-versus-host disease (GVHD) occurs in patients who have had bone marrow transplants. The donor bone marrow produces antibodies directed against the patient's normal tissue, which can cause a variety of systemic problems involving the skin, gastrointestinal tract, lungs, and liver. The eye is a common site of involvement, manifested by eyelid erythema and thickening, conjunctival inflammation, and symptoms of dry eye due to lacrimal gland dysfunction (Figure 27–16). Patients with GVHD are usually treated systemically with corticosteroids or cyclosporine. Ophthalmic treatment includes frequent use of ocular lubricants and occlusion of the lacrimal puncta to improve tear retention.

PIGMENTED CONJUNCTIVAL LESIONS

Conjunctival Nevi

Conjunctival nevi are relatively common in children. They most frequently present as pigmented lesions near the corneal limbus. They vary in color from amelanotic to dark brown. They may be flat or slightly elevated. They frequently have a cystic component that is visible on slit lamp examination, which is highly diagnostic (Figure 27–17A). They may also develop in other parts of the conjunctiva, including the caruncle (Figure 27–17B). They are usually relatively stable in size, but may change at the time of puberty. The potential for malignant transformation of conjunctival nevi in children is extremely low, but excisional biopsy may be indicated should abnormal growth occur.

Nevus of Ota (Oculodermal Melanocytosis)

Nevus of Ota is characterized by diffuse, patchy, gray-blue discoloration of the sclera (Figure 27–18A). The eyelid and periocular skin is hyperpigmented, following the distribution of the ophthalmic and maxillary branches of the trigeminal nerve (Figure 27–18B). Nevus of Ota occurs most frequently in patients of Asian descent, and is more common in females. The visual acuity is normal, but patients are at increased risk for the development of glaucoma[4] and malignant melanoma. Regular ophthalmic examinations are recommended for affected patients.

Nevus of Ota should be distinguished from scattered small patches of increased scleral pigmentation that are relatively common in African American and Asian patients (Figure 27–19). They cause no ocular problems.

Axenfeld Loops

The anterior sclera is innervated by the long posterior ciliary nerves. These nerves occasionally form small loops through the sclera that are visible as small pigmented nodules on the episcleral surfaces. They are benign.

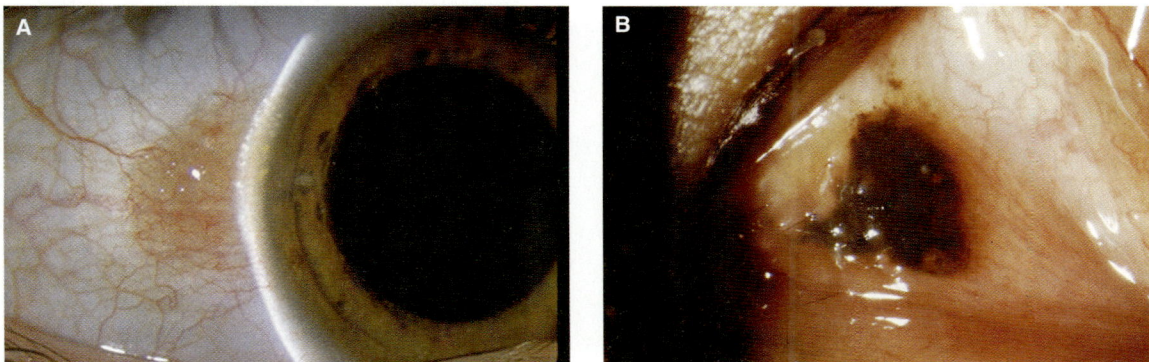

FIGURE 27–17 ■ Conjunctival nevi. (A) Lightly pigmented nevus adjacent to cornea. The lesion is slightly thickened and has a characteristic cystic appearance. (B) Heavily pigmented nevus of left caruncle.

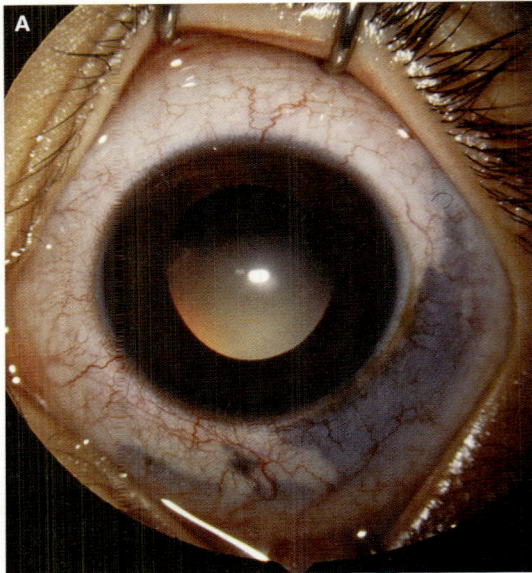

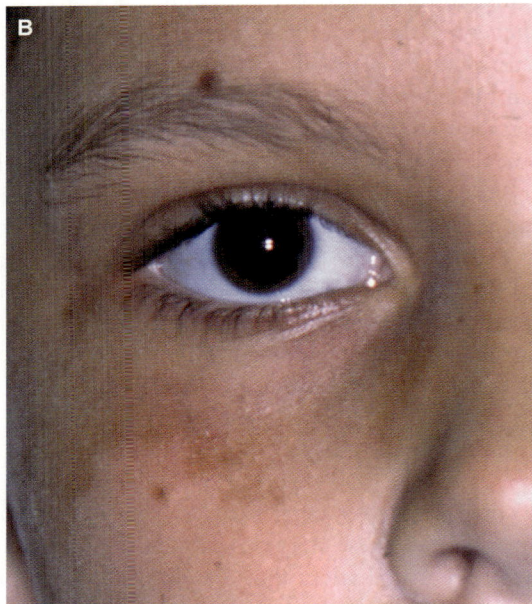

FIGURE 27–18 ■ Oculodermal melanocytosis. (A) Dark patch of scleral pigmentation. (B) Periocular pigmentation involving eyelids.

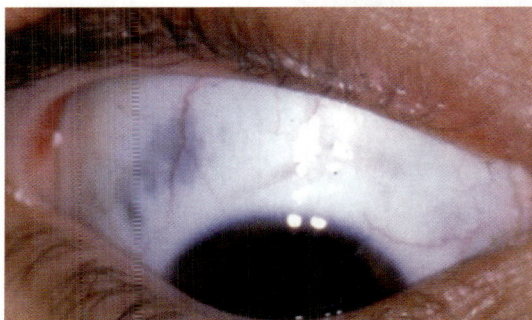

FIGURE 27–19 ■ Normal variant—patchy areas of increased scleral pigmentation.

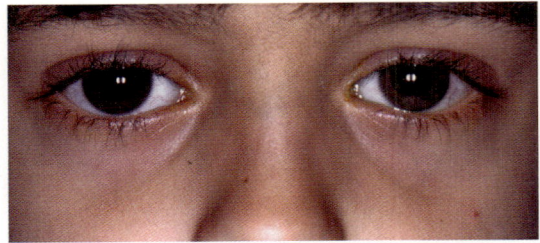

FIGURE 27–20 ■ Mild discoloration of lower eyelids in a patient with allergies ("allergic shiners").

ALLERGY-RELATED CONJUNCTIVAL DISORDERS

Allergic Conjunctivitis

Allergic conjunctivitis is a common pediatric ophthalmic problem. Most patients have a history of other atopic diseases, including eczema, reactive airway disease, or allergic rhinitis. Allergic conjunctivitis presents with symptoms of ocular irritation, excess tearing, and itching. The symptoms are typically worse during the spring and fall. The symptom of itching is highly suggestive of allergy. If the child is old enough to reliably articulate this symptom, and differentiate it from nonspecific irritation, it is very helpful in establishing a diagnosis.

Clinically, patients with acute allergic conjunctivitis may have a fairly unremarkable examination. The conjunctiva may be injected and chemotic, but there is no marked follicular or papillary reaction. Some patients develop discoloration of the lower eyelids (allergic shiners) (Figure 27–20). Chronic allergic conjunctivitis may cause papillary changes on the tarsal conjunctiva (Figure 27–21).

The treatment of allergic conjunctivitis is similar to the systemic treatment of allergies. Avoidance of specific

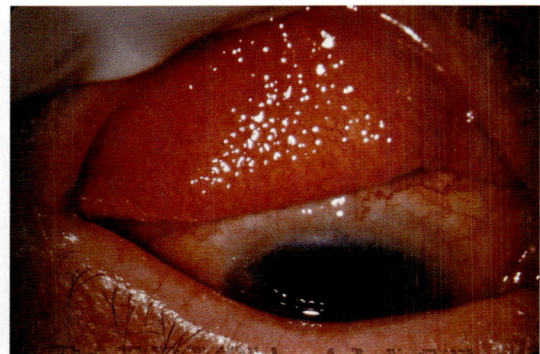

FIGURE 27–21 ■ Chronic allergic conjunctivitis with papillary reaction of tarsal conjunctiva. (Photograph contributed by Anthony Lubniewski, MD.)

Table 27–2.

Topical Allergy Medications

- Over-the-counter antihistamines
- Mast-cell stabilizers
- H_1-receptor agonists
- Combination medication
- Anti-inflammatories
  □ Corticosteroids
  □ Topical nonsteroidals
  □ Cyclosporine

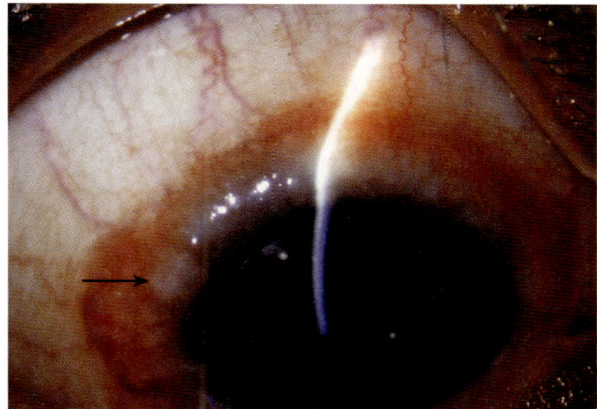

FIGURE 27–23 ■ Limbal vernal conjunctivitis. Note gelatinous thickening of conjunctiva at corneal limbus, with white-centered nodules (Horner-Trantas dots) (arrow).

allergens is most useful, but this may not be practical. Oral allergy medication is often better tolerated than drops in children, although it may be less effective in treating the ocular symptoms. Several topical medications are available, including over-the-counter antihistamines/vasoconstrictors and prescription mast cell stabilizers, H_1-receptor antagonists, nonsteroidal anti-inflammatories, or combinations thereof (Table 27–2). In severe cases, topical corticosteroids or cyclosporine may be used, but patients using these medications require ophthalmic monitoring due to potential side effects.

Vernal Keratoconjunctivitis

Vernal keratoconjunctivitis (VKC) is a specific form of allergic conjunctivitis with characteristic features. It is more common in males, and most patients have a history of atopic disease. It usually occurs in the spring and fall. Patients present with photophobia, intense itching, and thick mucoid discharge. There are 2 clinical presentations. The *palpebral* form primarily involves the inner (tarsal) surface of the upper eyelid. Changes vary from mild thickening to multiple, large flat papules (Figure 27–22).

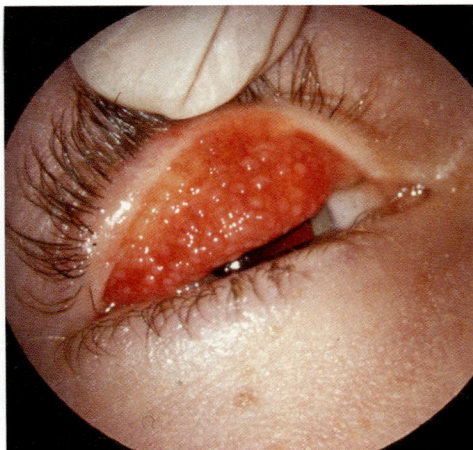

FIGURE 27–22 ■ Palpebral vernal conjunctivitis. Diffuse papillary reaction of upper tarsal conjunctiva.

The *limbal* form presents with similar symptoms, but the clinical appearance is different. In limbal VKC, thickening of the conjunctiva occurs at the corneal limbus. Patients develop gelatinous nodules with white centers (*Horner-Trantas dots*) (Figure 27–23). Some patients develop corneal epithelial defects (*shield ulcers*). Initial treatment with a combination mast cell stabilizer and H_1-receptor antagonist may provide relief. In patients with persistent symptoms, topical cyclosporine is usually effective, although this usually requires a custom-made drop with a higher concentration than that in the commercially available form.

EYELID LESIONS WITH CONJUNCTIVAL CHANGES

Blepharitis

Blepharitis is a condition in which the meibomian glands of the eyelids are predisposed to obstipation, such that the normal lipid products they produce do not flow freely into the tear lakes. Because the anterior lipid layer of the tear film is important for decreasing evaporation of the underlying aqueous tear layer, the tears tend to evaporate rapidly, leading to symptoms of dry eye. Blepharitis is very common in adults. It is less common in children, and it often is not recognized when it does occur.[5] It may be associated with *rosacea*.

Patients with blepharitis complain of ocular irritation and an ocular foreign body sensation. They frequently have crusts and matter on their eyelids in the morning. Because the normal rate of blinking decreases with concentration, such as during reading a book, the rapid evaporation of tears may lead to blurred vision. A historical clue suggesting blepharitis is that the blurred vision is not present immediately when reading begins,

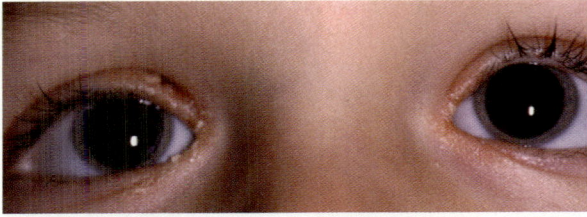

FIGURE 27–24 ■ Blepharitis with bilateral thickening and crusting of medial eyelids.

but develops after reading for a few minutes. On examination, crusts are usually visible within the eyelashes. The eyelid margin is erythematous and may be thickened (Figure 27–24). Plugging of the meibomian gland orifices is often visible on the eyelid margin. An increased oily component of the tear film and accelerated tear evaporation are found on slit lamp examination. Patients with more advanced disease may have punctate lesions on the cornea, and some develop peripheral corneal scarring and vascularization.

Treatment of blepharitis is performed in a stepwise fashion (Table 27–3). During routine examinations, many patients incidentally are noted to have mild blepharitis. If the cornea is not involved and the patients are asymptomatic, no treatment is necessary. Patients with mild or moderate symptoms are initially treated with eyelid hygiene techniques. These include warm soaks to the eyelid margins, followed by gentle scrubbing

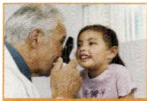

Table 27–3.

Step-wise Treatment of Symptomatic Blepharitis

- Lubrication with artificial tears
  - Used as needed
  - Does not treat underlying problem
  - Often not well tolerated in young children
- Eyelid hygiene
  - Warm compresses
  - Baby shampoo scrubs
- Topical antibiotics at bedtime
  - May decrease production of toxins by bacteria of eyelid
- Oral antibiotics
  - Erythromycin (young children)
  - Doxycycline (older children with mature dentition)
- Flaxseed oil
- Topical corticosteroids
  - Usually produces rapid improvement
  - Associated with potential complications
    - Increased intraocular pressure
    - Secondary infection
    - Cataracts
    - Requires monitoring by ophthalmologist

with a mild baby shampoo. The warm soaks cause dilation of the meibomian gland orifices and liquefaction of the obstipated lipids. The baby shampoo breaks down lipids and improves the flow of the oil. Although blepharitis is not caused by infection, bacteria on the eyelid margins may secrete toxins that exacerbate the condition. Therefore, topical antibiotics may be used on the eyelids, usually at bedtime. If the symptoms persist, oral antibiotics (erythromycin for young children, and tetracycline or doxycycline for older patients with mature dentition) or flaxseed oil supplements may be used. If the cornea has significant involvement, judicious use of topical corticosteroids often is beneficial, but careful ophthalmic follow-up is necessary to monitor for infections and potential side effects.

CONJUNCTIVAL MASS LESIONS

Dermolipoma (Lipodermoid)

Dermolipomas are choristomas that are present at birth, but often not noticed until later in childhood. They are composed of adipose and connective tissue. They are associated with Goldenhar syndrome, but in most patients they are an isolated abnormality. Dermolipomas are located beneath the lateral conjunctiva in the temporal fornix, and are usually not visible unless the eye moves medially. They have a smooth, slightly yellow, elevated appearance (Figure 27–25). Dermolipomas rarely cause any clinical problems and usually do not require treatment. If surgery is considered, care must be taken because the lesions may extend posteriorly and involve the extraocular muscles and orbital tissue. Usually only the anterior portion of a dermolipoma is removed.

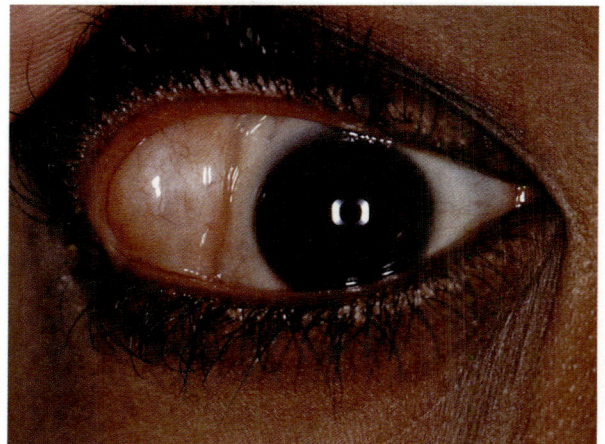

FIGURE 27–25 ■ Conjunctival dermolipoma. Elevated fleshy lesion of lateral conjunctiva.

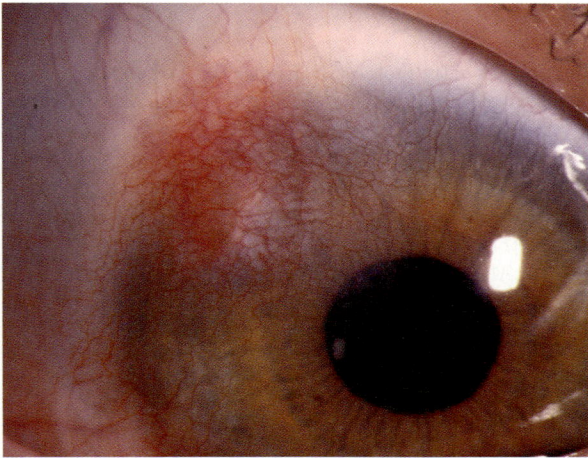

FIGURE 27–26 ■ Conjunctival lacrimal choristoma extending onto peripheral cornea.

Ectopic Lacrimal Gland

These are rare choristomatous lesions that present on the conjunctiva in infancy. They have a pink, elevated, vascular appearance. They are usually located adjacent to the cornea (Figure 27–26). They usually do not cause visual problems, but excisional biopsy may be indicated to establish a diagnosis.

Conjunctival Papilloma

Conjunctival papillomas are caused by human papillomavirus. They present as pedunculated or sessile, fleshy, vascularized lesions of the tarsal or bulbar conjunctiva. Pedunculated lesions are attached to the conjunctiva by a stalk of tissue. They have a lobulated appearance with multiple small blood vessels. Sessile lesions are most commonly found on the bulbar conjunctiva. They have a flat base and multiple small red dots (capillaries) on their surface. Conjunctival papillomas may spontaneously resolve. If they do not, surgical excision may be considered, but they have a tendency to recur.

Synthetic Fiber Granuloma ("Teddy Bear Granuloma")

These lesions may arise from an inflammatory reaction to synthetic fibers that get caught in the conjunctival space between the eyeball and the lower eyelid (Figure 27–27A). These occur most commonly in young children who sleep with toys or blankets made of synthetic material (Figure 27–27B). The diagnosis is established by histological examination, which reveals granulomatous inflammation and birefringence under polarized light. Removal of the lesion and the source of the material is curative.

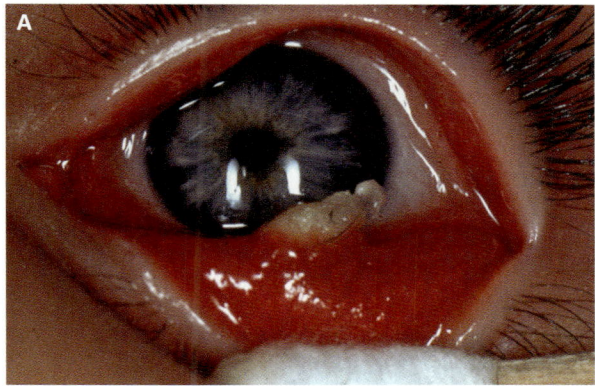

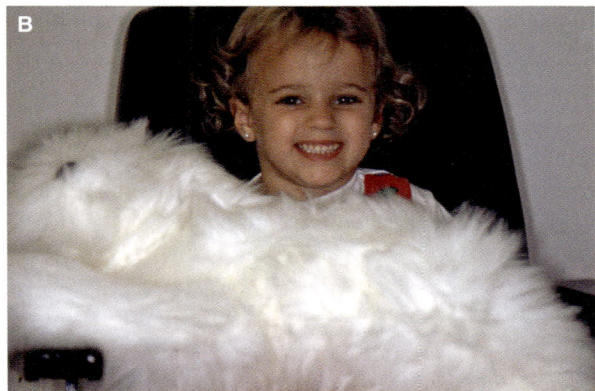

FIGURE 27–27 ■ Teddy-bear granuloma. (A) Lower tarsal conjunctiva. Hairs are adherent to the lesion. (B) The source of the synthetic material causing the teddy-bear granuloma. (Figures A and B are reprinted with permission from Lueder GT, Matsumoto B. Synthetic fiber granuloma. *Arch Ophthalmol.* 1995;113:848–849. Figures 1 and 2. Copyright American Medical Association. All rights reserved.)

CONJUNCTIVAL TRAUMA

Subconjunctival Hemorrhage

Hemorrhages within the conjunctiva may occur for a variety of reasons. Most frequently they result from minor trauma, a Valsalva maneuver, or following ocular surgery. They are often quite striking because the red blood is visible through the clear conjunctiva against the white background of the sclera. They are bright red and flat, and may extend to cover a large portion of the sclera (Figure 27–28).

Subconjunctival hemorrhages are benign and resolve spontaneously. They sometimes acquire a yellow tinge as they resolve due to degradation of hemoglobin. They usually occur in healthy people, but may be a sign of hypertension or a bleeding diathesis. Patients with spontaneous subconjunctival hemorrhages should be checked for these disorders.

Conjunctival lacerations may occur as a result of trauma. If they are isolated to the conjunctiva, most heal without sequela. Topical antibiotics are usually used to

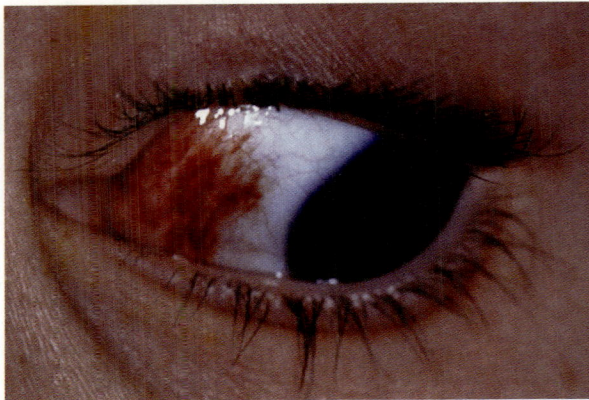

FIGURE 27–28 Subconjunctival hemorrhage. Note focal area of bright red blood. The remainder of the conjunctiva looks normal.

prevent secondary infections. Patients with conjunctival lacerations should be evaluated carefully to rule out scleral lacerations or a perforating ocular injury, which would require surgical intervention.

REFERENCES

1. Pomeranz HD, Storch GA, Lueder GT. Pediatric meningococcal conjunctivitis. *J Pediatr Ophthalmol Strabismus.* 1998;36:161–163.
2. Sotozono C, Ueta M, Koizumi N, et al. Diagnosis and treatment of Stevens-Johnson syndrome and toxic epidermal necrolysis with ocular complications. *Ophthalmology.* 2009;116:685–690.
3. Blatt AN, Vogler L, Tychsen L. Incomplete presentations in a series of 37 children with Kawasaki disease: the role of the pediatric ophthalmologist. *J Pediatr Ophthalmol Strabismus.* 1996;33:114–119.
4. Teekhasaenee C, Ritch R, Rutnin U, Leelawongs N. Glaucoma in oculodermal melanocytosis. *Ophthalmology.* 1990;97:562–570.
5. Jones SM, Weinstein JM, Cumberland P, Klein N, Nischal KK. Visual outcome and corneal changes in children with chronic blepharokeratoconjunctivitis. *Ophthalmology.* 2007;114:2271–2280.

CHAPTER 28

Diseases of the Cornea

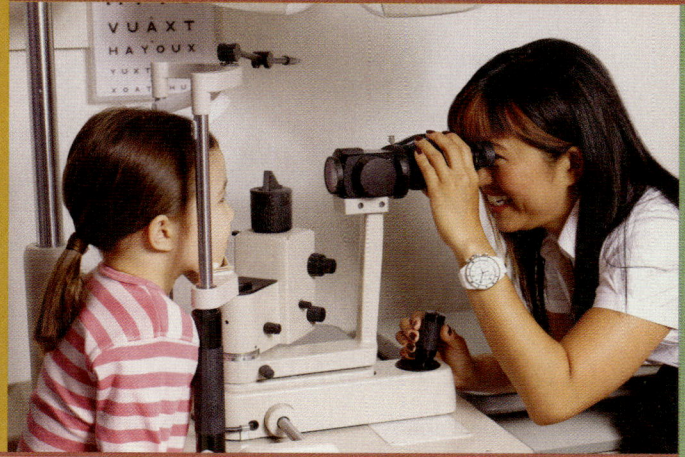

DEFINITIONS AND EPIDEMIOLOGY

The cornea is the clear structure at the front of the eye. When it is functioning normally it is not visible, just as a clean window is not visible as you look through it. The cornea and the lens focus light rays on the retina. The cornea has a rich supply of sensory nerves from the fifth cranial nerve (V1), and injuries or dysfunction of the cornea may therefore be quite painful. Corneal abnormalities in children are rare, but important due to their potentially severe effects on vision.

ANATOMY AND EMBRYOLOGY

The cornea is approximately 0.5 mm thick. It has 5 layers (Figure 28–1). The anterior layer is the corneal epithelium, a cellular layer that can regenerate rapidly (which is why corneal abrasions usually heal quickly). Beneath the epithelium is the thin, acellular Bowman's membrane. The bulk of the cornea is composed of the stroma, which is formed by a regular pattern of collagen fibers that allow light rays to transmit clearly. Descemet's membrane lies posterior to the stroma. It is another very thin acellular layer. The corneal endothelium lines the back of the cornea. The endothelium functions as a pump to keep excess fluid from accumulating in the stroma. It is critical in maintaining corneal clarity.

The normal corneal diameter is approximately 10 mm in newborns and increases to 12 mm in adults. The normal cornea has no blood vessels, which is another reason the cornea is clear and light rays can be focused through it. Because there are no blood vessels in the cornea, nutrition must be obtained via the tears anteriorly and the aqueous humor posteriorly.

Embryology

The cornea begins to form embryologically during the fourth week of gestation when the lens vesicle separates from the surface ectoderm. The ectoderm forms 2 layers. The innermost layer secretes collagen that forms the corneal stroma. Mesenchymal cells derived from the neural crest then migrate across the posterior surface of the cornea to form the endothelium.

PATHOGENESIS

The cornea must be clear and regular to focus light properly, and therefore most corneal diseases affect vision due to opacification. The rich supply of nerves to the corneal epithelium may cause significant discomfort in patients with corneal diseases.

Corneal diseases result from a variety of causes, including infection, trauma, metabolic diseases, developmental anomalies, inherited dystrophies, and as secondary effects of other ocular problems, such as glaucoma or tear film insufficiency.

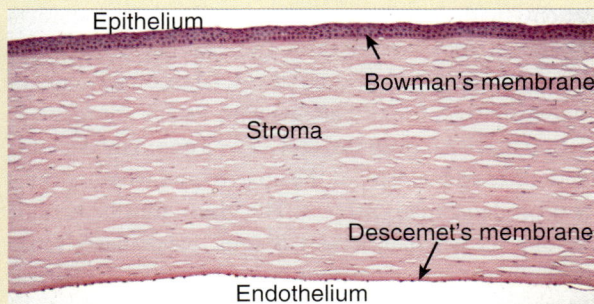

FIGURE 28–1 ■ Normal cornea. The layers are (1) epithelium, (2) Bowman's membrane, (3) stroma, (4) Descemet's membrane, and (5) endothelium. (Photograph contributed by Morton Smith, MD.)

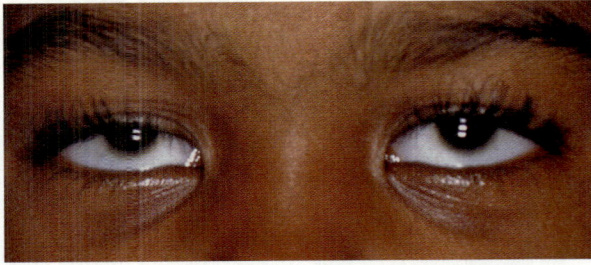

FIGURE 28–2 ■ Microcornea. The corneas are small relative to the size of the eyeball.

CLINICAL PRESENTATION

Many corneal abnormalities present with visible clouding of the cornea. The opacities may be localized or diffuse. If the corneal epithelium is involved, ocular discomfort will usually be present. In children, this typically is manifest by light sensitivity, excess tearing, and squinting of the eyes in bright light.

Depending on the etiology, corneal opacification may be accompanied by other signs or symptoms. Traumatic or infectious lesions, for instance, will usually have associated ocular inflammatory changes, such as conjunctival or eyelid erythema and swelling. Patients with metabolic diseases usually have systemic manifestations of the underlying disorder. The specific findings for different diseases are described in the following sections.

The normal corneal diameter at birth is approximately 10 mm. *Microcornea* is present if a newborn's corneal diameter is less than 9 mm (Figure 28–2), and *megalocornea* if the diameter is greater than 12 mm (Figure 28–3). These disorders can be familial, and may be associated with other ocular abnormalities. If isolated, ocular function may be otherwise normal.

CORNEAL DISORDERS

Infantile

The diagnosis of most infantile corneal lesions is based on the morphology of the opacity, as well as the patient's history and associated systemic abnormalities. Infantile

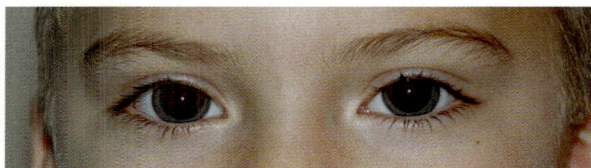

FIGURE 28–3 ■ Megalocornea. Bilateral corneal diameters are 14 mm (normal is 12 mm or less).

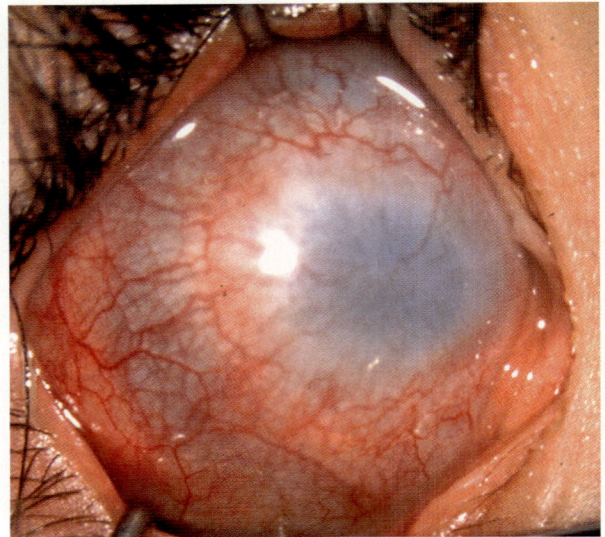

FIGURE 28–4 ■ Sclerocornea. A white opacity spreads across the entire cornea. The dark area centrally is the iris, which cannot be seen in detail due to the corneal opacity.

corneal opacities may cause profound amblyopia, similar to that which occurs in patients with infantile cataracts. Prompt diagnosis and treatment is needed to maximize the patients' visual potential.

Sclerocornea

Sclerocornea presents at birth with extension of the white sclera onto the corneal surface (Figure 28–4). The scleralization does not always cover the entire cornea, and clear areas may be present centrally. Most patients have other ocular abnormalities. Corneal transplantation may be indicated if the opacity involves the central cornea, but the visual prognosis is guarded.

Peter's anomaly

Peter's anomaly results from disruption of the central corneal endothelium. The appearance is the opposite of sclerocornea, in that the peripheral cornea is usually clear in Peter's anomaly, and there is a central circular area of corneal clouding. Strands of iris tissue often are attached at the border of the opacity (Figure 28–5). Patients with Peter's anomaly may also have cataracts (Figure 28–6). In severe cases, the lens may be adherent to the corneal defect (Figure 28–7). Glaucoma occurs in approximately 50% of patients with Peter's anomaly.

The visual prognosis for Peter's anomaly depends on the size and density of the opacity, and whether cataracts or glaucoma is present. The vision may be good if the opacity is small. Larger lesions, particularly those involving the lens, have poor vision potential. Unilateral Peter's anomaly is usually an isolated defect. Bilateral lesions are more likely to be associated with systemic abnormalities.

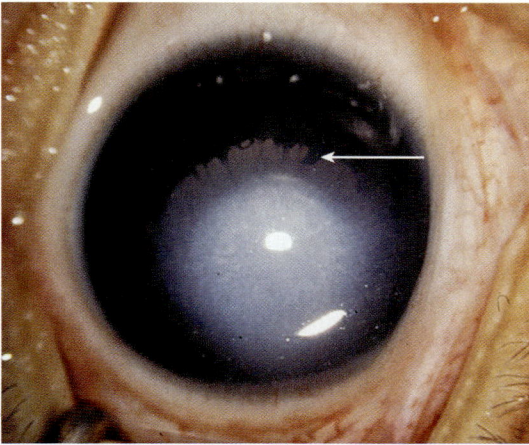

FIGURE 28–5 ■ Peter's anomaly. Note the central area of corneal clouding, with strands of iris tissue (arrow) attached to the posterior border of the anomaly.

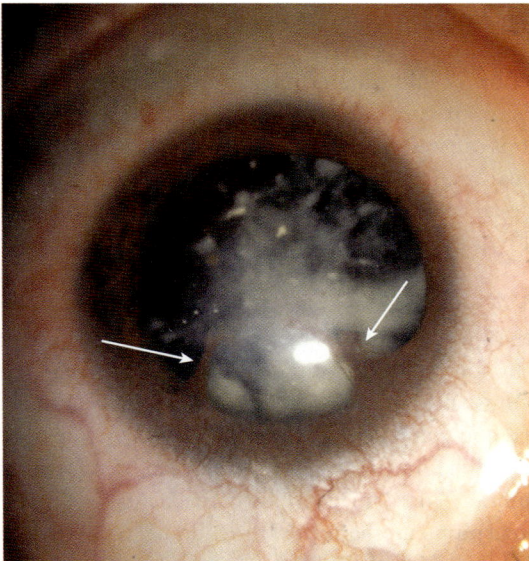

FIGURE 28–6 ■ Peter's anomaly plus cataract. Strands of iris tissue are visible attaching to the border of the corneal opacity (arrows).

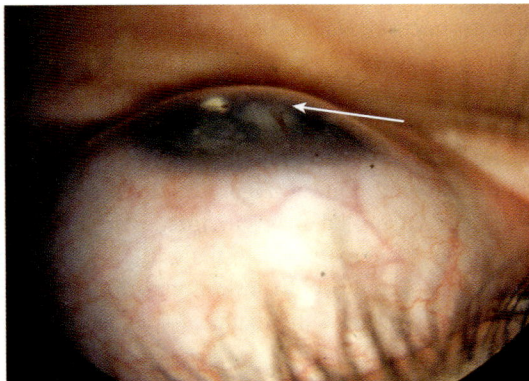

FIGURE 28–7 ■ Peter's anomaly plus cataract. The lens is adherent to the posterior surface of the cornea (arrow).

Anterior segment dysgenesis

Anterior segment dysgenesis includes a spectrum of abnormalities of the cornea and iris. The mildest form is *posterior embryotoxon*, in which Schwalbe's line (the anterior edge of the trabecular meshwork) is anteriorly displaced. Schwalbe's line cannot usually be seen, but it is visible in patients with posterior embryotoxon as a thin white strip at the peripheral cornea (Figure 28–8A and B). Posterior embryotoxon itself does not cause visual problems. It is a common feature of *arteriohepatic dysplasia (Alagille syndrome)*.

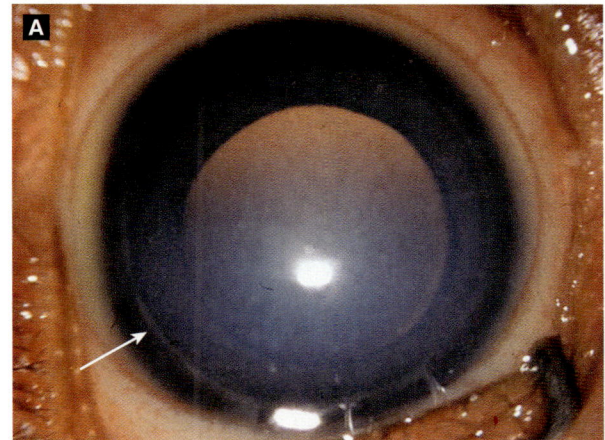

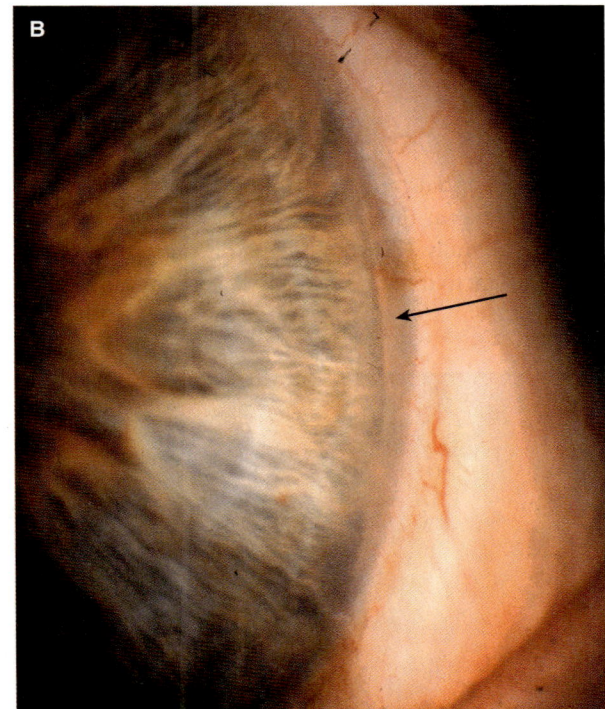

FIGURE 28–8 ■ Posterior embryotoxon. (A) The white line in the peripheral cornea (arrow) can sometimes be visualized with a penlight. Note that this patient with anterior segment dysgenesis also has a cloudy cornea. (B) Slit lamp view of a less prominent posterior embryotoxon (arrow).

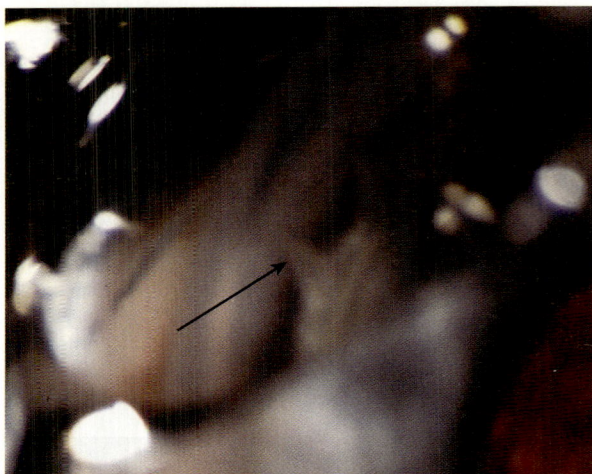

FIGURE 28–9 ■ Axenfeld-Rieger anomaly. Gonioscopic view of iris strands attaching to trabecular meshwork (arrow).

Axenfeld-Rieger syndrome is a more severe form of anterior segment dysgenesis, in which posterior embryotoxon is accompanied by strands of iris to the anteriorly displaced Schwalbe's line, and variable degrees of iris hypoplasia (Figure 28–9). Glaucoma develops in approximately 50% of patients.

Different genetic causes of Axenfeld-Rieger syndrome have been identified, including mutations of the *PITX2* and *FOXC1* genes. It is usually transmitted as an autosomal dominant disease. Systemic manifestations may include dental, umbilical, and cardiac abnormalities.

Corneal dermoid

Corneal dermoids are choristomas that present as elevated nodules at the junction of the cornea and sclera inferotemporally (Figure 28–10). They are usually not large enough to directly block vision, but they may cause

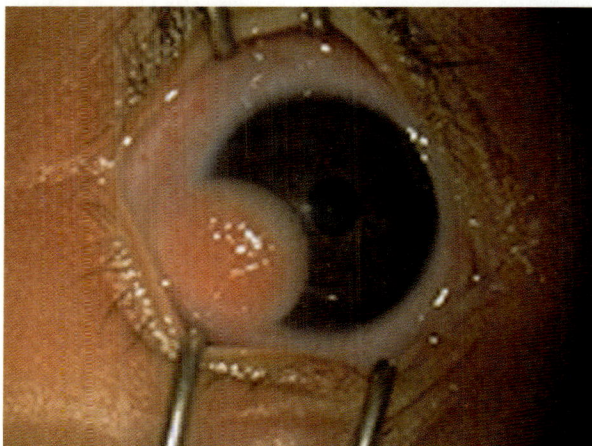

FIGURE 28–10 ■ Corneal dermoid.

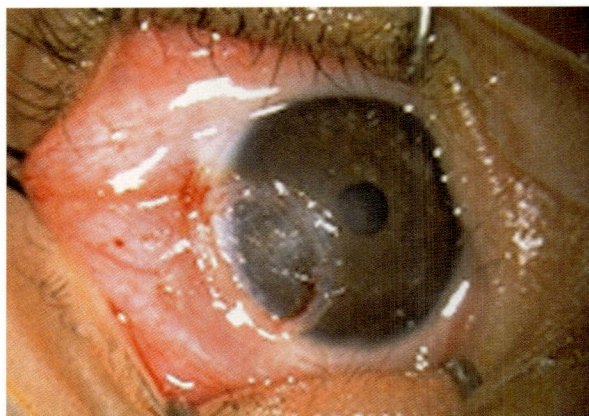

FIGURE 28–11 ■ Intraoperative photograph of corneal dermoid excision.

amblyopia secondary to induced astigmatism. They may be isolated or occur in association with *Goldenhar syndrome*. In addition to dermoids, other ocular abnormalities in Goldenhar syndrome include upper eyelid colobomas and Duane retraction syndrome. Surgical excision of corneal dermoids may be performed if the lesions cause decreased vision or irritation, or to improve appearance (Figure 28–11). Even with successful removal, patients usually have persistent astigmatism and require continued treatment for amblyopia.

Forceps injury

Corneal forceps injuries occur due to compression of the eye by forceps during difficult deliveries. Affected newborns usually have associated bruising and swelling of the eyelid and periocular tissue (Figure 28–12A). The corneal opacities in forceps injuries result from tears in Descemet's membrane and damage to the corneal endothelium. The normal pump mechanism of the endothelium is disrupted and fluid accumulates in the corneal stroma, producing clouding. The corneal clouding is usually diffuse in the immediate postpartum period, and hemorrhages may be visible (Figure 28–12B).

As the cornea heals and the endothelial pump regains its function, *Haab striae* become visible. These are parallel lines at the edges of the breaks in Descemet's membrane (Figure 28–12C). In forceps injuries they are oblique, following the same angle as the forceps. Haab striae are also common in infantile glaucoma, but in glaucoma they are curvilinear (Figure 28–13, see discussion below). The corneal damage in forceps injuries often causes marked astigmatism, and patients are at high risk for amblyopia. Careful ophthalmic monitoring with patching and glasses increases the chances for a good outcome.

Infections

Corneal opacities may result from intrauterine or postpartum infections. A leading cause of congenital corneal

FIGURE 28–13 ■ Corneal changes in infantile glaucoma. (A) Bilateral enlarged corneas. (B) Curvilinear Haab striae in infantile glaucoma (arrow). The cornea is mildly cloudy.

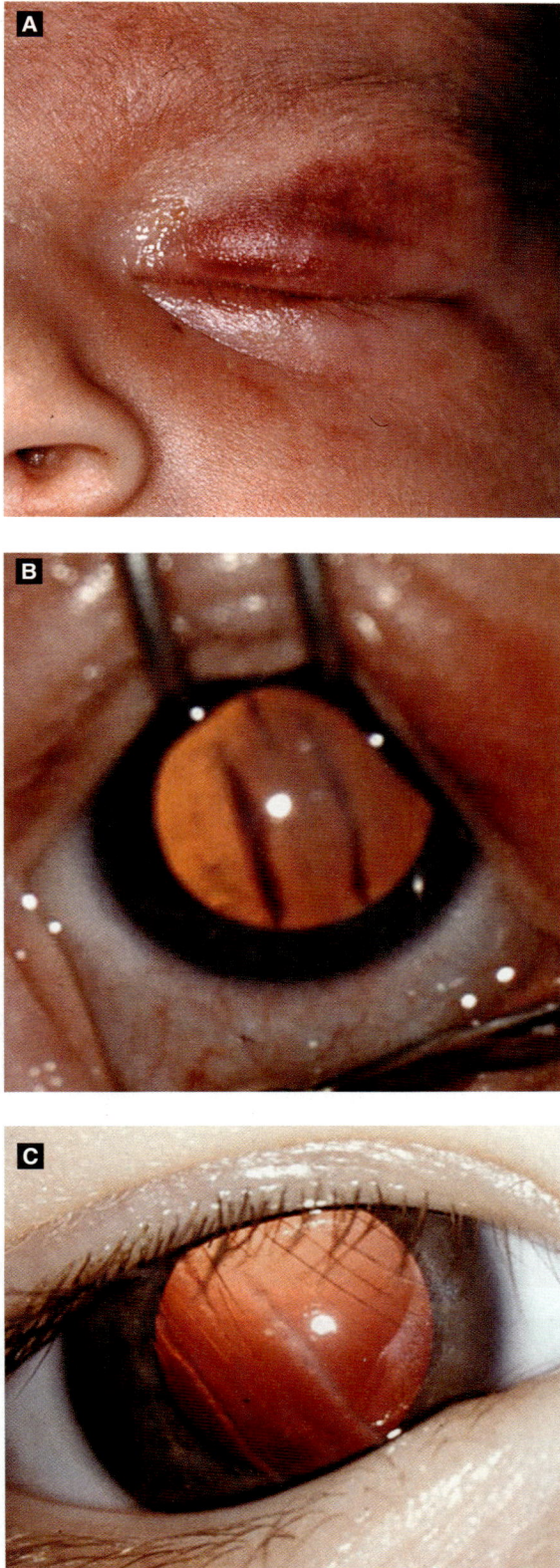

FIGURE 28–12 ■ Corneal forceps injury. (A) Patients usually present with associated bruising and swelling of the eyelids due to the forceps. (B) Initial appearance of cornea in the newborn period. Note clouding of the cornea and linear corneal hemorrhages (following the path of forceps compression). (C) Late appearance. Linear Haab striae (due to linear tears in Descmet's membrane).

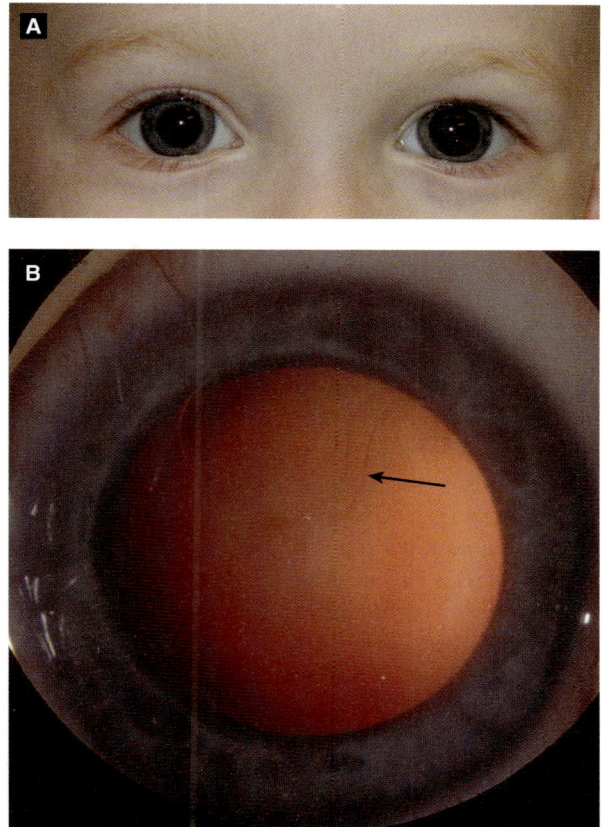

infections is *ophthalmia neonatorum*, in which organisms are usually acquired during passage through the birth canal. Most forms of ophthalmia neonatorum present primarily as conjunctivitis, without direct corneal involvement. *Neisseria gonorrhoea*, however, may directly infect the cornea, leading to potentially severe consequences such as ocular perforation. Affected infants are also at risk for systemic infection, including sepsis and arthritis. Prompt systemic antibiotic treatment is indicated.

Neonatal *herpes simplex virus* (HSV) may affect the cornea, as well as the conjunctiva, retina, and lens. Corneal involvement may include the corneal epithelium or stroma. Infants with congenital HSV have a high risk of disseminated disease and systemic complications. Intravenous treatment with antiviral medication, such as acyclovir, is required.

Inherited corneal dystrophies

These are rare disorders that present with cloudy corneas in infancy. Patients with *congenital hereditary endothelial dystrophy* (CHED) have diffusely thick and opacified corneas. The appearance may be similar to that of

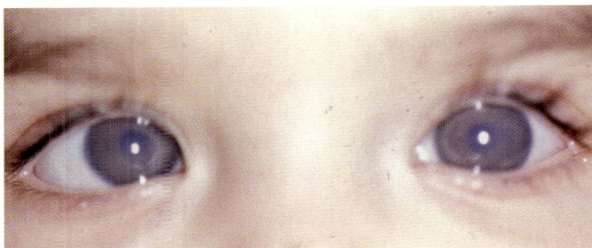

FIGURE 28–14 ■ Bilateral corneal clouding secondary to congenital hereditary endothelial dystrophy. The patient also has sensory strabismus

infantile glaucoma (Figure 28–14). *Congenital hereditary stromal dystrophy* (CHSD) presents with clouding of the stroma. This is distinguished from CHED by a normal corneal thickness and normal corneal epithelium. CHED occurs in autosomal recessive and autosomal dominant forms. CHSD is autsomal dominant.

Inherited corneal dystrophies are rare, and establishing a diagnosis may be difficult. A detailed slit lamp examination is helpful, which usually requires sedation in an infant. The corneal clouding in these disorders may be difficult to distinguish from changes due to infantile glaucoma (see next section). The thickened cornea may result in artificially high readings of intraocular pressure, which further complicates the assessment. The presence of Haab striae confirms the diagnosis of glaucoma, but these are not always present. In some patients, serial monitoring for abnormal eye growth and glaucomatous optic nerve changes may be necessary to differentiate these disorders. If the patient requires a corneal transplant, histological evaluation of the cornea may provide a diagnosis.

Glaucoma

One of the most common causes of infantile corneal clouding is glaucoma. The increased intraocular pressure in glaucoma interferes with the normal pump mechanism of the corneal endothelium, which leads to edema and thickening of the corneal stroma. Because infants' sclera is distensible (unlike adults), the pressure may also cause enlargement of the eyeball. This results in an enlarged corneal diameter (Figure 28–13A). *Haab striae* are commonly seen. Because they are caused by centrifugal stretching, the Haab striae in glaucoma are typically curved (Figure 28–13B), unlike the linear Haab striae seen in forceps injuries (Figure 28–12C). Treatment of infantile glaucoma is discussed in Chapter 32.

Older Children

Systemic diseases

Progressive corneal abnormalities may occur in several systemic diseases. In these disorders, the corneal changes are usually not present at birth.

Mucopolysaccharidoses and mucolipidoses These metabolic disorders are characterized by abnormal accumulation of glycosaminoglycans. There are at least 8 forms of mucopolysaccharidoses (MPS). Systemic abnormalities include involvement of the central nervous system, extremities, ears, liver, spleen, and lungs. The diagnosis is often first suspected based on the physical appearance, which includes coarse facial features and short, thick hands (Figure 28–15A and B). Bone marrow transplantation may improve the systemic problems, and may have beneficial effects on the ocular complications.[1]

Ocular manifestations of MPS include dysfunction of the optic nerve and retina. Corneal clouding is the most common associated ocular abnormality. Depending on the disorder, the corneal changes usually develop during the first few years of life, and they provide clinical clues to the diagnosis. The earliest changes are usually seen in mucolipidosis IV, in which opacities may develop within the first 2 months of life. Changes

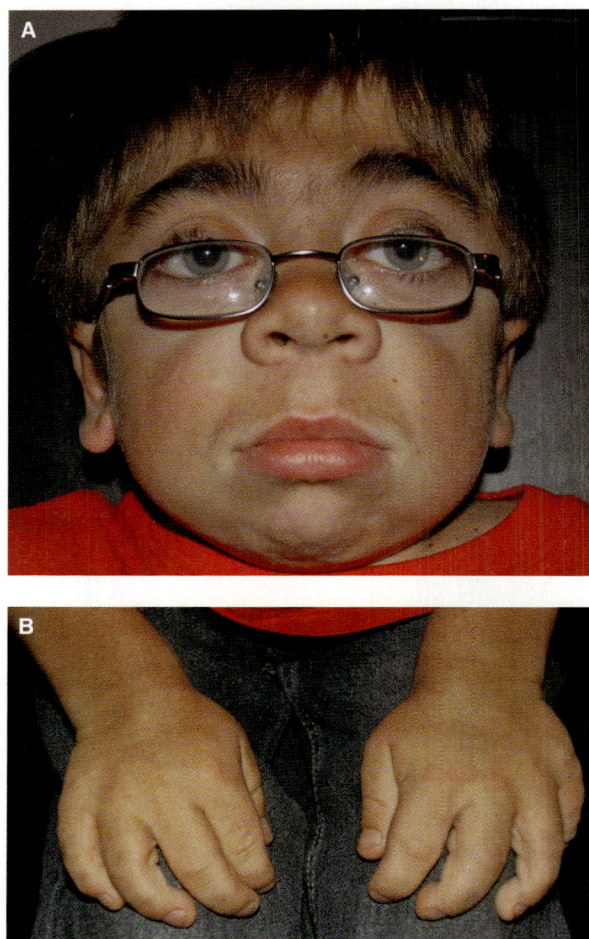

FIGURE 28–15 ■ Systemic findings in mucopolysaccharidosis type 1-H (Hurler syndrome). (A) Coarse facial features. (B) Thickened, short hands.

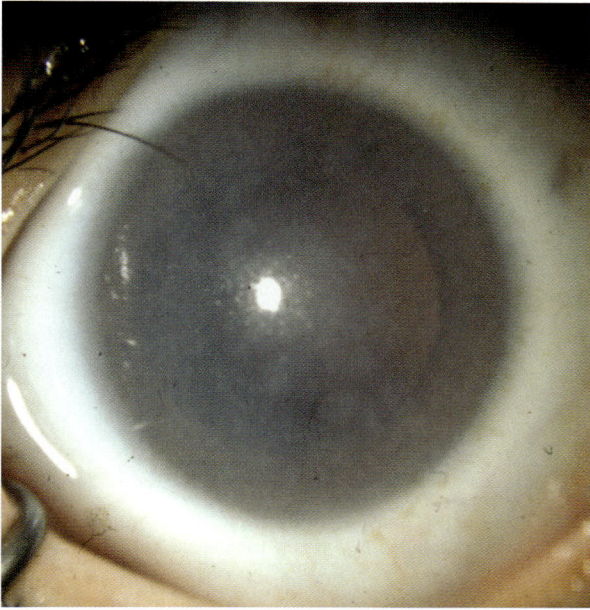

FIGURE 28–16 ■ Corneal clouding in MPS 1-H (Hurler syndrome).

are usually seen within 6 months in MPS 1-H (Hurler syndrome) (Figure 28–16) and within 12 to 24 months in MPS HIS (Hurler-Scheie syndrome). Corneal transplantation may improve visual function.

Cystinosis Corneal crystals are a prominent feature of the infantile form of cystinosis, and may assist in the diagnosis. The pathognomonic abnormality is discrete iridescent crystals that are usually present by 1 year of age. They begin in the peripheral and anterior portions of the cornea, and gradually spread to include the entire corneal width and depth (Figure 28–17). The deposits are also present in the conjunctiva and ciliary body. They usually produce marked photophobia. Systemic manifestations

include renal and bone disease (*Fanconi disease*). Topical cysteamine drops may be used in patients who have symptomatic corneal lesions. These drops, however, are difficult to obtain, require very frequent instillation, and are of variable efficacy. In practice, most patients do not continue their use due to these problems.

Hepatolenticular degeneration (Wilson disease) This is an autosomal recessive disorder of copper metabolism that affects the liver, kidneys, and basal ganglia. Copper deposition in the peripheral cornea may produce a *Kayser-Fleischer* ring, with a brownish appearance in peripheral Descemet's membrane. Kayser-Fleischer rings do not cause any visual problems. Most patients are referred to ophthalmologists to look for this finding to assist in the diagnosis of patients with liver disease.

Inflammatory disease Children with chronic ocular inflammatory diseases (most frequently *juvenile idiopathic arthritis*) may develop *band keratopathy* (Figure 28–18). These are superficial deposits of calcium that begin at the peripheral cornea medially and temporally. They may spread across the central corneal surface. Minor accumulations are asymptomatic, but more severe deposits may cause ocular irritation and interfere with vision.

Patients with band keratopathy benefit from treatment of the underlying ocular inflammation. This does not cause the band keratopathy to resolve, but may halt its progression. If patients with band keratopathy have significant problems due to decreased vision or ocular irritation, the excess calcium may be removed

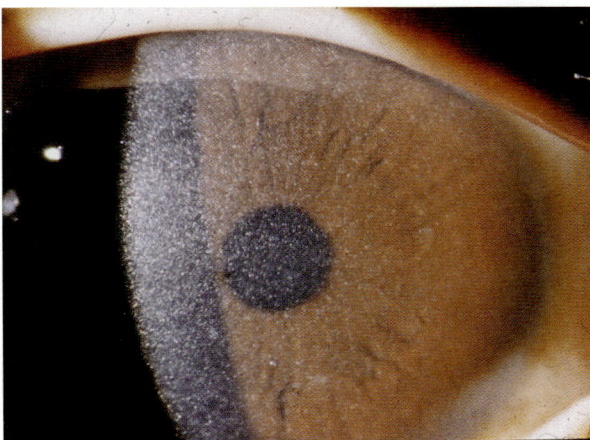

FIGURE 28–17 ■ Cystinosis. Diffuse iridescent corneal crystal deposits, involving all layers of cornea.

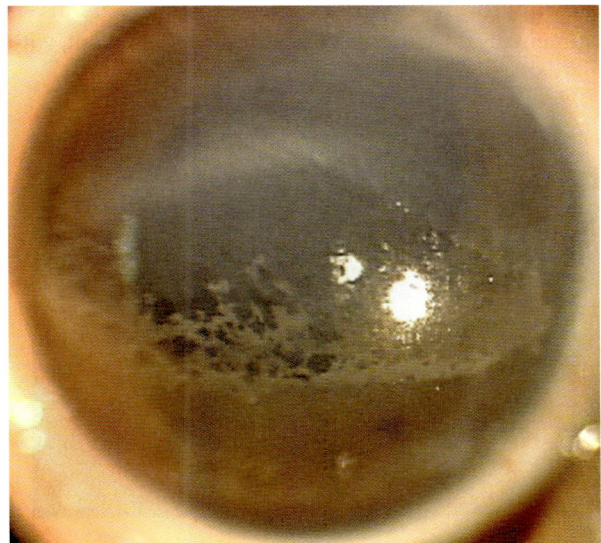

FIGURE 28–18 ■ Band keratopathy. Corneal calcium deposits produce lacy opacities.

by chelation. In children this is performed under anesthesia. The corneal epithelium is removed, and the cornea is treated with EDTA swabs, which removes the calcium. Patients are usually quite uncomfortable postoperatively until the epithelium regrows, and the calcium deposits may recur.

Familial dysautonomia (Riley-Day syndrome)

This is a rare autosomal recessive disease associated with autonomic and sensory nerve dysfunction. Systemic findings include absent fungiform papillae of the tongue and decreased deep tendon reflexes. The corneal problems in familial dysautonomia may be severe due to the combination of decreased tear formation and decreased corneal sensation. Because the patients cannot feel their corneas, they have decreased blinking and ocular protection mechanisms. They are at high risk for developing corneal infections and ulcerations.

Fabry disease (angiokeratoma corporis diffusum)

Fabry disease is an X-linked recessive sphinglipidosis caused by a deficiency of α-galactosidases A. Systemic manifestations include renal dysfunction, skin lesions, and dysethesias in the extremities. The cornea has a distinctive appearance, known as *cornea verticillata*, characterized by whorled deposits of sphingolipid in the basal layer of the cornea epithelium (Figure 28–19). Cornea verticillata may also occur as a side effect of treatment with *amiodarone* (Figure 28–20) and *chloroquine*.

Tyrosinemia (Richner-Hanhart syndrome)

Tyrosinemia type II is an autosomal recessive disorder of tyrosine metabolism. It presents in early childhood with painful hyperkeratotic lesions on the hands and feet. Approximately half of affected patients are developmentally delayed. Eye symptoms are prominent, with

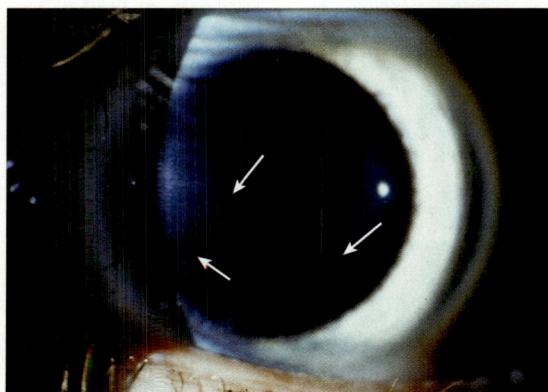

FIGURE 28–20 ■ Cornea verticillata due to amiodarone toxicity. (Photograph contributed by Anthony Lubniewski, MD.)

marked photophobia and excess tearing. These symptoms are caused by corneal *pseudodendrites*, which clinically appear similar to the dendrites seen in herspes simplex keratitis (Figure 28–21). The 2 are differentiated by bilateral involvement, lack of improvement with antiviral medication, and absence of fluorescein staining in the pseudodendrites of tyrosinemia.

Vitamin A deficiency Vitamin A has an important role in ocular function. Vitamin A deficiency due to malnutrition is a major cause of blindness in underdeveloped countries. In developed nations, deficiency may result from malabsorption due to gastrointestinal dysfunction (in cystic fibrosis or following small bowel resection, for example). Ocular manifestations include *xerophthalmia* (dryness) of the cornea and keratiniza-

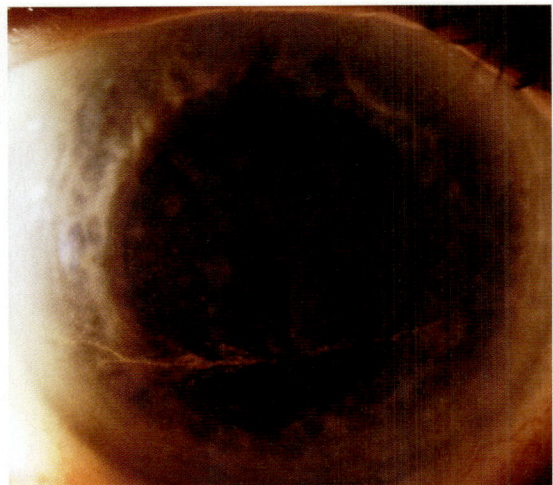

FIGURE 28–19 ■ Cornea verticillata in Fabry disease. Note subtle whorled corneal opacities (arrows). (Photograph contributed by Anthony Lubniewski, MD.)

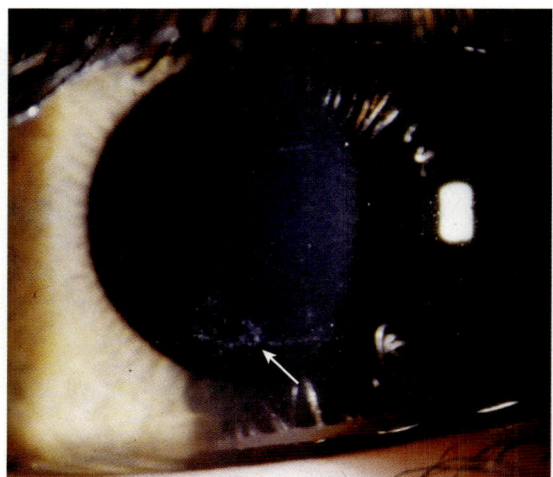

FIGURE 28–21 ■ Pseudodendrites (arrow) in a patient with tyrosinemia.

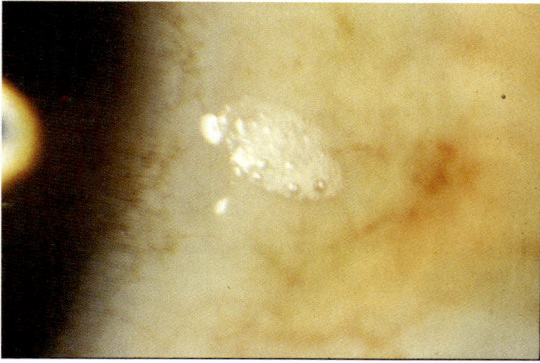

FIGURE 28–22 ■ High-magnification slit lamp photograph of Bitot's spots (leratinization of the conjunctiva) in a patient with vitamin A deficiency due to malabsorption.

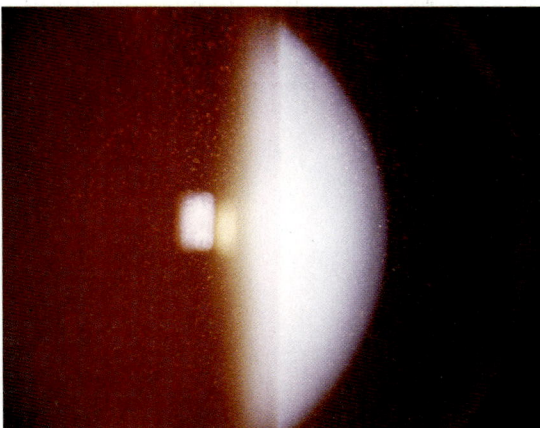

FIGURE 28–24 ■ Schnyder's crystalline corneal dystrophy, high-magnification slit lamp view. Note the fine needle-like crystalline corneal deposits.

tion of the conjunctiva (Bitot spots) (Figure 28–22). The corneal abnormalities predispose patients to infection, which may exacerbate vision loss. The vitamin A deficiency also disturbs retinal photoreceptor function, leading to symptoms of night blindness. In the absence of associated malnutrtion, the ocular symptoms usually improve when vitamin A levels are restored to normal.

Corneal dystrophies

Unlike CHSD and CHED, which present in infancy, other inherited corneal dystrophies do not present until later in childhood or adulthood. These conditions are all rare. Those that may initially manifest in childhood include the following:

Meesman dystrophy (juvenile epithelial dystrophy) develops early in life. It affects the corneal epithelium, causing accumulations of small cysts (Figure 28–23). The clinical effects are mild.

Macular dystrophy is an autosomal recessive disorder that presents before age 10 years. It begins in the corneal stroma with focal grayish opacities. These opacities progress, and dysfunction of both the epithelium and endothelium may occur.

Schnyder crystalline corneal dystrophy is an autosomal dominant disorder that may be present within the first few years of life. It is characterized by needle-shaped crystal deposits in the anterior corneal stroma (Figure 28–24).

Posterior polymorphous dystrophy may be inherited in autosomal recessive or dominant forms. It is uncommon, but occurs more frequently than the other dystrophies discussed above. It is characterized by dysfunction of the corneal endothelium and Descemet's membrane. With slit lamp examination gray opacities, vesicles, or bands of abnormal tissue of the posterior cornea are seen (Figure 28–25). Some patients develop distortion of the iris.

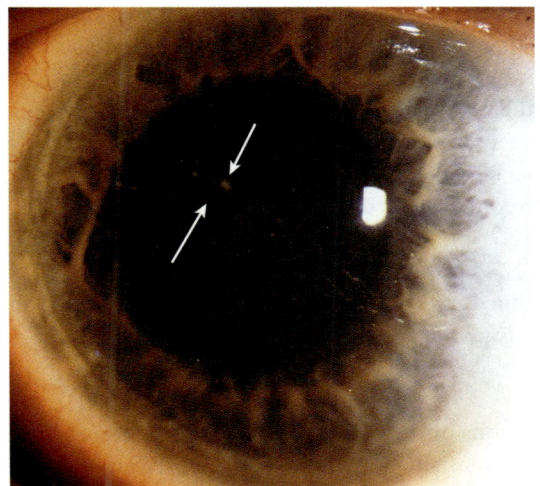

FIGURE 28–23 ■ Meesman corneal dystrophy, slit lamp view with retroillumination. Multiple small epithelial cysts are visible to the left of the slit beam. (Photograph contributed by Anthony Lubniewski, MD.)

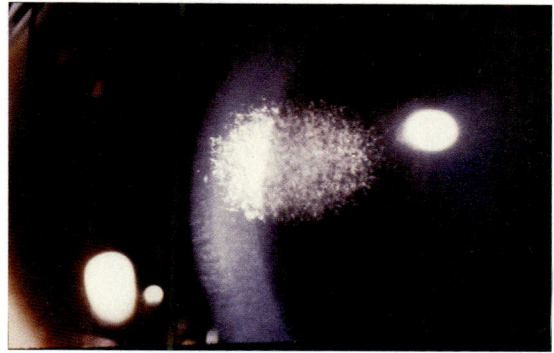

FIGURE 28–25 ■ Posterior polymorphous corneal dystrophy. Note bands of corneal endothelial tissue with scalloped edges (arrow). (Photograph contributed by Anthony Lubniewski, MD.)

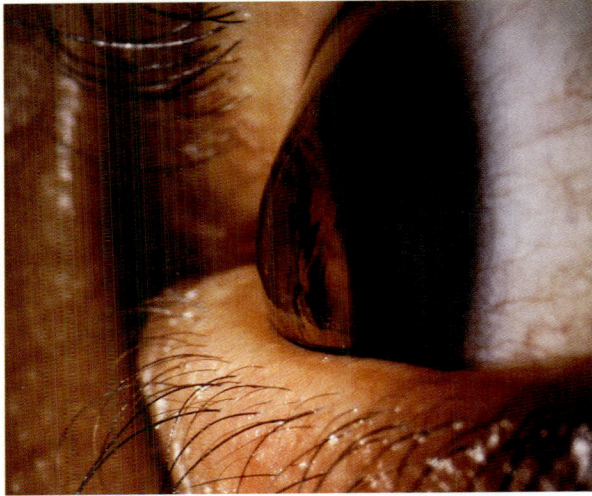

FIGURE 28–26 ■ Keratoconus. Note "sagging" appearance of cornea, with inferior bulge over the lower eyelid. (Photograph contributed by Anthony Lubniewski, MD.)

Ectatic disorders

Ectatic disorders are characterized by abnormal thinning of the cornea with secondary changes in the shape due to protrusion.

Keratoglobus This is a very rare ectatic disorder that presents in infancy with diffuse thinning of the cornea, which has a globular appearance. Patients frequently have blue sclera. The cornea is fragile and prone to perforation. Keratoglobus is associated with Ehlers-Danlos type VI.

Keratoconus Keratoconus is the most common ectatic disorder. It usually begins in adolescence and progressively worsens. In keratoconus, the central cornea is thinned, which causes sagging of the inferior portion of the cornea (Figure 28–26). The initial symptoms are usually blurred vision due to irregular astigmatism. Patients may develop tears in Descemet's membrane, which produces edema and opacification of the central cornea (*acute hydrops*). Keratoconus is more common in patients with atopic disease and Leber's congenital amaurosis, which is presumed due to frequent eye rubbing in these disorders. It is also more common in patients with Trisomy 21 (Figure 28–27). For patients with significant vision loss due to keratoconus, the prognosis for corneal transplantation is good.

Infections

Infections of the cornea (*keratitis*) are serious problems that potentially threaten vision. Prompt evaluation and treatment are necessary to minimize this risk.

Bacterial and fungal infections Bacterial and fungal infections of the cornea are unusual, and typically

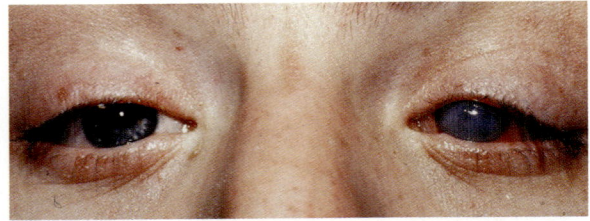

FIGURE 28–27 ■ Left corneal clouding due to hydrops in a patient with keratoconus and Trisomy 21.

are associated with some underlying corneal problem. They present with marked conjunctival injection and corneal clouding. Severe infections may cause a *hypopyon*, a layering of pus in the anterior chamber (Figure 28–28). The 2 most common etiologies are trauma and contact lens wear. Traumatic injuries, such as corneal foreign bodies, may disrupt the corneal epithelium, which predisposes the cornea to infection. The risk of fungal keratitis is increased if the trauma is associated with organic material, such as a tree branch or lake water. Patients who wear contact lenses also are at risk for developing bacterial corneal ulcers, particularly if they do not care for their lenses properly. Although bacterial conjunctivitis is common in children, the cornea is rarely directly involved.

Children with infected corneal lesions require prompt evaluation to establish a diagnosis. Corneal scrapings for bacterial and fungal cultures and stains are ideally done before instituting topical antibiotic therapy. Patients are treated initially with instillation of antibiotic drops every 30 to 60 minutes. Broad-spectrum fortified drops, with high concentrations of antibiotics such as vancomycin and tobramycin, are used while waiting for culture results. Fungal keratitis may be difficult to treat, particularly if the infection extends to the deep cornea.

Syphilis In some cases of congenital syphilis, patients do not become symptomatic until later in childhood.

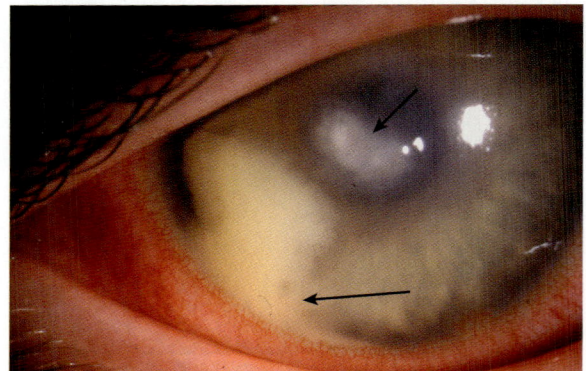

FIGURE 28–28 ■ Corneal bacterial infection (small arrow) with hypopyon (pus in anterior chamber) (large arrow).

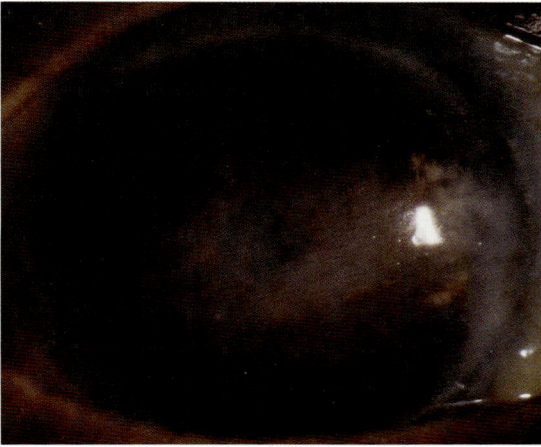

FIGURE 28–29 ■ Interstitial keratitis in a patient with syphilis. (Photograph contributed by Anthony Lubniewski, MD.)

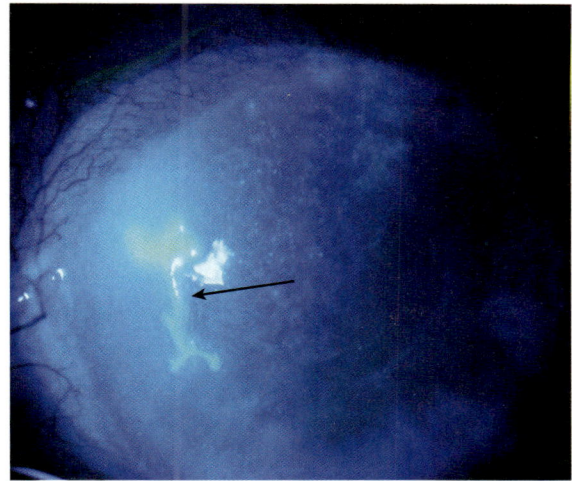

FIGURE 28–31 ■ Corneal dendrite (arrow) secondary to HSV, stained with fluorescein. (Photograph contributed by Anthony Lubniewski, MD.)

Interstitial keratitis is an immune-related lesion that may not begin until as late as the teen years (Figure 28–29). Patients present with symptoms of eye pain and redness, most commonly bilateral. The corneal changes include progressive opacification and vascularization of the stroma. Patients frequently have other manifestations of congenital syphilis. *Hutchinson triad* is the association of peg-shaped teeth, sensory deafness due to eighth nerve involvement, and interstitial keratitis. Systemic treatment of syphilitic infections is necessary to decrease the risk of these complications.

Viral infections

Herpetic keratitis Herpes simplex virus (HSV) is a common cause of corneal infections. This may affect the epithelium or stroma. Primary HSV infection often involves the conjunctiva and periocular skin, with typical vesicular lesions on the eyelid (Figure 28–30). If the cornea is involved in primary HSV, it usually is limited to epithelial disease. This classically presents with dendritic lesions with bulbs on the end (Figure 28–31). Less commonly, inflammatory changes of the peripheral cornea develop (Figure 28–32). More severe involvement may lead to large (geographic) ulcers. Patients typically complain of foreign body sensation, photophobia, and blurred vision. The conjunctiva is often injected.

Recurrent HSV infections occur in approximately 25% of patients due to reactivation of virus in the trigeminal nerve ganglia. Recurrences may manifest as the same type of dendritic lesions seen in primary infection, but may also cause corneal stromal keratitis. Interstitial keratitis causes opacities in the corneal stroma, without active epithelial disease. Disciform lesions may be associated with epithelial edema and iritis. Chronic corneal scarring may persist after the active infection resolves (Figure 28–33).

The diagnosis of corneal HSV infections is usually made based on the clinical appearance. Antigen and

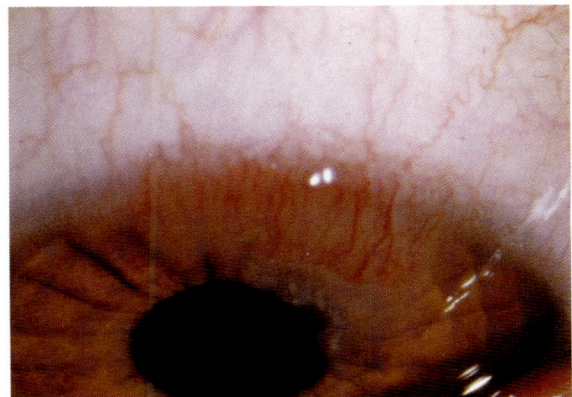

FIGURE 28–30 ■ Primary HSV infection causing vesicular reaction of periocular skin.

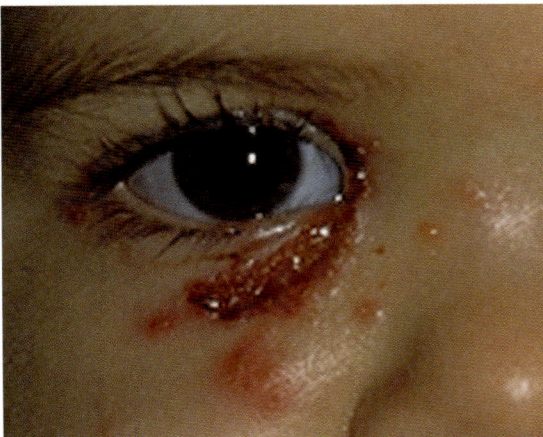

FIGURE 28–32 ■ Peripheral corneal HSV infection.

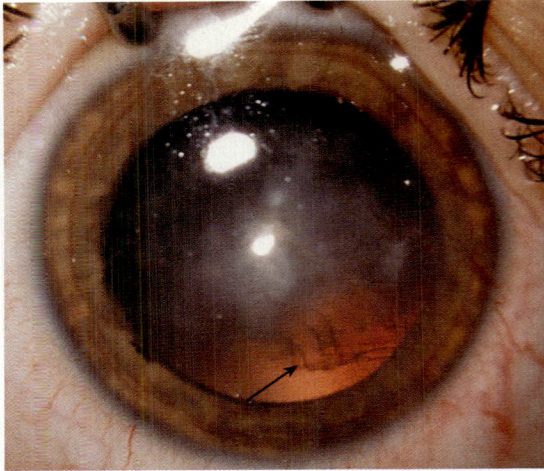

FIGURE 28-33 ■ Central corneal scar secondary to chronic HSV infection. The scar is vascularized, with blood vessels visible in the peripheral cornea (arrow).

PCR testing are sometimes used if the diagnosis is not certain. Treatment of HSV ocular infection depends on the nature of the eye involvement. Treatment is recommended if the cornea is involved. Although topical medications such as vidaribine and trifluridine are available, systemic treatment with oral acyclovir is often the best treatment. The use of oral medication is usually better tolerated than frequent eye drops in children, and acyclovir is effective for both treating acute corneal involvement and preventing recurrent ocular disease.[2]

Epstein-Barr virus Epstein-Barr virus infections are the cause of infectious mononucleosis. Affected patients may develop distinctive disc-shaped corneal opacities (*nummular keratitis*) (Figure 28–34). This is usually self-limited and treatment is not required.

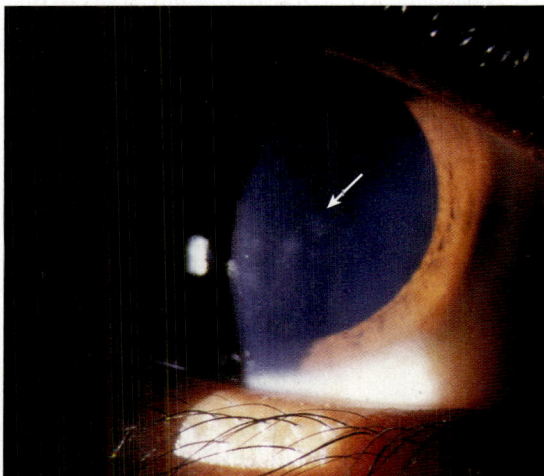

FIGURE 28-34 ■ Nummular keratitis (coin-shaped opacities) (arrow) due to Epstein-Barr virus infection.

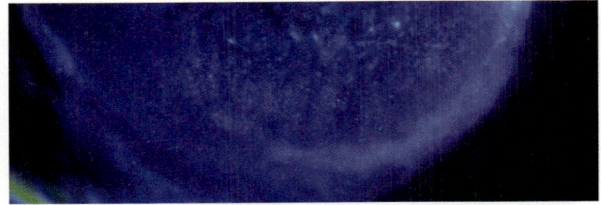

FIGURE 28-35 ■ High-magnification slit lamp photograph of inferior corneal irritation spots (superficial punctate keratitis), stained by fluorescein. (Photograph contributed by Anthony Lubniewski, MD.)

Dry eyes

Patients with abnormal tear function may develop corneal problems due to inadequate lubrication. This may occur for a variety of reasons. Primary dysfunction of the lacrimal gland in children is unusual, but may occur in disorders such as familial dysautonomia. Eyelid malposition or inflammation (blepharitis) may interfere with tear function. Children who have undergone bone marrow transplantation may develop *graft-versus-host disease*, which commonly affects the lacrimal gland.

The symptoms of dry eyes are similar in these disorders. These include ocular irritation, light sensitivity, intermittent blurred vision, and a foreign body sensation in the eyes. On examination, microscopic irritation spots of the cornea are visible with fluorescein staining (*superficial punctate keratitis*) (Figure 28–35). Artificial tear lubricating drops can be used for treatment, but are often difficult to use in children. Occlusion of the lacrimal puncta with either punctal plugs (Figure 28–36) or cau-

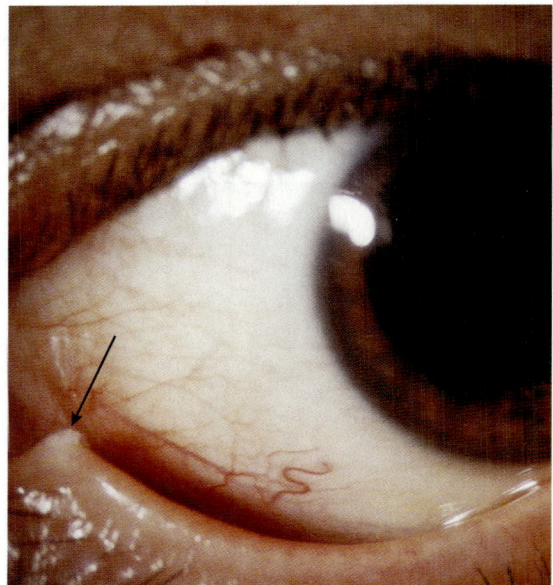

FIGURE 28-36 ■ Punctal plug (arrow) in a patient with dry eyes. The plug is inserted into the puncta, and the top lays flat against the eyelid. (Photograph contributed by Anthony Lubniewski, MD.)

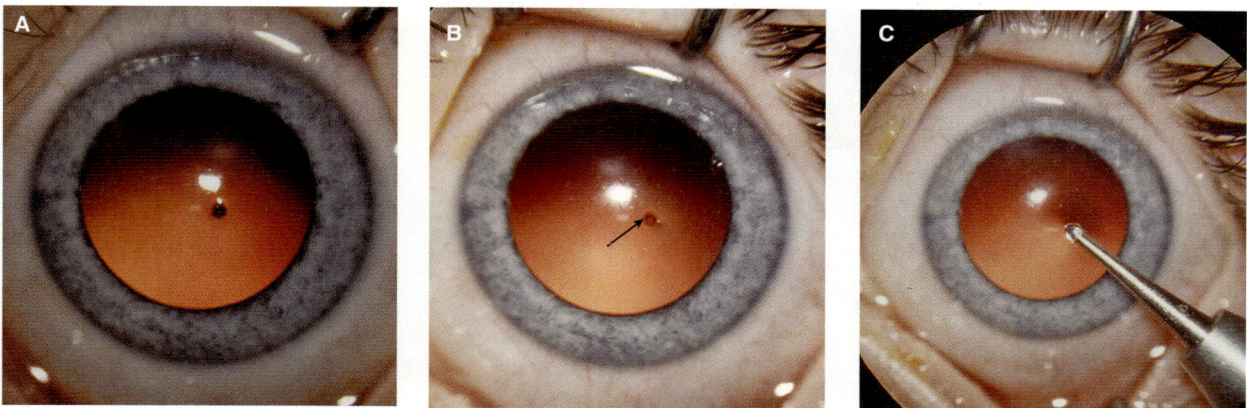

FIGURE 28–37 ■ Small metallic corneal foreign body. (A) The foreign body is often most easily seen in retroillumination. (B) A rust ring (arrow) remains after removal of the metallic foreign body. (C) A corneal burr is used to remove the rust ring.

tery may provide relief by allowing the tears that are produced to stay in place longer and provide lubrication.

Corneal trauma

Corneal trauma in children usually results from a corneal abrasion, a foreign body, or a penetrating ocular injury:

Corneal abrasion or foreign body Corneal abrasions and foreign bodies usually present with the acute onset of eye pain and conjunctival redness. In most patients the history is straightforward, with the patient reporting development of symptoms while playing or working with something that gets into the eyes. In infants and young children, the episode may be unwitnessed.

On examination, corneal abrasions are diagnosed by uptake of fluorescein in the area of the abrasion, which produces fluorescence when viewed with a blue light. Corneal foreign bodies are usually visible on examination, either with a penlight or with slit lamp (Figure 28–37A). However, some may be difficult to visualize, particularly clear glass or plastic.

Uncomplicated corneal abrasions are treated with topical antibiotic ointment. Most resolve within 24 to 48 hours. Superficial corneal foreign bodies can often be removed with a cotton-tipped applicator after placement of topical anesthetic drops. Patients should be referred to an ophthalmologist if there are signs of corneal infection (cloudiness surrounding the area of the abrasion or foreign body) (Figure 28–38), a foreign body that cannot be removed, or an abrasion that does not heal within 48 hours. Metallic foreign bodies may produce a rust ring in the cornea, requiring removal with a burr (Figure 28–37B and C).

Blunt trauma Blunt injuries to the cornea may cause dysfunction of the corneal endothelium, resulting in corneal edema. Folds on the inner layer of the cornea

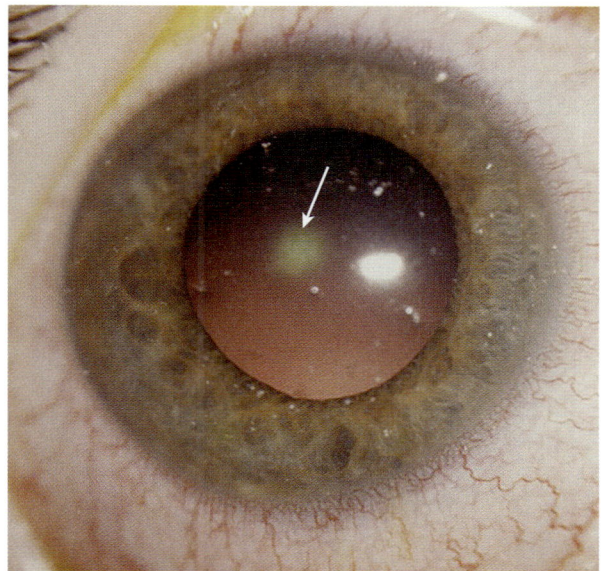

FIGURE 28–38 ■ Corneal foreign body after patient was struck by a tree branch. The presence of corneal clouding (arrow) at the site of the foreign body suggests infection, and prompt referral to an ophthalmologist is indicated.

may be visible on slit lamp examination (Figure 28–39). This type of injury usually improves with time.

Corneal laceration Corneal lacerations usually result from injury to the eye with a sharp object, but may also occur with a direct blunt injury (Figure 28–40A). If a corneal laceration is suspected, a metal protective shield should be placed over the eye (but not in direct contact with the eye) and the patient should be referred to an ophthalmologist immediately. If associated retinal injuries are not present, visual recovery may be good (Figure 28–40B). Some injuries are so severe that repair is not possible (Figure 28–41). A rare disorder, *sympathetic ophthalmia*, may

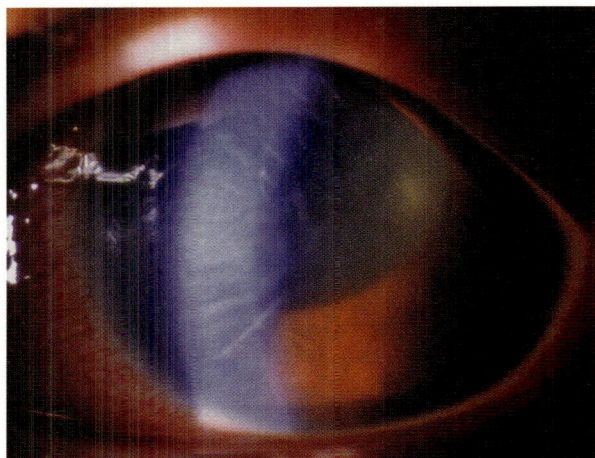

FIGURE 28–39 ■ Linear corneal endothelial folds and edema following blunt injury.

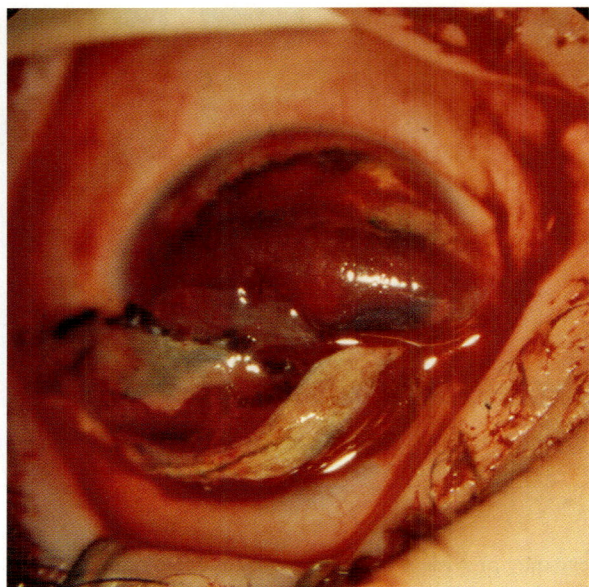

FIGURE 28–41 ■ Severe corneoscleral laceration with iris prolapse and disruption of intraocular contents.

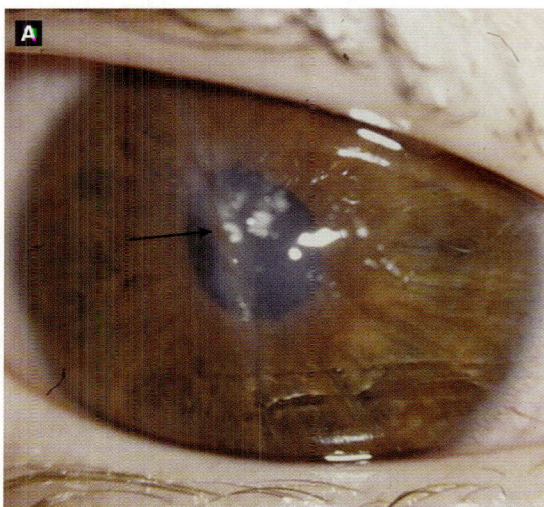

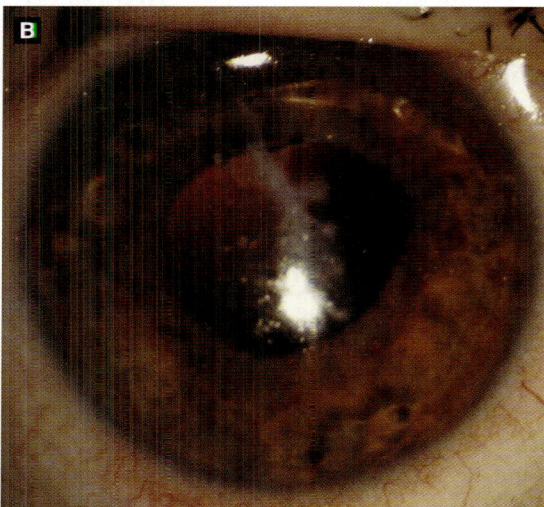

FIGURE 28–40 ■ Penetrating corneal injury. (A) Central laceration (arrow) from sharp object. (B) Well-healed scar after repair. Visual acuity returned to 20/20.

occur in patients with severe injuries. In sympathetic opthalmia, an autoimmune reaction develops in the normal eye, with uveitis that potentially may cause loss of vision. For this reason, eyes with severe injuries and no reasonable expectation for visual recovery are often surgically removed (enucleated).

REFRACTIVE SURGERY

Patients with moderate refractive errors, primarily near-sightedness, may undergo surgical procedures to reduce or eliminate the need for glasses. This is a very common elective procedure in adults. In corneal refractive surgery, the corneal shape is changed so that the light rays are focused properly on the retina. This can be performed by laser or incisional surgery. Refractive surgery may also be performed by insertion of intraocular lenses to change the eye's focus.

In general, children are not considered candidates for refractive surgery for 2 reasons. First, the shape of the eye changes continuously during childhood, so that even successfully performed surgery will become gradually ineffective due to normal growth of the eye. Second, the healing patterns of childrens' corneas differ from those of adults, and are less predictable. In some settings, however, refractive surgery in children may be a reasonable treatment option. One of these is disabled children with marked refractive errors who cannot wear spectacles due to behavioral problems.[3] Another is children with severe unilateral amblyopia due to asymmetric refractive errors.[4]

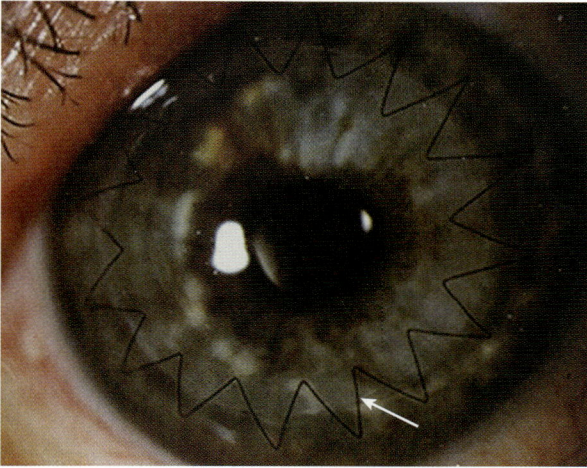

FIGURE 28–42 ■ Corneal transplant (penetrating keratoplasty) with excellent clarity. The fine suture used to sew the transplant to the host is visible (arrow) in a stellate configuration for 360°.

CORNEAL TRANSPLANTATION

Corneal transplantation (penetrating keratoplasty) may be used to treat corneal opacities that do not respond to other treatments. In a corneal transplant, a trephine is used to remove the cornea from the host, and a donor cornea is sewn into the eye (Figure 28–42). There are several issues that make corneal transplantation more complicated in infants and young children when compared with adults. First, the small size and increased elasticity of the infant cornea make the procedure technically challenging. Second, one of the greatest risks of corneal transplantation is rejection of the transplant, leading to opacification. The active immune systems of children increase this risk. Third, even successfully transplanted corneas may have large degrees of astigmatism, which increases the risk for amblyopia. Fourth,

continuous application of corticosteroid drops is often necessary to prevent rejection, and these drops have the potential for deleterious side effects, such as increasing intraocular pressure. Fifth, transplants are not typically performed in the presence of active inflammation, infection, or persistently elevated intraocular pressure, which may prolong the period of decreased vision while waiting for a transplant, thus worsening the amblyopia. Finally, patients with corneal transplants require meticulous follow-up, which usually necessitates frequent examinations under anesthesia in infancy.

A new transplantation technique, Descemet stripping endothelial keratoplasty (DSEK), has been developed in which just the corneal endothelium, rather than the entire cornea, is transplanted. The surgery is performed through a small incision. The patient's endothelium is scraped off and removed. A sheet of donor endothelium is rolled with a special instrument, placed in the eye, and unfolded. This technique shows promise, and may eliminate some of the problems noted above, but DSEK has not been studied extensively in children.

REFERENCES

1. Summers CG, Purple RL, Krivit W et al. Ocular changes in the mucopolysaccharidoses after bone marrow transplantation. *Ophthalmology.* 1989;96:977–985.
2. Schwartz GS, Holland EJ. Oral acyclovir for the management of herpes simples virus keratitis in children. *Ophthalmology.* 2000;107:278–282.
3. Tychsen L, Packwood E, Hoekel J, Lueder G. Refractive surgery for high bilateral myopia in children with neurobehavioral disorders: clear lens extraction and refractive lens exchange. *JAAPOS.* 2006;10:357–363.
4. Paysse EA, Coats DK, Hussein MAW, Hamill MB, Koch DD. Long-term outcomes of photorefractive keratectomy for anisometropic amblyopia in children. *Ophthalmology.* 2006;113:169–176.

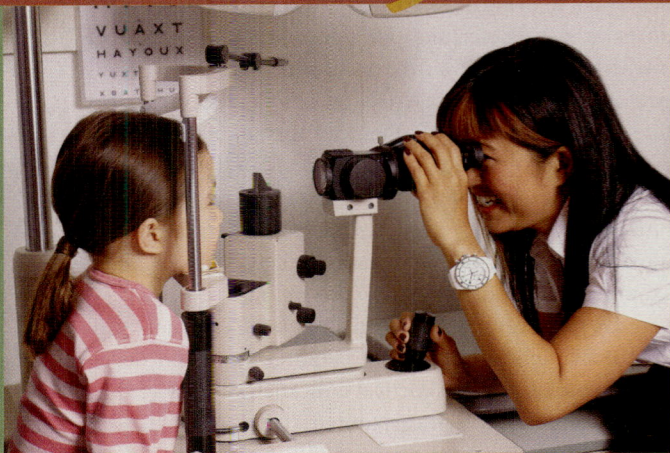

CHAPTER 29

Disorders of the Iris and Pupil

ANATOMY AND EMBRYOLOGY

The iris is a structure composed of connective tissue and blood vessels that lies just anterior to the lens. The central opening in the iris forms the pupil. The color of the iris is determined by pigmented cells within the stroma. Pigment may accumulate in these cells during the first year of life, and the color of the iris often changes during this time. The posterior layer of the iris is deeply pigmented. It extends slightly onto the anterior surface at the edge of the pupil.

The size of the pupil is variable. It changes in response to neural input to the smooth muscles within the iris. The dilator muscle of the iris is stimulated by sympathetic pathways. The chain of neurons responsible for dilation begin in the hypothalamus and synapses in the thoracic vertebra (first-order neuron), then passes out of the spinal column, across the pulmonary apex to synapse in the superior cervical ganglion (second-order neuron), then along the internal carotid plexus and through the cavernous sinus to join with the ophthalmic division of cranial nerve V and travel to the dilator muscle (third-order neuron) (Figure 29–1). The iris sphincter muscle is innervated by the parasympathetic system. These neurons originate in the Edinger-Westphal subnucleus of the third cranial nerve and travel along the inferior division of the nerve to the ciliary ganglion (preganglionic fibers), then to the iris sphincter through the short ciliary nerves (postganglionic fibers). These pathways mediate pupil constriction to light and near.

Embryology

At 6 weeks of gestation the iris begins to form in association with the *tunica vasculosa lentis*. This is a network of blood vessels that extends through mesenchymal

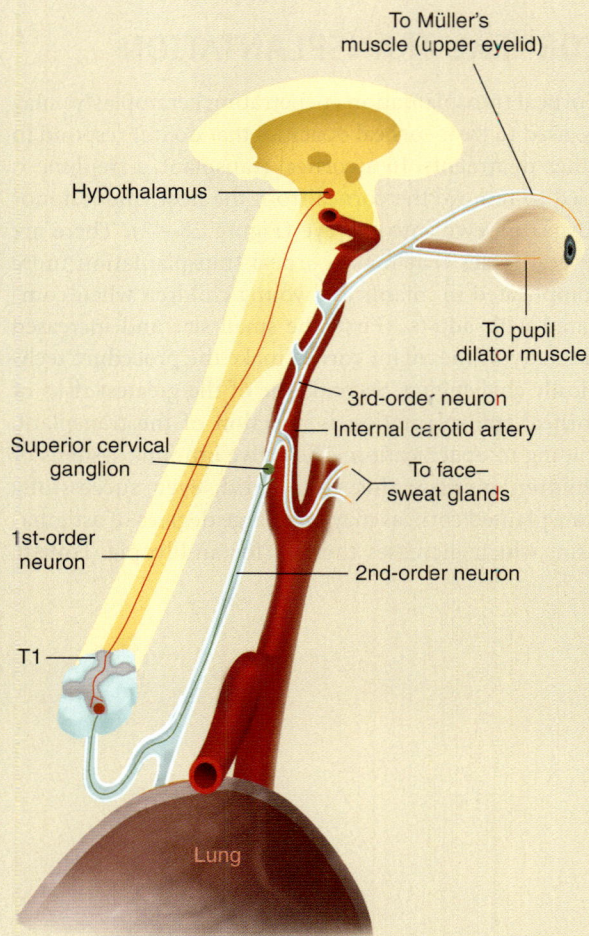

FIGURE 29–1 ■ The sympathetic pathway for iris dilator muscles (pupil dilation). The first-order neuron begins in the hypothalamus, travels through the spinal cord, and synapses in the thoracic vertebrae. The second-order neuron travels over the pulmonary apex and synapses in the superior cervical ganglion. The third-order neuron travels adjacent to the internal carotid artery, then through the cavernous sinus to reach the eye. Damage anywhere along this pathway may cause Horner syndrome.

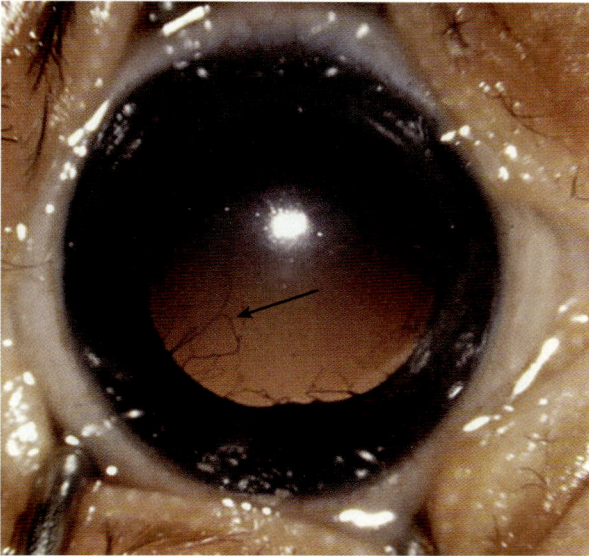

FIGURE 29–2 ■ Physiological regressing iris vessels (tunica vasculosa lentis) in a premature infant (arrow).

tissue on the anterior surface of the developing lens. The muscles of the iris sphincter begin to develop at around 3 months' gestation, followed at 6 months by formation of the dilator muscles. The iris stroma forms from neural crest cells. The posterior pigmented epithelium and muscles form from neuroectoderm. Much of the iris remains incompletely formed at birth, including pigmentation of the anterior layer and formation of the dilator muscles. This is why the iris often appears somewhat hypoplastic, even in normal newborns. During normal embryogenesis the tunica vasulosa lentis resorbs in the pupillary opening by birth. Remnants of the membrane may be seen in premature infants (Figure 29–2).

Abnormalities of the iris in children are relatively uncommon.

PATHOGENESIS

Abnormalities of the iris and pupil may occur in a variety of conditions. These include developmental abnormalities, structural changes, iris masses, changes associated with systemic diseases, inflammation, and neurological abnormalities that affect the pupils.

CLINICAL PRESENTATION

Iris abnormalities are usually detected by an abnormal appearance. These include changes in shape or size of the pupil, iris color, or lesions on the iris. Some iris disorders affect vision, but many do not. The latter are first noted by families or physicians (during a penlight examination or by noting an abnormality of the red reflex).

IRIS DISORDERS

Structural Abnormalities of the Iris

Congenital abnormalities of size

The pupil may be abnormally small or large at birth. *Microcoria* describes a small pupil, typically less than 2 mm. Primary microcoria occurs as a result of dilator muscle insufficiency. Generally, pupil openings smaller than 1.5 mm do not allow for adequate image formation, and may require surgical enlargement. Microcoria may occur as an isolated finding, or may be associated with systemic disorders, including Lowe syndrome, Marfan syndrome, and congenital rubella (Figure 29–3A). If the

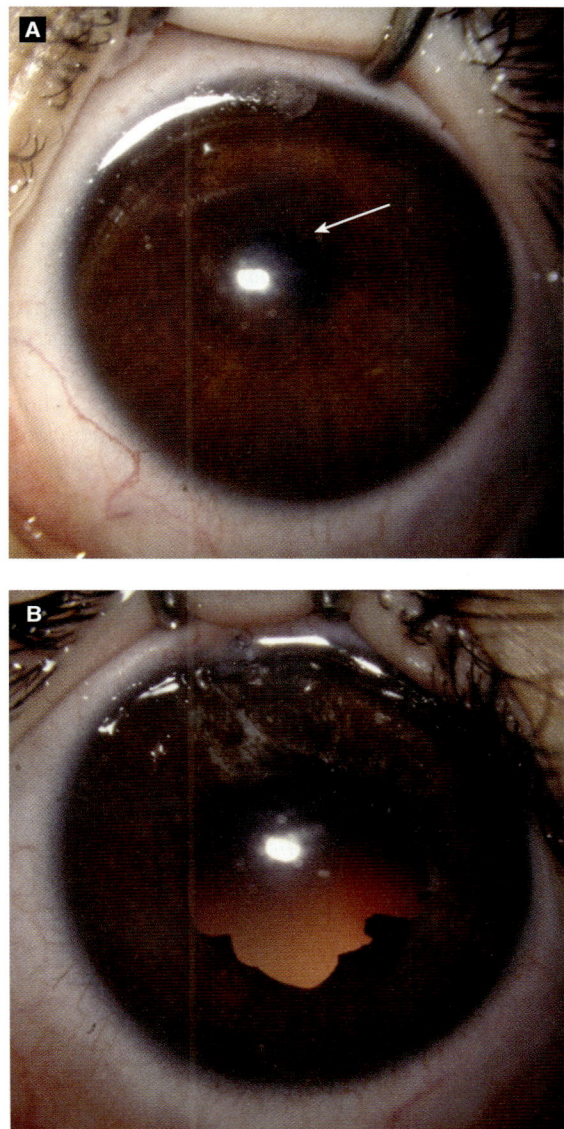

FIGURE 29–3 ■ (A) Microcoria (small pupil) in a patient with Marfan syndrome. A few strands of iris tissue are attached to the lens (arrow). (B) Appearance after pupilloplasty (surgery to enlarge pupillary opening).

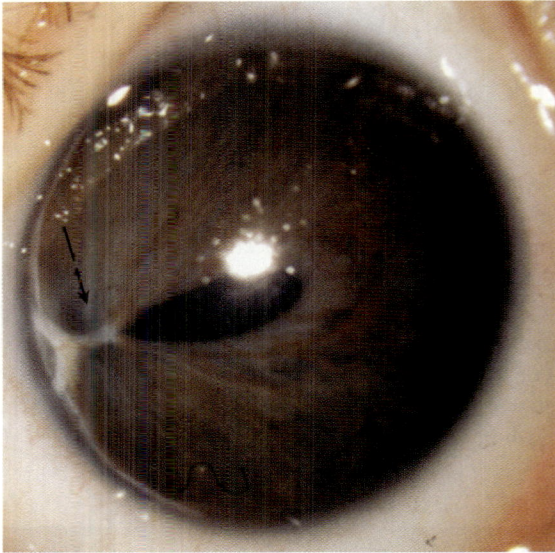

FIGURE 29–4 ■ Congenital corectopia. The pupil is distorted due to a band of fibrous tissue (arrow).

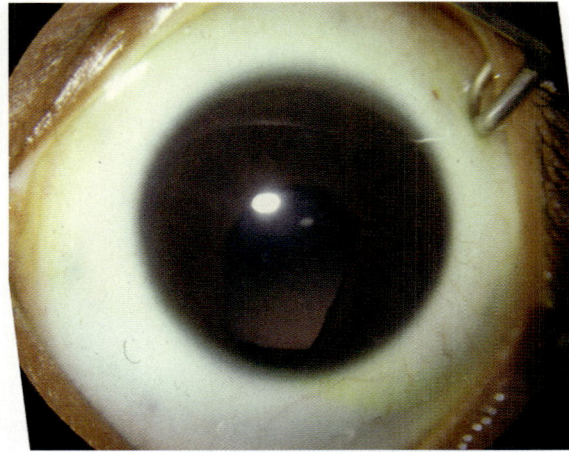

FIGURE 29–5 ■ Iris coloboma, left eye.

pupillary opening is so small that visual images cannot be properly formed, surgery to enlarge the opening is indicated. In this surgery, the pupil is enlarged by making cuts through the margin of the pupil (Figure 29–3B).

Congenital mydriasis is a condition in which the pupils are large and poorly reactive at birth. This sometimes occurs in association with congenital cardiac disease. If there are significant symptoms (e.g., photophobia), treatment with iris constricting medication (pilocarpine) or surgical reduction of the pupillary opening may be indicated.

Congenital abnormalities of shape or location

An abnormal shape of the iris is called *corectopia*. This may occur as a primary defect (Figure 29–4), or in association with lens subluxation.

Iris coloboma Iris colobomas occur as a result of incomplete closure of the embryonic fissure during formation of the eye. Because the inferonasal quadrant is the last area of the fissure to close, this is the typical location of iris colobomas (Figure 29–5). Colobomas may be isolated to the iris, or may be associated with colobomas of the lens, retina or optic nerve. Large colobomas are often associated with underdevelopment of the entire eye (*microphthalmos*), and may be accompanied by lens subluxation (Figure 29–6). Iris colobomas may occur in association with many systemic abnormalities, including Trisomy 13 and CHARGE syndrome (Coloboma, Heart defects, Atresia of nasal choanae, growth Retardation, Genitourinary and Ear anomalies).

Persistent tunica vasculosa lentis During embryological development, the normal network of vessels in the pupillary opening usually regresses by the time of birth. Residual vessels may be seen in normal infants who are born prematurely (Figure 29–2), and small remnants are visible in many normal individuals (Figure 29–8). Very prominent vessels are sometimes present at birth, which may regress spontaneously (Figure 29–7A and B). Larger bands of tissue may extend from the iris and attach to the lens capsule, causing distortion of the iris. Rarely, these remnants are large enough that they may interfere with vision (*persistent pupillary membrane*), in which case surgical removal may be indicated (Figure 29–9A and B).

Heterochromia Iridis

The color of the iris is determined by pigment cells within the stroma. During the first year of life, pigment accumulation may change the color. In most

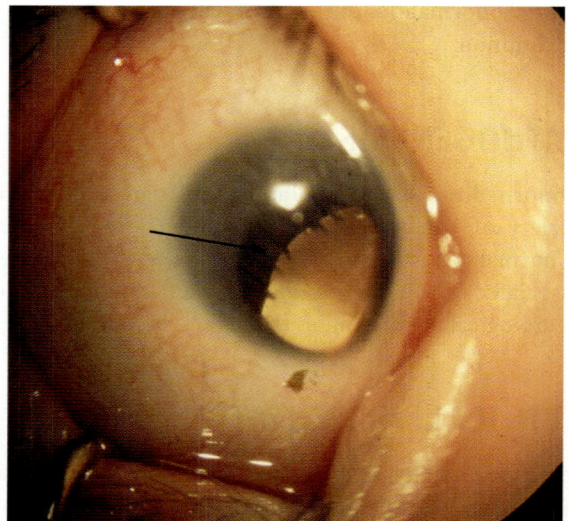

FIGURE 29–6 ■ Iris coloboma and lens subluxation (the arrow points to the inferonasally displaced lens border, with attached elongated ciliary processes), right eye.

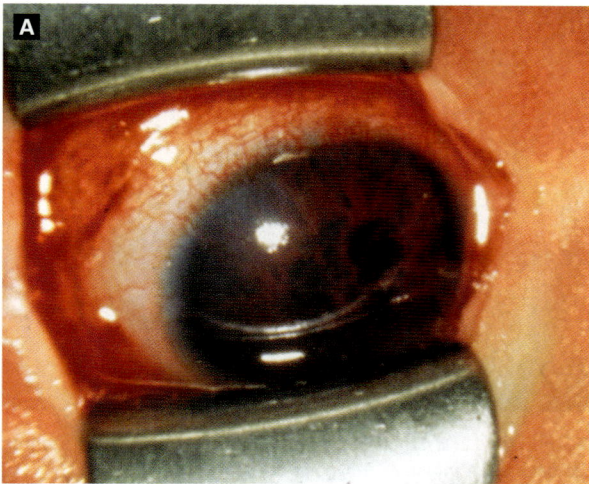

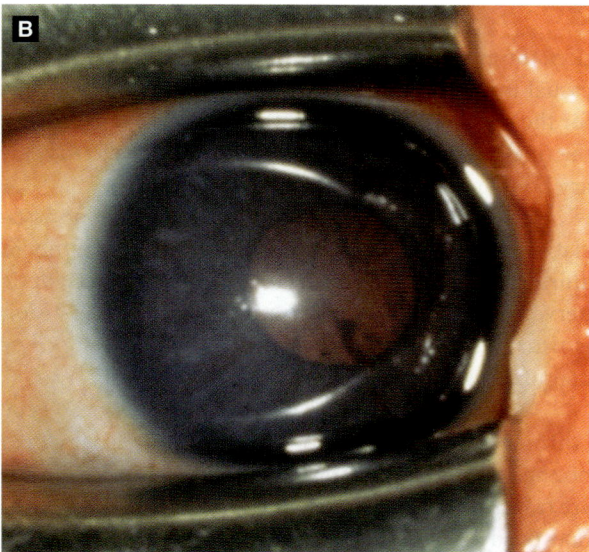

FIGURE 29–7 ■ (A) Marked persistent tunica vasculosa lentis in a 1-day-old infant. (B) Significant reduction in abnormal vessels by day of life 4.

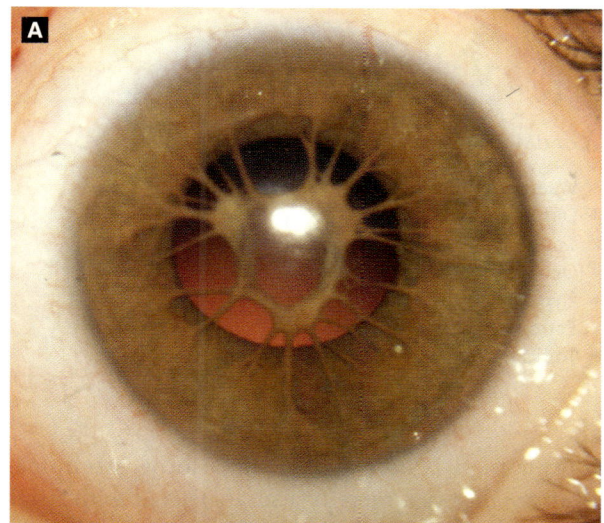

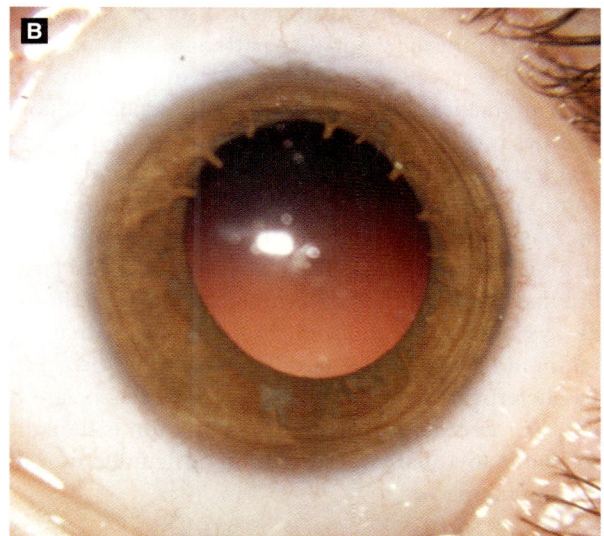

FIGURE 29–9 ■ (A) Prominent persistent pupillary membrane, interfering with vision. (B) Appearance after surgical removal of membrane.

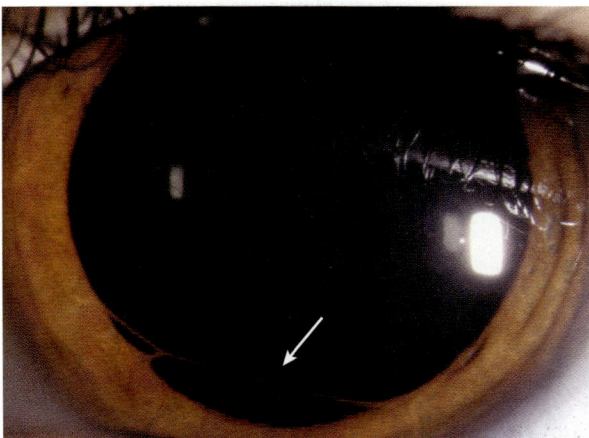

FIGURE 29–8 ■ Small persistent pupillary membrane (arrow). This produces no visual problems.

people, the 2 pupils have the same color. *Heterochromia* is present if the color of the 2 irises is different (Figure 29–10). This may occur in association with a number of ocular or systemic conditions (Table 29–1). These include *Waardenburg syndrome* (Figure 29–11),

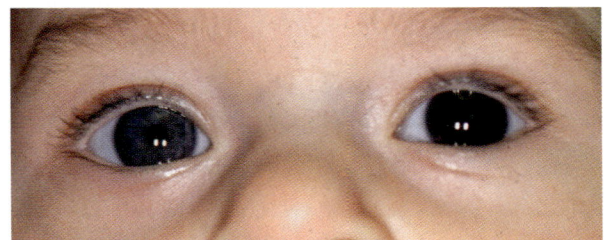

FIGURE 29–10 ■ Congenital iris heterochromia.

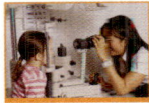

FIGURE 29–12 ■ Whorl pattern of abnormal skin pigmentation on the back of an infant with hypomelanosis of Ito.

hypomelanosis of Ito, and congenital Horner syndrome. *Waardenburg syndrome* is also associated with focal areas of decreased hair pigmentation and hearing loss. *Hypomelanosis of Ito* is a sporadic disorder characterized by an unusual whorl-like pattern of skin pigmentation (Figure 29–12). Central nervous system and limb anomalies occur in some patients. Ocular abnormalities include heterochromia, cataracts, and abnormal retinal pigmentation. *Iris nevi* are relatively common in children, and present as focal areas of increased pigment against the lighter normal iris stroma (Figure 29–13). The size is variable, and large lesions may mimic heterochromia. Iris nevi are almost always benign in children, but evaluation may be required if they change (similar to nevi on the skin). Iris heterochromia has been reported in association with *Hirschsprung disease*. This association is thought to be due to a shared perturbation of neural crest cell development.

Aniridia

Aniridia is a congenital, bilateral condition in which the iris is severely underdeveloped. The term aniridia is a misnomer, because almost all affected patients have at least a rudimentary stump of iris tissue, although this may not be visible without gonioscopy. On examina-

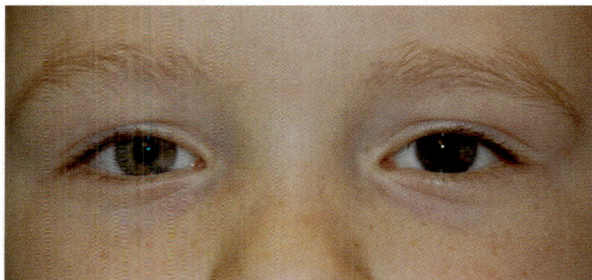

tion, the entire lens is visible (Figure 29–14A and B). On casual inspection the edge of the lens may be mistaken for the pupillary opening. With slit lamp magnification, the fine suspensory fibers that attach the lens to the ciliary body may be visualized.

Aniridia has important ocular and systemic associations. Ocular abnormalities that occur commonly in aniridia include corneal surface disease, cataracts, optic nerve and foveal hypoplasia, and glaucoma. The vision is usually significantly decreased. Infants develop nystagmus early in life.

Aniridia is caused by mutations of the *PAX6* gene (chromosome 11p13), and may occur in heritable and nonheritable forms. Approximately two-thirds of cases are transmitted as an autosomal dominant disorder, and one-third are sporadic. Wilms tumor occurs in approximately one-third of sporadic cases, because the Wilms tumor gene (*WT1*) is contiguous with the aniridia gene.

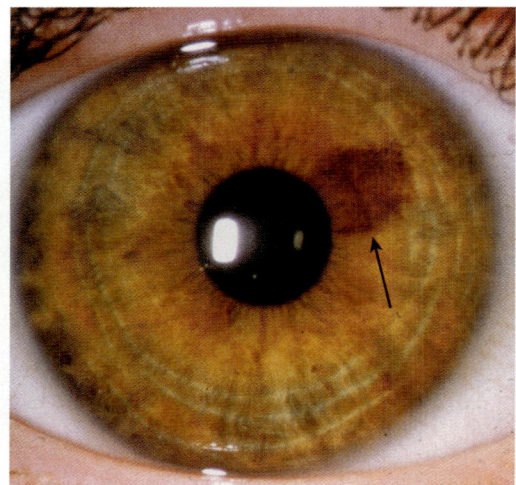

FIGURE 29–11 ■ Heterochromia in a patient with Waardenburg syndrome.

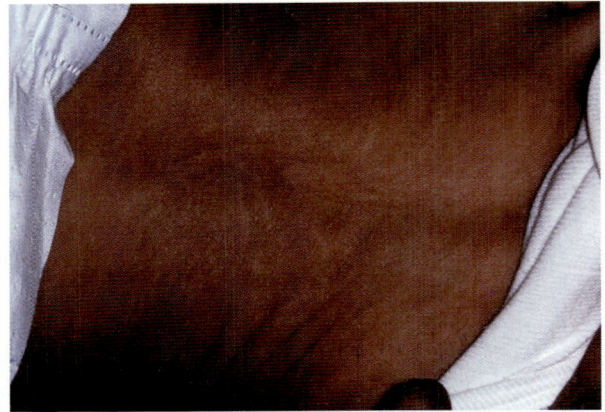

FIGURE 29–13 ■ Small iris nevus (arrow). These lesions are almost always benign in children.

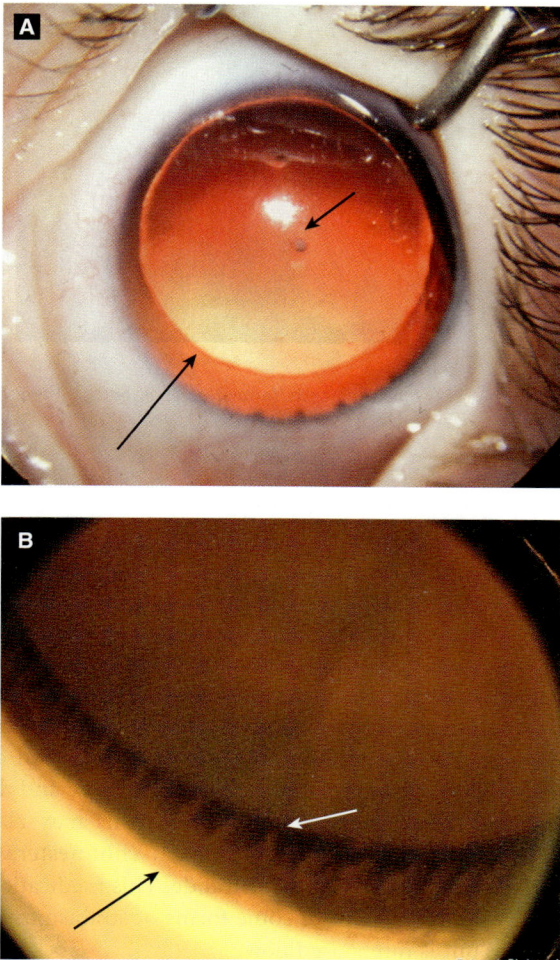

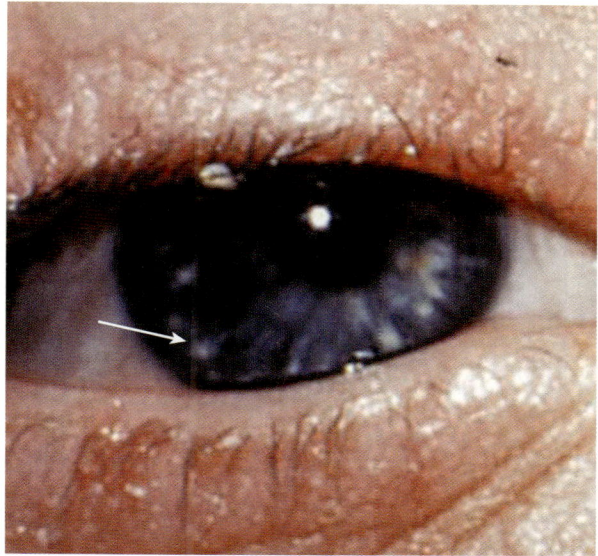

FIGURE 29–15 ■ Brushfield spots (arrow) in a patient with Trisomy 21.

FIGURE 29–14 ■ (A) Aniridia. The edge of the lens is visible for 360° (long arrow). A small cataract is present in the center of the lens (short arrow). (B) Gonioscopic view in aniridia. The ciliary processes (short arrow) are visible adjacent to the edge of the lens. The tan stripe (long arrow) is the normal trabecular meshwork.

tan-colored, and appear as small, stuck-on lesions on the iris surface (Figure 29–16). They increase in number and size with age. They are present in approximately 10% of patients with neurofibromatosis at 1 year of age, and in more than 90% of patients by adulthood. They do not cause visual problems, but are important diagnostic finding that may help in the evaluation of patient with neurofibromatosis.

Iris mammilations

Iris mammilations usually appear as bilateral, multiple, small, slightly elevated lesions on the iris surface (Figure 29–17). Their color is the same as the underlying normal iris. They do not produce any visual problems. Iris

Mutations of this location may also produce the WAGR complex (Wilms tumor, aniridia, genitourinary abnormalities, and mental retardation). If genetic testing of children with sporadic aniridia identifies tumors in the *WT1* gene, regular monitoring for Wilms tumor with renal ultrasonography is indicated.

Iris Lesions

Brushfield spots

Children with Trisomy 21 often have small, white spots on the iris that result from hyperplasia of the stroma (Figure 29–15). They are nonprogressive and do not cause any visual dysfunction.

Lisch nodules

Lisch nodules are small hamartomas that occur on the iris in patients with *neurofibromatosis*. They are usually

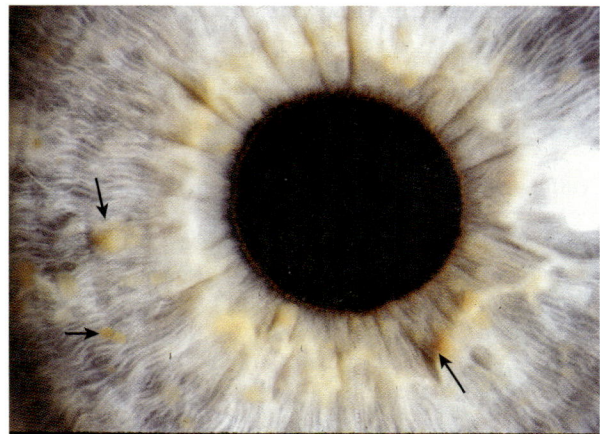

FIGURE 29–16 ■ Multiple small Lisch nodules in a patient with neurofibromatosis. They are the small, tan-colored nodules on the anterior surface of the blue background iris. The arrows point to some of the lesions.

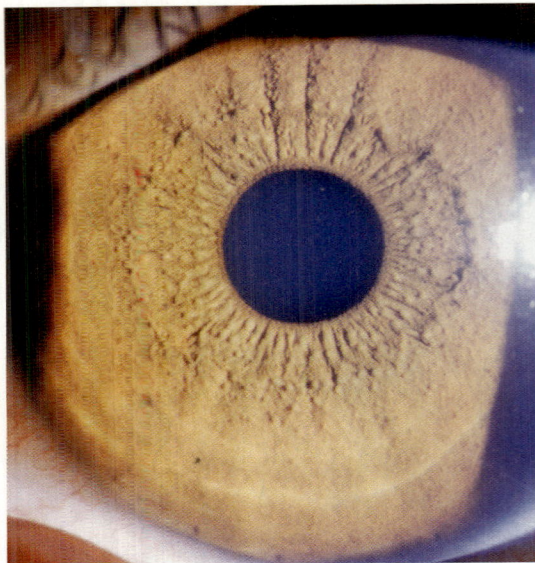

FIGURE 29–17 ■ Iris mamillations. These are differentiated from Lisch nodules by their smaller size and same color as the background iris.

mamillations need to be differentiated from Lisch nodules, because they are not diagnostic of neurofibromatosis (Table 29–2). Lisch nodules are distinguished by their irregular distribution, difference in color from the underlying iris, and stuck-on appearance.

Juvenile xanthogranuloma

Iris lesions in patients with juvenile xanthogranuloma (JXG) may occur as an isolated finding or in conjunction with skin lesions. They may appear as yellow-reddish, elevated lesions on the iris surface, or as diffuse thickening of the iris. Spontaneous bleeding from these lesions may occur, and JXG is one of the most common causes of spontaneous hyphemas in infants. Glaucoma may result from the bleeding or from accumulation of JXG cells in the trabecular meshwork. Treatment

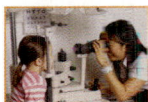

FIGURE 29–18 ■ Small iris cysts (arrow) at pupil border. These do not cause visual problems.

options for intraocular JXG that is causing complications include topical or systemic corticosteroids and low-dose radiation.

Iris cysts

Iris cysts may present in different fashions. Small cysts of the pigment epithelium may appear as small irregularities at the pupil margin in newborns (Figure 29–18). They are most commonly noted during evaluation of the red reflex. These lesions are nonprogressive and do not cause visual problems. Similar lesions may also develop following the use of topical cholinesterase inhibitors such as phospholine iodide. This medication was used for treatment of some forms of strabismus in the past, but is rarely used now.

Primary cysts of the iris stroma may present as elevated areas on the iris surface. They may enlarge and cause complications, including glaucoma and amblyopia due to obstruction of vision (Figure 29–19).

Congenital iris ectropion (ectropion uveae)

In this condition, heavily pigmented cells from the posterior pigmented iris epithelium migrate onto the anterior iris surface at the pupil. It presents with dark pigment at

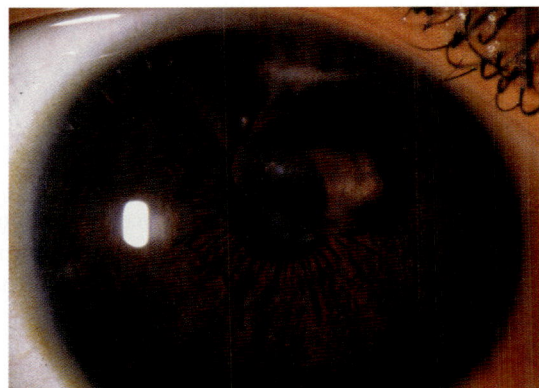

Table 29–2.

Differentiating Iris Mammilations from Lisch Nodules

	Lisch Nodules	Iris Mammilations
Diagnostic significance	Pathognomonic for neurofibromatosis	None
Change with age	Increased size and number	No change
Distribution	Irregular	Symmetric
Size	Small to large	Small
Color	Usually tan	Same color as background iris
Location	Appear "stuck on" top of iris	Within iris stroma itself

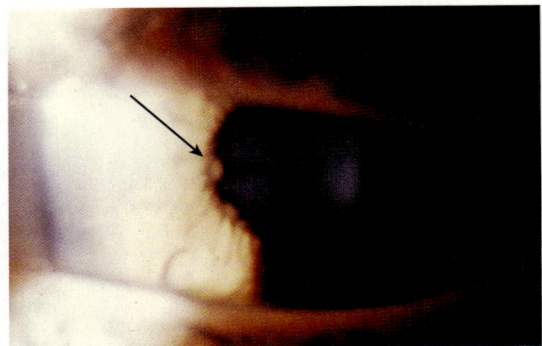

FIGURE 29–19 ■ Iris cyst obstructing most of pupil.

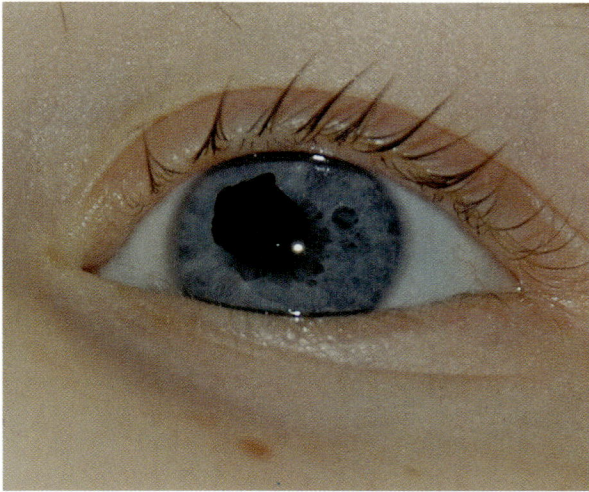

FIGURE 29–20 ■ Congenital ectropion uveae in a patient with neurofibromatosis. The dark, irregular lesion extends onto the surface of the iris from the pupil.

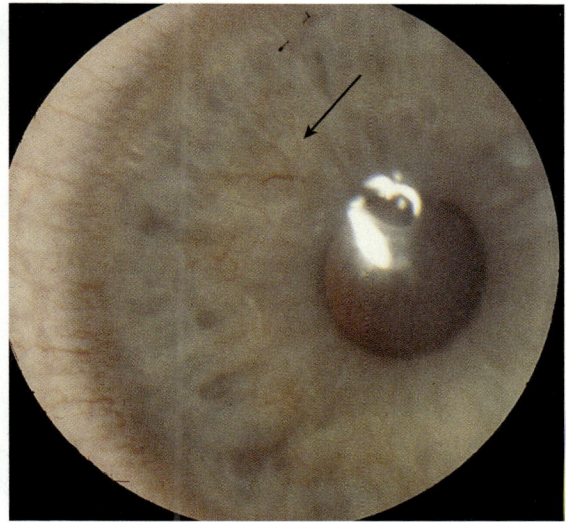

FIGURE 29–21 ■ Leukemic iris infiltrates. The vascular, creamy lesions (arrow) are present on the anterior iris.

the pupil margin with irregular borders (Figure 29–20). It may occur as an isolated abnormality or in association with other abnormalities of the anterior segment, in which case there is a risk of glaucoma. It is sometimes seen in patients with neurofibromatosis type 1.

Iris tumors

Iris tumors in children are very rare. Primary or metastatic lesions may occur. As discussed above, iris nevi are fairly common in children. They present as flat, pigmented areas that do not disturb the underlying iris architecture. Malignant transformation of iris nevi in children almost never occurs.

Medulloepitheliomas (diktyomas) are rare tumors that arise in the ciliary body in children. They usually present due to distortion of the adjacent iris. These lesions may be malignant and may metastasize. Enucleation (removal) of the eye may be necessary for treatment.

Metastatic iris lesions may occur with pediatric malignancies, but they are rare. The iris may be a site of leukemia recurrence, because chemotherapeutic agents penetrate into the eye poorly (Figure 29–21).

If an iris tumor is suspected, fine needle biopsy may be performed to establish a diagnosis.

Iris Abnormalities Due to Other Ocular Diseases

Ocular Trauma

Trauma to the iris may cause damage to the sphincter or dilator muscles, resulting in an irregularly-shaped pupil (corectopia), small pupil (miosis), or large pupil (mydriasis). This may be limited to specific areas of the iris, which can be visualized as sectoral zones of poor

constriction on slit lamp examination. Pupillary dysfunction that is present in the immediate posttraumatic period often improves with time, but sometimes the damage is permanent. It usually does not interfere with vision, although some patients with traumatic mydriasis may have symptoms of photophobia.

More severe blunt trauma may cause *iridodialysis*, in which the base of the iris separates from its peripheral attachments to the sclera (Figure 29–22). Patients with this type of injury frequently have other manifestations of trauma, such as traumatic cataract or retinal detachments. Corectopia may be present in penetrating ocular injuries in which the iris prolapses through the wound (Figure 29–23).

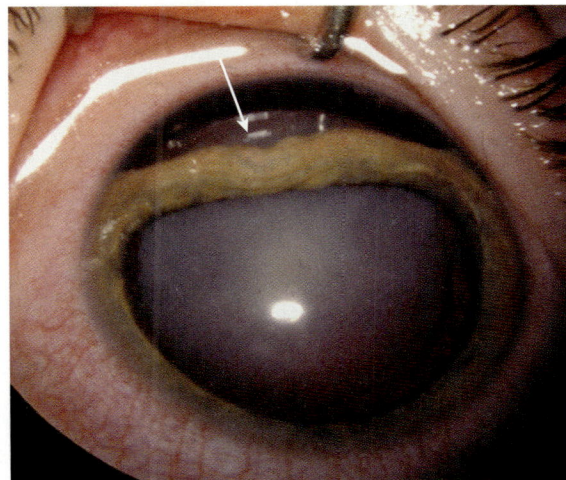

FIGURE 29–22 ■ Traumatic iridodialysis. The base of the iris has separated from its attachment to the wall of the eye (arrow). The patient also has a traumatic cataract.

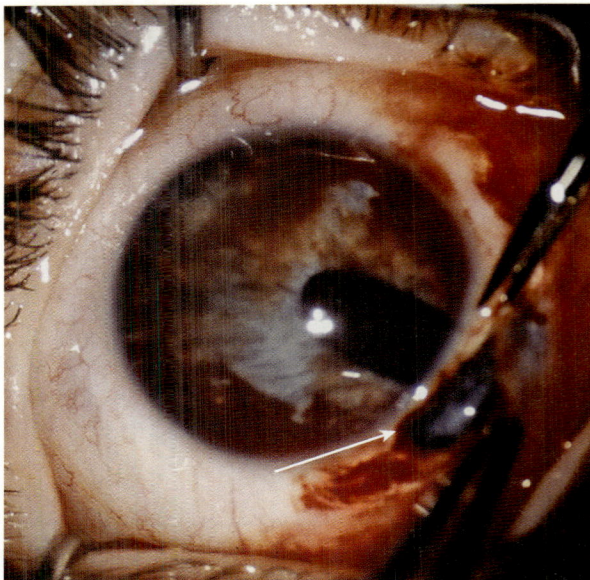

FIGURE 29-23 ■ Penetrating ocular injury, with iris protruding through wound (arrow). The eye is being held by surgical forceps.

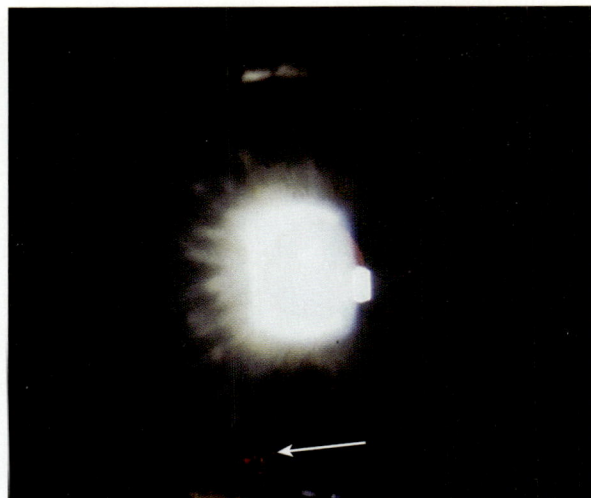

FIGURE 29-25 ■ Iris transillumination defects, high-magnification slitlamp view. The light is shined directly into the pupil and the transillumination defects are visible as glowing red areas (arrow) in the peripheral iris.

Ocular trauma may also cause bleeding from blood vessels within the iris, causing blood to enter the anterior chamber of the eye (*hyphema*). This is discussed in Chapter 32.

Retinopathy of Prematurity

In advanced retinopathy, dilation of the ocular vasculature may include the vessels of the iris (*iris plus disease*) (Figure 29–24). The presence of these vessels on the iris

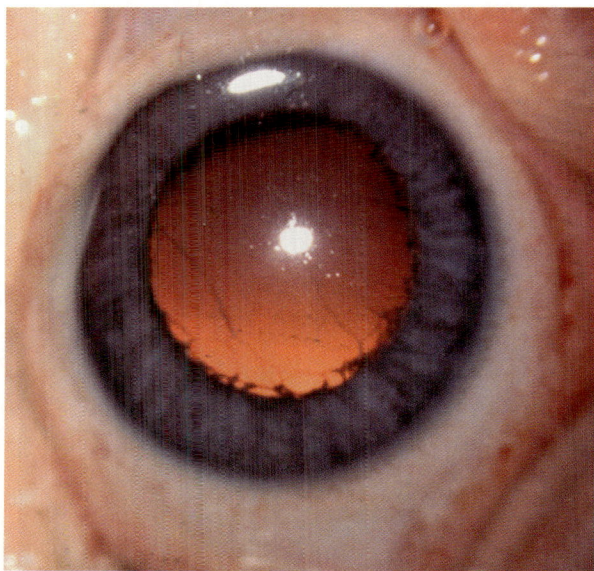

FIGURE 29-24 ■ Iris plus disease in a patient with retinopathy of prematurity. The abnormal vessels are visible on the edge of the pupil and on the iris surface itself.

is almost always associated with significant changes within the retinal vasculature itself. The iris abnormalities may interfere with pupil dilation, making laser treatment more difficult.

Iris Transillumination Defects

These are caused by areas of decreased pigment within the iris stroma. They are usually not visible on direct examination, because light reflects off the normal anterior iris surface. They may be visualized by shining a light directly into the pupil (Figure 29–25), or by holding a transilluminating light against the sclera. Transillumination defects in children are most commonly seen in children with albinism, and are helpful in establishing this diagnosis. They may also occur in association with ocular trauma or inflammation.

Iritis/Ocular Inflammation

The most common ocular inflammatory disease that causes secondary iris changes is *juvenile idiopathic arthritis* (JIA). Inflammation may cause scar tissue (synechia) to form between the iris and the lens capsule (Figure 29–26). This may produce areas of irregular dilation or fixed pupils.

JIA usually presents in early childhood. Patients may have isolated arthritis, isolated ocular inflammation, or both. The systemic and ocular inflammations often occur independently of one another. A strikingly unusual feature of JIA-associated iritis is the frequent absence of pain. Unlike most patients with iritis, who experience marked ocular discomfort, patients with JIA may have severe intraocular inflammation that is not is based on risk factors that increase the likelihood that patients will develop iritis, which include female gender, pauciarticular arthritis, and positive antinuclear antibodies in the blood (Table 29–3).[1]

Other Causes of Iritis in Children

Tubulointerstitial nephritis and uveitis In this disorder, patients usually present in the second decade with bilateral iritis. Females are more commonly affected. Systemic symptoms due to interstitial nephritis include malaise, weight loss, fatigue, and fever. The symptoms due to renal disease usually (but not always) precede the development of iritis. Renal evaluation reveals decreased creatinine clearance and elevated urinary β-2 microglobulins.

Intermediate uveitis (pars planitis) The primary site of ocular inflammation in this form of uveitis is the pars plana (the anterior border of the retina). It is usually idiopathic, but may occur with several systemic diseases, including sarcoidosis, multiple sclerosis, syphilis, tuberculosis, and Lyme disease. Patients present with inflammatory cells in the anterior chamber and/or vitreous cavity. Collections of white blood cells are often present at the pars plana inferiorly, a finding referred to as *snowbanking*. The vision may be affected due to edema within the retina, retinal detachments, and cataracts.

Sarcoidosis Sarcoidosis may occur in children, and is associated with a form of iritis characterized by thickened deposits on the corneal endothelium and iris. Unlike adults with sarcoidosis, who usually have pulmonary involvement, children are more likely to develop skin nodules and arthritis. Elevated angiotensin-converting enzyme (ACE) levels may be

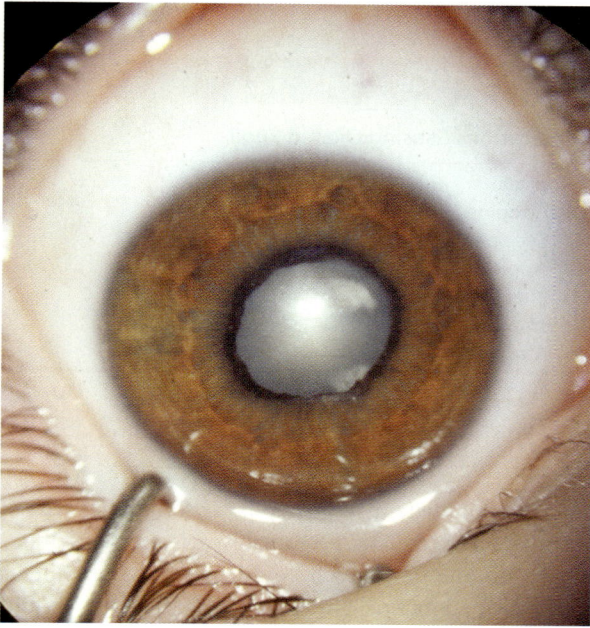

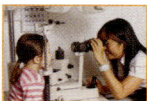

FIGURE 29–26 ■ Juvenile idiopathic arthritis (JIA). Dense cataract and scarring of iris to anterior lens capsule secondary to iritis. Note that the remainder of the eye does not appear inflamed, which is a characteristic feature of JIA-associated iritis.

painful. The disease is often not detected until the visual acuity is affected by cataracts or abnormal pupil reactions due to iris scarring are noted.

Because Juvenile idiopathic arthritis (JIA)-associated iritis is often asymptomatic and the potential visual consequences are severe, children with this diagnosis require routine ophthalmological examinations to monitor for iritis. The frequency of these examinations

Table 29–3.

Recommended Frequency of Ophthalmologic Examinations in Children With JIA

Type	ANA	Age at Onset, y	Duration of Disease, y	Risk Category	Eye Examination Frequency, mo
Oligoarthritis or polyarthritis	+	≤6	≤4	High	3
	+	≤6	>4	Moderate	6
	+	≤6	>7	Low	12
	+	>6	≤4	Moderate	6
	+	>6	>4	Low	12
	−	≤6	≤4	Moderate	6
	−	≤6	>4	Low	12
	−	>6	NA	Low	12
Systemic disease (fever, rash)	NA	NA	NA	Low	12

ANA = antinuclear antibodies; NA = not applicable.
Recommendations for follow-up continue through childhood and adolescence.
Source: Reprinted with permission from Pediatrics. 2006;117(5):1843–1845 (Copyright 2006 by the AAP.[1]).

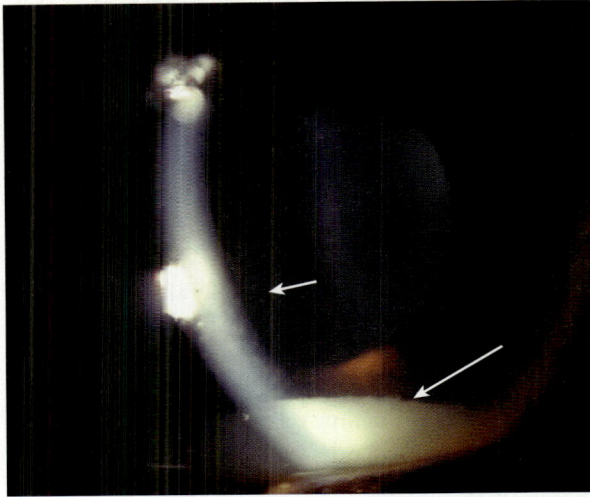

FIGURE 29–27 ■ Pseudoiritis secondary to retinoblastoma. The material layering out in the anterior chamber (long arrow) is a collection of tumor cells. Individual cells circulating in the anterior chamber are visible in the slit lamp beam (short arrow). (Reprinted with permission from *Arch Pediatr Adolesc Med*. 2001;155:519–520. Figure 1. Copyright American Medical Association. All rights reserved.)

present, but this finding may be difficult to interpret, because children tend to have higher ACE levels than adults. For these reasons, sarcoidosis may be difficult to distinguish from JIA in young children. If conjunctival nodules are present, a biopsy may reveal diagnostic noncaseating epithelioid granulomas. Systemic treatment for sarcoidosis usually includes corticosteroids or other immunosuppressive agents.

Pseudoiritis Rarely, retinoblastoma may present with tumor cells in the anterior chamber. These cells are white and may be mistaken for iritis. If a large number of cells are present, they may visible on penlight examination. They may layer out in the anterior chamber, creating an appearance similar to a hypopyon, but without the marked ocular inflammation associated with infection (Figure 29–27).

PUPIL DISORDERS

Assessment of abnormal pupils requires identification of the onset of the disorder, whether the changes are constant or variable, and whether both eyes are symmetrically affected.

Bilateral, Symmetric Changes

Infants may be born with small or large pupils, as noted above in the section on microcoria and congenital mydriasis. Acquired changes may also occur.

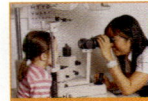

Table 29–4.

Medications Causing Dilated Pupils

- Topical:
  - Atropine
  - Cyclopentolate
  - Tropicamide
  - Phenylephrine
- Systemic:
  - Atropine

Normal variant

Intermittent bilateral large pupils are sometimes seen in normal children. This presumably arises from sympathetic stimulation, which could occur if the child is excited or agitated. The pupils in this case should respond to light normally.

Medications

Systemic medications that have sympathetic effects can produce dilated pupils (Table 29–4). Topical medications could produce the same finding, but they would have to be placed in both eyes.

Dorsal midbrain syndrome (Parinaud syndrome)

Dorsal midbrain syndrome results from lesions in the midbrain. The most common etiologies in children are pineal tumors and congenital aqueductal stenosis. Affected patients have bilateral mid-dilated pupils that do not react to light, but which do constrict when the patient attempts to focus at near (*light-near dissociation*). Other signs include limited upward gaze, decreased voluntary convergence, and a form of nystagmus in which the eyes converge and retract when the patient attempts to look up quickly (*convergence-retraction nystagmus*).

Argyll Robertson pupils

In this condition the pupils are small and do not react to light, but do have a preserved near response. They are a manifestation of tertiary syphilis.

Anisocoria (see also Chapter 18)

Most pupillary abnormalities are noticed because one pupil is smaller than the other. In this condition, the evaluation begins with a determination of which pupil is abnormal—the smaller or larger pupil. If the anisocoria is worse in dim light, this implies a weakness of the dilator muscle of the smaller pupil. If the anisocoria is worse in bright light, this implies a weakness of the sphincter muscle of the larger pupil. If one of the pupils does not respond at all, this suggests pharmacological dilation (with atropine drops, for example), structural damage to the iris muscles (usually from trauma), or adhesions of the iris to the lens (secondary to trauma or inflammation).

Diagnosis of anisocoria

Anisocoria greater in dim light

Physiological anisocoria Intermittent pupil asymmetry of up to 0.5 mm may be seen in normal patients. Physiological anisocoria is a benign condition in which the difference between the pupil sizes exceeds this amount. The anisocoria is more noticeable in dim light. The hallmark of this condition is variability, with the pupils sometimes appearing equal. This condition may be inherited.

Horner syndrome This is a common cause of anisocoria in children. Horner syndrome results from an interruption of the sympathetic pathway affecting the iris Associated findings include ptosis and abnormal sweating on the affected side of the face. If the problem develops early in infancy, patients may also have heterochromia (Figure 29–28). In Horner syndrome the smaller pupil is abnormal. Because it cannot dilate well, the anisocoria is greater in dim light. The anisocoria in physiological anisocoria is also most noticeable in dim light. It is important to distinguish this from Horner syndrome, because physiological anisocoria is benign, whereas Horner syndrome may be a manifestation of serious underlying problems such as neuroblastoma.

Diagnosis of Horner syndrome The diagnosis of Horner syndrome can be established by pharmacological testing (Table 29–5). Available agents include topical cocaine, apraclonidine, and hydroxyamphetamine. In Horner syn-

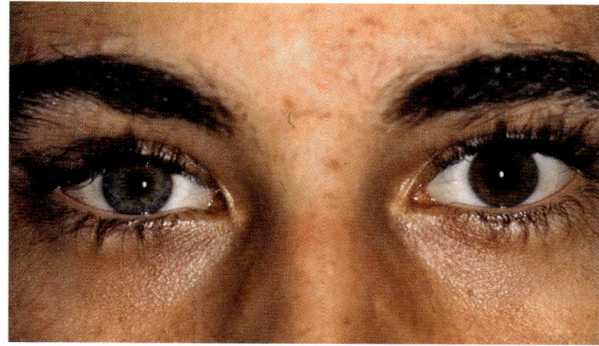

FIGURE 29–28 ■ Right Horner syndrome in a patient with congenital cardiac disease. The Horner syndrome developed following insertion of a central line in the right cervical area. In addition to unequal pupil size and mild ptosis, the patient also has heterochromia (unequal pupil color).

drome, the interruption of the sympathetic pathway results in lack of release of norepinephrine by the presynaptic vesicles at the iris dilator muscle. Cocaine blocks the reuptake of norepinephrine by the presynaptic vesicles, so the normal pupil should dilate when it is instilled. Because the nerve in patients with the Horner syndrome does not release norepinephrine, the pupil does not change in response to topical cocaine. Therefore, the anisocoria should increase if cocaine is instilled in both eyes of a patient with Horner syndrome (because the normal eye responds and the Horner eye does not) (Figure 29–29A and B), whereas both pupils will dilate in a patient with physiological anisocoria (Figure 29–30A and B). In practice, the use of this test is limited by the availability of topical cocaine and an often-equivocal endpoint.

Apraclonidine drops are α-adrenergic agonists. They are relatively weak, so they normally have little effect on normal pupils. However, in Horner syndrome, the

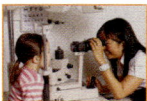

Table 29–5.

Medications Used in the Diagnosis of Horner Syndrome

Medication	Mechanism of Action	Effect on Smaller Pupil	Other
Cocaine	Prevents reuptake of norepinephrine	Pupil does not dilate	
Hydroxyamphetamine	Stimulates release of presynaptic norepinephrine	Third-order neuron—pupil does not dilate First- or second-order neuron—pupil dilates	
Apraclonidine	Weak α-adrenergic agonist	First few weeks after onset—no effect Later—pupil dilates (reversal of anisocoria) due to supersensitivity	Risk of respiratory depression in infants

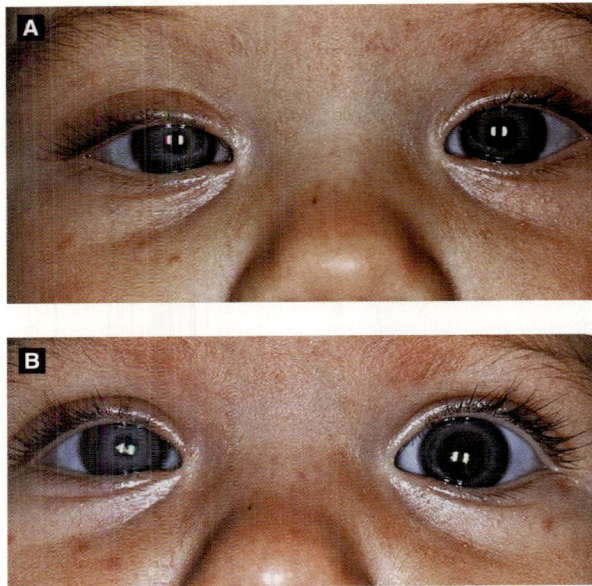

FIGURE 29–29 ■ Cocaine testing in Horner syndrome. (A) Right Horner syndrome. Note small pupil and mild ptosis on right. (B) After instillation of cocaine in both eyes the normal left pupil dilates and the right pupil does not, confirming the diagnosis of Horner syndrome.

postsynaptic receptors develop adrenergic supersensitivity, and reversal of the anisocoria after placement of apraclonidine in both eyes provides an easily identifiable confirmation of the diagnosis (Figure 29–31A and B). The supersensitivity takes time to develop, however, and false-negative results may occur early in the course of Horner syndrome. *Apraclonidine drops are usually not used in infants due to potential side effect of respiratory depression.*

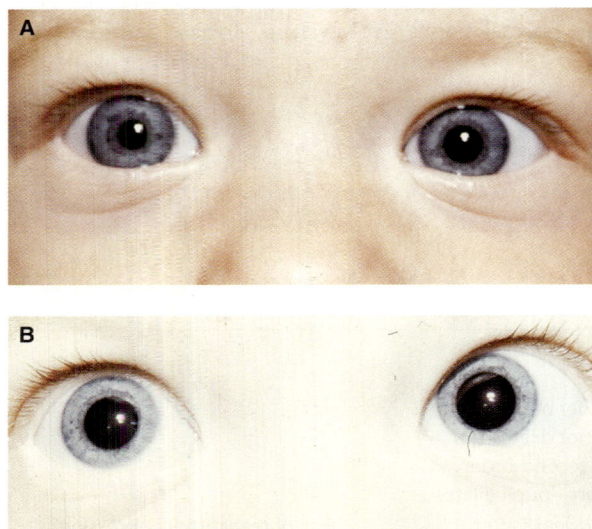

FIGURE 29–30 ■ Cocaine testing in physiological anisocoria. (A) The right pupil is smaller than the left. Note absence of ptosis. (B) Both pupils dilate after instillation of cocaine, confirming the diagnosis of physiological anisocoria.

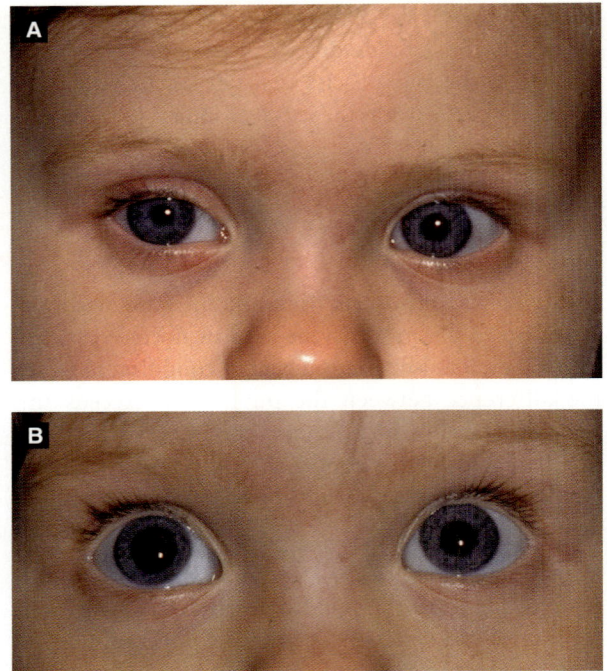

FIGURE 29–31 ■ Apraclonidine testing in Horner syndrome. (A) Congenital right Horner syndrome. Note mild ptosis and smaller pupil on right. (B) The anisocoria reverses (the right pupil becomes larger) after placement of apraclonidine drops, due to adrenergic supersensitivity. This confirms the diagnosis of Horner syndrome.

The third pharmacological agent used in the diagnosis of Horner syndrome is hydroxyamphetamine, which can be helpful in localizing the site of interruption of the sympathetic pathway. Hydroxyamphetamine works by directly causing release of norepinephrine from presynaptic vesicles. If the lesion causing Horner syndrome affects the first- or second-order neuron, the presynaptic vesicles of the third-order neuron should be intact, and the pupil should dilate in response to hydroxyamphetamine. If the third-order neuron is damaged, no neurotransmitter will be released and the pupil should not change (Figure 29–32A and B).

Evaluation of patients with Horner syndrome If a diagnosis of Horner syndrome is established, an evaluation may be necessary to identify the cause. If the lesion is congenital, it is usually benign, although some cases of neuroblastoma present in infancy. Congenital Horner syndrome may result from a difficult delivery, presumed secondary to damage to the cervical region, but often there is no such history and the infants are otherwise normal.

The development of acquired Horner syndrome requires an evaluation to search for the cause, unless the etiology is clearly recognized (for example, if the Horner syndrome develops immediately following a surgical procedure involving an area along the sympathetic chain). Neuroblastoma is a common etiology, and

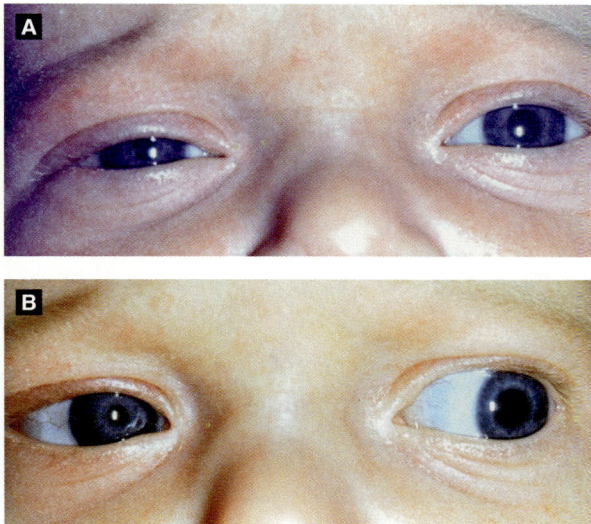

FIGURE 29–32 ■ Hydroxyamphetamine testing in Horner syndrome. (A) The infant had a right Horner syndrome secondary to cervical injury during a forceps-assisted delivery. Note the ptosis and smaller pupil on the right. The diagnosis had been previously confirmed by testing with cocaine drops. (B) The ptosis and anisocoria persist after placement of hydroxyamphetamine drops in both eyes, indicating that the patient had third-order neuron damage, consistent with the history of cervical injury.

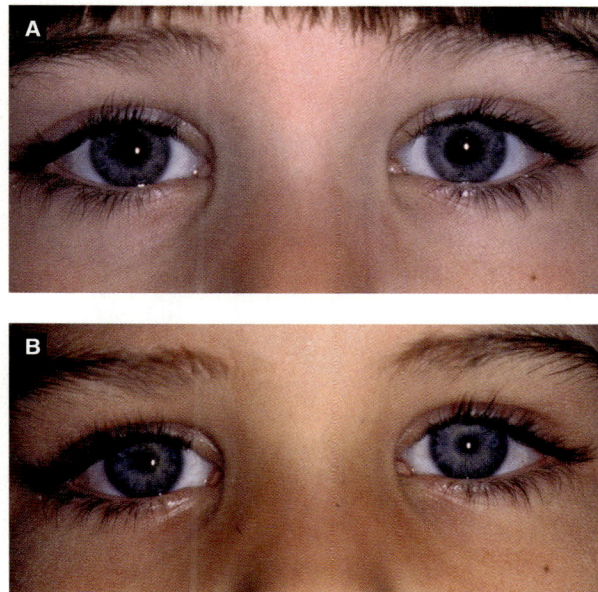

FIGURE 29–33 ■ (A) Adie's tonic pupil, left eye. (B) The diagnosis is confirmed by constriction of the left pupil to dilute pilocarpine. A normal pupil does not react to the dilute medication, but the pupil in Adie's is supersensitive because of denervation.

blood tests for metabolic byproducts of the tumor are indicated (e.g., urine vanillylmandelic acid). Because the sympathetic pathway may be affected at any site, magnetic resonance imaging of the head, neck, and thorax should also be performed.[2]

Damage to the cervical portion of the sympathetic chain may also occur due to surgical manipulation or during attempts at vascular access in the neck.

Anisocoria greater in bright light This finding implies that the sphincter muscle of the larger pupil is dysfunctional.

Pharmacological This may occur due to unilateral use of medication that dilates the pupil (Table 29–4). If the medication has long-lasting effect, such as atropine, the pupil will not react to light or applications of drops that would normally cause constriction (e.g., pilocarpine).

Adie tonic pupil This is an acquired condition in which the pupil responds poorly and irregularly to light. It is more common in females and is usually unilateral. It occurs most commonly in young adults, but may be seen in older children. It results from damage to the parasympathetic fibers. The postganglionic fibers

become supersensitive, and the diagnosis may be established by a constriction response to dilute pilocarpine (Figure 29–33A and B). Systemic features include decreased deep tendon reflexes.

Third cranial nerve palsy The third cranial nerve innervates the iris sphincter, and therefore the pupil is usually dilated in third cranial nerve palsies. In some infants with congenital third nerve palsies, however, the affected pupil may be smaller in the affected eye. This is usually accompanied by ptosis and strabismus. Acute third nerve palsies in children require prompt evaluation.

REFERENCES

1. Cassidy J, Kivlin J, Lindsley C, Nocton J, the Section on Rheumatology, the Section on Ophthalmology. Ophthalmologic examinations in children with juvenile rheumatoid arthritis. *Pediatrics.* 2006;117:1843–1845.
2. Mahoney NR, Liu GT, Menacker SJ, Wilson MC, Hogarty MD, Maris JM. Pediatric Horner syndrome: etiologies and roles of imaging and urine studies to detect neuroblastoma and other responsible mass lesions. *Am J Ophthalmol.* 2006;142:651–659.

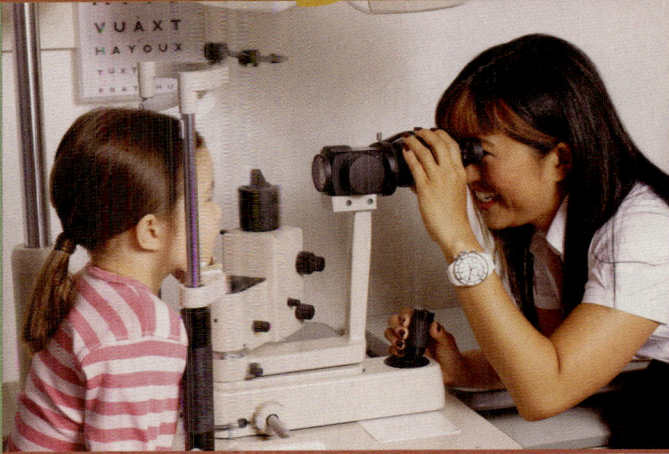

CHAPTER 30

Disorders of the Lens

DEFINITIONS AND EPIDEMIOLOGY

The lens is the normally clear structure that is located just posterior to the iris. The primary function of the lens is to focus light rays on the retina. The lens is attached to the ciliary body by zonules. These zonules produce tension in response to contraction of the ciliary muscle. The ciliary muscle is circular, so that when it contracts its diameter becomes smaller (Figure 30–1). This decreases the tension on the lens zonules, and the lens becomes more spherical. This is known as *accommodation*, which is what allows the eye to focus at near. As people age, the lens becomes progressively stiffer.

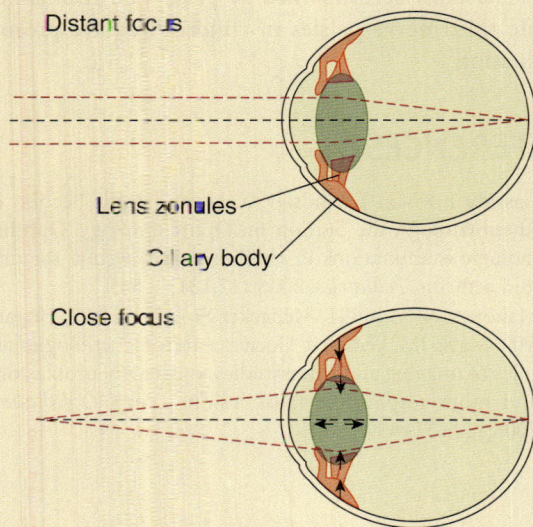

Because of this, the ability to focus at near gradually deteriorates, to the point that almost all people require reading glasses during the fourth decade of life.

The lens consists of the *anterior and posterior lens capsules*, which are basal lamina produced by the lens epithelium. The lens epithelium lines the inner capsule. The epithelial cells at the equator of the lens continue to divide and produce lens fibers throughout life. The central portion of the lens (the *nucleus*) is formed by birth, and the surrounding portion of the lens (the *cortex*) is produced postnatally (Figure 30–2). The cytoplasm of lens cells contains *crystallins*, which produce the light-focusing properties of the lens.

Cataracts are present if the lens is not clear. Cataracts may range from mild to severe, and their effect on vision can range from minimal to profound. Cataracts are very common in adults as they age, but they are uncommon in children. However, they do represent a significant cause of visual morbidity in children, accounting for approximately 10% of childhood vision impairment.

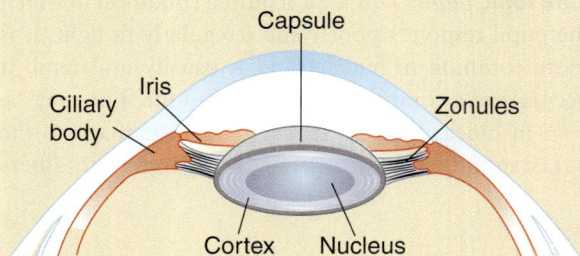

FIGURE 30–1 ■ Focusing of the lens is controlled by the ciliary body. (Top) When the ciliary body is relaxed the lens is thinner and focuses light rays from distant objects. (Bottom) When the ciliary muscle contracts, the lens zonules loosen, and the lens assumes a more spherical shape. This allows the lens to focus on near objects.

FIGURE 30–2 ■ Lens anatomy. The lens is composed of the inner nucleus, surrounding cortex, and outer capsule. The lens is attached to the ciliary body by the lens zonules. The iris in front of the lens forms the pupil.

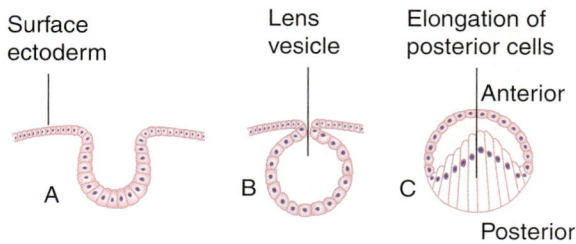

FIGURE 30–3 ■ Lens embryology. (A) The lens begins as an out-pouching of cells from the surface ectoderm. (B) The invaginated tissue separates from the ectoderm and forms the circular lens vesicle. (C) Cells from the posterior lens vesicle elongate to fill the vesicle, creating the embryonic nucleus.

In addition to cataracts, rare lens disorders include *aphakia* (absence of the lens), *microspherophakia* (an abnormally small, round lens), *ectopia lentis* (decentration of the lens), and *lens coloboma* (a partial defect in the periphery of the lens due to absence of adjacent zonules, usually associated with colobomas of the iris and retina)

Embryology

The lens initially develops as a thickening of the surface ectoderm overlying the optic vesicle. This tissue invaginates and separates to form the circular lens vesicle. The outer portion of this vesicle becomes the lens capsule. The cells on the posterior surface of the vesicle elongate and fill the vesicle, which becomes the embryonic nucleus (Figure 30–3). Epithelial lens cells at the equator then divide and produce secondary lens fibers, which gradually move toward the center to form the Y-sutures. These cells continue to proliferate throughout life.

The embryological formation of the lens is analogous to rings on a tree, with continuous layering of lens fibers. Because of this, the timing of intrauterine disturbances of lens growth can be inferred by the location of the abnormality: early disturbances create central lens opacities and later disturbances affect the peripheral lens.

PATHOGENESIS

Cataracts are considered visually significant if they substantially interfere with ability of the lens to focus light. There are a wide variety of etiologies and appearances of cataracts. They may be unilateral or bilateral. They may be present at birth or develop later in life. Unilateral infantile cataracts are usually sporadic and often have no identifiable etiology. Bilateral infantile cataracts are more likely to be associated with other disorders. Approximately one-third of bilateral infantile cataracts are hereditary, approximately one-third are associated with systemic diseases, and approximately one-third are idiopathic. Cataracts in older children may be idiopathic, but are more likely to have an identifiable cause,

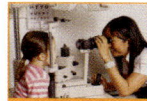

Table 30–1.

Systemic Diseases Associated With Cataracts (Partial list)

- Chromosomal abnormalities
  □ Trisomy 21
  □ Trisomy 18
  □ Trisomy 13
  □ Multiple other deletions, translocations
- Infectious diseases
  □ Herpes simplex virus
  □ Toxoplasmosis
  □ Rubella
  □ Syphilis
  □ Cytomegalovirus
  □ Varicella
- Metabolic disorders
  □ Galactosemia (and associated disorders)
  □ Diabetes mellitus
- Renal disorders
  □ Lowe syndrome
  □ Alport syndrome
- Parathyroid disorders
  □ Hypoparathyroidism
  □ Pseudohypoparathyroidism
- Muscoloskeletal disorders
  □ Chondrodysplasia
  □ Myotonic dystrophy
- Other
  □ Cockayne syndrome
  □ Fabry disease
  □ Hallermann-Streiff syndrome
  □ Rothmund-Thomson syndrome
  □ Incontinentia pigmenti

such as trauma, external beam radiation, or medications (such as corticosteroids).

Heritable cataracts are most commonly inherited as an autosomal dominant trait, but autosomal recessive and X-linked forms also occur. A large number of genetic mutations have been identified in patients with familial cataracts. Currently there are over 350 entities associated with cataracts in the Online Mendelian Inheritance in Man database. The age at which inherited cataracts appear varies from infancy to young adulthood.

Many systemic disorders are associated with cataracts, particularly those that present in infancy. These include metabolic diseases, chromosomal aberrations, and congenital infections (Table 30–1). Infants with bilateral cataracts require a medical evaluation to search for these problems (discussed below) (Table 30–2).

Unilateral ectopia lentis is often related to ocular trauma. Bilateral ectopia lentis may occur as an isolated finding, but is often associated with one of several specific systemic disorders (discussed below) (Table 30–3).

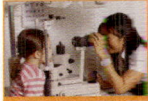

Table 30–2.

Evaluation for Patient With Bilateral Infantile Cataracts

- General physical examination for other abnormalities
- Chromosomes
- TORCH titers
- Urine reducing substances, galactose-1-phosphate uridyl transferase, galactokinase
- Urine amino acids
- Serum calcium, phosphorus, and glucose
- Serum ferritin

In addition to their direct effects on vision, cataracts and other lens disorders in children may also cause visual loss due to amblyopia. This is particularly true in young infants with unilateral cataracts. The onset of amblyopia in this setting is rapid and profound, and early intervention is necessary to maximize the chance for a good visual outcome.

CLINICAL PRESENTATION

Cataracts are most commonly noted in infants and young children by their interference with the red reflex. Dense cataracts may appear as white opacities in the normally black pupil, which may be directly visible to the parents (Figure 30–4). Cataracts are usually best detected by an abnormality of the red reflex (Figure 30–5).

If cataracts are not visualized directly, they may cause other problems that ultimately lead to their detection. Infants with bilateral significant cataracts cannot fixate normally, and nystagmus develops at 2 to 4 months of age. Infants and young children with unilateral cataracts generally ignore the poor vision in the affected eye, and they can function normally by using only the good eye. They may develop strabismus due to the poor vision, which is sometimes the first abnormality that brings the cataract to attention.

The appearance of cataracts is highly variable. The opacities can occur anywhere from the front surface of the

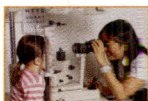

Table 30–3.

Disorders Associated With Ectopia Lentis

- Marfan syndrome
- Homocystinuria
- Weill-Marchesani syndrome
- Sulfite oxidase deficiency

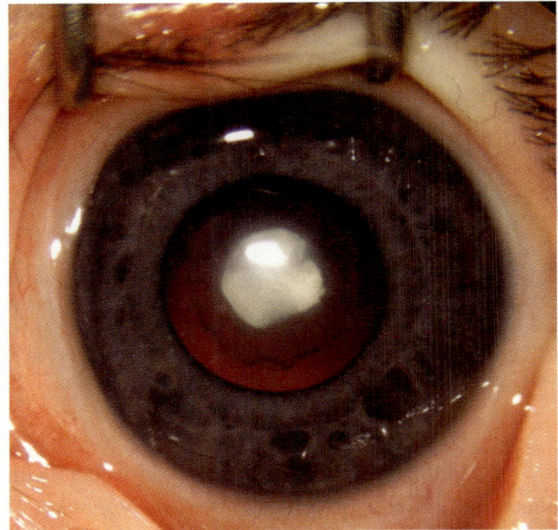

FIGURE 30–4 ■ Dense white infantile cataract, noted by parents at birth.

lens to the back of the lens. The appearance of these various morphologies may assist in the differential diagnosis.

DIFFERENTIAL DIAGNOSIS BASED ON CATARACT MORPHOLOGY

Beginning at the front of the lens and moving posteriorly:

Anterior Polar Cataracts

Anterior polar cataracts are small, white opacities on the anterior surface of the lens (Figure 30–6). They are present at birth and may be unilateral or bilateral. They are not progressive and are usually small enough that they do not directly interfere with vision. However, affected patients have an increased risk of amblyopia due to asymmetric refractive errors.

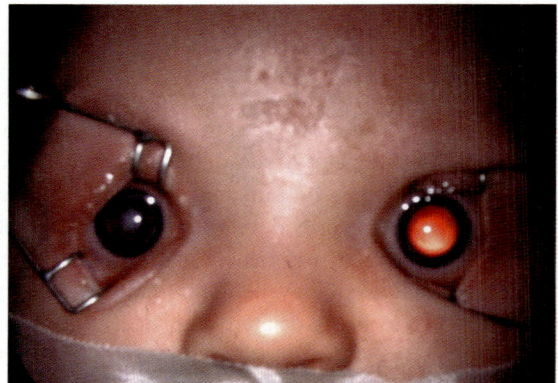

FIGURE 30–5 ■ Abnormal red reflex, right eye, secondary to infantile cataract.

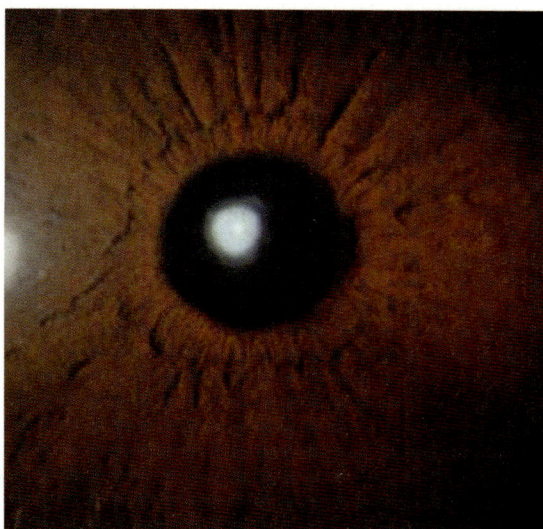

FIGURE 30–6 ■ Small anterior polar cataract. The white opacity is on the front surface of the lens.

FIGURE 30–7 ■ Autosomal dominant nuclear cataracts. (A) Daughter. (B) Mother.

Nuclear Cataracts

These cataracts affect the central portion of the lens, usually resulting from a perturbation of lens formation early in its embryological development. These may be inherited as an autosomal dominant trait (Figure 30–7A and B). The effect on vision depends on the density of the opacity.

Lamellar Cataracts

Lamellar cataracts affect one or more layers in the mid-periphery of the lens, and are therefore larger than nuclear cataracts. These develop during a later stage of lens formation than nuclear cataracts.

Posterior Subcapsular Cataracts

These appear as irregular white opacities on the back surface of the lens. These may be present at birth, but are more frequently acquired. Traumatic cataracts and corticosteroid-induced cataracts are most commonly of this type. External beam radiation may also cause posterior subcapsular opacities (Figure 30–8).

Posterior Lenticonus

These uncommon cataracts result from weakness of the posterior lens capsule. They are usually not present at birth, but develop later during childhood. They are characterized by progressive posterior outpouching of the capsule and subsequent opacification of this area (Figure 30–9A and B). Because they are not present at birth, the prognosis for improvement in vision after surgery is better in this type of cataract.

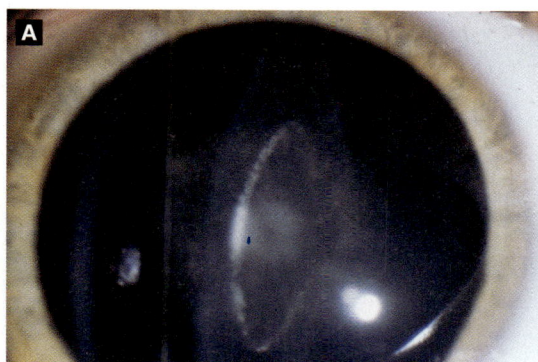

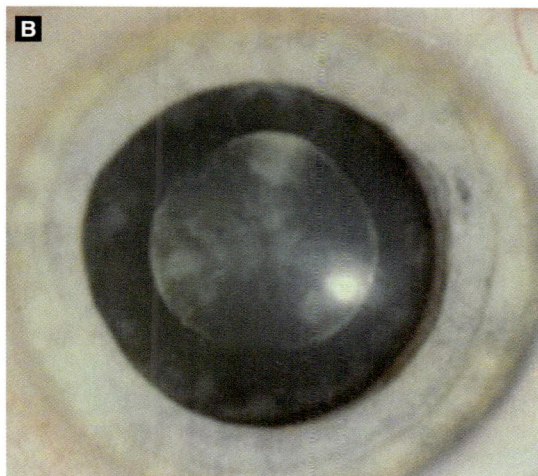

Persistent Fetal Vasculature

This condition, previously known as *persistent hyperplastic primary vitreous*, results from incomplete regression of the hyaloid artery. The hyaloid artery is the blood vessel that is normally present during embryological development of the eye. It extends from the optic nerve to the posterior

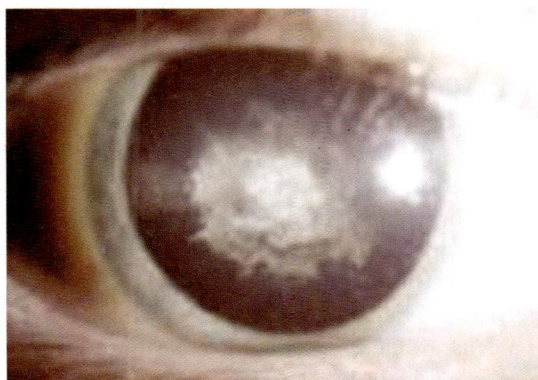

FIGURE 30–8 ■ Posterior subcapsular cataract following external beam radiation for retinoblastoma. The opacity is on the posterior surface of the lens.

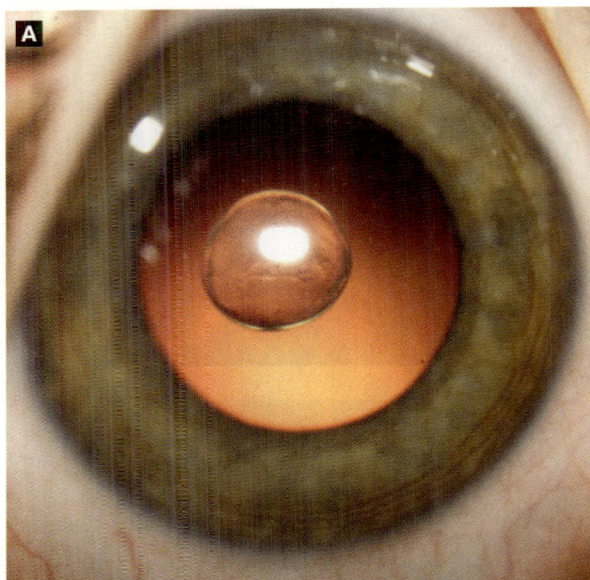

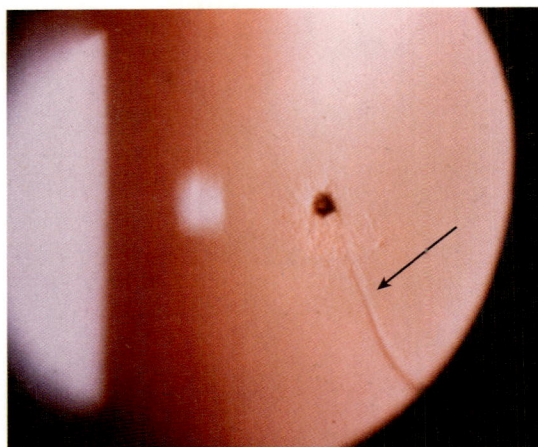

FIGURE 30–10 ■ Mittendorf dot, high-magnification slit lamp view. The small lens opacity on the posterior surface of the lens is seen in retroillumination. Note the thin remnant of the hyaloid artery attached to the lens (arrow).

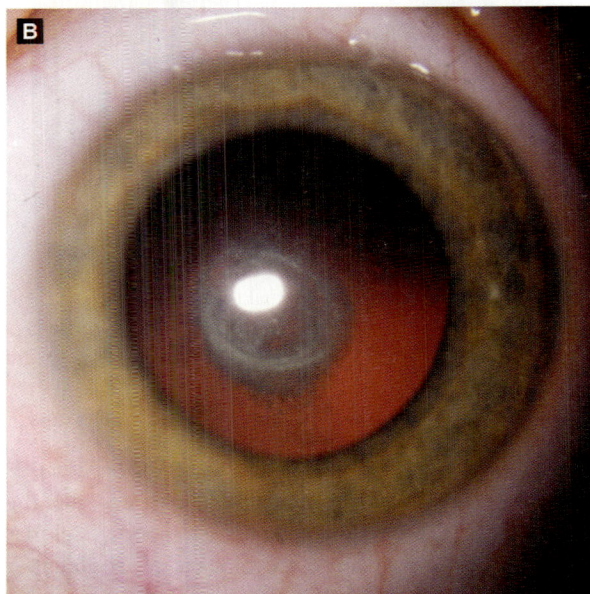

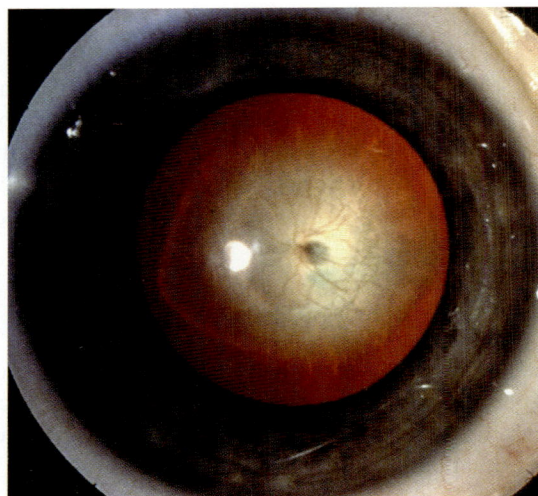

FIGURE 30–11 ■ Vascularized plaque on posterior lens capsule due to persistent fetal vasculature.

FIGURE 30–9 ■ Posterior lenticonus. (A) Early changes. The central defect is an outpouching of the posterior surface of the lens capsule. (B) Progressive opacification of lens defect.

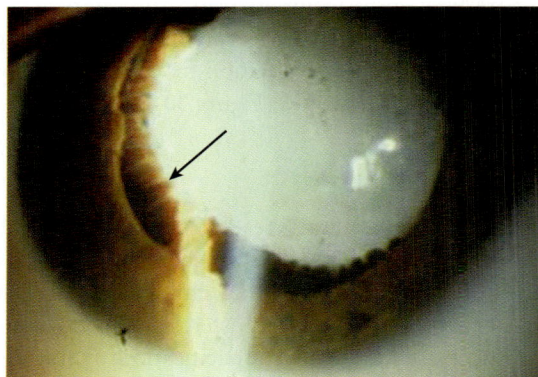

FIGURE 30–12 ■ Dense white cataract and contraction of ciliary processes (arrow) due to persistent fetal vasculature.

surface of the lens, and supplies blood to support these developing structures. It usually regresses by birth. If the hyaloid artery does not regress, it may produce a variety of ocular abnormalities. The most mild of these is a *Mittendorf dot*, a small opacity on the posterior surface of the lens that does not cause visual problems (Figure 30–10). In persistent fetal vasculature (PFV), patients typically have a dense, white, vascularized plaque on the posterior lens capsule (Figure 30–11). This may contract such that the ciliary processes are visible (Figure 30–12).

A thick stalk of tissue (formed by the persistent hyaloid vessel) may be present in patients with PFV

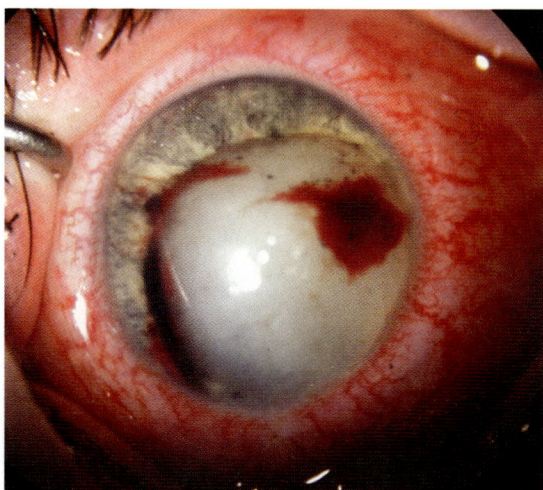

FIGURE 30–13 ■ Total (complete dense white) cataract following trauma. Note associated iris damage and intraocular hemorrhage.

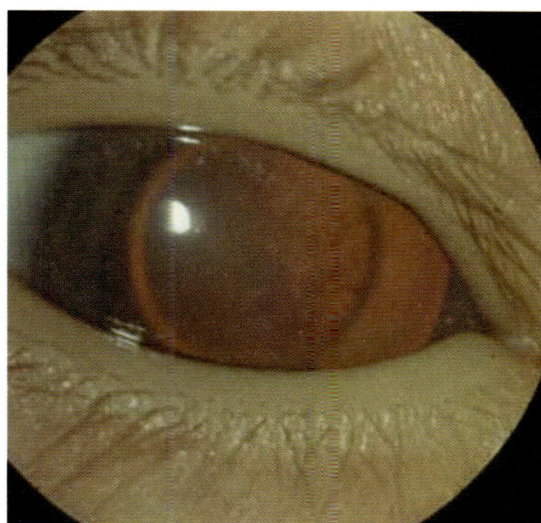

FIGURE 30–14 ■ Oil-droplet cataract in a patient with galactosemia.

between the optic nerve and the lens, and distortion of the retina may occur. The eyes are usually smaller than normal (microphthalmic), and there is a high risk of glaucoma. The visual prognosis of PFV is worse than other forms of cataracts, but good results can sometimes be obtained with early treatment, particularly if there is no retinal involvement.

Total Cataract

A total cataract is present if the entire lens is white. Infantile cataracts may present in this fashion. Another common etiology is ocular trauma, particularly if the lens capsule is disrupted (Figure 30–13). The leakage of material from within the lens may cause inflammation and glaucoma. Total cataracts typically reduce vision to the point that patients can only perceive light. Early surgery is necessary to preserve vision and prevent secondary damage caused by inflammation.

DIFFERENTIAL DIAGNOSIS BASED ON SYSTEMIC DISEASE

A large number of systemic diseases are associated with cataracts, including chromosomal disorders, syndromes, and metabolic abnormalities (Table 30–1). The lens opacities in many of these are nonspecific, but the appearance of some cataracts may suggest certain diagnoses.

Galactosemia

Galactosemia is a metabolic disorder in which patients are unable to convert galactose into glucose. Systemic abnormalities include hepatomegaly and developmental delay. Cataracts occur in galactosemia due to accumulation of galactose and galactitol within the lens. This creates an osmotic gradient, with inflow of fluid and progressive opacification. The classic ocular finding in galactosemia is the *oil-droplet cataract* in the center portion of the lens, which develops within the first few weeks of life (Figure 30–14). This cataract may be reversible with early institution of an appropriate diet. Galactokinase deficiency is a variant of galactosemia in which the primary abnormality is cataract formation. In practice, cataracts due to galactosemia are now rarely seen due to newborn screening and early initiation of dietary treatment for this disorder.

Myotonic dystrophy

This disorder is associated with delayed relaxation of contracted muscles, facial and eyelid weakness, and cardiac conduction defects. Patients with myotonic dystrophy may develop a distinctive polychromatic cataract with iridescent crystals in the lens cortex.

Hepatolenticular degeneration (Wilson disease)

This disorder results from abnormal copper metabolism. The classic ocular abnormality found in this disease is the *Kayser-Fleischer ring*, a reddish-brown discoloration on the peripheral posterior surface of the cornea. Patients may also develop *sunflower cataracts*, stellate deposits of reddish-brown material in the anterior lens that resemble a sunflower.

Alport syndrome

Alport syndrome is an inherited disorder associated with renal dysfunction and deafness. It is usually inherited

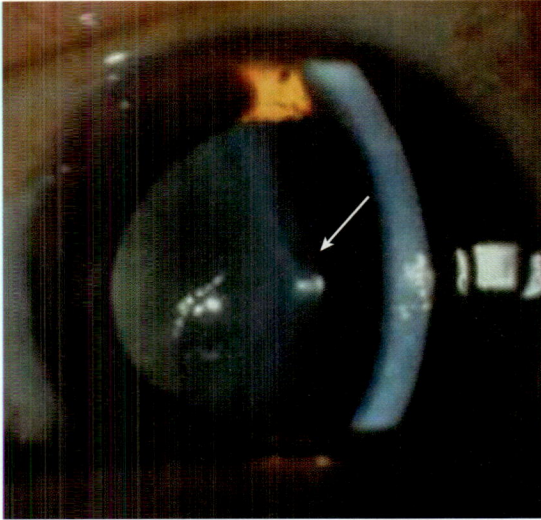

FIGURE 30–15 ■ Anterior lenticonus, which may occur in Alport syndrome. The vertical white line on the right is the slit beam on the corneal surface. Note the irregularity of the slit lamp beam on the lens surface (arrow) caused by a bulge in the anterior capsule.

in an X-linked fashion. Anterior lenticonus (a localized bulging of the central anterior surface of the lens) and cataract may occur (Figure 30–15).

Lowe syndrome (oculocerebral syndrome)

This is an X-linked disorder associated with renal dysfunction and developmental delay. Patients with Lowe syndrome may develop an unusual disciform flat cataract. It is one of very few disorders in children that present with concomitant cataracts and glaucoma.

Congenital infections

Any of the TORCH infections (toxoplasmosis, rubella, cytomegalovirus, herpes simplex virus), as well as congenital varicella and syphilis, may cause infantile cataracts. The infection most specifically associated with cataracts is rubella. Systemic manifestations of congenital rubella include cardiac abnormalities, developmental delay, and hearing loss. Ocular abnormalities include glaucoma, retinopathy, and cataracts. The cataract associated with congenital rubella is usually nuclear, and the surrounding lens cortex may be liquefied (Figure 30–16).

TRAUMATIC CATARACTS

Cataracts in children often result from ocular trauma. They may be caused by blunt or penetrating injuries. They are often associated with other ocular injuries, such as hyphema, iris damage, and retinal detachment

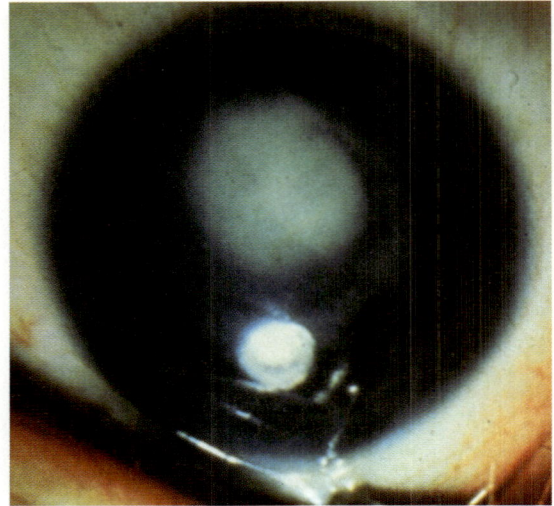

FIGURE 30–16 ■ Cataract due to congenital rubella infection.

(Figure 30–17). The cataracts may be present at the time of initial evaluation, or develop later (usually in the first few weeks following the injury).

ECTOPIA LENTIS

In ectopia lentis, the lens is displaced due to weakness of the lens zonules. This may be an isolated abnormality or be caused by ocular trauma (Figure 30–18) or excessive eye growth in infantile glaucoma. The amount of lens subluxation is variable, ranging from minimal to marked

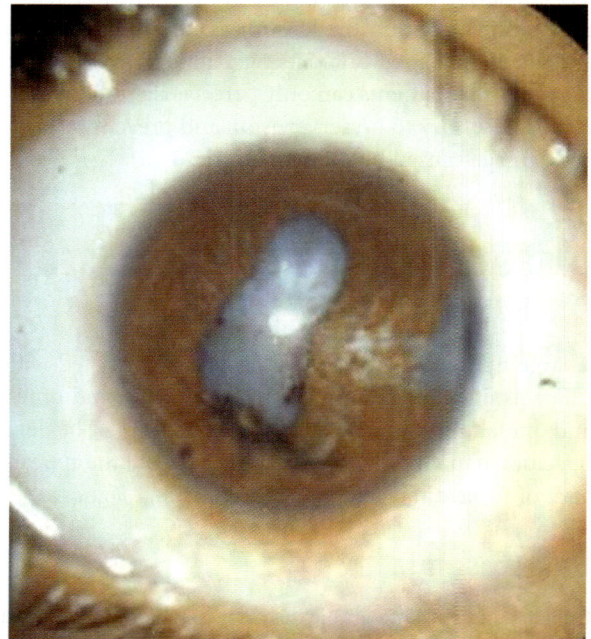

FIGURE 30–17 ■ Dense traumatic cataract. Note associated iris injury.

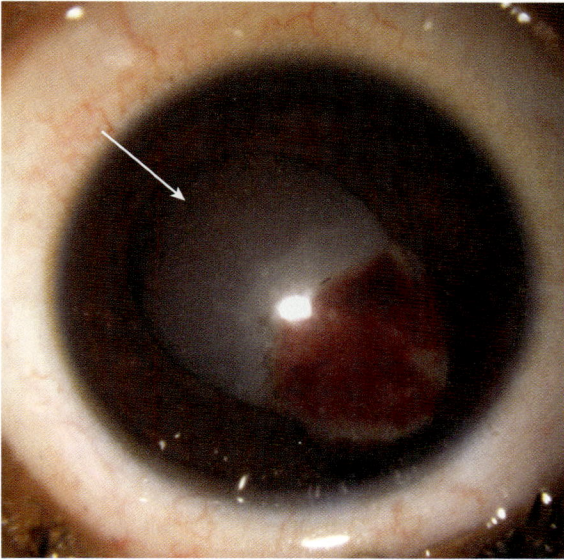

FIGURE 30–18 ■ Mild lens subluxation (arrow shows edge of lens) associated with dense traumatic cataract, intraocular hemorrhage, and iris damage.

FIGURE 30–19 ■ Variable degrees of lens subluxation. (A) Minimal. The lens zonules are normally not visible, even following pupil dilation. They are visible (arrow) in this patient, who has mild superior lens dislocation. (B) The lens edge is easily visualized (arrow) through the pupil in this patient with more marked subluxation.

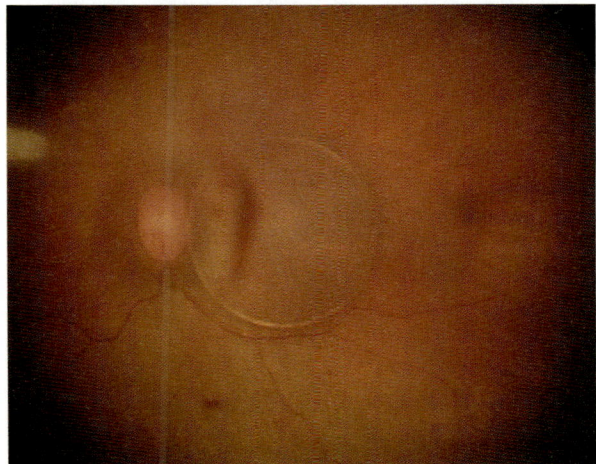

(Figure 30–19A and B). In severe cases the lens may be completely separated from the lens zonules and be displaced into the vitreous cavity (Figure 30–20).

Ectopia lentis is associated with several systemic diseases.

Marfan Syndrome

Marfan syndrome is an autosomal dominant disorder of connective tissue caused by mutations of the fibrillin gene. Patients have a distinct appearance. They are tall, have wide arm spans, and have long, thin fingers (Figure 30–21). Systemic manifestations include dilation of the aortic root and chest deformities.

Approximately 80% of patients with Marfan syndrome have ocular problems. The most common is ectopia lentis, with the lens usually displaced upward (Figure 30–22A and B). The lens dislocation may be present at birth, and may be progressive. Other ocular abnormalities include small pupils, visible fluctuations of iris tissue with movement (iridodonesis), and retinal detachments.

Homocystinuria

Homocystinuria is an autosomal recessive disorder of homocystine metabolism, most commonly caused by abnormalities of the cystathionine-β-synthase enzyme. The general clinical appearance is similar to Marfan syndrome. Affected patients are tall and have long limbs and digits. Unlike Marfan syndrome, patients with homocystinuria may be developmentally delayed. Thrombotic disease is a frequent complication of this

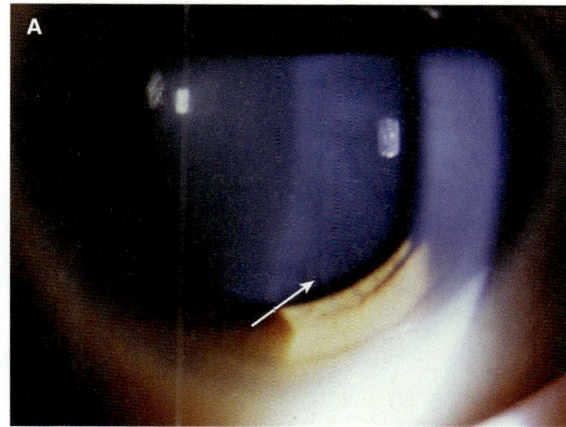

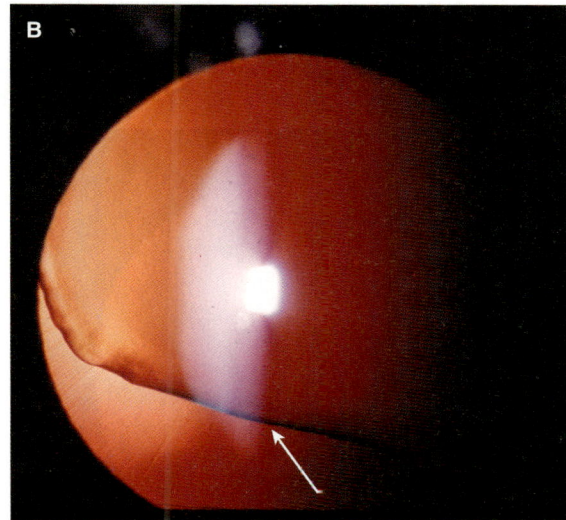

FIGURE 30–20 ■ The lens is completely dislocated (luxated) into the vitreous cavity, and is located just anterior the optic nerve and macula.

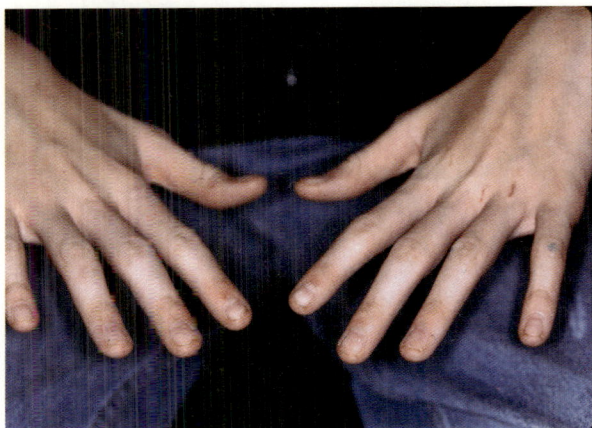

FIGURE 30–21 ■ Long, thin digits in a patient with Marfan syndrome.

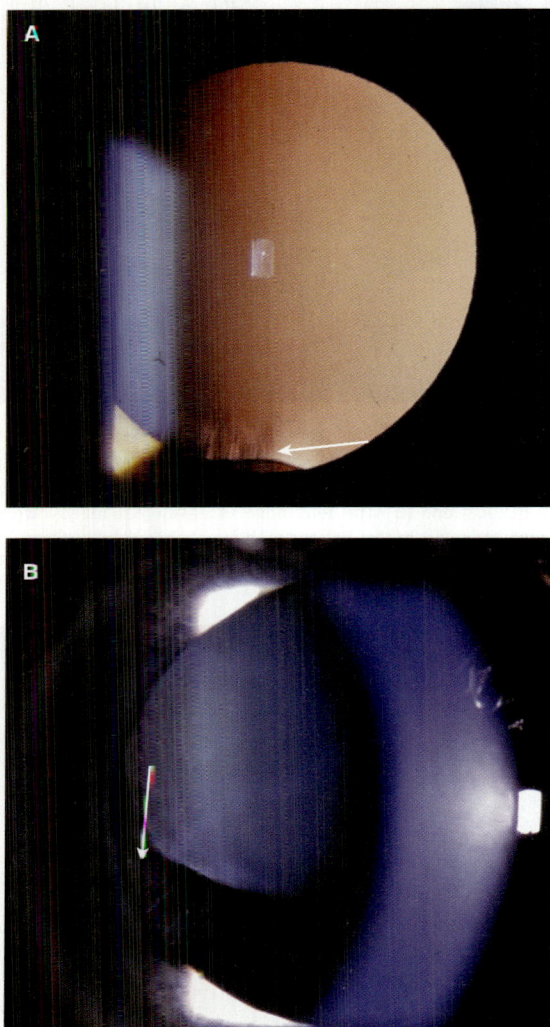

FIGURE 30–22 ■ Lens subluxation (ectopia lentis) in a patient with Marfan syndrome. (A) View of lens through pupil. Very mild subluxation, with inferior edge of lens visible. Lens zonules can be seen attached to lens periphery (arrow). (B) Progressive subluxation, with edge of lens near central visual axis. Lens zonules are visible (arrow).

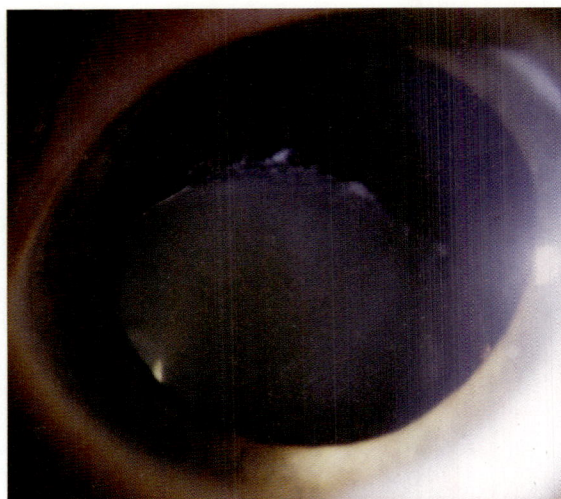

FIGURE 30–23 ■ Homocystinuria. Inferior lens subluxation and disruption of lens zonules.

disorder. Lens dislocation occurs frequently in homocystinuria (Figure 30–23), including dislocation of the entire lens into the vitreous cavity or anterior chamber.

Sulfite Oxidase Deficiency

This is a rare metabolic disorder that causes significant neurological problems in early childhood. Lens dislocation is a frequent finding.

Weill-Marchesani Syndrome

Patients with this disorder have systemic features that are essentially the opposite of Marfan syndrome. They tend to be short and have short limbs and fingers. The lenses in this disorder may have a characteristic round, small appearance (*microspherophakia*). The lens may obstruct the iris such that the flow of fluid between the ciliary body and anterior chamber is blocked, producing closed angle glaucoma.

DIAGNOSIS

Diagnostic Tests

Cataracts

Infants who are born with bilateral cataracts require evaluation due to the potential association between the cataracts and systemic disorders. A recommended evaluation is as follows (Table 30–2):

■ General physical examination for other systemic abnormalities
■ Careful family history, specifically for inherited cataracts or systemic diseases associated with cataracts

- Complete ophthalmological examination for associated abnormalities
- Chromosome analysis (Trisomy 13, Trisomy 13 Trisomy 21, other translocations, deletions, duplications)
- TORCH (Toxoplasmosis, Rubella, Cytomegalovirus Herpes) titres and tests for syphilis
- Screening for disorders of galactose metabolism urine for reducing substances, galactose-1-phosphate uridyl transferase, galactokinase
- Screening for other metabolic disorders: urine amino acids, serum calcium, phosphorus, and glucose
- Screening for hyperferritinemia: serum ferritin

Ectopia lentis

- Marfan syndrome: cardiac ultrasonography, fibrillin gene mutation screening
- Homocystinuria: urine screening for disulfides
- Sulfite oxidase deficiency: measurement of sulfite oxidase activity in skin fibroblasts

TREATMENT

The treatment of lens disorders is dependent on the age of the child and the degree to which the abnormality affects vision. A good outcome is dependent on 3 things:

1. successful surgical removal of the lens opacity
2. replacement of the lens focusing power
3. treatment of amblyopia.

The risk of amblyopia is greatly increased in younger children, and the younger the child, the greater the risk. *Unilateral cataracts in particular are highly amblyogenic in newborns. They need to be removed within 4 to 6 weeks of age to maximize the potential for good vision.*[1] Bilateral cataracts may also cause amblyopia in newborns, but the time frame for optimal removal in this setting extends to 2 to 3 months.[2] The risk of amblyopia in patients with acquired cataracts decreases as children get older, but persists until ages 5 years or more.

If an older child presents with a unilateral cataract, the prognosis for improvement is dependent on the age at which the opacity developed. If it has been present since early infancy, the prognosis is poor even if the surgery itself is successful, because of amblyopia. If the child has had a period of normal visual development and subsequently develops a cataract (such as might occur with trauma), the prognosis is much better.

Surgical Treatment for Cataracts

Surgery for cataracts is indicated when the potential benefits of surgery outweigh the potential risks. In many cases the decision is straightforward. Mild lens opacities, such as anterior polar cataracts, do not interfere with formation of visual images and do not require removal. Dense total cataracts profoundly affect vision, and surgery for these is almost always indicated. Most patients lie between these extremes, and a decision regarding surgery is based on an objective assessment of the lens opacity by the ophthalmologist and a measurement of the patient's vision.

Objective assessment of the degree to which a cataract affects vision is based on slit lamp examination and evaluation of the red reflex, with either a direct ophthalmoscope or a retinoscope. The severity of the lens opacity can be further assessed by noting the degree to which it interferes with visualization of the retina, because the cataract affects the ability of the examiner to see into the eye as well as the patient's ability to see out of the eye. If a poor red reflex is present and the retina cannot be seen clearly, surgery is recommended. Because of the difficulty in quantifying vision loss in young children, the examiner's assessment is the primary basis for a decision regarding surgery in infants.

In older children in whom the vision can be measured, cataract surgery is usually indicated if the vision is 20/40 or less. The potential for vision improvement also depends on whether the rest of the eye is normal. Children who have cataracts and retinal disorders have a worse prognosis, because the retinal problems will persist after the cataract is removed.

Surgical treatment of cataracts consists of removing the lens opacity. There are 3 portions of the lens that are handled separately:

- The first is the anterior capsule, the elastic anterior layer of the lens. A circular opening is created in this, which allows access to the inner portion.
- The second is the lens cortex and nucleus. This inner lens material is usually very soft in children, and is removed by aspiration through a special handpiece (Figure 30–24).
- The third portion is the posterior capsule, the elastic layer on the back surface of the lens. In infants and young children a circular opening is created in this (Figure 30–25), because if it is not removed there is a very high incidence of postoperative opacification (secondary cataract). A portion of the vitreous gel is also removed to decrease the risk of secondary cataract formation. In older children and adults, the posterior capsule may be left in place.

If an intraocular lens is used, it is usually positioned in front of the posterior capsule, in the same space the original lens occupied (within the capsular bag) (Figure 30–26). In infants in whom an intraocular lens is not placed during the initial operation, but

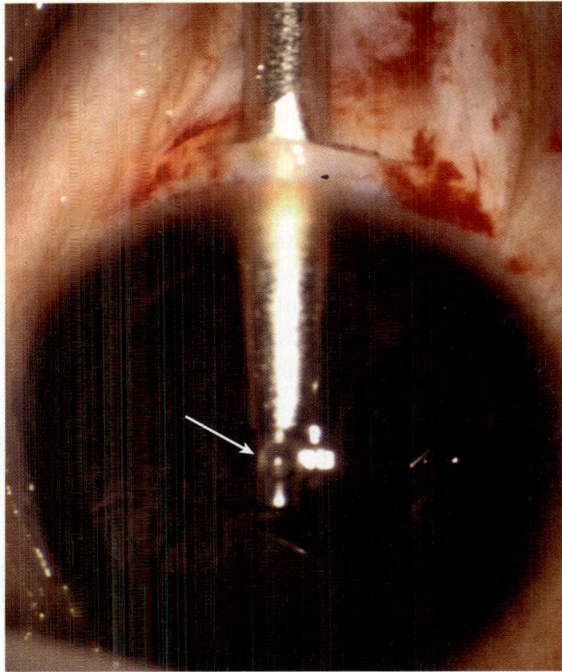

FIGURE 30–24 ■ Cataract surgery. The instrument is inserted through a small incision. The lens material is aspirated through the opening in the instrument (arrow).

in whom later intraocular lens implantation is anticipated, central circular openings in the anterior and posterior capsules provide a clear space for formation of visual images. The periphery of the lens capsule is left intact to serve as future support for an intraocular lens (like a doughnut, with a central opening and intact rim).

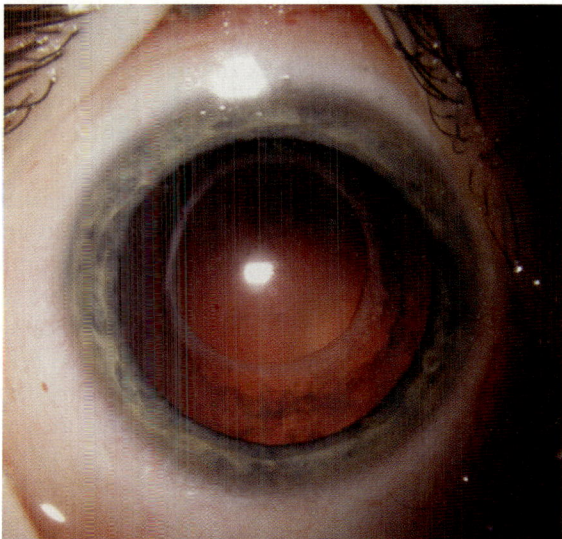

FIGURE 30–25 ■ A circular opening has been created in the posterior capsule of the lens. This photograph was taken before secondary placement of an intraocular lens.

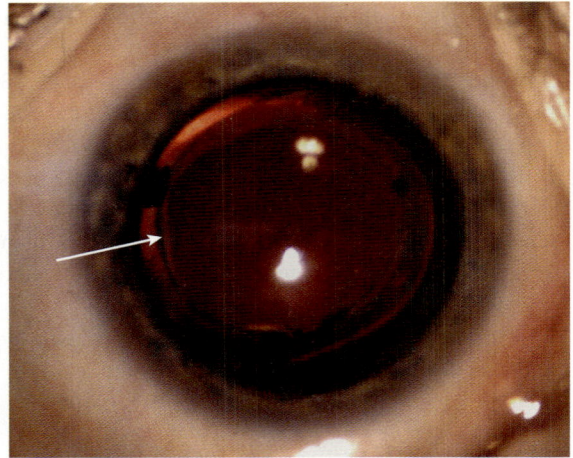

FIGURE 30–26 ■ Same patient as Figure 30–25 after implantation of intraocular lens. The arrow points to the edge of the artificial lens.

Replacement of the Lens Focusing Power

The lens' primary function is to focus light on the retina. If a cataract is removed, this focusing power must be replaced to restore vision. Options for this include glasses, contact lenses, and intraocular lenses. Intraocular lenses are usually the best option in older children, because they most closely restore the eye to its natural state. Many patients require glasses in addition to the intraocular lens to fine-tune the focusing, but these glasses are of normal thickness (unlike the very thick glasses required if an intraocular lens is not used). Because the intraocular lens has only one power, a bifocal is needed in order for patients to focus at near.

Intraocular lenses are not usually placed in early infancy, for 2 reasons. First, the incidence of complications related to intraocular lenses, such as glaucoma, lens displacement, and inflammation, is much higher in the first few months of life. Second, the eye grows rapidly during the first 1 to 2 years of life, and this growth affects the refraction. Intraocular lenses are not adjustable, and a lens that focuses correctly in a 1-month-old child will be substantially overpowered by the time the child is 2. Therefore, most infants with unilateral cataracts are treated with contact lenses for the first few years of life, after which an intraocular lens can be implanted during a second surgery (secondary intraocular lens implantation). Glasses are also an option for replacing focusing power, but they are very thick, which causes distortion (Figure 30–27A and B). They are most useful in infants who have had bilateral cataract removal.

Surgical Treatment for Ectopia Lentis

The considerations for treatment of children with subluxed lenses are similar to those for cataracts. In ectopia (the peripheral lens capsule) is off-center and unstable, and therefore the intraocular lens cannot be safely placed in its normal location.

Amblyopia

Ongoing treatment for amblyopia is critical in children with lens disorders, particularly infants with unilateral opacities. Patching is often necessary during the first several years of life to achieve the best possible vision.

Complications of Lens Surgery

There are several potential complications of lens surgery:

- *Amblyopia* is a major cause of vision loss in children with cataracts. This is most frequently the cause of no or minimal improvement in vision in patients with a good surgical result.
- *Strabismus* is very common in children with cataracts, even those with good visual outcomes. Approximately 80% to 90% of children with unilateral infantile cataracts develop strabismus.
- *Secondary cataracts* are opacities that develop after lens surgery, due to reproliferation of lens epithelial cells or scar tissue in the anterior vitreous (Figure 30–28). Secondary cataracts have the same visual consequences as the initial cataract. They can be removed with a laser or additional intraocular surgery.
- *Glaucoma* occurs frequently in children following cataract surgery, particularly in patients with infantile

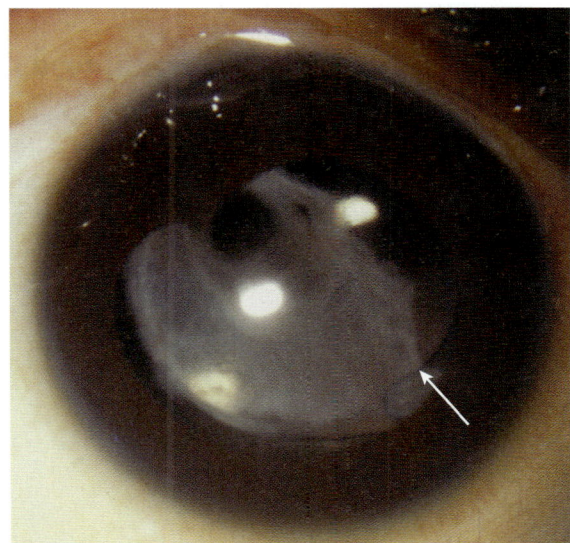

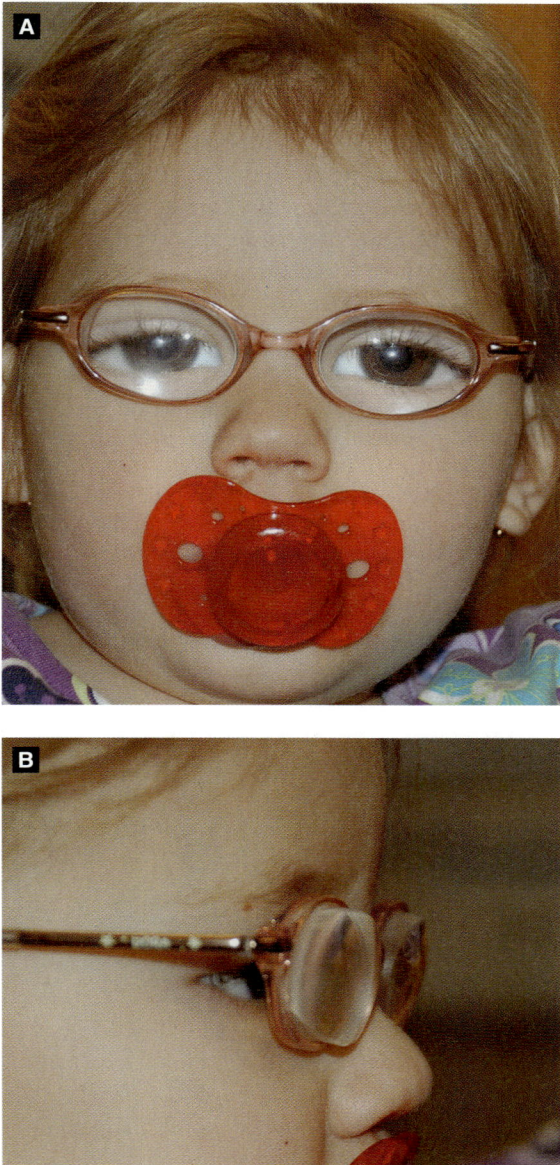

FIGURE 30–27 ■ Glasses (pseudophakic spectacles) used during first 2 years of life in a patient with bilateral infantile cataracts. Secondary placement of intraocular lenses is planned at age 2 years. (A) Note the magnified appearance of the eyes due to the high lens power. (B) Note the marked thickness of the lenses.

lentis the lens itself is clear, but the vision may be impaired due to its eccentric location. Mild subluxation usually does not cause problems, but progressive lens dislocation creates visual blur due to distortion and astigmatism caused by viewing through the peripheral portion of the lens. This worsens as the edge of the lens approaches the central visual axis.

Surgical treatment of ectopia lentis consists of removing the lens, including the anterior and posterior lens capsules. Most patients require contact lenses or glasses. Intraocular lens placement is problematic because the structure that normally supports an intraocular lens

FIGURE 30–28 ■ Secondary cataract. An opacity has formed on the posterior lens capsule following cataract removal and intraocular lens implantation. The arrow points to the edge of the intraocular lens.

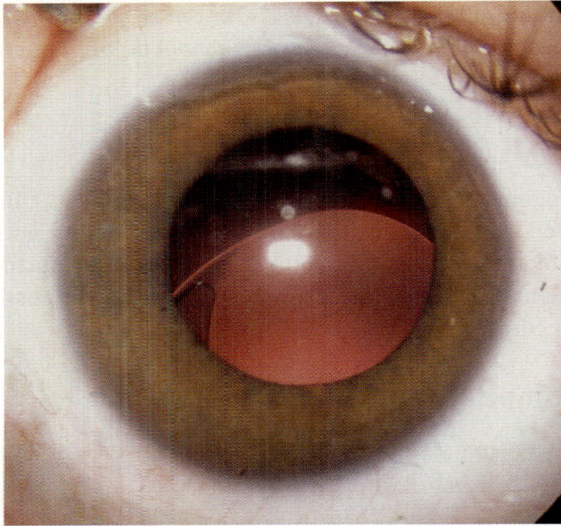

FIGURE 30–29 ■ The intraocular lens has shifted inferiorly.

cataracts. It often does not develop for several years. Continued monitoring for glaucoma is necessary as children who have had cataract surgery get older.

- *Problems with lens:* Intraocular lenses may shift out of position (Figure 30–29) or the power may be incorrect, necessitating repositioning or replacement.
- *Other:* Retinal detachments, corneal opacities, and infections are also potential complications of cataract surgery, but these are uncommon in children.

REFERENCES

1. Birch EE, Stager DR. The critical period for surgical treatment of dense congenital unilateral cataract. *Invest Ophthalmol Vis Sci.* 1996;37:1532–1538.
2. Birch EE, Cheng C, Stager Jr DR, Weakley Jr DR, Stager Sr DR. The critical period for surgical treatment of dense congenital bilateral cataracts. *JAAPOS.* 2009;13:67–71.

CHAPTER 31

Disorders of the Retina

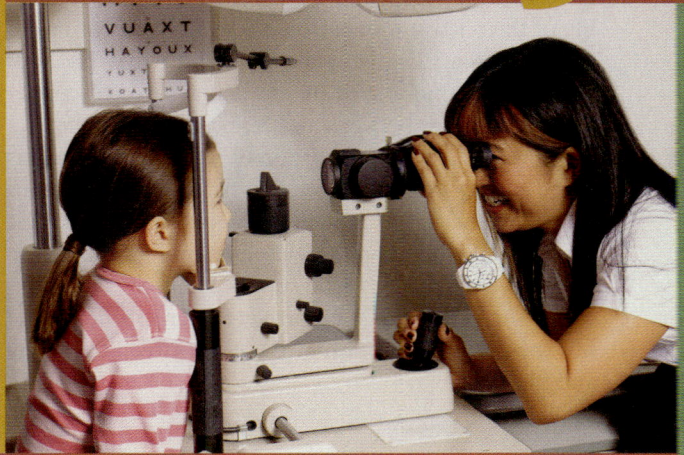

ANATOMY AND EMBRYOLOGY

The retinal is a multilayered structure that lines the inside of the back of the eye. Light rays are focused on the retina by the cornea and lens. When they reach the retina, they cause chemical reactions in the deepest layer of the retina, the *rods and cones (photoreceptors)*. This creates an impulse that is transmitted through the middle layer of the retina (the bipolar cells) to the inner portion (the ganglion cells) (Figure 31–1). The ganglion cells then travel and coalesce in the posterior portion of the eye to form to the optic nerve, which transmits the impulses to the brain. The retina is analogous to the film in a camera, in that it senses and changes in reaction to light.

The cones are responsible for discriminating fine visual detail and color. They are concentrated in the *macula*, which is the central portion of the retina between the vascular arcades. At the center of the macular is the fovea, visible as a focal area of increased pigment (Figure 31–2). This is the area of highest visual discrimination. It is used when reading or watching objects. The rods are more sensitive to dim light. They are concentrated in the peripheral retina. They are primarily responsible for peripheral vision.

On a molecular level, the perception of light is based on chemical reactions that occur in the outer layer of the photoreceptors. In the rods, photons are absorbed by rhodopsin molecules. This causes a reaction that results in release of glutamate (a neurotransmitter), which initiates a sequence of cellular connections that ultimately stimulates the ganglion cells and is transmitted to the brain via the optic nerve. The cones have a similar response, but there are 3 separate opsin molecules

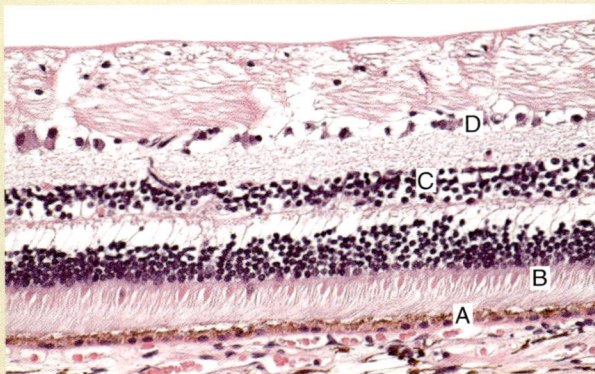

FIGURE 31–1 ■ Photomicrograph of retina. (A) Retinal pigment epithelium. (B) Photoreceptors, (C) Bipolar cells, (D) Ganglion cells. (Photo contributed by Morton Smith, MD.)

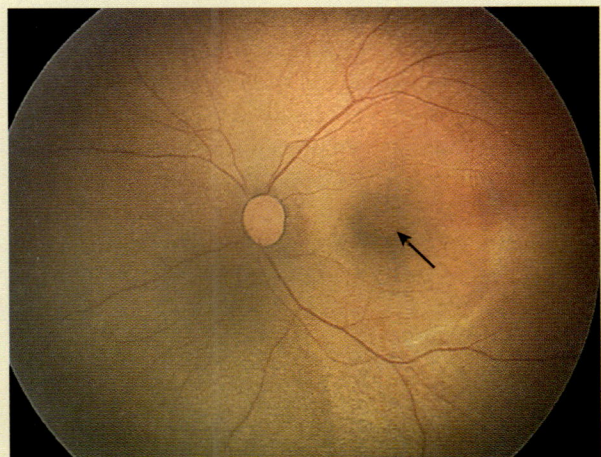

FIGURE 31–2 ■ Normal posterior retina and optic nerve. The arrow points to normal fovea.

that respond to different wavelengths of light. The apparent color of an object results from central processing of the relative inputs from these 3 types of cones.

The retina is highly metabolically active. The rods and cones are nourished by the retinal pigment epithelium, which lies between the retina and the choroidal blood vessels. The inner portion of the retina receives its blood supply from the blood vessels that line the retina. The retina itself is transparent. The red reflex that is visible during ophthalmoscopy and in photographs results from light reflecting off the blood supply within the choroid.

The vitreous is the normally clear substance that fills the posterior portion of the eye between the retina and the lens.

Embryology

The retina develops from neuroectodermal cells in the inner layer of the optic cup. This process begins during the first month of development. The outer layer of the cup becomes the retinal pigment epithelium, and the inner layer develops into the neurosensory retina. Within the retina itself, the inner ganglion cells develop first. Beginning at the sixth week of gestation, they migrate to the optic stalk to form the optic nerve. The rods and cones develop from the outer layer of neuroblastic tissue, with the outer segments of the cones differentiating at 5 months and the rods at 7 months. Overall, the differentiation of the retina begins in the central, posterior portion of the retina, then spreads to the peripheral portion. The process of retinal cell maturation continues after birth. This is why retinoblastoma tumors, which affect developing retinal cells, form in the posterior retina in newborns, and in the peripheral retina as children age.

The vitreous goes through 3 stages of development. The primary vitreous forms between the first and second months of gestation. It consists of vascular and mesenchymal cells between the lens vesicle and inner surface of the optic cup. The secondary vitreous develops between the second and third month. It is an avascular structure that gradually replaces the primary vitreous. The tertiary vitreous forms during the third and fourth month by condensation of fibrils in the area of the future lens zonules. The vitreous is supplied by the hyaloid artery during development. This structure normally regresses by the time of birth.

EPIDEMIOLOGY

Retinal disorders are uncommon in children. Many are untreatable or only partially treatable, and therefore they are an important cause of visual morbidity. Several retinal abnormalities have specific findings that help in

Table 31–1.

Diseases With Specific Retinal Findings That Suggest a Diagnosis

- Egg yolk—Best disease
- Lacunae—Aicardi syndrome
- Cherry-red spot—metabolic diseases
- Retinal necrosis and hemorrhage—Cytomegalovirus
- Astrocytic hamartoma—Tuberous sclerosis

establishing a diagnosis (Table 31–1). These are described later the chapter.

PATHOGENESIS

Retinal disorders may occur from a variety of causes, including congenital defects (e.g., coloboma), vascular abnormalities (e.g., retinopathy of prematurity [ROP]), infections, tumors, trauma, and metabolic diseases. These are discussed in the following sections.

CLINICAL PRESENTATION

The degree to which retinal abnormalities affect vision varies depending on the disorder, but many cause marked visual loss. Similar to most other ocular problems in children, unilateral abnormalities may be difficult to detect, because the children function well if the vision is good in the other eye. The vision loss may not be noticed until the child has a vision test or if the child occludes the normal eye (e.g., when rubbing the eye). Strabismus may develop in eyes with unilateral vision loss, and this may be the first sign of a problem. In some lesions, such as retinoblastoma or large colobomas, an abnormality of the red reflex may be noted. If the vision loss is bilateral, decreased vision will usually be evident. In infants, significant bilateral vision loss initially manifests as nystagmus that develops within the first 2 to 3 months of life.

CONGENITAL STRUCTURAL RETINAL DEFECTS

Retinal Coloboma

Similar to iris colobomas, retinal colobomas occur as a result of incomplete closure of the embryonic fissure during formation of the eye. The fissure normally comes together in the inferonasal quadrant of the eye, and this is the location of most retinal colobomas. They appear as white defects, because the sclera is directly visible due

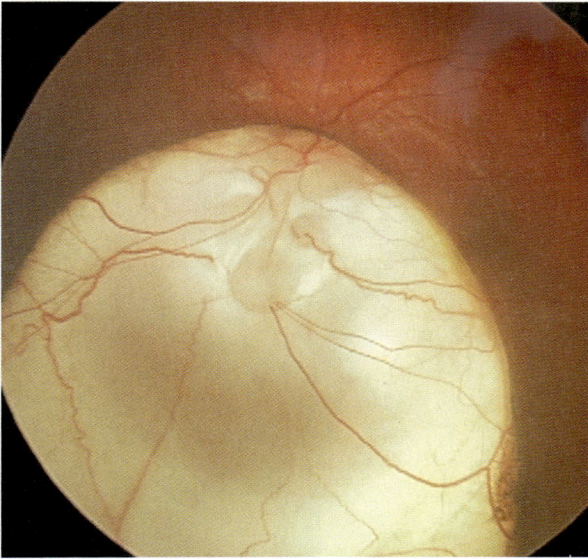

FIGURE 31–3 ■ Large retinal and optic nerve coloboma, left eye.

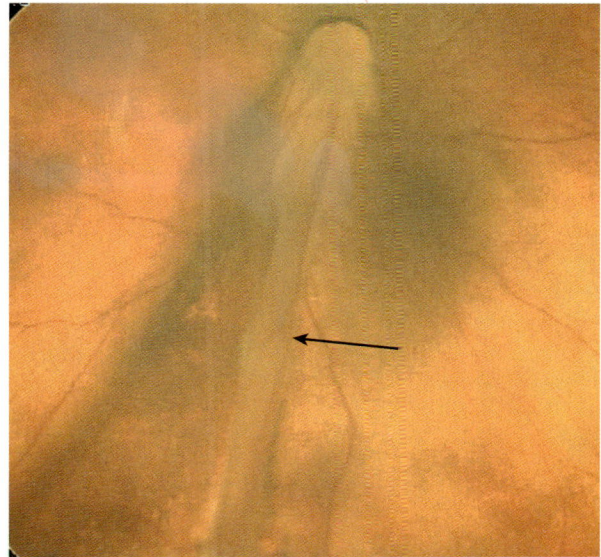

FIGURE 31–4 ■ Congenital retinal fold (arrow), right eye.

to the absence of normal retina and retinal pigment epithelium. They can vary from small focal defects inferior to the optic nerve to large defects that encompass the optic nerve and posterior retina (Figure 31–3).

The visual prognosis for retinal colobomas is primarily dependent on whether the fovea is involved.[1] If a clear foveal reflex is present, most patients will have good vision, even if the remainder of the coloboma is large. Conversely, even small defects may have significant effects on vision if they are located directly in the fovea.

Colobomas may occur as isolated findings or may be associated with systemic disorders, such as CHARGE (Coloboma, Heart defects, Atresia choanae, Retardation of growth, Genitourinary anomalies, and Ear anomalies) syndrome. Colobomas are not progressive. Retinal detachments may occur at the edge of the coloboma. These are difficult to treat.

Congenital Retinal Fold

Congenital retinal folds are rare anomalies in which a fold of retinal tissue extends from the optic nerve to the retinal periphery, usually in the inferotemporal portion of the eye (Figure 31–4). These may be inherited in an autosomal dominant fashion. They are usually associated with marked vision loss, and are not amenable to treatment.

Persistent Fetal Vasculature

Persistent fetal vasculature (PFV) (previously known as *persistent hyperplastic primary vitreous*) results from incomplete regression of the hyaloid blood vessel during embryological development. The most common ocular complication of PFV is a cataract (see Chapter 30).

A stalk of tissue is often visible extending to the optic nerve and retina (Figure 31–5). If the stalk causes significant distortion of the retinal tissue, visual loss may occur. The cataract in most patients with PFV can be successfully removed, and the presence of retinal defects is therefore usually the most important factor in determining the patient's visual prognosis.

Aicardi Syndrome

Aicardi syndrome is an X-linked disorder that has very distinctive retinal changes. It typically occurs only in females, as it is lethal in males. There is often a history of

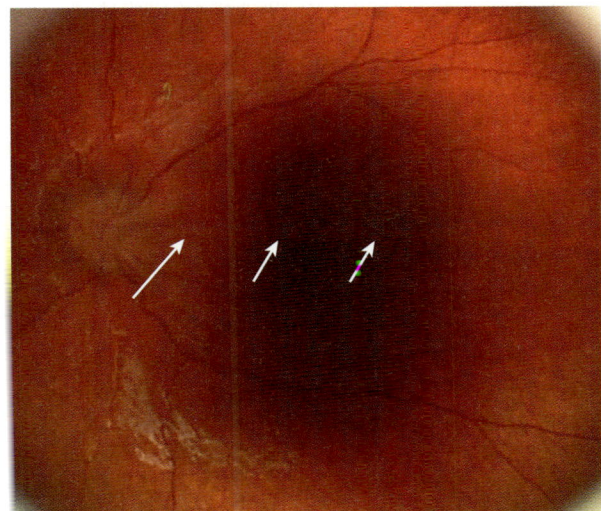

FIGURE 31–5 ■ Thin stalk of persistent fetal vascular tissue (arrows) extending through the vitreous to the optic nerve head.

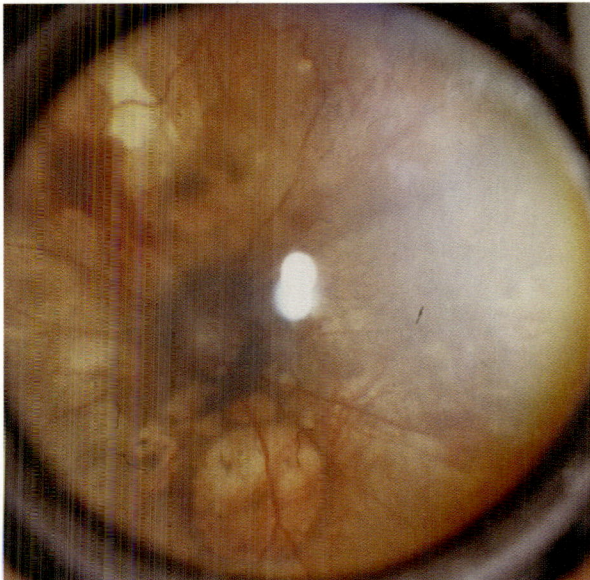

FIGURE 31–6 ■ Aicardi syndrome. Note multiple lacunar, hypopigmented retinal defects.

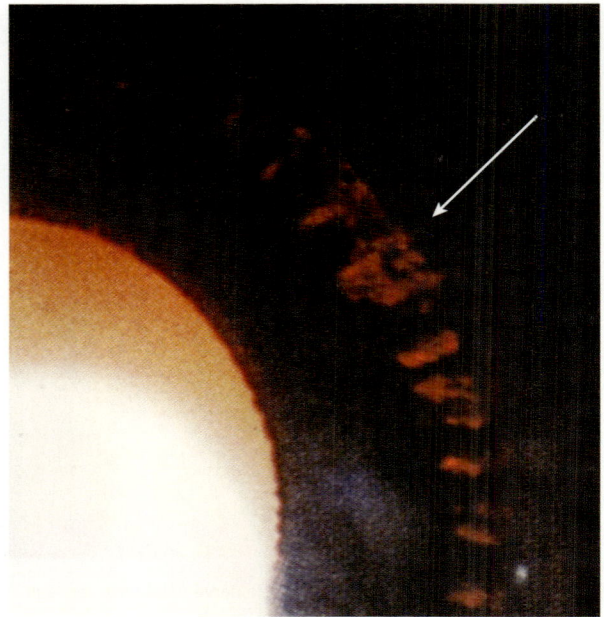

FIGURE 31–7 ■ Iris transillumination defects, high-magnification slit lamp view. Light is directed through the center of the pupil (lower left) and transillumination defects are visible in the peripheral iris (arrow).

maternal spontaneous abortions because of this. Systemic findings include absence of the corpus callosum, developmental delay, and seizures. Retinal findings consist of multiple round depigmented areas (lacunae), primarily in the posterior portion of the retina (Figure 31–6).

Albinism

Patients with albinism have a number of ocular abnormalities but the primary vision problems result from underdevelopment of the fovea. Albinism may be associated with systemic manifestations of decreased pigment (*oculocutaneous albinism* [OCA]), or the changes may be isolated to the eye (*ocular albinism*). Patients usually present in the neonatal period with decreased vision and nystagmus. Patients with OCA are easily identified by their decreased skin and hair pigment. Patients with ocular albinism often have slightly decreased, but not markedly abnormal, systemic pigment. Ocular examination findings in both forms of albinism consist of transillumination defects of the iris (Figure 31–7), decreased peripheral retinal pigmentation, and hypoplasia of the fovea (Figure 31–8).

The diagnosis of albinism can be established by genetic testing and a characteristic abnormality of visual evoked potentials. In normal patients, approximately half of the optic nerve fibers connect to each occipital lobe. In patients with albinism, a greater-than-normal number of fibers from each eye decussate and connect to the contralateral occipital lobe (Figure 2–9). Visual acuity in patients with albinism usually is in the 20/100 to 20/200 range.

Foveal Hypoplasia

The fovea is the structure at the center of the posterior retina that is responsible for fine visual discrimination. It is usually visualized as an area of increased pigment with a bright light reflex centered between the retinal vascular arcades. The retinal blood vessels arc around the fovea in an organized fashion, and the fovea itself is

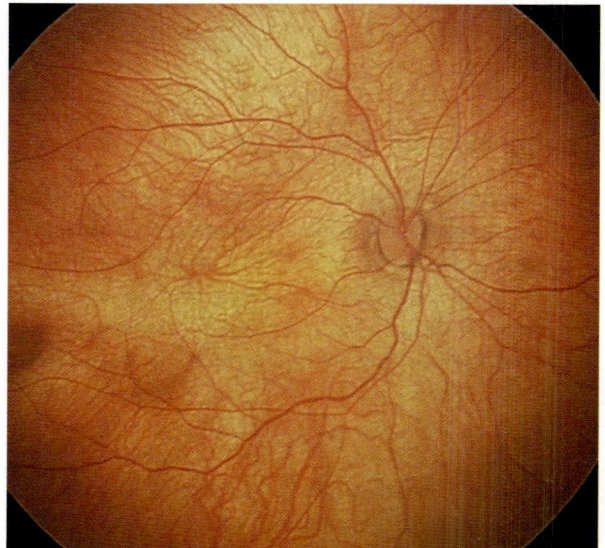

FIGURE 31–8 ■ Albinism. Note generalized decreased pigment and absence of normal foveal pigment and light reflex.

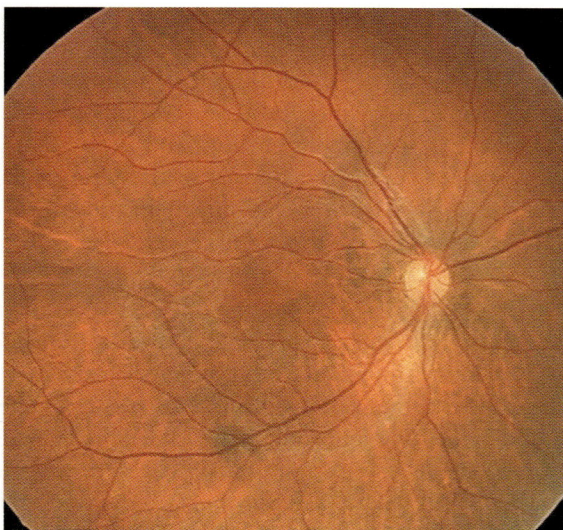

FIGURE 31–9 ■ Foveal hypoplasia in a patient with aniridia. Note absence of normal foveal pigment and light reflex.

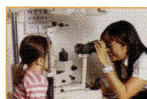

Table 31–2.		
ROP Screening Guidelines		
Gestational Age at Birth (wk)	**Chronological Age at First Examination (wk)**	**Postmenstrual Age at First Examination (wk)**
22	9	31
23	8	31
24	7	31
25	6	31
26	5	31
27	4	31
28	4	32
29	4	33
30	4	34

Timing of first eye examination based on gestational age at birth.
Source: Reprinted with permission from reference 3

avascular. In foveal hypoplasia, the normal foveal reflex is missing and the retinal blood vessels are not organized around the fovea.

The abnormal foveal anatomy causes decreased vision in patients with foveal hypoplasia. The most common disorder that causes foveal hypoplasia is ocular albinism (see above). It is also a feature of aniridia (see Chapter 29) (Figure 31–9). Rarely it may occur as an isolated abnormality. If this is the case, it is important to recognize foveal hypoplasia as the cause of decreased vision. Because the examination findings are fairly subtle, affected patients may be suspected of having amblyopia or factitious visual loss unless the retina is carefully examined.[2]

ABNORMALITIES OF VASCULAR DEVELOPMENT

Retinopathy of Prematurity

ROP is a disorder of retinal vascular development that occurs in premature infants. Normal retinal vascular development begins at 16 weeks of gestation. The vessels start in the posterior portion of the eye at the optic nerve and grow toward the retinal periphery. When infants are born prematurely, the blood vessels stop growing for a period. When growth resumes, most children develop normal vessels. In some infants, however, abnormal neovascular tissue develops. This tissue may proliferate and cause bleeding and traction, which can progress to retinal detachment. ROP is a major cause of morbidity in premature infants. The risk increases with decreasing birth weight and gestational age, occurring almost exclusively in infants born at 30 weeks gestation or less.

Screening for ROP

Regular ophthalmic monitoring of premature infants is required to identify and treat ROP when high-risk features are present. Guidelines have been published that describe the recommended age at initial screening and appropriate follow-up (Table 31–2).[3] If retinal detachments occur, they are very difficult to treat and the visual outcome is usually poor. Therefore, the goal of treatment is to halt the progression of disease before this occurs. The presence of *plus disease* is a key indicator of risk. Plus disease describes increased tortuosity and dilation of the posterior blood vessels (Figure 31–10), which reflects the abnormal retinal vascular development.

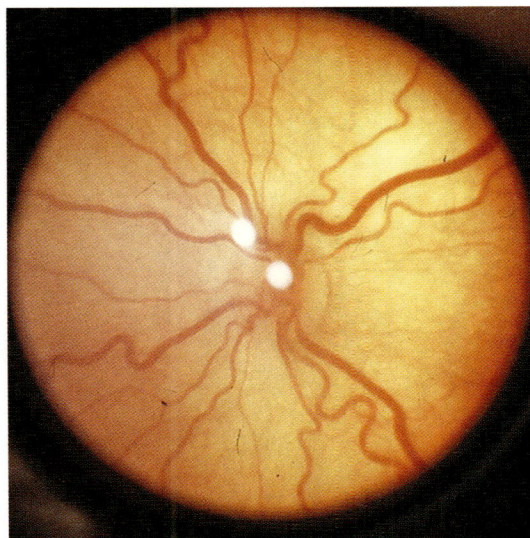

FIGURE 31–10 ■ ROP with plus disease. The posterior retinal blood vessels are dilated and tortuous.

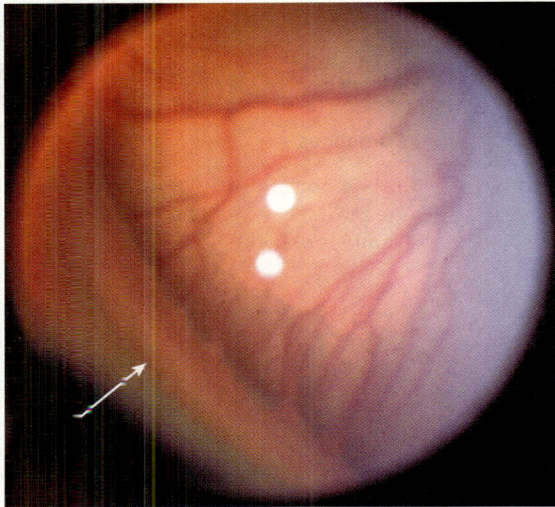

FIGURE 31–11 ■ Stage 3 retinopathy of prematurity. An elevated area of retinal tissue with abnormal vessels is present at the juncture between the vascular and avascular retina (arrow). Some of the retinal blood vessels are being elevated from the retinal surface due to traction

In addition to plus disease, ROP is classified using a standardized system by *stage* and *zone*. The stage of ROP describes the type of abnormality present at the juncture of the posterior vascularized retina and the peripheral nonvascularized retina. Stage 1 is a demarcation line at this site. Stage 2 is an elevated ridge. Stage 3 is present when abnormal neovascular vessels begin to grow from the ridge (Figure 31–11). The presence of stage 3 (in addition to plus disease) is a high-risk factor. If the disease continues, patients may develop retinal

detachments (stage 4—partial retinal detachment, and stage 5—complete retinal detachment).

The zone of ROP describes the location (Figure 31–12). Zone 1 is the most posterior portion of the retina, zone 2 is the middle portion, and zone 3 is the peripheral retina. The more posterior the abnormality, the higher the risk of vision loss due to the proximity of the abnormal vessels to the macula and fovea.

Treatment of ROP

The aim of treatment is to prevent retinal distortion and detachment by stopping the abnormal vascular activity before these complications occur. Multicenter studies have identified the following high-risk factors in ROP: the presence of any plus disease or stage 3 disease in zone 1, or the presence of stages 2 or 3 and plus disease in zone 2. Treatment for patients with ROP is indicated when they develop these findings on examination.[4]

The peripheral retina in patients with ROP produces vascular endothelial growth factor (VEGF), which stimulates the growth of abnormal vessels. Treatment consists of ablation of the peripheral, nonvascularized retina with laser or cryotherapy (Figures 31–13 and 31–14). The goal is to decrease production of VEGF and induce regression of the abnormal vessels. Multicenter trials have shown that treatment is effective, but not all patients respond. Some patients develop scars in the fovea after treatment, which may impair visual acuity (Figure 31–15). If patients develop progressive retinal detachments, retinal surgery (such as vitrectomy) may be indicated. However, once the posterior retina has detached the visual outcomes are usually

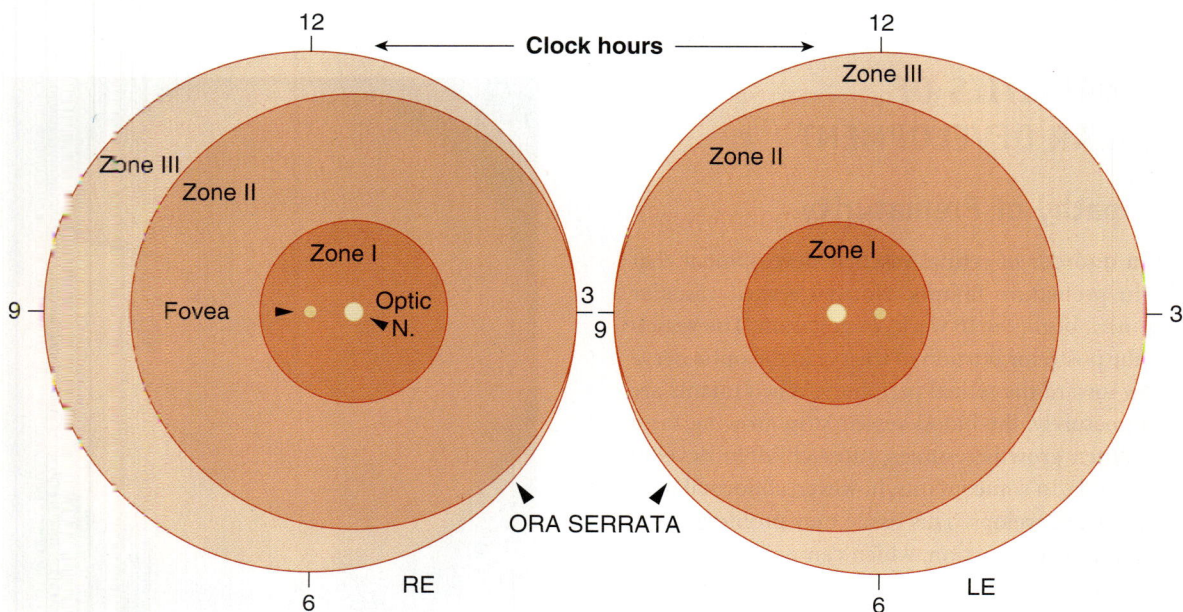

FIGURE 31–12 ■ Standard diagram for documenting retinopathy of prematurity. Zone 1 is defined by a circle centered on the optic nerve with a radius twice the distance from the optic nerve to the fovea. Zone 2 is defined by a circle centered on the optic nerve that extends to the nasal ora serrata (edge of retina). Zone 3 is the remaining temporal retina.

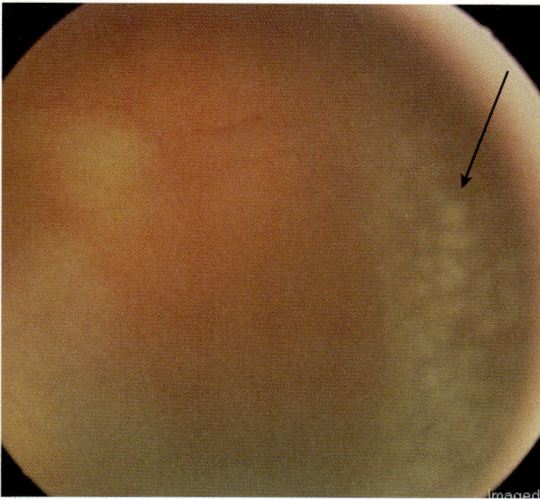

FIGURE 31–13 ■ ROP. Laser scars in peripheral retina (arrow) immediately after treatment.

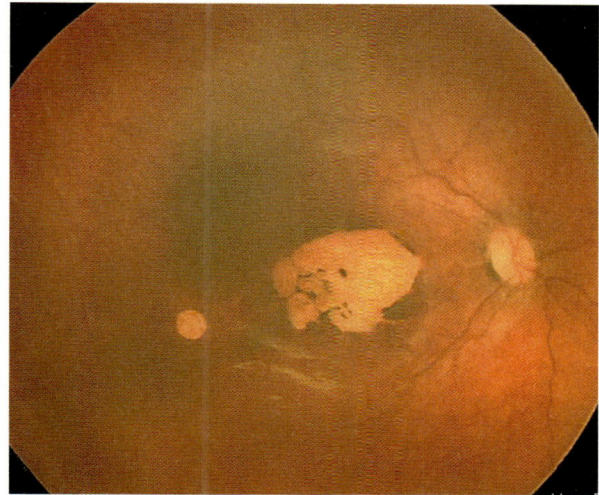

FIGURE 31–15 ■ ROP. Scar in fovea following peripheral laser treatment.

poor, even if the retina is successfully reattached. For this reason, efforts are made to treat the disorder before this occurs. Recently, anti-VEGF injections into the vitreous cavity have been reported to induce regression of ROP, but large-scale studies of this treatment have not been performed.

Beyond the neonatal period, infants with ROP are at risk for other ocular problems, including strabismus, amblyopia, and refractive errors. They may also experience vision problems due to associated central nervous system morbidities, such as intraventricular hemorrhages and periventricular leukomalacia (Figure 31–16).

Other Disorders of Peripheral Retinal Vascularization

A number of other rare disorders have peripheral retinal vascular changes that appear similar to those seen in

ROP, including neovascularization and retinal detachment. These include the following:

■ *Norrie disease.* An X-linked disorder characterized by the retinal abnormalities, hearing loss, and developmental delay.
■ *Familial exudative vitreoretinopathy (FEVR).* An autosomal dominant disorder caused by mutation of the

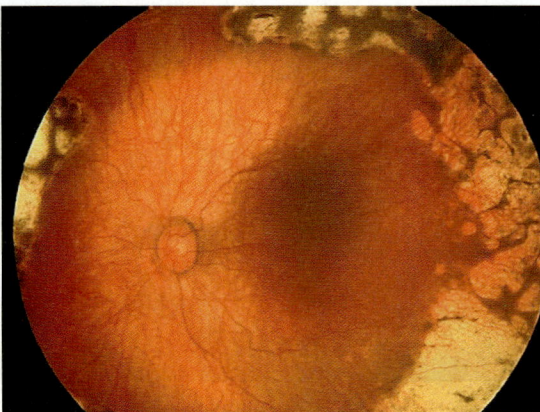

FIGURE 31–14 ■ ROP. Appearance of peripheral retinal scars several months after laser treatment.

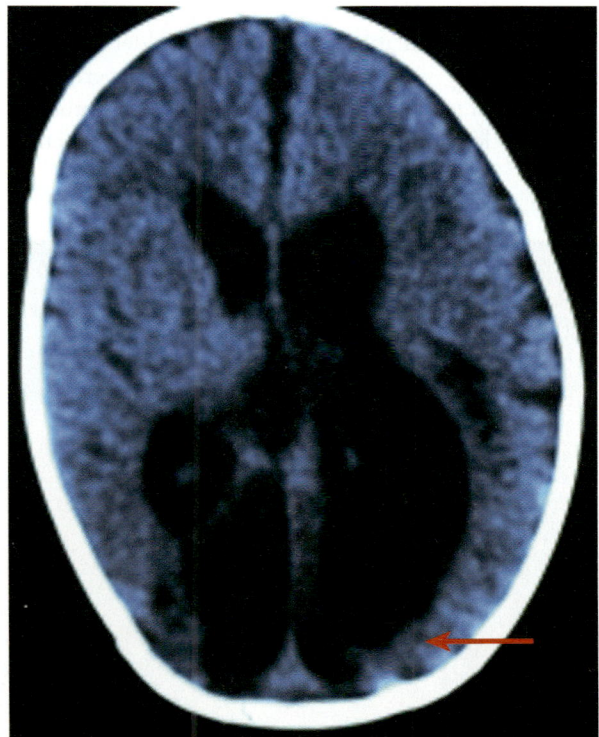

FIGURE 31–16 ■ Computed tomography scan showing enlarged ventricles following intraventricular hemorrhage, with volume loss in occipital lobes (arrow).

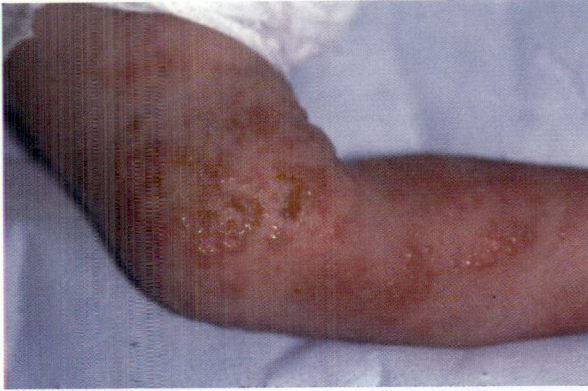

FIGURE 31–17 ■ Right leg of neonate with vesicular lesions due to incontinentia pigmenti.

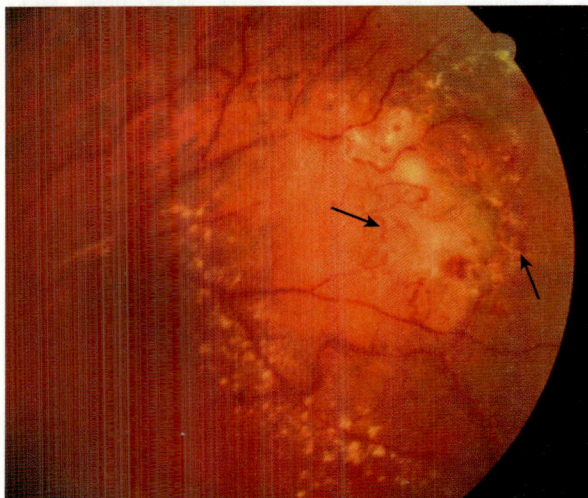

FIGURE 31–19 ■ Coat's disease. Retinal detachment (left) and subretinal lipid deposits involving fovea.

FEVR gene on chromosome 11. The peripheral retinal findings are very similar to those in ROP, but the patients are not premature and other family members are affected.

■ *Incontinentia pigmenti.* An X-linked disorder that is usually lethal in males. Affected patients develop bullous erythematous skin lesions in the neonatal period (Figure 31–17), followed by verrucous changes, and subsequently hyperpigmented macules. Developmental delay and dental changes occur in some patients. Approximately one-third of patients develop retinal changes similar to ROP. Many patients also develop cataracts.

■ *Coat's disease.* Coat's disease is an idiopathic disorder of retinal vasculature that occurs in older children. It is usually unilateral. In Coat's disease, peripheral abnormal telangiectatic retinal blood vessels proliferate and leak exudative fluid (Figure 31–18). This may

produce large collections of yellow subretinal fluid and retinal detachments (Figure 31–19). Treatment consists of attempts to eradicate the abnormal telangiectatic vessels, with either laser or cryotherapy. The appearance of Coat's disease may be similar to retinoblastoma and is in the differential diagnosis of this tumor (Figure 31–20).

■ *Von-Hippel-Lindau disease (VHL).* This is an autosomal dominant disorder in which patients develop vascular tumors of the retina and central nervous system. Systemic manifestations include renal cell

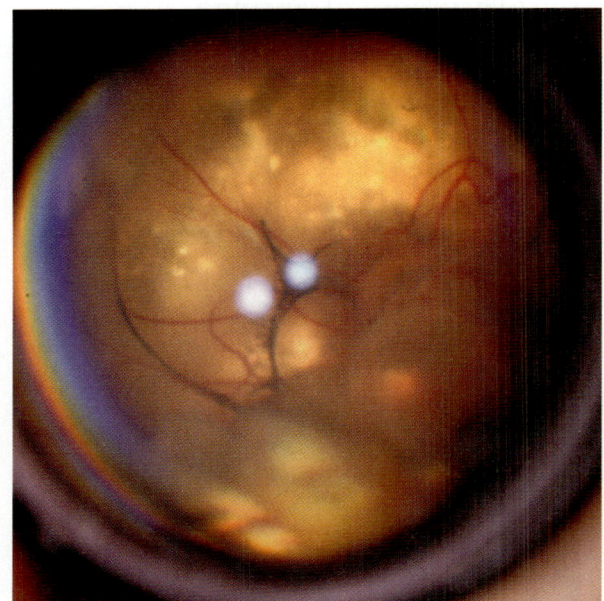

FIGURE 31–18 ■ Coat's disease. Peripheral retinal telangiectasias (arrows) with lipid exudates.

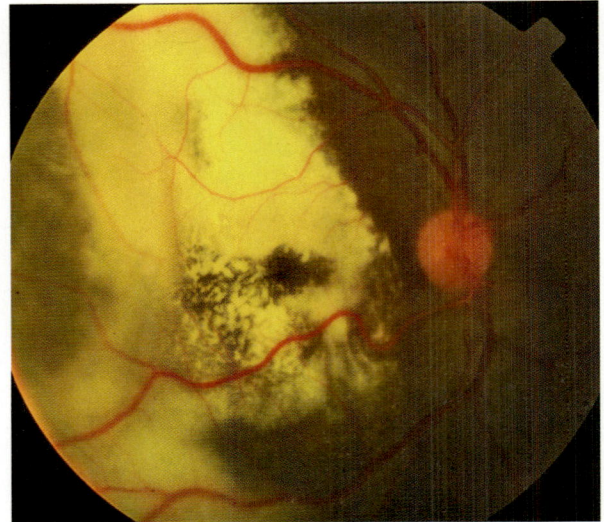

FIGURE 31–20 ■ Coat's disease. Clinical appearance may be similar to retinoblastoma.

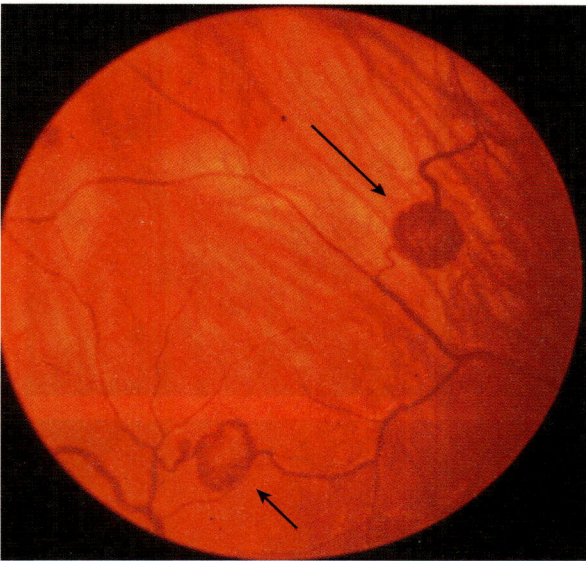

FIGURE 31–21 ■ Von Hippel-Lindau disease. Peripheral retinal angiomas (arrows).

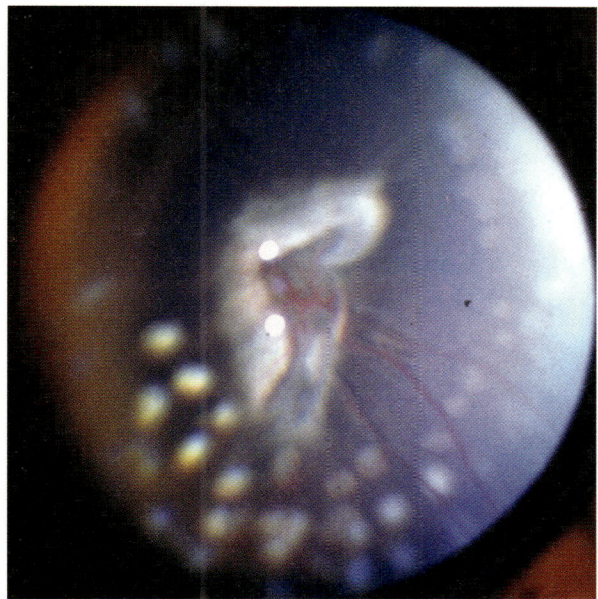

FIGURE 31–22 ■ Peripheral retinal abnormality ("sea fan") in patient with sickle retinopathy, surrounded by multiple laser treatment spots.

carcinoma, pheochromocytoma, and lesions in multiple other organs. The retinal lesions usually do not develop until young adulthood, but sometimes present during the teen years. These retinal angiomas gradually enlarge and are associated with dilation of the feeding and draining arteries and veins (Figure 31–21). The lesions can be treated, and therefore periodic ophthalmic monitoring of patients with VHL is recommended.

■ *Diabetes mellitus.* Patients with diabetes mellitus are at risk for developing retinal vascular abnormalities, including neovascularization of the peripheral retina and macular edema. The risk increases with the duration of disease and decreases with improved glycemic control. It usually does not develop until 10 to 15 years following diagnosis, and therefore almost never in the first decade of life. Annual monitoring by an ophthalmologist should be performed beginning 5 years after diagnosis or after age 10 years whichever is later.[5]

■ *Sickle cell disease.* Patients with sickle cell disease may develop peripheral retinal abnormalities secondary to decreased vascular perfusion. This is caused by arteriolar occlusion induced by sickling of the abnormal red blood cells. Patients with hemoglobin SC disease and sickle thalassemia have the highest risk of retinal complications. The most severe of these is retinal neovascularization induced by ischemia, with an underlying mechanism similar to that of ROP. If untreated, this may progress and cause vitreous hemorrhage and retinal detachments. Laser treatment is used to treat these lesions (Figure 31–22).

INFECTIOUS DISEASES

Many infectious diseases can affect the retina, either as congenital or acquired infections. Retinal involvement in herpes simplex virus (HSV) and cytomegalovirus (CMV) infection is usually confined to infants with congenital infections or older patients with immune deficiencies.

Herpes Simplex Virus

Congenital HSV is usually acquired during passage through the birth canal. Infants may have systemic involvement, including the skin, central nervous, liver, lungs, and eyes. There is a significant mortality in infants with disseminated disease. Ocular findings include conjunctivitis and keratitis. If the retina is involved, patients may develop massive retinal necrosis with marked visual loss. Treatment includes systemic medication, such as acyclovir.

Cytomegalovirus

CMV is the most common congenital infection in humans. The majority of patients are asymptomatic. Systemic manifestations of congenital CMV include liver, hematological, hearing, and central nervous system abnormalities. Ophthalmic manifestations include retinochoroiditis, which is characterized by focal areas of retinal necrosis and hemorrhages (Figure 31–23). Infants with systemic involvement and older immunocompromised children with CMV are usually treated with ganciclovir.

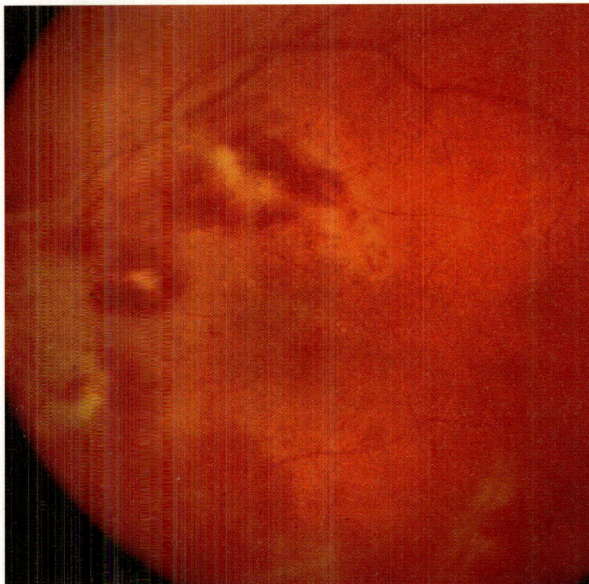

FIGURE 31–23 ■ CMV retinitis, with foci of hemorrhage and retinal necrosis (white areas).

Syphilis

Congenital syphilis may cause a wide variety of systemic and ocular problems. Ocular abnormalities may develop in infancy or later in childhood. Retinal involvement consists of chorioretinitis, which may appear similar to retinitis pigmentosa.

Toxoplasmosis

Toxoplasmosis is caused by *Toxoplasma gondii*, an obligate intracellular parasite. It is usually acquired by exposure to cats or through contaminated meat or drinking water. Systemic infection may cause flulike symptoms, which may not be identified as due to *Toxoplasma*. Congenital infections are associated with liver, spleen, central nervous system, and ocular involvement. Cysts may remain dormant for prolonged periods or they may rupture, producing inflammation due to release of tachyzoites.

Ocular toxoplasmosis most commonly is characterized by inactive circumscribed pigmented retinal scars. If the lesions reactivate, focal areas of retinitis with inflammation and overlying vitritis are seen (Figure 31–24A and B). The infection is usually self-limited, but reactivation may occur. Treatment is generally reserved for active lesions that may impair vision, such as those in the fovea. Various treatment regimens have been described, which usually include a combination of antimicrobials for the infection and corticosteroids to decrease inflammation. In some studies, prenatal treatment of infants whose mothers are affected has been shown to improve visual outcomes.

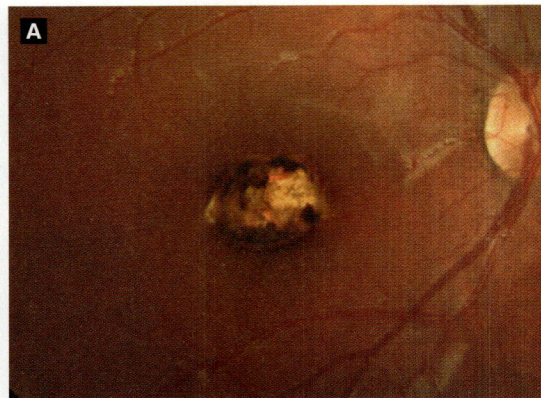

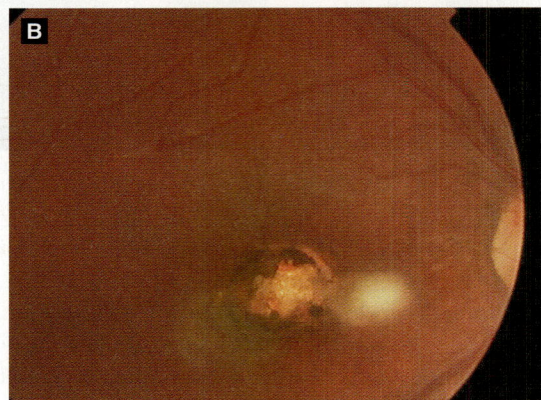

FIGURE 31–24 ■ Toxomplasmosis. (A) Inactive foveal scar. (B) Reactivated retinitis with focus of inflammation adjacent to original scar. (Photographs contributed by Alan Richards, MD.)

Rubella

The incidence of rubella in the United States is now very low due to successful immunization programs. Systemic involvement includes cardiac, hearing, and central nervous system abnormalities. Ocular findings include cataracts and glaucoma. Retinal manifestations include pigmentary changes that may mimic retinitis pigmentosa. The spotty areas of pigmentation are sometimes described as salt-and-pepper retinopathy (Figure 31–25).

Lymphocytic Choriomeningitis Virus

This disorder is transmitted by exposure to rodents. Systemic manifestations primarily involve the central nervous system, including hydrocephalus, microcephaly, calcifications, and developmental delay. Ocular manifestations consist of chorioretinal scars, primarily in the posterior retina. The appearance of these scars may be similar to those seen in toxoplasmosis and Aicardi syndrome.

Toxocariasis

This disease is caused by *Toxocara canis*, a parasite that is acquired through exposure to dog or cat feces or unclean

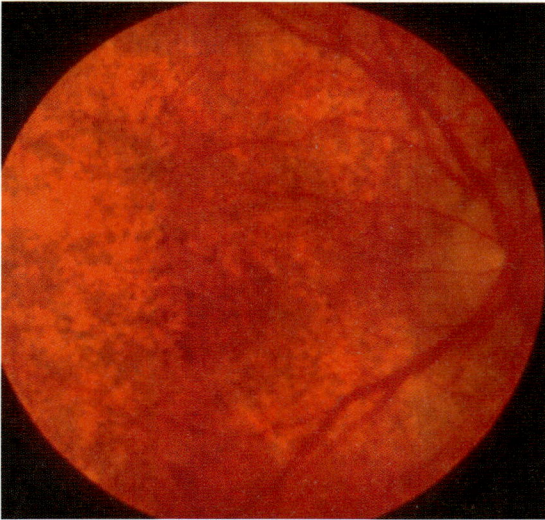

FIGURE 31–25 ■ Salt-and-pepper retinopathy due to congenital rubella.

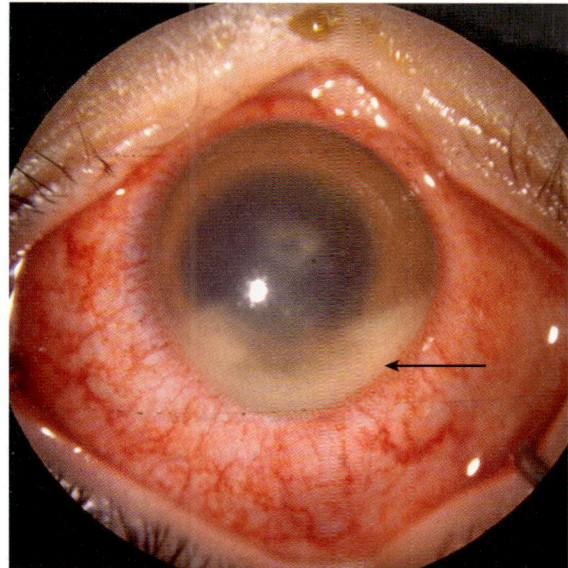

FIGURE 31–27 ■ Intense ocular inflammation with layered pus in anterior chamber (arrow) (hypopyon) due to bacterial endophthalmitis.

food. Systemic involvement includes *visceral larval migrans*, usually in infants and toddlers. It may present with flulike symptoms. Ocular involvement includes focal retinal granulomas, associated with inflammation and bands of traction tissue (Figure 31–26). Treatment is indicated if the vision is threatened, but may be complicated by induction of a marked inflammatory response.

Bacterial Endophthalmitis

This is a rare and potentially devastating infection of the vitreous and retina. It most commonly occurs as a result of penetrating ocular injury or as a complication of

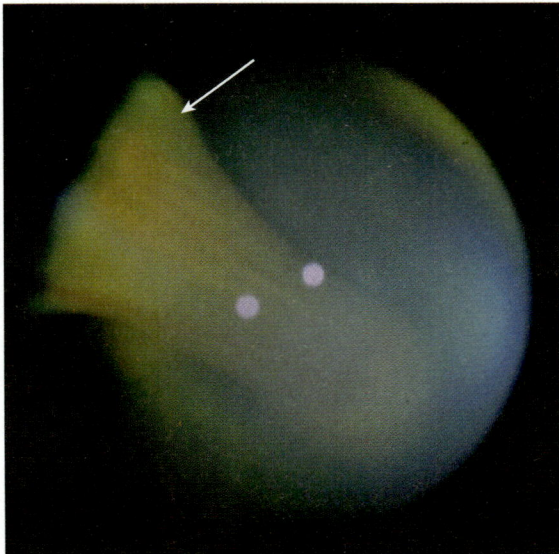

FIGURE 31–26 ■ Toxocariasis. Band of scar tissue extending to peripheral retinal granuloma (arrow).

ophthalmic surgery. Rarely, endogenous endophthalmitis may develop in patients with endocarditis or other systemic disease. It presents with marked ocular inflammation. A *hypopyon* (a collection of pus in the anterior chamber) is often present (Figure 31–27). Prompt treatment with systemic and intravitreal antibiotics is usually necessary if vision is to be preserved.

INHERITED DISORDERS OF RETINAL FUNCTION

Retinitis Pigmentosa

Retinitis pigmentosa (RP) includes a large number of inherited disorders characterized by dysfunction of the retinal photoreceptors (rods and cones). Patients with RP typically develop pigmentary changes in the retina, with clumps of hyperpigmented tissue that appear like bone spicules (Figure 31–28). The diagnosis of RP is established by measurement of the electrical function of the retina with an *electroretinogram (ERG)*.

Leber Congenital Amaurosis

Leber congenital amaurosis (LCA) is a congenital form of RP that is inherited in an autosomal recessive fashion and that affects both rods and cones. It presents within the first few months of life with poor or absent visual fixation and nystagmus. Poorly reactive pupils and marked farsightedness are usually present. The retina initially appears normal, but most patients develop pigmentary changes with age. The diagnosis is established

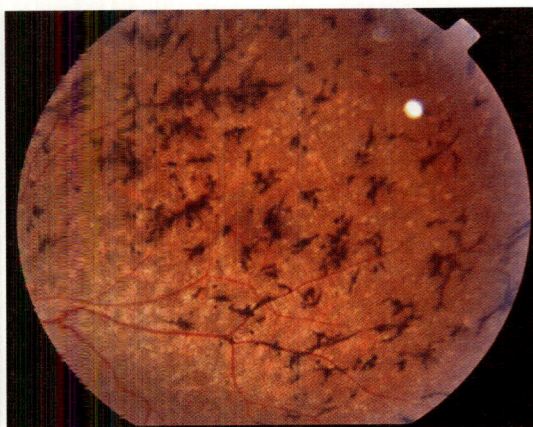

FIGURE 31–28 ■ Retinitis pigmentosa. Bone-spicule pigmentation in peripheral retina.

by a nonrecordable ERG, which is present in infancy. LCA is usually an isolated ocular disorder, but may be associated with systemic disorders, including renal and central nervous system abnormalities.

A number of genetic mutations have been identified in patients with LCA. A dog model has shown some improvement with gene therapy, and early human trials have shown an initial improvement in visual function.[6]

Systemic Disorders Associated with Retinitis Pigmentosa

Retinitis pigmentosa is a feature of several diseases with other systemic manifestations. In addition to RP, *Bardet-Biedl syndrome* is associated with developmental delay, extra digits on the hands and feet, obesity, and hypogonadism. *Usher syndrome* is associated with sensorineural hearing loss.

Stargardt Disease (Juvenile Macular Degeneration)

This disease is usually inherited in an autosomal recessive pattern. Affected patients present with unexplained vision loss, usually during the second decade. It is caused by a mutation of the retina-specific ATP-binding transporter protein (ABCR). The retina often initially appears normal, and the child may be suspected of malingering. Progressive foveal changes develop with time, which is described as a "beaten metal" appearance of the macula (Figure 31–29). Some patients have a characteristic dark appearance of the choroid on fluorescein angiography of the retina.

Neuronal Ceroid Lipofuscinosis (Batten Disease)

This is a group of autosomal recessive disorders in which abnormal deposits develop in neuronal lysosomes.

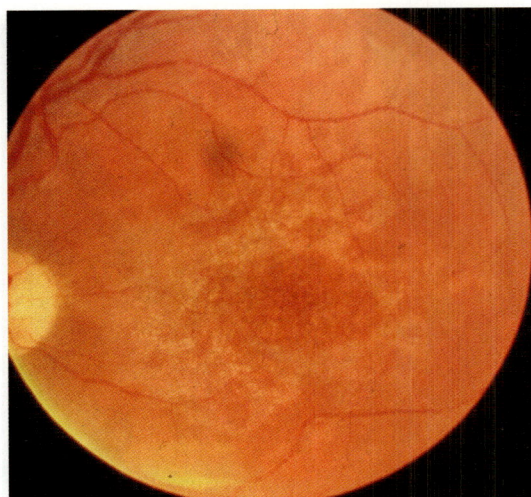

FIGURE 31–29 ■ Macular abnormality in Stargardt disease, described as a "beaten metal" appearance.

There are several childhood forms, which present with decreased vision, developmental delay, and seizures. Ophthalmic findings include optic nerve atrophy and pigmentary deposits within the retina. Genetic testing can establish the diagnosis.

Disorders Associated With Cherry-red Spots

Cherry-red spots may be seen in a number of rare metabolic disorders, including Tay-Sachs, Niemann-Pick, sialidosis, and Sandhoff disease. The appearance is due to accumulation of abnormal material in the ganglion cells surrounding the fovea (Figure 31–30). Because the fovea itself does not contain ganglion cells, it has a red

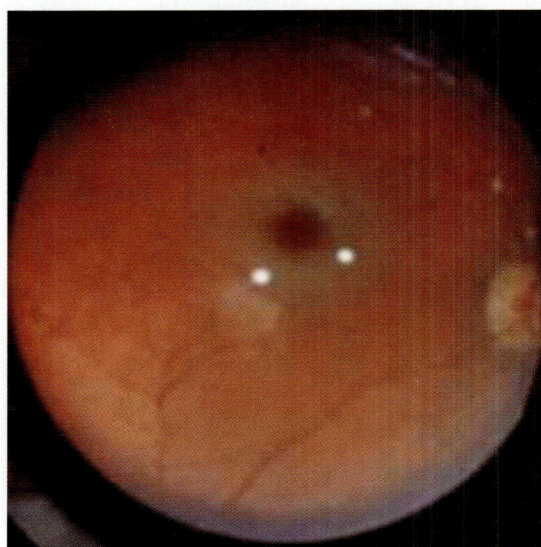

FIGURE 31–30 ■ Retinal cherry-red spot.

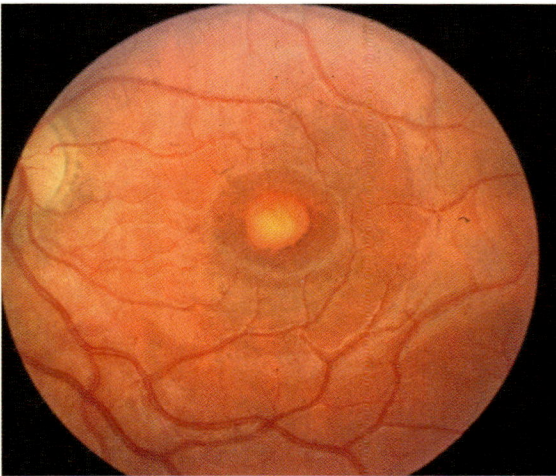

FIGURE 31–31 ■ Best's disease with egg yolk appearance of foveal lesion.

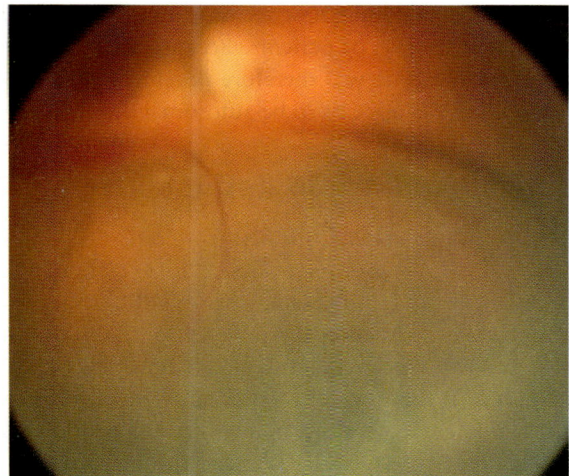

FIGURE 31–32 ■ Peripheral retinal detachment due to juvenile X-linked retinoschisis (the lower portion of the photograph is an elevated, detached retina with a blood vessel visible on the surface).

appearance in contrast to the milky-white appearance of the surrounding abnormal ganglion cells.

Other Inherited Disorders of Retinal Function

A large number of these disorders exist. Most are very rare.

- *Best vitelliform dystrophy.* An autosomal dominant disorder caused by mutation of the vitelliform macular dystrophy gene. It presents in older children with a distinctive yellow cystic structure in the macula that may look like an egg yolk (Figure 31–31). The diagnosis is established by an abnormal electrooculogram, which reflects dysfunction of the retinal pigment epithelium.
- *Achromatopsia (rod monochromatism).* This is a very rare disorder characterized by absent cone function. Infants present in a similar fashion to LCA, with minimal fixation and nystagmus in early infancy. They are usually photophobic. The diagnosis is established by absence of cone responses on an ERG.
- *Congenital stationary night blindness.* This is a less severe form of congenital RP that may be inherited in any form. Infants typically present with nystagmus in the first few months of life, but visual function is not markedly impaired. The diagnosis is established by characteristic ERG changes.
- *Juvenile retinoschisis.* Juvenile retinoschisis is an X-linked disorder in which the inner layers of the retina separate. This occurs initially in the fovea. Older patients may develop peripheral retinal detachments (Figure 31–32). Patients often have progressive vision loss. A characteristic ERG abnormality (a decreased scotopic b-wave with preserved a-wave) is diagnostic.
- *Joubert syndrome.* Joubert syndrome is a congenital disorder characterized by maldevelopment of the ce-

bellar vermis, identified on imaging studies by the "molar tooth sign." It frequently presents with abnormal breathing in infancy. Other systemic features include hypotonia, ataxia, and developmental delay. Some patients with Joubert syndrome have a congenital form of retinal dystrophy that presents with poor visual responses and nystagmus in infancy. Ocular motor apraxia is a common feature.

RETINOBLASTOMA

Epidemiology and Molecular Biology of Retinoblastoma

Retinoblastoma (RB) is rare, occurring in approximately 1:20,000 births, but it is the most common primary intraocular tumor in children. It results from mutations of the retinoblastoma gene, and may be inherited in either a sporadic or familial form. The retinoblastoma gene is important in regulating the cell cycle. In order for tumors to develop, both retinoblastoma genes must be dysfunctional, resulting in tumors due to unregulated cell growth. In patients with sporadic disease, the 2 RB genes are mutated in a single retinal cell, which then grows to a single tumor. In patients with heritable disease, the patients are born with a mutation in one of the genes, and therefore all cells in the body carry this mutation. Typically, second mutations develop in several retinal cells, and the average patient ultimately develops 6 to 8 separate retinal tumors.

Clinically, the heritable form of the disease appears to be transmitted as an autosomal dominant trait. On a molecular level, however, it is actually an autosomal recessive disorder, because both genes must be altered for tumors to develop. These second mutations occur in approximately 90% of patients. Because most patients who carry the gene will therefore develop tumors, the disease clinically appears to be autosomal dominant.

Clinical Findings in Retinoblastoma

Retinoblastoma arises from maturing retina cells, and usually develops within the first 2 to 3 years of life. Unless there is a family history of retinoblastoma and the patient is being monitored by an ophthalmologist, most tumors will grow undetected until they cause symptoms. If the tumor becomes large enough it produces leukocoria, an abnormal white reflex within the eye (Figure 31–33A and B). If the tumor affects the central vision, patients may develop strabismus. Rarely, retinoblastoma may present with a clinical picture suggestive of orbital cellulitis or iritis. Early detection and treatment of retinoblastoma improves the prognosis. This is why the red reflex should be monitored during well-child examinations, and patients with abnormalities should be referred for prompt evaluation.

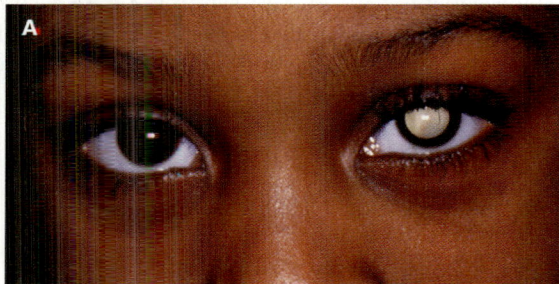

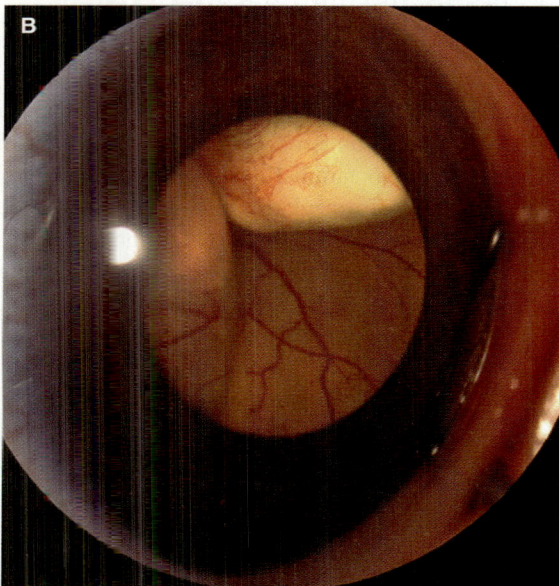

FIGURE 31–34 ■ Retinoblastoma in posterior retina. The view of the optic nerve is blocked by the tumor (arrow).

Clinically, retinoblastoma appears as a cream-colored mass arising from the retina (Figure 31–34). Large tumors often have associated retinal detachment due to leakage of fluid from abnormal blood vessels. The presence of fine vitreous seeds overlying the tumor is a very specific diagnostic sign (Figure 31–35). Notably, there is usually no associated retinal scarring, traction, or cataract. The absence of these findings is helpful in distinguishing RB from inflammatory disorders and other retinal diseases associated with tractional detachments.

The lesion that can most closely resemble retinoblastoma is an *astrocytic hamartoma* (Figure 31–36), which occurs in some patients with *tuberous sclerosis* (TS) (discussed later in chapter). The associated systemic

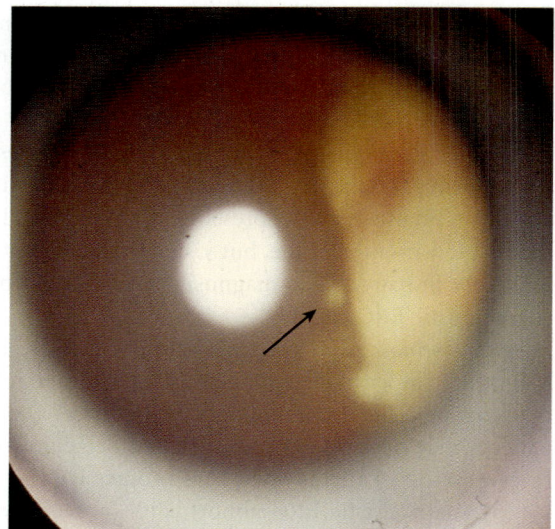

FIGURE 31–33 ■ (A) Leukocoria due to large retinoblastoma. (B) Large tumor visible through pupil.

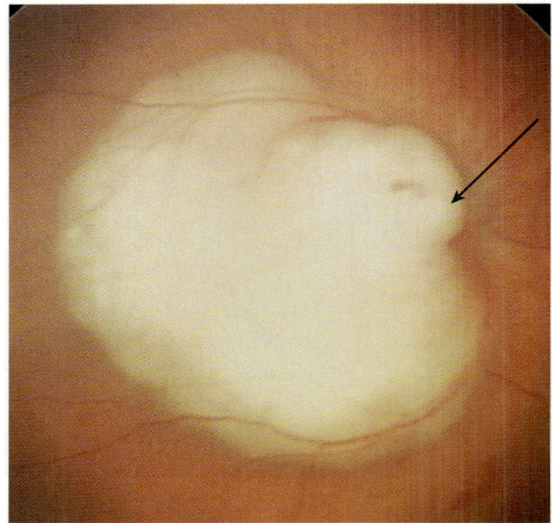

FIGURE 31–35 ■ Retinoblastoma. Vitreous seeds (arrow) adjacent to large tumor.

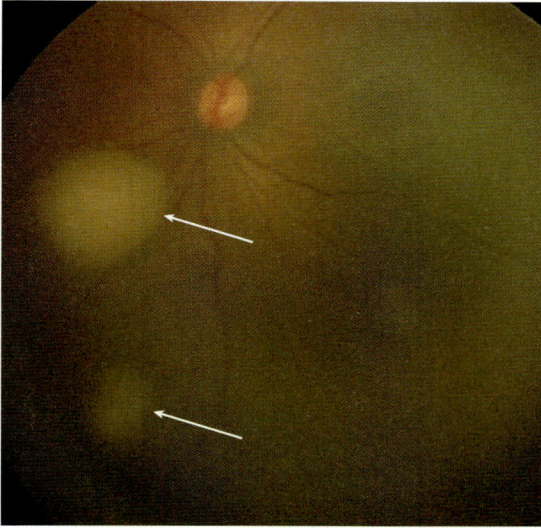

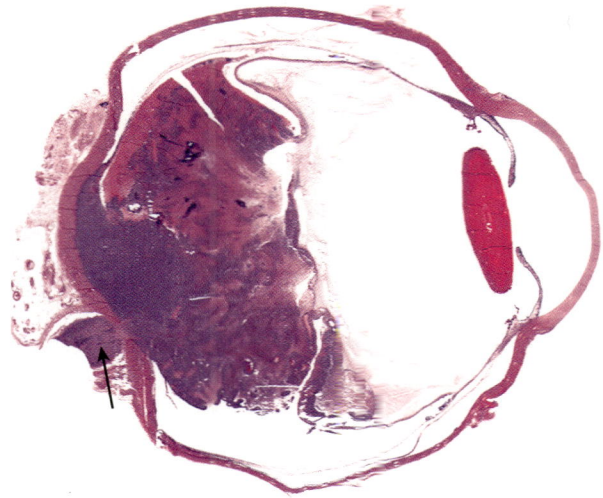

FIGURE 31–37 ■ Histopathological findings in retinoblastoma. Dark blue areas indicate tumor, and extension is seen in optic nerve (arrow). (Photograph contributed by Morton Smith, MD.)

findings in TS usually make this diagnosis straightforward. Astrocytic hamartomas usually do not grow, nor do they impair visual function. In rare cases, fine needle biopsy may be indicated to establish a diagnosis, but this is usually not indicated due to the risk of systemic dissemination of tumor.

In patients with large retinal masses, particularly if retinoblastoma is suspected, imaging studies are usually performed. Most large retinoblastomas are calcified, and the presence of calcification on computed tomography is highly specific. Magnetic resonance imaging may be used to look for evidence of extraocular extension or associated pineal tumors.

Treatment of Retinoblastoma

The treatment of retinoblastoma depends on the size and laterality of the tumor. The primary goal of treatment is to preserve life, and the secondary goal is to preserve vision. If RB spreads beyond the eye, treatment is very difficult and the mortality is high.

Patients with unilateral retinoblastoma usually develop large tumors before a diagnosis is made, and the potential for useful vision is poor. If the other eye is normal, the child will function normally. Therefore, enucleation (surgical removal of the eye) is usually recommended. Rarely, unilateral retinoblastoma is detected when the tumors are small enough that they can be successfully treated and some vision preserved. This usually occurs because a pediatrician notices an abnormal red reflex during a well-child evaluation.[7]

When patients are enucleated, the prognosis is excellent if the tumor is found to be confined to the eye. The primary methods of metastases for RB are direct

extension along the optic nerve and through the layers of the eye. For this reason, as long an optic nerve section as possible is obtained during the surgical removal of the eye. If histopathological examination of the eye reveals no signs of spread and the central nervous system imaging is normal, no additional treatment is necessary. If tumor extension into the optic nerve or through the walls of the eye is found (Figure 31–37), then lumbar puncture and bone marrow studies are performed. Children with these high-risk findings are usually treated with chemotherapy, although there are no large-scale studies that demonstrate whether or not this is beneficial. If tumor is found at the cut end of the optic nerve, local external beam radiation is usually performed.

If the patient has bilateral tumors, efforts are made to preserve some vision. This usually consists of carboplatin-based chemotherapy to shrink the tumors, with adjuvant treatment with retinal laser or cryotherapy (Figure 31–38A and B). External beam radiotherapy (EBRT) or local plaque radiotherapy is sometimes used, but usually avoided due to potential complications. The main complication of EBRT is an increase of second nonocular tumors. Patients with bilateral retinoblastoma have a germline mutation of the RB gene that predisposes them to second tumors, and this risk is substantially increased in patients who receive EBRT.[8] Other complications of EBRT in young patients with retinoblastoma include cataracts and malformation of the orbit due to interference with normal bone growth.

Genetic Testing for Retinoblastoma

Patients with germline mutations of the retinoblastoma gene are at risk for additional tumors. These include pineal tumors, osteogenic sarcoma, and a number of

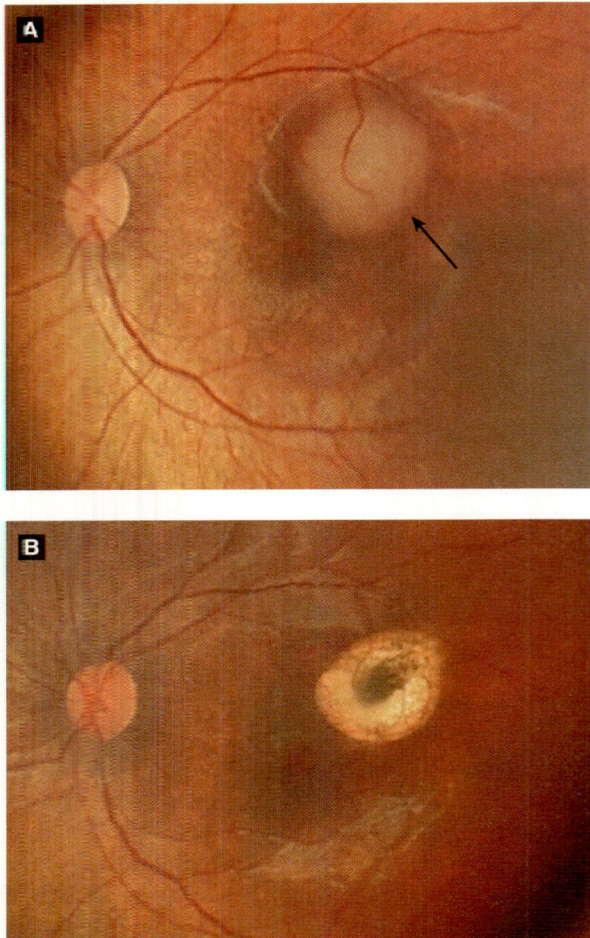

FIGURE 31-38 ■ Retinoblastoma. (A) Before treatment (arrow). (B) Flat chorioretinal scar after successful laser treatment.

other unusual malignancies. All patients with bilateral RB have germline mutations. Most patients with unilateral tumors have sporadic RB, but approximately 10% have germline mutations. The siblings and offspring of patients with germline mutations are at risk for developing RB and may require monitoring with examinations under anesthesia because of this risk.

Genetic testing is available that can usually identify with high specificity which patients have germline mutations and which have sporadic tumors. This information is valuable in determining whether patients require serial monitoring under anesthesia and whether their siblings or offspring require evaluation.

RETINAL HEMORRHAGE

Retinal hemorrhages may occur as a result of systemic or ocular diseases. Except for birth-related hemorrhage, their presence usually indicates the need for further investigation.

Parturition-related Hemorrhage

Retinal hemorrhages are a common finding immediately after birth, occurring in 30% to 40% of infants. They are most common following vacuum-assisted delivery, but also may occur following normal vaginal deliveries and occasionally following caesarean section. They vary from scattered posterior hemorrhages to diffuse bleeding in all quadrants of the eye. They usually resolve without sequela during the first few weeks of life.

Nonaccidental Trauma

Retinal hemorrhages are a frequent finding in children who have been victims of child abuse, with reported incidences ranging from 20% to 80%. They are often associated with intracranial hemorrhages and other signs of abuse. The hemorrhages may occur in any layer of the retina and vitreous hemorrhage may also occur.

The presence of retinal hemorrhages is an important finding in the evaluation of patients suspected of abuse. The absence of retinal hemorrhages neither confirms nor rules out nonaccidental injury because not all children with shaking injuries develop retinal hemorrhages. Diffuse multilayered retinal hemorrhages, particularly in the absence of external signs of trauma, are highly suspicious for nonaccidental injury (Figure 31–39). In severe cases of shaking injury the layers of the retina may split (retinoschisis). This produces a dome-shaped elevation overlying the macula, often with folds of retinal tissue bordering the lesion (Figure 31–40). Blood

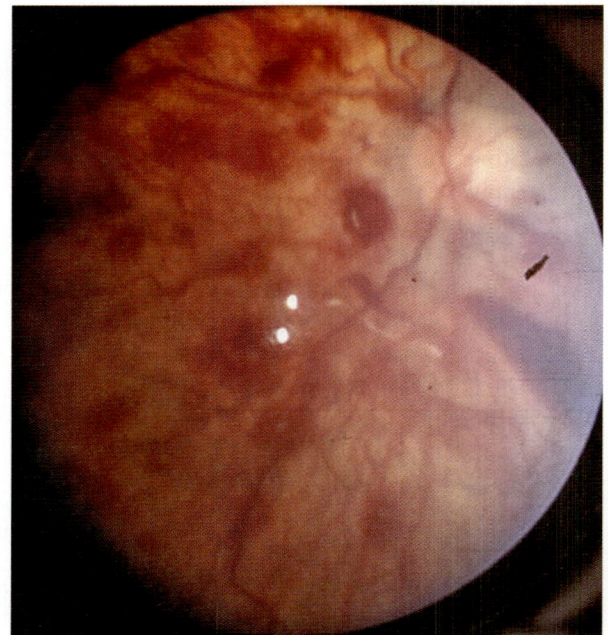

FIGURE 31-39 ■ Nonaccidental injury. Multiple hemorrhages in posterior retina.

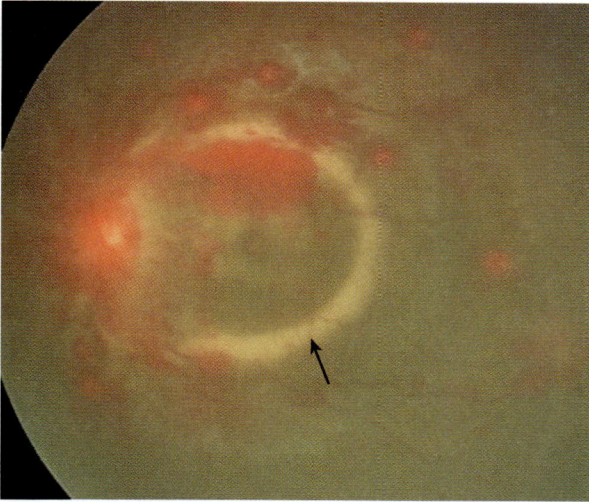

FIGURE 31–40 ■ Nonaccidental injury. Retinoschisis cavity with perimacular folds (arrow).

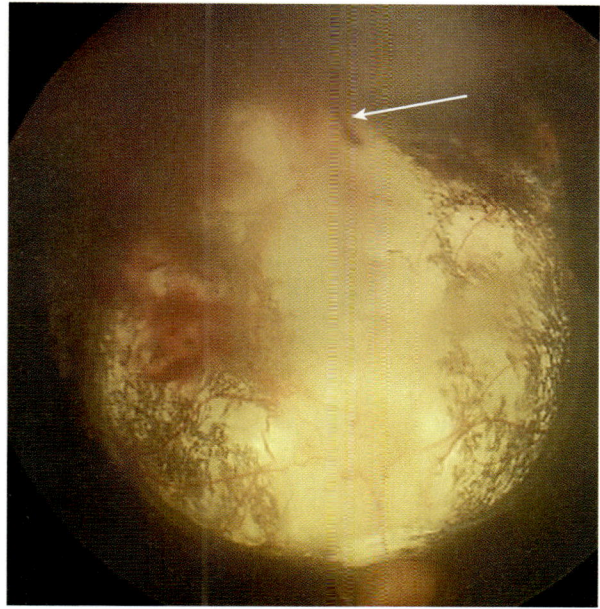

FIGURE 31–41 ■ Retinal and vitreous hemorrhage following blunt trauma in a patient with a coloboma (the white area is the coloboma). Strands of blood are present in the vitreous (arrow).

layering may occur within this cavity, with the position of the blood dependent on how the patient's head is positioned. This finding has been very rarely reported in infants with severe crush head injuries. In the absence of such a history and associated findings, retinoschisis cavities are essentially pathognomonic for nonaccidental injuries.

Other Causes of Retinal Hemorrhage

Retinal hemorrhages from other causes in children are rare. They may occur due to bleeding diatheses, massive intracranial hemorrhage (such as rupture of an aneurysm), malignancy (especially leukemia), overwhelming infection, and some rare metabolic disorders (glutaric aciduria). Children with retinal hemorrhages in whom abuse is suspected should be evaluated for these possibilities.

OTHER RETINAL TRAUMA

Some ocular trauma, particularly direct injuries to the globe, may cause retinal detachments or vitreous hemorrhage (Figure 31–41). The symptoms of these injuries are *floaters*, which the patient describes as small objects that float across the patient's vision; *photopsias*, which the patient perceives as small flashes of light in the peripheral visual field; and decreased peripheral vision. If these symptoms are present, prompt evaluation by an ophthalmologist is indicated because early repair of retinal detachments improves the prognosis for vision.

Less severe ocular trauma may cause *commotio retinae*. This produces focal areas of whitening within the retina due to damage to the outer layer of the retina.

Commotio usually resolves without sequela, but patients need to be evaluated for associated retinal injuries.

Patients with chronic retinal detachments from any cause, including trauma, may develop *phthisis bulbi*. This results in progressive shrinkage and atrophy of the eye (Figure 31–42). Most phthisical eyes are completely blind. Treatment is usually indicated due to the abnormal appearance of the eye. If the shrunken eye is not painful, a scleral shell may be fit, similar to that used following an enucleation (Figure 31–43). Phthisical eyes often become painful, in which case enucleation of the eye is indicated.

COLOR VISION ABNORMALITIES

Color vision results from central visual system analysis of the inputs from the 3 different cone photoreceptor opsin molecules. These 3 cone opsins are sensitive to

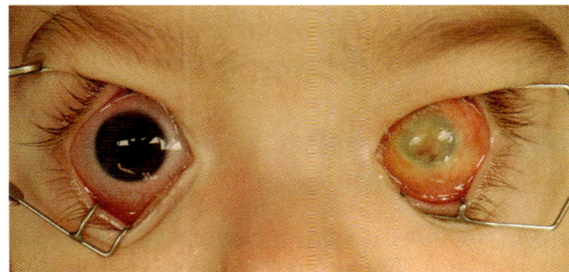

FIGURE 31–42 ■ Phthisis, left eye, secondary to chronic retinal detachment. Note that the left eye is smaller than the right. The cornea is cloudy and the anterior segment is disorganized.

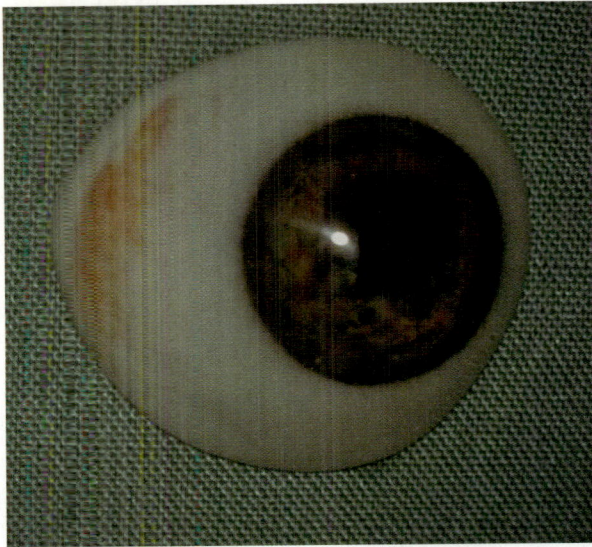

FIGURE 31–43 ■ Ocular prosthesis. These can be fit over a phthisical eye to create a more normal appearance.

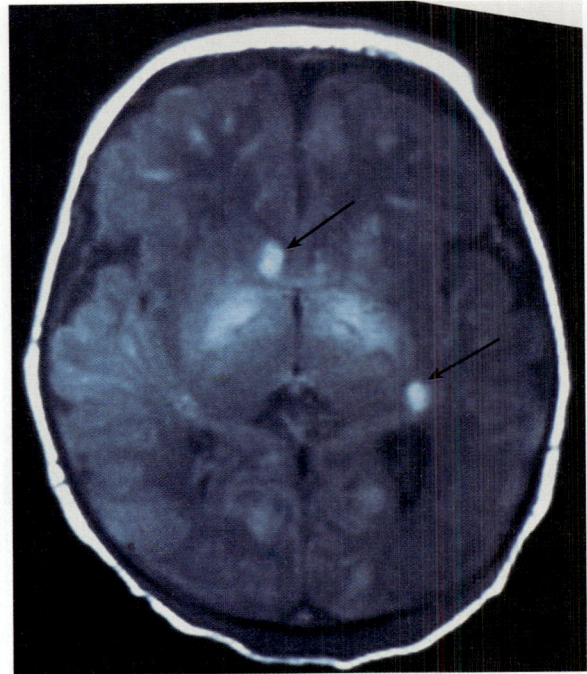

FIGURE 31–44 ■ Tuberous sclerosis. Magnetic resonance imaging demonstrating cortical lesions (arrows).

different wavelengths of light (blue, green, and red). The genes for the green and red opsins are located adjacent to one another on the X chromosome.

Inherited color vision defects are common in males, occurring in approximately 7% of men and less than 1% of women. These usually involve abnormalities of the red and green opsins, and are X-linked. They produce a range of difficulty discriminating colors, depending on the specific genetic defect. In general, red-green color deficiency does not cause significant educational or vocational difficulties. There are certain occupations, however, in which abnormal color discrimination could limit job performance, such as an electrician who must distinguish color-coded wires within a cable.

In contrast to inherited color vision abnormalities, acquired retinal abnormalities may cause difficulty distinguishing colors in the blue-yellow spectrum. This type of problem rarely occurs in children.

OTHER SYSTEMIC DISEASES ASSOCIATED WITH SPECIFIC RETINAL ABNORMALITIES

Tuberous Sclerosis (Bourneville disease)

TS is an autosomal dominant phakomatosis. Most cases represent new mutations. Systemic abnormalities include developmental delay, seizures, and tumors of the central nervous system, kidney, and heart (Figure 31–44). Characteristic skin lesions include ash-leaf spots,

adenoma sebaceum, and subungual fibromas (Figure 31–45A and B).

Approximately one-third to one-half of patients with TS have retinal astrocytic hamartomas. In young patients these are typically smooth, elevated grayish nodules that are found in the posterior retina (Figure 31–46).

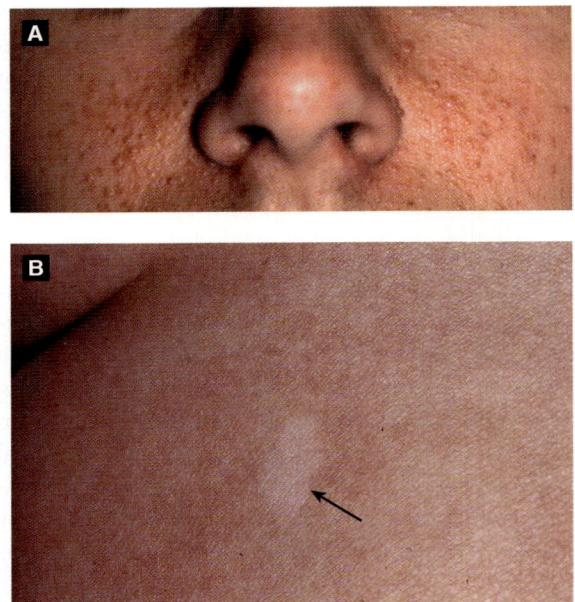

FIGURE 31–45 ■ Tuberous sclerosis. (A) Adenoma sebaceum, (B) ash-leaf spot (arrow).

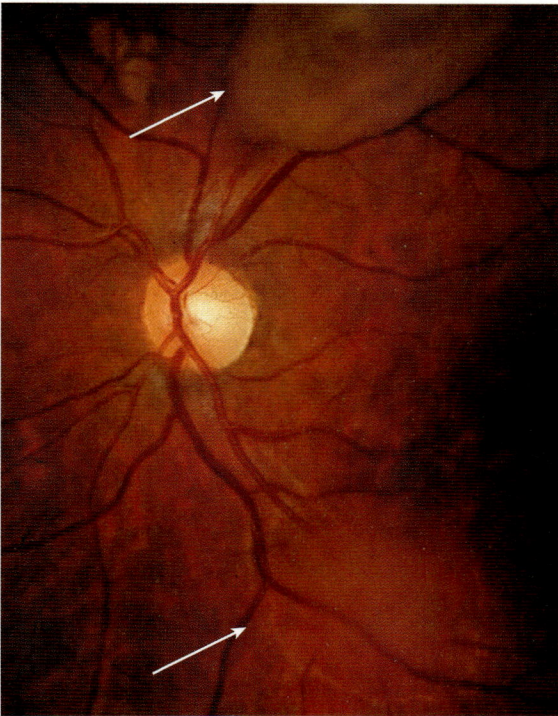

FIGURE 31–46 ■ Tuberous sclerosis. Retinal astrocytic hamartomas (arrows), with appearance similar to retinoblastoma.

As discussed in the section on retinoblastoma earlier in this chapter, the appearance of these lesions may be similar to small retinoblastoma tumors. However, the associated clinical abnormalities in TS usually make the diagnosis straightforward. In older patients, astrocytic hamartomas tend to have an irregular lobulated surface (Figure 31–47). The retinal lesions in TS may grow with age, but they almost never produce any visual problems. They are primarily important in terms of establishing a diagnosis.

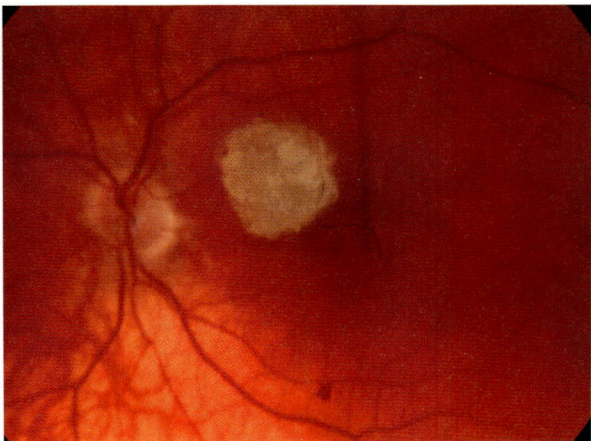

FIGURE 31–47 ■ Tuberous sclerosis. Retinal astrocytic hamartoma with lobulated appearance, more commonly seen in older affected children.

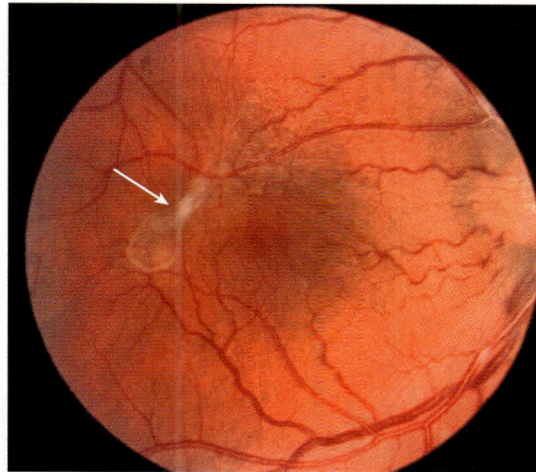

FIGURE 31–48 ■ Neurofibromatosis type 2. Epiretinal membrane (arrow). Note distortion of retinal blood vessels on right side of figure, caused by traction from the membrane.

Neurofibromatosis Type 2

Neurofibromatosis type 2 (NF2) is much less common than neurofibromatosis type 1 (see Chapter 33 – Optic Nerve). NF2 is inherited in an autosomal dominant fashion. Patients uniformly develop acoustic neuromas. They do not have iris Lisch nodules. Posterior subcapsular cataracts may occur.

A specific retinal abnormality associated with NF2 is an *epiretinal membrane* (Figure 31–48). These arise on the inner retinal surface and may cause a wrinkled appearance of the retina when they contract. Epiretinal membranes occur relatively commonly in adults, particularly the elderly. They may occur as an isolated abnormality or in association with other ocular problems, such as trauma or inflammation. They are rare in children, and the presence of an epiretinal membrane in the absence of another ocular abnormality that could explain its presence should alert the physician to the possible diagnosis of NF2.

Chronic Granulomatous Disease

Chronic granulomatous disease (CGD) is a disorder of phagocytosis that is usually inherited in an X-linked fashion. Patients develop severe recurrent infections in multiple organ systems. Patients may develop retinal pigment epithelial scarring along the course of the retinal blood vessels (Figure 31–49). The etiology of these retinal abnormalities is unknown.

Familial Adenomatous Polyposis (Gardner Syndrome)

This is an autosomal dominant disorder in which affected individuals develop polyps in the colon with a high

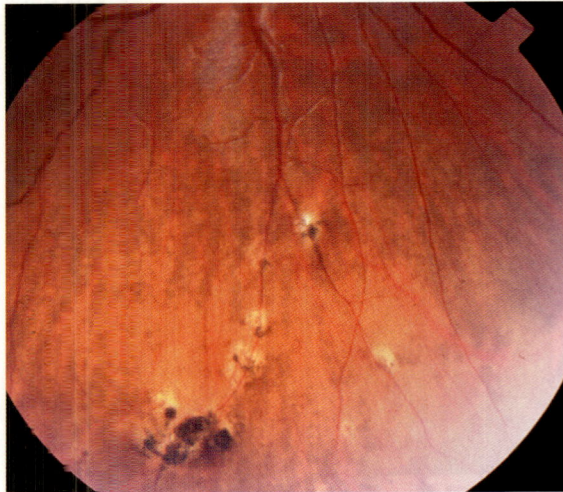

FIGURE 31–49 ■ Chronic granulomatous disease. Pigmented perivascular lesions.

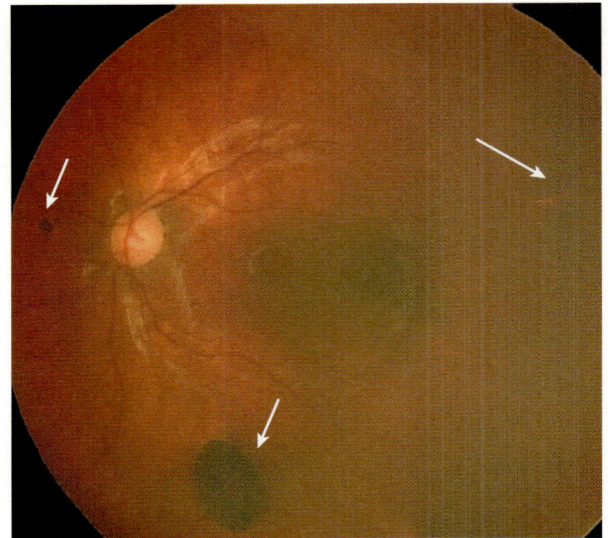

FIGURE 31–50 ■ Retinal findings in a patient with familial adenomatous polyposis (Gardner syndrome), with areas of congenital hypertrophy of the retinal pigment epithelium (arrows).

potential for malignant conversion. *Congenital hypertrophy of the retinal pigmented epithelium* is a fairly common retinal finding in normal individuals, characterized by circular areas of dark retinal pigmentation. Patients with Gardner syndrome develop similar lesions, but they are increased in number and have an ovoid appearance (Figure 31–50). This retinal finding may be useful in identifying patients in families with Gardner syndrome who are at risk for the development of colon cancer.

REFERENCES

1. Olsen TA, Summers CG, Knobloch WH. Predicting visual acuity in children with colobomas involving the optic nerve. *J Pediatr Ophthalmol Strabismus.* 1996;33:47–51.
2. Yang LLE, Lambert SR. Reappraisal of occlusion therapy for severe structural abnormalities of the optic disc and macula. *J Pediatr Ophthalmol Strabismus.* 1995;32:37–41.
3. American Academy of Pediatrics, Section on Ophthalmology, American Academy of Ophthalmology, American Association for Pediatric Ophthalmology and Strabismus. Screening examination of premature infants for retinopathy of prematurity. *Pediatrics.* 2006;117:572–576.
4. Early Treatment for Retinopathy of Prematurity Cooperative Group. Revised indications for the treatment of retinopathy of prematurity. Results of the early treatment for retinopathy of prematurity randomized trial. *Arch Ophthlamol.* 2003;121:1684–1696.
5. Screening for retinopathy in the pediatric patient with type 1 diabetes mellitus. *Pediatrics.* 2005;116:270–273.
6. Maguire AM, High KA, Auricchio A, et al. Age–dependent effects of RPE65 gene therapy for Leber's congenital amaurosis: a phase 1 dose-escalation trial. *Lancet.* 2009;374: 1597–1605.
7. Lueder GT. The effect of initial recognition of abnormalities by physicians on outcome of retinoblastoma. *JAAPOS.* 2005;9:383–385.
8. Roarty JD, McLean IW, Zimmerman LE. Incidence of second neoplasms in patients with bilateral retinoblastoma. *Ophthalmology.* 1988;95:1583–1587.

CHAPTER 32

Glaucoma

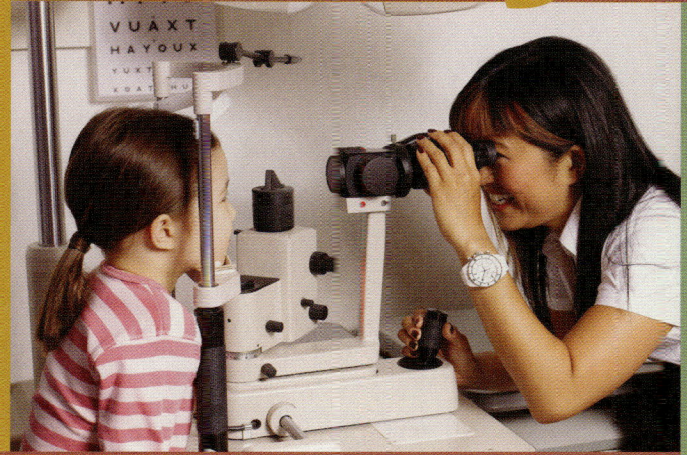

DEFINITIONS AND EPIDEMIOLOGY

Glaucoma is a disorder characterized by damage to the optic nerve that, if untreated, leads to progressive loss of vision. In children it is almost always caused by increased intraocular pressure (IOP). Glaucoma is one of the leading causes of visual loss in adults, but is rare in children. Estimates of the incidence of primary infantile glaucoma range from 1 in 2,500 to 1 in 22,000.

Glaucoma may be classified as *primary* or *secondary*. Primary glaucoma is caused by an underlying disorder of aqueous fluid outflow from the eye. Secondary glaucoma occurs due to a variety of ocular defects that lead to increased IOP.

Glaucoma may also be classified as *open angle* or *closed angle* (Figure 32–1). This refers to whether or not the trabecular meshwork is visible when viewed with a *goniolens*, an instrument that allows the examiner to visualize the fluid outflow pathways. Open angle glaucoma is much more common. In this condition, the pressure increases due to resistance within the outflow pathways, usually caused by microscopic alterations within the trabecular meshwork. In closed-angle glaucoma, access to the trabecular meshwork is blocked. This is usually caused by forward movement of the iris. This may occur for a variety of reasons, including a mass growing behind the iris (e.g., retinoblastoma), scarring of the pupil margin causing fluid to build up behind the iris and push it forward (as may occur in iritis), or in patients with very small eyes (nanophthalmos).

PATHOGENESIS

Normal ocular pressure is maintained by a balance of fluid (aqueous humor) production by the ciliary body and fluid outflow through the trabecular meshwork

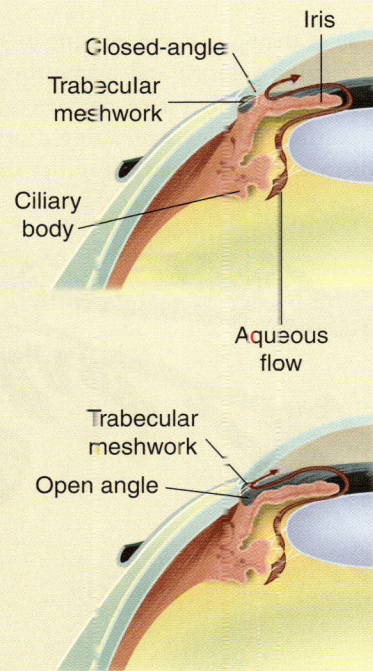

FIGURE 32–1 ■ Fluid in the eye is produced by the ciliary body. It flows around the iris and drains into the trabecular meshwork. Top: In closed-angle glaucoma, the fluid cannot reach the trabecular meshwork, usually because the iris tissue moves forward and obstructs the flow. Bottom: In open-angle glaucoma, microscopic obstruction is present within the trabecular meshwork itself, which impedes flow, resulting in increased intraocular pressure.

(Figures 32–2 and 32–3A and B). Glaucoma virtually always results from obstructed outflow, rather than fluid overproduction. When the IOP is elevated, the optic nerve is damaged by compression against the sclera, resulting in loss of the ganglion cells that form the optic nerve. This initially affects the upper and lower fibers on

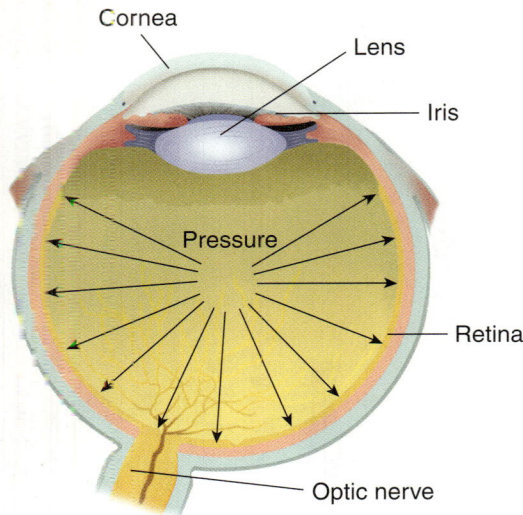

FIGURE 32–2 ■ Glaucoma causes increased intraocular pressure, which in children may result in enlargement of the eye and damage to the optic nerve.

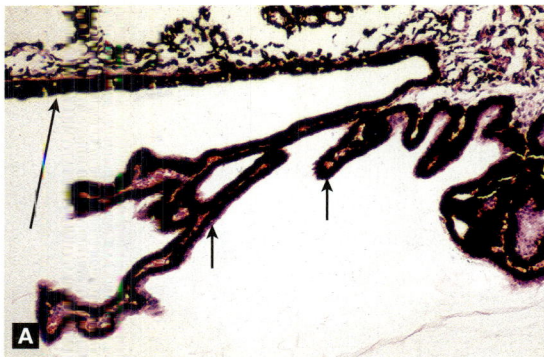

FIGURE 32–4 ■ Congenital glaucoma, right eye. Note that the right eye and cornea are much larger (buphthalmos) than the left.

the lateral side of the optic nerve, causing loss of vision in an arcuate pattern above and below the center of vision. If untreated, progressive constriction of the visual field occurs, ultimately affecting central vision late in the disease. Patients may not notice the periph-

eral loss initially, and therefore they may remain asymptomatic until substantial damage has occurred.

One of the main differences between adults and children with glaucoma is due to decreased scleral rigidity in children. In adults the sclera is rigid and nondistensible. Therefore, the effect of pressure is entirely directed to the optic nerve, and changes in the nerve may be the only visible sign of the disorder. In infants and young children, however, the sclera can enlarge. This may produce visible abnormal growth of the eye (*buphthalmos*) and enlargement of the cornea (Figure 32–4). Tears in Descemet's membrane (*Haab stria*) may develop due to the stretching (Figure 32–5), leading to edema of the cornea. The corneal edema is the cause of the epiphora and light sensitivity frequently seen in infants with glaucoma. The beneficial effect of scleral distensibility is that improvement in optic nerve cupping may be seen in infants with successful treatment (Figure 32–6A and B), whereas the cupping never improves in adults, even if the IOP is lowered.

In primary glaucoma, there is an underlying defect of the trabecular meshwork that inhibits normal

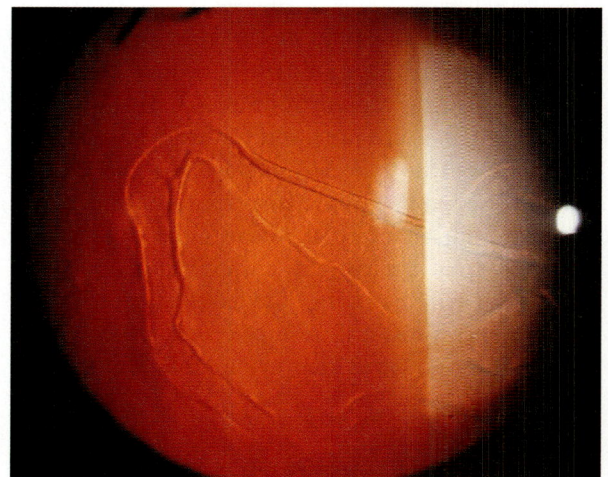

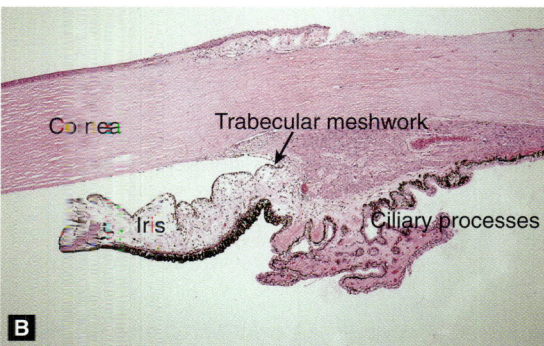

FIGURE 32–3 ■ Histology of normal structures responsible for IOP. (A) Ciliary processes (short arrows). These structures lie just posterior to the iris (long arrow). They produce aqueous fluid that flows forward around the pupil into the anterior chamber. (B) Anterior chamber angle. The fluid exits through the trabecular meshwork (arrow). The other structures are labeled. (Photographs contributed by Morton Smith, MD.)

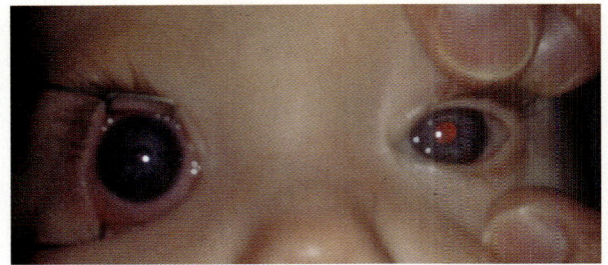

FIGURE 32–5 ■ Haab striae of cornea, slit lamp view with retroillumination. These curvilinear breaks in Descemet's membrane occur due to stretching caused by increased intraocular pressure.

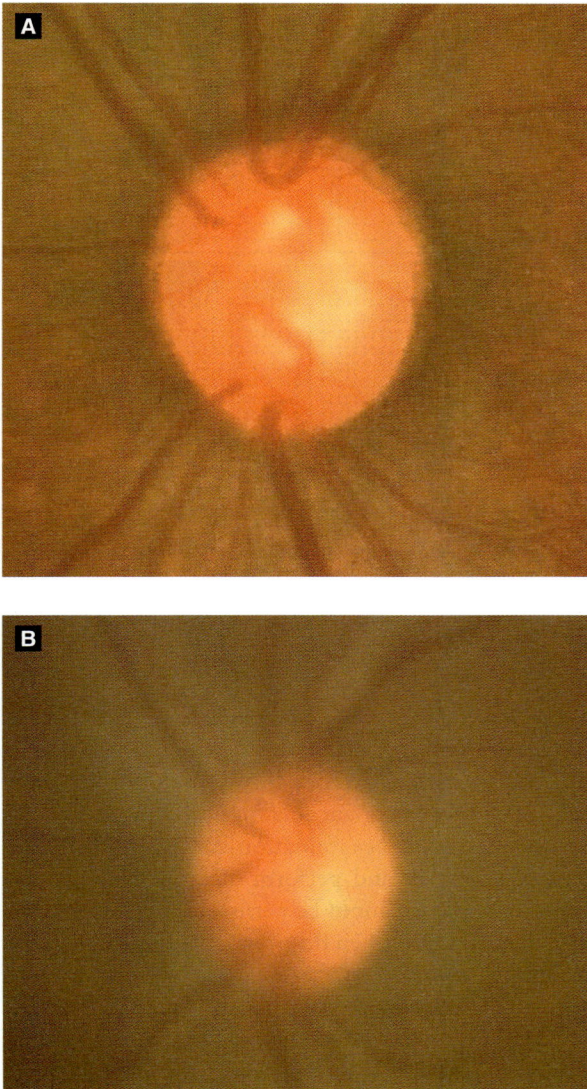

FIGURE 32–6 ■ Reversal of optic nerve cupping following treatment of infantile glaucoma. (A) Enlarged cup:disc ratio before surgery. (B) Improved cupping following successful surgery.

outflow of fluid, with a resultant increase in pressure. Secondary glaucoma may occur as a result of other ocular defects. Examples include blockage of the normal outflow due to forward displacement of the iris from a retinal tumor, or abnormal resistance to outflow due to vascular abnormalities in patients with Sturge-Weber syndrome (SWS).

Primary infantile glaucoma is usually sporadic, but can be inherited in an autosomal recessive pattern. Mutations of the *CYP1B1* gene on chromosome 2p21 have been identified as a cause of this disorder. Other genetic abnormalities associated with glaucoma include mutations of the *MYOC* gene in autosomal dominant juvenile glaucoma, and mutations of the *PITX2* and *FOXC1* genes in patients with anterior segment dysgenesis syndromes.

CLINICAL PRESENTATION

Glaucoma may occur acutely, subacutely, or insidiously, depending on how rapidly the pressure rises. Most infants with glaucoma present subacutely. Increased pressure in the eye produces a variety of effects, some of which are visible and some of which are not. In infants and young children, the entire eye enlarges (*buphthalmos*, from the Greek "ox eye"). This enlargement is most noticeable if only one eye is affected, because of the contrast with the normal eye (Figure 32–4). The eye appears to bulge from the orbit, and the space between the eyelids may appear larger than normal. Enlargement of the cornea increases the portion of the cornea visible between the eyelids. In severe cases the cornea may fill the entire space between the eyelids (Figure 32–7).

The increased IOP also causes dysfunction of the corneal endothelium, resulting in thickening and edema that creates a cloudy or ground-glass corneal appearance. Curvilinear Haab stria may sometimes be seen with a penlight, but usually a slit lamp is required for visualization (Figure 32–5). In severe cases of infantile glaucoma, the lens zonules stretch, and subluxation of the lens may occur.

The end result of glaucoma is damage to the optic nerve, which can be visualized with an ophthalmoscope as an increase in the cup:disc ratio. Abnormal growth of the eye in children with glaucoma may also cause myopia (nearsightedness) due to an increase in the length of the eye. In the typical subacute presentation of infants, most children will have light sensitivity (photophobia), excess tearing (epiphora), and squeezing of the eyelids (blepharospasm) due to corneal irritation. Decreased vision and nystagmus may be noted in severe bilateral cases.

Acute presentations of glaucoma occur if the rise in IOP is marked and rapid. Approximately 25% of infants with primary infantile glaucoma are born with enlarged and cloudy corneas. The prognosis in such infants is poor. In older children, most cases of acute glaucoma are secondary to other ocular problems, such

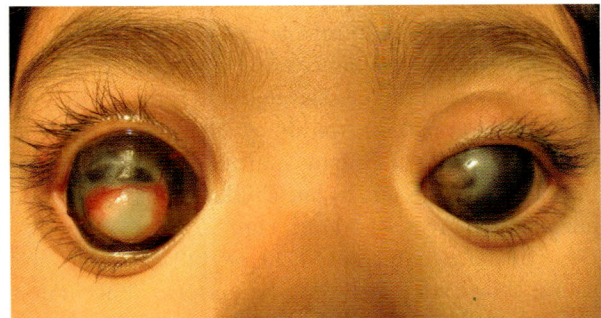

FIGURE 32–7 ■ Severe untreated infantile glaucoma with marked buphthalmos and corneal scarring, right greater than left.

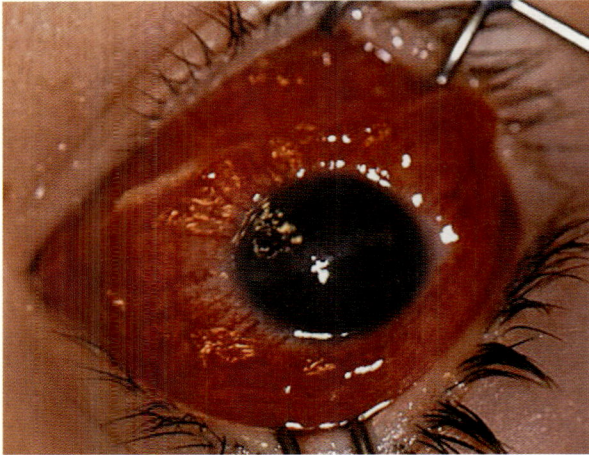

FIGURE 32–3 ■ Acute glaucoma due to rapid marked rise in IOP.

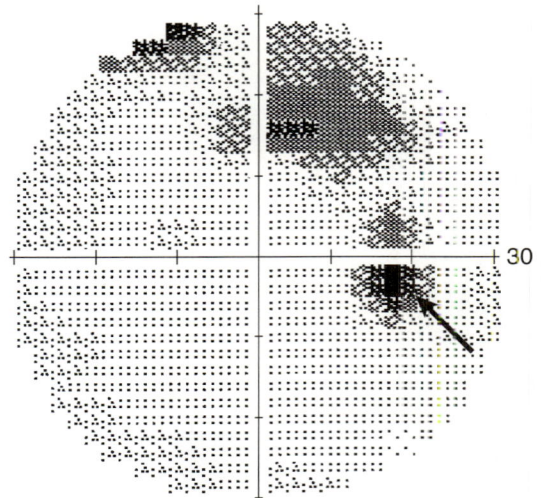

FIGURE 32–9 ■ Typical visual field changes in glaucoma, right eye. The field loss occurs in an arcuate pattern from the blind spot (arrow), which represents the loss of ganglion cells that form the optic nerve.

as trauma or ocular tumors. If the pressure rises rapidly to high levels (usually >40 mm Hg), the eye becomes acutely painful, the cornea becomes cloudy, the conjunctiva is usually injected, and the vision is decreased (Figure 32–8). Nausea and vomiting frequently develop when the pressure is this high.

Glaucoma in older children and adults often presents insidiously. If the pressure is not high enough to produce symptoms of acute glaucoma, but is high enough to cause damage to the optic nerve, patients are often initially asymptomatic. The nerve damage first affects the peripheral vision, which may go unnoticed until it progresses to near the center of vision. This is why glaucoma, particularly in adults, is sometimes referred to as "the sneak thief of sight." On examination, the IOP is elevated, and the cup:disc ratios are enlarged. Formal visual field testing shows peripheral loss in an arcuate pattern (Figure 32–9). This testing is often not possible in children due to the degree of cooperation and concentration required.

DIAGNOSIS

The diagnosis of glaucoma requires a detailed ophthalmic examination. Vision is assessed in the standard fashion for children. In infants and young children, the remainder of the assessment often necessitates examination under anesthesia. Elevated IOP is the underlying final common pathway for almost all glaucoma in children. Normal IOP in infants is around 12 mm Hg. This increases with age, and by late childhood and adulthood normal pressure is 10-20 mm Hg.

In practice, measurement of IOP in infants and young children often cannot be performed accurately when they are awake. Although the measurements are taken after use of topical anesthetic drops, the proximity of the instrument to the eye usually provokes anxiety. When the children forcefully close their eyes, this squeezing artificially raises the IOP. Therefore, most young children with glaucoma (or in whom glaucoma is suspected) require examination under anesthesia to measure the IOP and perform other portions of the examination that cannot be performed accurately with the patient awake. When the pressure is measured under anesthesia, there is also a potential for inaccurate readings due to effects of anesthetic agents on the IOP. Therefore, the pressure is measured as soon as the child is adequately sedated, preferably before placement of an endotracheal tube or laryngeal mask.

Other features of the glaucoma evaluation include measurement of the corneal diameter, assessment of corneal clarity, and slit lamp examination. Measurement of the refractive error may reveal abnormal myopia (nearsightedness) due to enlargement of the eye.

The anterior chamber angle is not visible directly, but can be viewed with a *goniolens*. This is a mirrored lens that is placed directly on the cornea. By coupling the lens to the cornea via the tear film, the angle becomes visible (Figure 32–10A and B). Gonioscopy allows assessment of the anatomic configuration of the angle. This can differentiate between open-angle and closed-angle glaucoma. In infantile glaucoma, a membrane-like structure (Barkan's membrane) is sometimes visible overlying the trabecular meshwork (Figure 32–11).

Careful assessment of the optic nerve is important in diagnosing glaucoma. The nerve is visible with an opthalmoscope. The nerve is described by its *cup:disc ratio*. The white central portion of the nerve is the cup. There are no axons in this area. The peripheral orange

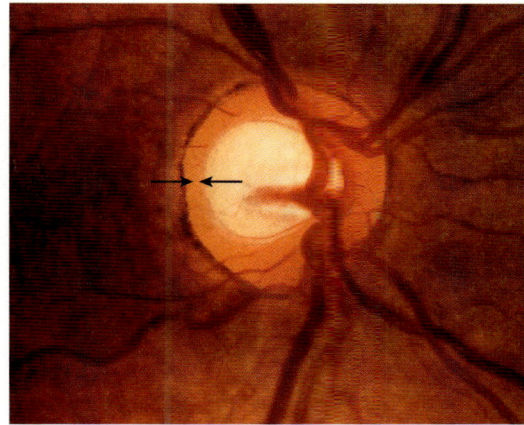

FIGURE 32–12 ■ Physiological cupping of right optic nerve (normal variant). Note the circular appearance of the cup, and the regular thickness of the nerve tissue on the lateral side of the disc (arrows).

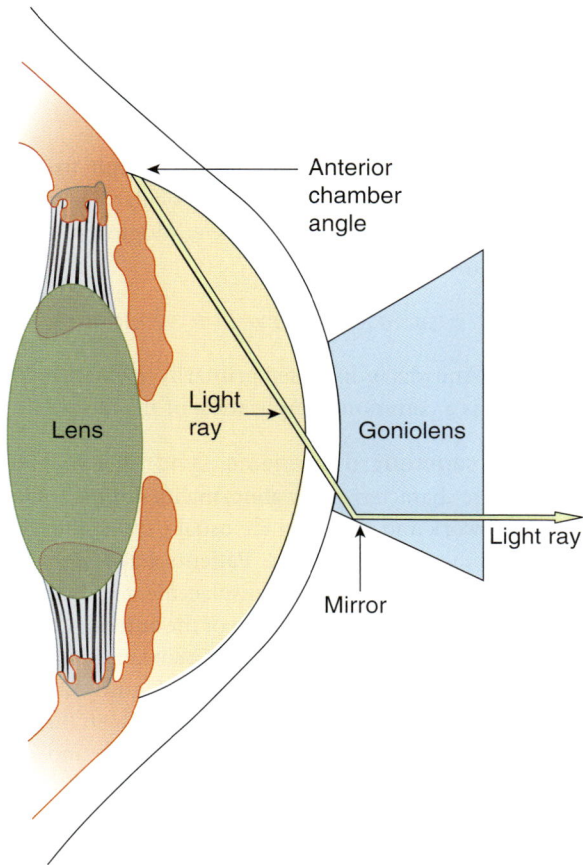

FIGURE 32–10 ■ Gonioscopy. The anterior chamber angle is not directly visible, but can be viewed through a gonioscope. The gonioscope is placed in contact with the cornea. It allows the light rays to be reflected so that the anterior chamber angle can be visualized.

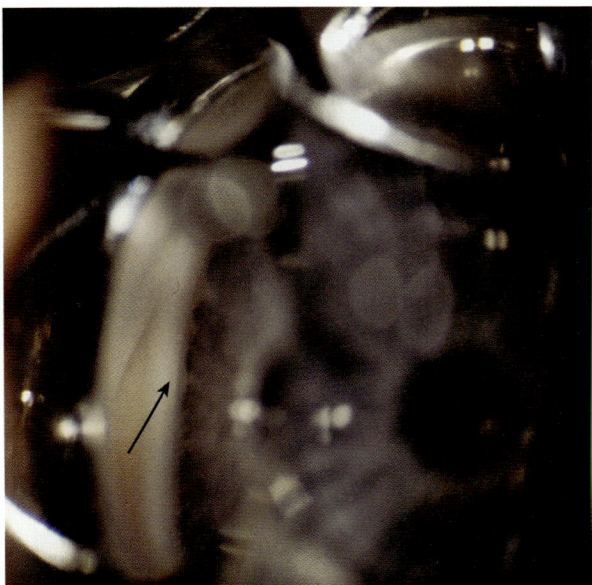

FIGURE 32–11 ■ Gonioscopic view of Barkan's membrane (arrow) in the anterior chamber angle in a patient with infantile glaucoma.

portion comprises the nerve fibers that transmit information to the brain. The normal cup:disc ratio in children is less than 0.3, and the cup:disc ratio of the 2 optic nerves is usually similar. A cup:disc ratio greater than 0.3 in an infant, or a significant difference in the cup:disc ratio between the 2 eyes raises the suspicion for glaucoma. The vertical ratio is usually larger than the horizontal ratio in glaucoma. The normal cup:disc ratio in older children, and particularly in patients with African American heritage, may be larger. Physiological cupping, in which the cup:disc ratio is larger than normal, but not associated with glaucoma, is characterized by a smooth, round cup (Figure 32–12). Older patients with glaucoma typically develop asymmetric notching of the cup, most prominent on the upper and lower portions on the lateral side of the nerve, and may develop hemorrhages around the optic nerve (Figure 32–13).

Other Tests

During examination under anesthesia, the length of the eye (axial eye length) can be measured with A-scan ultrasonography, and compared with standard nomograms. The corneal thickness can be measured with a *pachymeter*. The cornea is often thickened in patients with glaucoma, which may induce artifacts in the measurement of IOP. The significance of these changes has not yet been clarified. Photographs of the optic nerve may be taken while infants are under anesthesia and used to monitor for future changes.

In older children, formal visual field testing is an important component of monitoring glaucoma. The visual field loss in glaucoma typically first affects the periphery. Arcuate defects due to ganglion cell damage on the upper and lower portion of the temporal disc are classic findings (Figure 32–9). Optical coherence tomography can provide detailed measurements of the

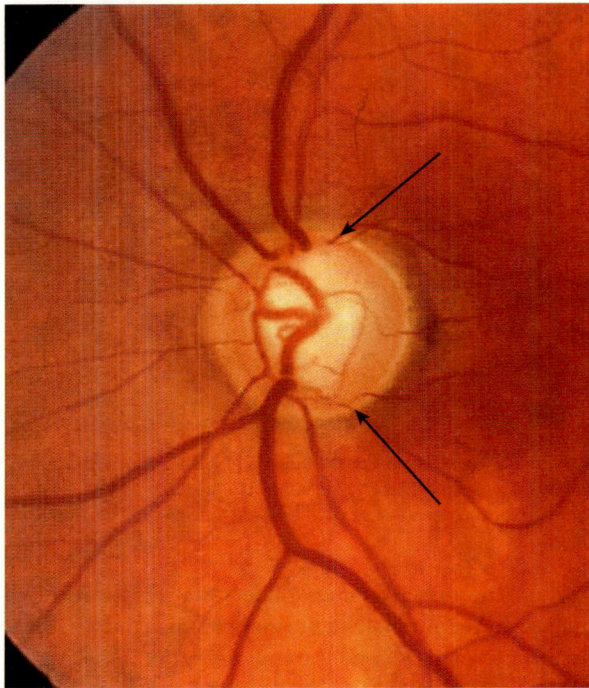

FIGURE 32-13 ■ Glaucomatous left optic nerve cupping. Note the vertical elongation of the cup:disc ratio, and notching (segmental loss of nerve fibers) on the upper and lower portions of the temporal portion of the nerve (arrows). These notches correspond to the arcuate visual field loss that occurs in patients with glaucoma.

optic nerve and ganglion cell layer in children who are old enough to cooperate for the imaging.

Monitoring

Glaucoma is a chronic (usually lifelong) disease. All of the parameters noted above are followed serially, looking for evidence of progressive damage, such as abnormal eye growth, optic nerve cupping, or visual field changes.

TYPES OF GLAUCOMA

Primary Glaucomas

Primary infantile glaucoma

Primary infantile glaucoma accounts for more than 50% of glaucoma in children. It is usually sporadic, but can occur as an autosomal recessive trait. The signs and symptoms result from enlargement of the globe, as discussed above. Approximately 80% of patients develop symptoms within the first year of life.

Juvenile open-angle glaucoma

Juvenile open-angle glaucoma has its onset later in childhood, usually after age 3 years. Because the eye itself in older children does not grow in response to pressure, juve-

nile glaucoma is similar to adult glaucoma, in that it may be asymptomatic until severe vision loss occurs.

Secondary Childhood Glaucomas

Secondary glaucoma in childhood may result from a variety of causes, including underlying ocular disorders, systemic diseases, and exogenous etiologies such as trauma or medication.

Glaucoma associated with ocular syndromes

Aniridia Aniridia is discussed primarily in Chapter 29. Glaucoma is a common complication of this disorder.

Anterior segment dysgenesis syndromes These disorders are characterized by abnormalities of the trabecular meshwork and iris. They are usually transmitted as an autosomal dominant trait. Patients have *posterior embryotoxon*, which is anterior displacement of Schwalbe's line (the anterior-most portion of the anterior chamber angle). This can be visualized with a slit lamp as a thin white band at the peripheral cornea (Figure 32–14). Bands of iris tissue may bridge the space between the iris and trabecular meshwork (Axenfeld anomaly), and iris defects may occur (Rieger anomaly) (Figure 32–15). Glaucoma occurs in approximately half of patients with Axenfeld-Rieger anomaly. Systemic abnormalities, including dental, genitourinary, and pituitary anomalies, may occur in Axenfeld-Rieger syndrome.

Peter's anomaly Peter's anomaly is characterized by a central defect in the corneal endothelium (see Chapter 28). Approximately half of patients with Peter's anomaly have glaucoma.

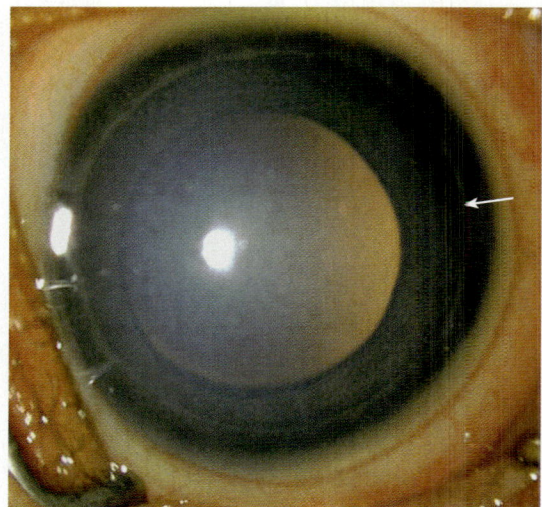

FIGURE 32-14 ■ Posterior embryotoxon (arrow) visible for 360° in the peripheral cornea in a patient with Axenfeld-Rieger syndrome. Note the clouding of the cornea due to glaucoma.

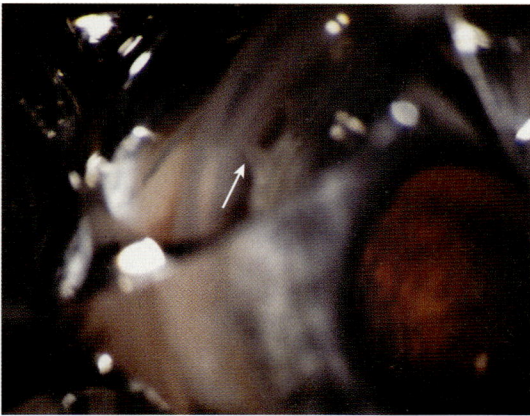

FIGURE 32–15 ■ Axenfeld-Rieger syndrome. Gonioscopic view of tissue bands (arrow) extending from peripheral iris across trabecular meshwork.

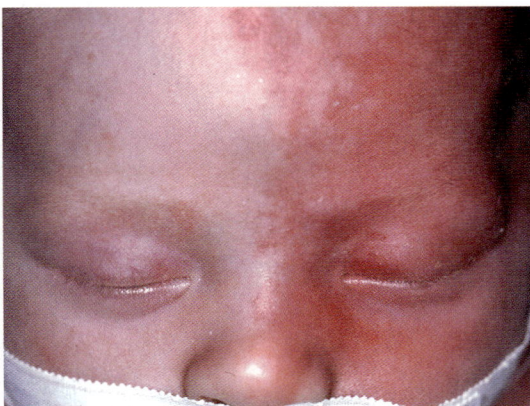

FIGURE 32–17 ■ Right leptomeningeal abnormalities (arrow) in a patient with Sturge-Weber syndrome.

Glaucoma associated with systemic diseases

Sturge-Weber syndrome (encephalofacial angiomatosis)

SWS is a sporadic disorder associated with nevus flammeus (port-wine stain) of the face (Figure 32–16). Patients may have leptomeningeal vascular abnormalities, in which case developmental delay and seizures can occur (Figure 32–17).

Glaucoma in SWS usually develops in patients whose port-wine stains involve the eyelids. The glaucoma most commonly results from increased venous pressure associated with the vascular abnormalities, which inhibits the outflow of fluid from the trabecular meshwork (Figure 32–18). Children with SWS may also have hemangiomas in the choroidal layer of the eye (Figure 32–19). They have an increased risk of hemorrhagic complications from glaucoma surgery.

Congenital rubella

The most notable ocular complication of congenital rubella is cataracts. Glaucoma may also occur.

Lowe syndrome (oculocerebrorenal syndrome)

Lowe syndrome is an X-linked recessive disease characterized by renal tubular dysfunction and mental retardation. Cataracts and glaucoma are commonly present.

Rubinstein-Taybi syndrome

Glaucoma may occur in this disorder (Figure 32–20A and B), which is associated with developmental delay, abnormal thumbs (Figure 32–21), and short stature.

Glaucoma associated with other ocular problems

Lens abnormalities

Abnormalities of lens shape (microspherophakia) or lens dislocation may cause glaucoma. These disorders are discussed in Chapter 30.

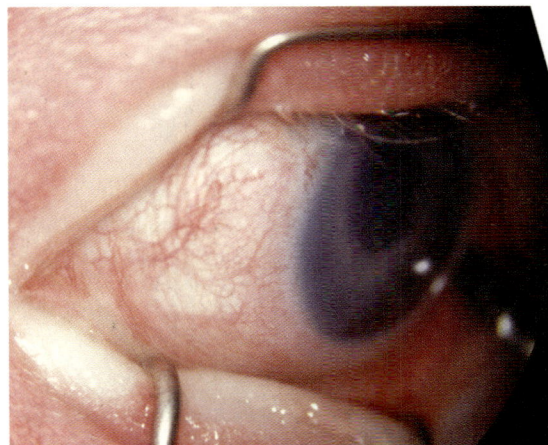

FIGURE 32–16 ■ Port-wine stain involving the left upper and lower eyelids in a patient with Sturge-Weber syndrome.

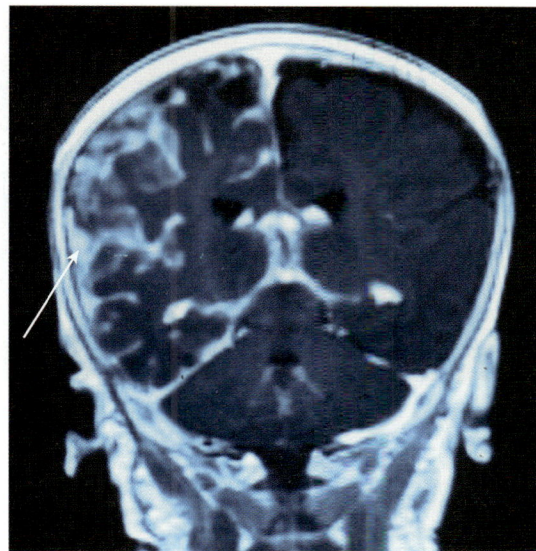

FIGURE 32–18 ■ Prominent episcleral blood vessels in a patient with Sturge-Weber syndrome.

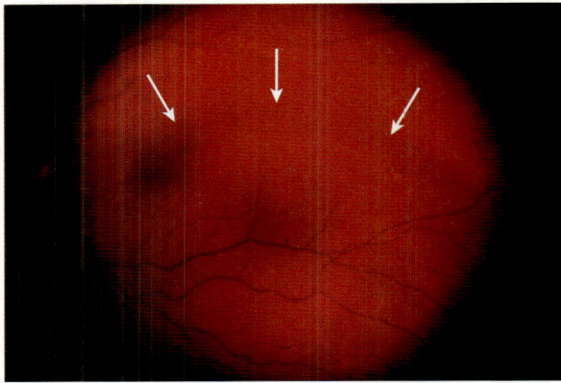

FIGURE 32–19 ■ Choroidal hemangioma in a patient with Sturge-Weber syndrome. The posterior retina, including the fovea, is elevated. The arrows point to the superior border of the hemangioma.

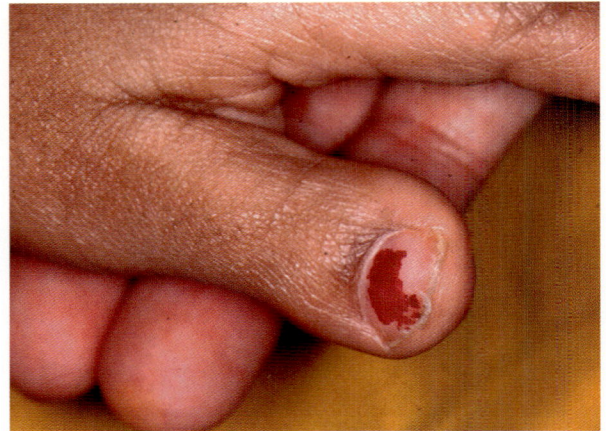

FIGURE 32–20 ■ Bilateral glaucoma damage to optic discs in a patient with Rubinstein-Taybi syndrome. The right optic nerve (A) has more severe cupping than the left (B).

FIGURE 32–21 ■ Broad, flat thumb in a patient with Rubinstein-Taybi syndrome (the patient is wearing red nail polish).

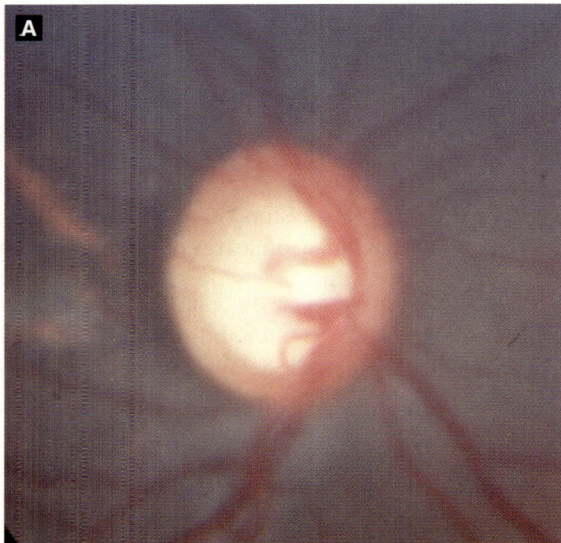

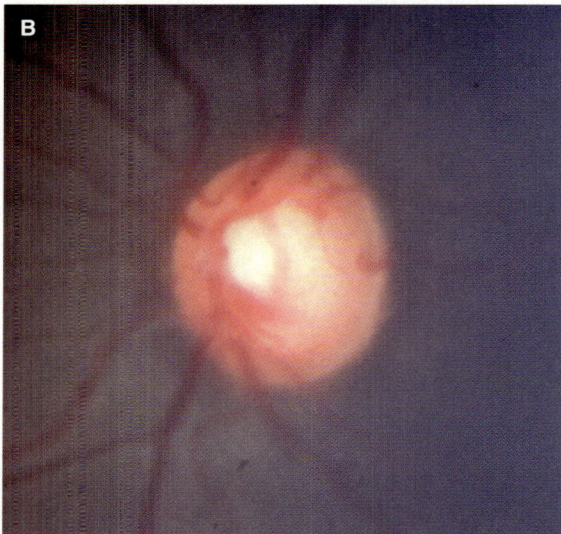

Retinal abnormalities A number of retinal abnormalities may produce forward displacement of the iris, causing secondary glaucoma due to blockage of fluid drainage from the eye (Figure 32–1). These include retinoblastoma and other tumors, retinopathy of prematurity, and persistent fetal vasculature.

Trauma Ocular trauma may produce glaucoma by different mechanisms.

Hyphema At the time of blunt injuries, bleeding may occur in the anterior chamber (*hyphema*). Hyphemas may vary from microscopic bleeding, in which blood cells are only visible with a slit lamp, to blood completely filling the anterior chamber (*8-ball hyphema*) (Figure 32–22). Most hyphemas are between these 2 extremes, and layered blood can be seen in the anterior chamber with a slit lamp (Figure 32–23).

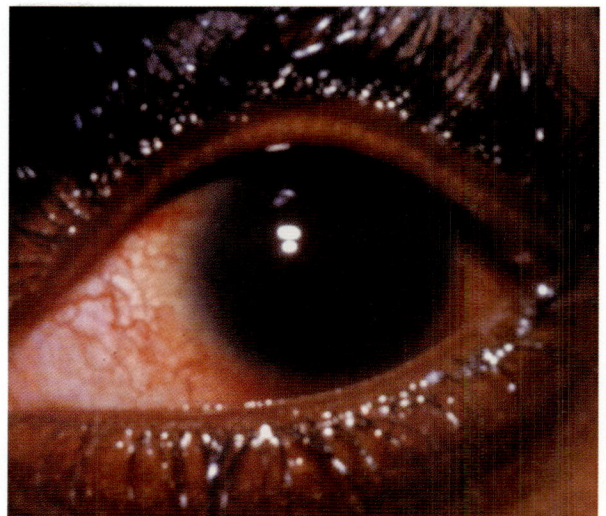

FIGURE 32–22 ■ Eight-ball hyphema. Blood completely fills the anterior chamber.

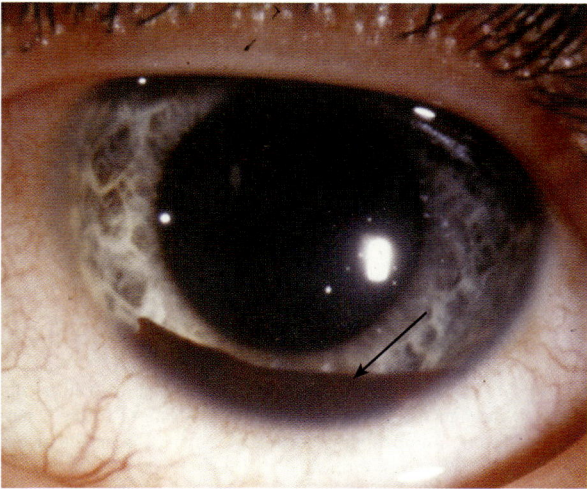

FIGURE 32–23 ■ Layered hyphema. Blood cells are layered in the inferior portion of the anterior chamber (arrow).

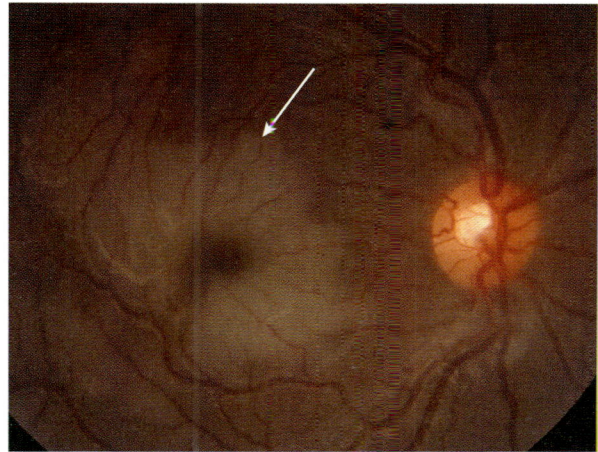

FIGURE 32–24 ■ Retinal artery occlusion in a patient with sickle cell trait. The occlusion occurred following a hyphema with persistently elevated intraocular pressure. The whitish area (arrow) reflects retinal edema surrounding the fovea.

Hyphemas require both acute and long-term care. Acutely, the blood within the anterior chamber may obstruct the outflow of aqueous humor through the trabecular meshwork, causing acute glaucoma. If the pressure is high enough, damage to the optic nerve may occur. Patients may also develop blood staining of the cornea. The pressure can sometimes be controlled with topical medications, but surgery to drain the blood may be indicated if the pressure remains high despite medication.

Patients with sickle cell trait are at particularly high risk for complications of hyphema. This is because sickling of red blood cells in the anterior chamber may occur due to hypoxia, which increases the risk of elevated IOP. This may cause occlusion of the retinal blood vessels, causing permanent loss of vision (Figure 32–24). Therefore, African American patients with hyphemas should be screened for sickle cell trait, and referred to an ophthalmologist promptly if the test is positive.

Traumatic angle recession In the long term, patients with blunt trauma and hyphemas may develop problems due to *angle recession*, in which the iris is displaced posteriorly and the ciliary body becomes visible on gonioscopy (Figure 32–25). Patients with angle recession are at risk of glaucoma, which may not develop until several years after the injury. They should be monitored annually by an ophthalmologist for this potential complication.

Iritis/uveitis Patients with iritis may develop either open-angle or closed-angle glaucoma. The open-angle form is more common. It results from inflammation and scarring within the trabecular meshwork, causing glaucoma due to impaired fluid outflow. Acute closed-angle glaucoma may also develop due to scarring of the

iris to the lens at the border of the pupil. The intraocular fluid that is made by the ciliary body gets trapped behind the pupil, which causes the iris to bulge forward and block the trabecular meshwork.

Glaucoma following infantile cataract removal (aphakic glaucoma) Patients with infantile cataracts are at increased risk of glaucoma, which typically does not develop until later in childhood. The reason that these

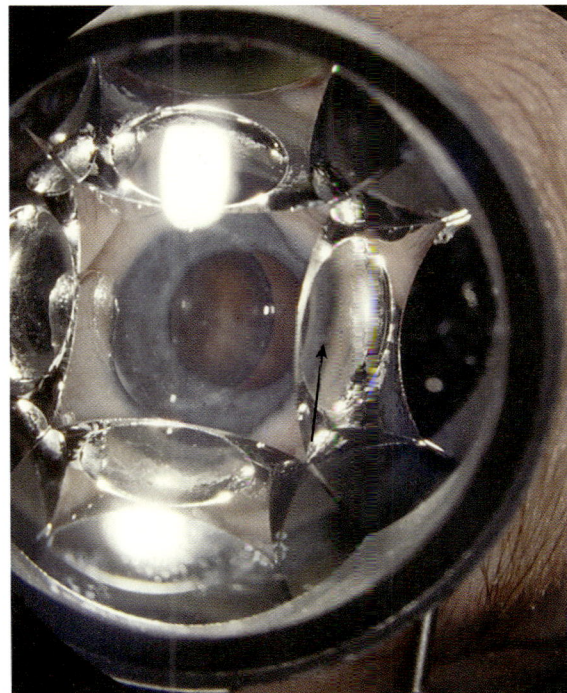

FIGURE 32–25 ■ Traumatic angle recession, gonioscopic view. The ciliary body is visible as a black band (arrow) posterior to the trabecular meshwork.

children develop glaucoma is not clear, but it is probably related to anatomic abnormalities of the anterior segment of the eye. Patients with infantile cataracts require long-term follow-up to monitor for this problem.

Pupillary block Pupillary block occurs when aqueous humor fluid cannot flow through the pupillary opening to gain access to the anterior chamber. This produces pressure behind the iris, which bows forward and blocks the trabecular meshwork. This is much more common in adults, but may occur in children with very small eyes (*nanophthalmos*), or in patients who have scar tissue that forms between the iris and lens.

Glaucoma associated with medication

Corticosteroids Some patients develop increased IOP in response to corticosteroid treatment, most commonly with topical eye drops. Because this may produce few symptoms, patients treated chronically with corticosteroids should have their IOP monitored periodically. In some disorders, such as iritis, topical corticosteroids are a common treatment, and it may be difficult to distinguish whether glaucoma is caused by the corticosteroid drops or the underlying disorder itself.

Topirimate Topirimate (Topomax) is an antiepileptic medication that has been associated with acute bilateral angle closure glaucoma. This complication results from effusion of fluid in the choroid and ciliary body that produces anterior displacement of the iris and lens. Patients typically present with acute bilateral eye pain and blurred vision within 1 month of beginning the medication. The condition resolves with discontinuation of the medication.

TREATMENT

Surgical Treatment

The treatment of primary infantile glaucoma is primarily surgical. Treatment is often difficult, and many patients require multiple surgeries. The initial surgical treatment usually consists of either *goniotomy* (Figure 32–26) or *trabeculotomy*. In these procedures, a sharp blade is used to create an opening in the trabecular meshwork, with the hope of increasing outflow and decreasing pressure. If unsuccessful, a *trabeculectomy* may be performed. In this procedure, a flap of scleral tissue is elevated adjacent to the anterior chamber, and an opening into the chamber is created beneath the flap (Figure 32–27). Fluid then flows around the flap into the surrounding conjunctiva, creating an elevated bleb (Figure 32–28). A common problem in children is that

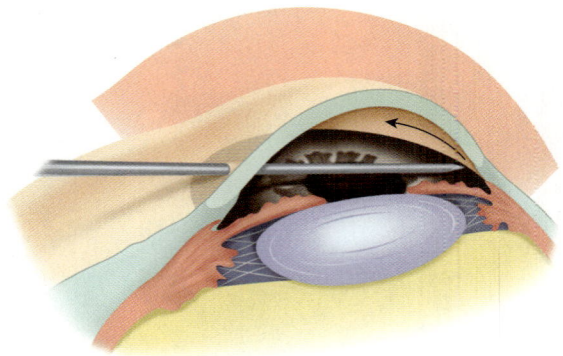

FIGURE 32–26 ■ Goniotomy surgery for glaucoma. A small needle is placed through the peripheral cornea and advanced to the trabecular meshwork. An opening is created by moving the needle across the trabecular meshwork (arrow).

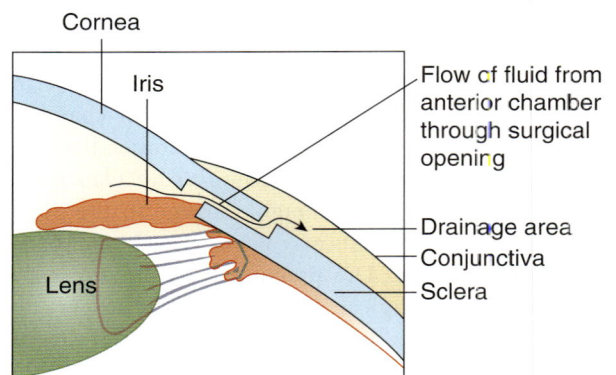

FIGURE 32–27 ■ Trabeculectomy surgery for glaucoma. A flap is dissected in the sclera, and fluid flows from the anterior chamber through the flap into the space beneath the conjunctiva.

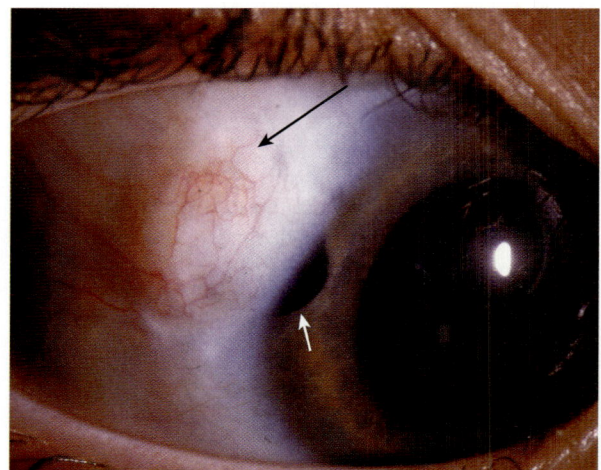

FIGURE 32–28 ■ Trabeculectomy bleb. An elevated bleb (long arrow) is present adjacent to the cornea, caused by diversion of fluid into the bleb from the anterior chamber. The black area in the iris (short arrow) is a peripheral iridectomy, where a portion of iris has been removed to facilitate flow of fluid from the eye.

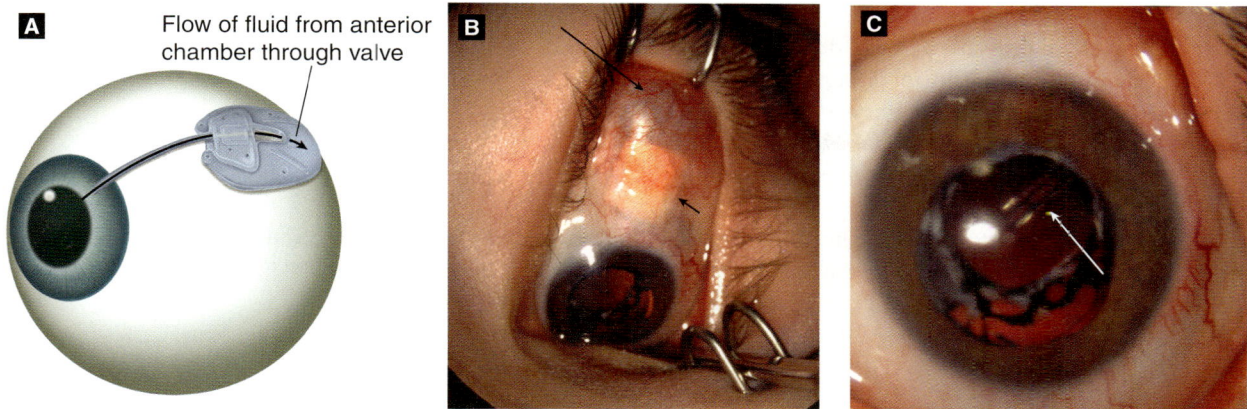

FIGURE 32–29 ■ A) Glaucoma tube shunt. (A) An Ahmed™ glaucoma valve is attached to the sclera and a tube is inserted into the anterior chamber. The fluid flows through the tube and out through the valve. (B) The tube is placed beneath the conjunctiva and is covered by a piece of donor sclera (short arrow) to prevent extrusion, and a bleb forms posteriorly over the plate (long arrow). (C) The tube is visible in the anterior chamber (arrow). Note that the patient has had cataract surgery and an intraocular lens is present.

the tissue scars, and the flow of fluid ceases. For this reason, antimetabolites such as Mitomycin C may be used in an attempt to prevent scarring and increase the success rate of surgery.

An alternative to trabeculectomy is placement of a glaucoma tube shunt. In this procedure, a plate is sewn to the sclera. A tube attached to the plate is placed into the anterior chamber. The aqueous flows through the tube to the plate and disperses, forming a bleb (Figure 32–29A–C).

The aim of the above glaucoma surgeries is to increase the outflow of fluid from the eye. If these fail, an alternative approach is to decrease fluid production by destroying portions of the ciliary body that create the aqueous humor. This can be performed using either laser or freezing treatment. *Transscleral cyclophotocoagulation* or *cryotherapy* can be performed from the outside of the eye, without the need for an incision. The laser or freezing probe is placed above the ciliary body, with the goal of destroying the cells through the sclera. Laser can also be applied directly to the ciliary processes by means of an endoscope (*endoscopic laser cyclophotocoagulation*) (Figure 32–30).

Medical Management

If the IOP remains elevated despite surgery, medical management may also be used. There are a number of topical agents available for use:

Beta-blockers: These agents work by decreasing aqueous humor production in the ciliary body. They have a long history of use in pediatric patients. They are contraindicated in patients with reactive airway disease and some patients with cardiac disease.

Carbonic anhydrase inhibitors: These also work by decreasing ciliary body fluid production. These agents are available in topical and systemic forms. Topical therapy has few side effects. Oral agents such as acetazolamide are sometimes used acutely to decrease pressure, and occasionally are used chronically. Side effects of systemic treatment include paresthesias, lethargy, and a metallic-taste sensation. Monitoring of electrolytes is usually required with chronic use.

Prostaglandin analogues: These agents work by increasing outflow of aqueous humor, although the exact mechanism by which this occurs is unknown. Peculiar side effects of these medications include darkening of the iris pigment and periocular skin, and eyelash hypertrichosis. An advantage of these medications is that once-daily dosing is used.

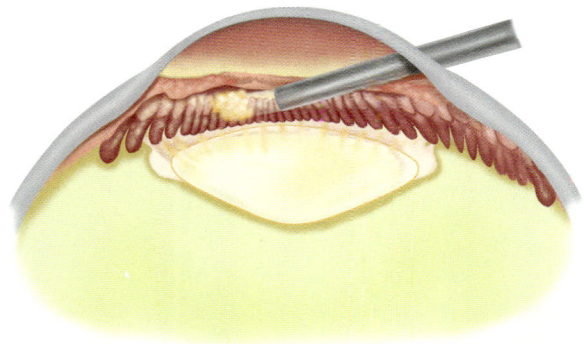

FIGURE 32–30 ■ Endoscopic laser cyclophotocoagulation. A small instrument containing an endoscope and a laser delivery system is inserted through the peripheral cornea and placed behind the iris. The ciliary processes are visualized with the endoscope, and the laser is used to photocoagulate the ciliary processes and decrease fluid production.

Alpha-2 adrenergic agonists: These medications may affect pressure by both decreasing aqueous production and increasing outflow. *The use of these agents in infants and young children is usually contraindicated due to a risk of central nervous system effects, including somnolence and respiratory depression.*

Hyperosmotic agents: These medications are used systemically to acutely decrease IOP in the face of marked IOP elevation. Patients require systemic monitoring for side effects due to their potential effects on systemic fluid redistribution and cardiac output. They are for short-term use only.

REFERENCE

1. Freedman SF. Central corneal thickness in children—does it help or hinder our evaluation of eyes at risk for glaucoma? *JAAPOS.* 2008;12:1–2.

CHAPTER 33

Disorders of the Optic Nerve

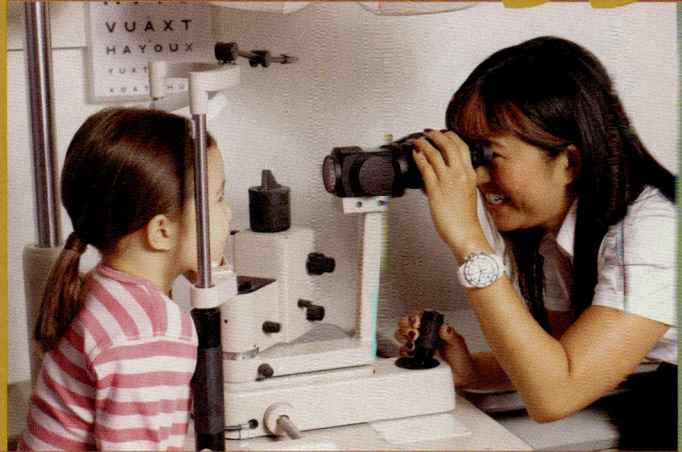

ANATOMY AND EMBRYOLOGY

The optic nerve is the structure at the back of the eye that carries visual information from the eye to the central nervous system (CNS). Approximately 120 million rods and cones sense light in the outer retina. This information is transmitted to approximately 1 million ganglion cells in the inner retina. These ganglion cells converge to form the optic nerve. The electrical impulses generated in the optic nerve are transmitted to the occipital lobe via the lateral geniculate nucleus. Posterior to the eye, the optic nerve is covered by a dural sheath and arachnoid membrane. This structure surrounds the nerve until it enters the brain, where it is contiguous with the subdural space (Figure 33–1).

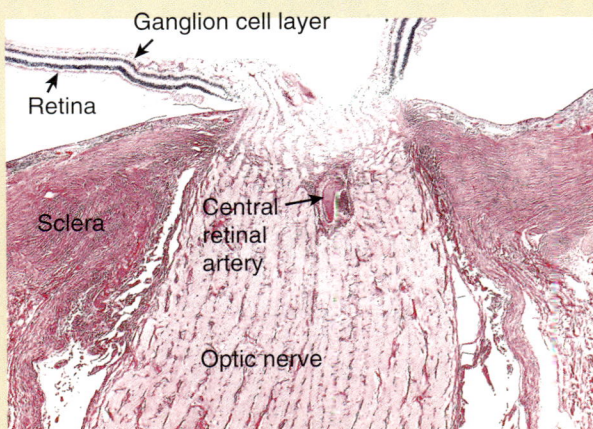

The only portion of the optic nerve that is visible on examination is the site where the nerve attaches to the eye at the posterior retina (Figure 33–2). The normal nerve has a central area through which the central retinal artery travels, branching into vessels lining the inner layer of the retina. The central portion is called the cup, and the entire area is called the disc. The *cup:disc ratio* describes the relationship between these 2 structures. The normal ratio ranges from 0.1 to 0.4, although larger cups may be normal in certain ethnic populations, particularly African Americans. Increased intraocular pressure may cause enlargement of the cup, and increased intracranial pressure (ICP) may cause edema and obscuration of the cup.

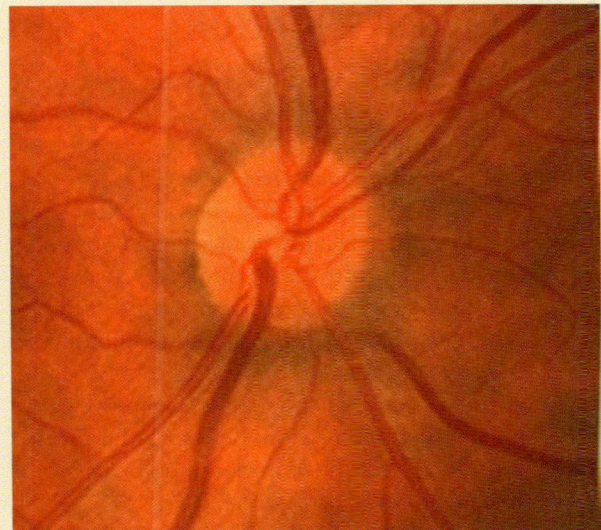

FIGURE 33–1 ■ Normal microscopic appearance of optic nerve as it exits the eyeball. The neurons of the inner ganglion cell layer of the retina combine to form the nerve. The sclera surrounds the nerve. A portion of the central retinal artery is visible in cross-section. The retina is artificially detached due to histological processing. (Photograph contributed by Morton Smith, MD.)

FIGURE 33–2 ■ Normal view of optic nerve as seen with ophthalmoscope. The cup:disc ratio of this nerve is 0.1.

Optic nerve problems in children occur infrequently. However, bilateral optic nerve hypoplasia (ONH) is one of the common causes of profound visual loss in infancy.

Embryology

The optic nerves form from the optic stalk, the structure that connects the embryonic forebrain and optic vesicle. It contains an outer layer of cells from the neural crest, which differentiates into the structures of the sheath that surround the optic nerve (pia, arachnoid, and dura). An inner neuroectodermal layer regresses and is replaced by ganglion cells that originate in the inner layer of the retina and travel through the optic nerve to the lateral geniculate body. At 4 months of gestation, almost 4 million ganglion cells are present within the nerve. This number decreases to 1 million by the time of birth. Myelinization of the optic nerve occurs late in gestation. It begins at the optic chiasm and travels forward, stopping at the juncture between the nerve and the eyeball.

PATHOGENESIS

Optic nerve problems may be caused by intrinsic abnormalities within the nerve itself, or may be secondary to problems within the eye or brain. Increased pressure within the eye (e.g., glaucoma) or inflammation (e.g., autoimmune, infectious) may damage the nerve. Increased ICP can be transmitted through the sheath to the optic nerve head, creating papilledema. Primary congenital malformations and inherited optic nerve disorders also occur.

CLINICAL PRESENTATION

Children with bilateral visually significant optic nerve abnormalities, such as ONH, present within the first few months of life with poor visual fixation, nystagmus, and decreased or absent pupillary responses.

Patients with increased ICP may experience systemic symptoms that include headache and vomiting. Papilledema itself initially causes minimal visual acuity changes. Formal visual field testing may show enlargement of the blind spot, but this is usually asymptomatic. Chronic increased pressure can lead to loss of vision. Symptoms of diplopia (due to sixth cranial nerve palsy) and transient visual obscurations (episodes of decreased vision lasting a few seconds) are common ocular complaints in patients with increased ICP.

Compression of the nerve may lead to decreased visual acuity. In children, however, if the compression causes unilateral visual loss and the vision is normal in the opposite eye, the decreased vision may go undetected for prolonged periods, because the children function well using only the vision in the normal eye. Sensory strabismus may develop if the decreased vision persists.

A very sensitive sign of unilateral optic nerve dysfunction is a *relative afferent pupillary defect (RAPD)*. This can be detected by the *swinging flashlight test*. The pupillary reactions are connected in the brain, so that a light that is shined into one eye normally causes equal constriction of both pupils. When the light is removed, both pupils dilate. If a light is swung back and forth between the 2 eyes, there should be an initial pupil constriction each time the light is shined into an eye. If one optic nerve is damaged, the abnormal pupil will still constrict when a light is shined into the normal pupil, because the neural pathway for this reaction does not travel through the damaged optic nerve. When the light is moved to the abnormal eye, the signal for constriction will be diminished because of the optic nerve problem. At the same time, a dilating signal is being sent from the normal eye, because the light has been removed from that eye. In the presence of optic nerve damage this dilating signal will be stronger than the weak constricting signal from the light in the abnormal eye. The pupil in the abnormal eye will therefore initially dilate, rather than constrict, when the light is shined into it (see also, Chapter 1, Figure 1–26).

Diseases that compromise the function of the optic nerve may interfere with color vision discrimination. Various methods of testing color vision are available, ranging from color test plates that can be used easily in the office, to sophisticated tests that require computer analysis. The ability of children to perform these tests varies with age and the degree of visual impairment. The color vision deficits in acquired diseases of the optic nerve and retina tend to be primarily in the blue-yellow spectrum, whereas inherited color vision defects, which affect approximately 7% of males, cause red-green discrimination difficulties.

OPTIC NERVE DISORDERS

Congenital Anomalies

Bergmeister's papilla

Bergmeister's papillae are benign remnants of the hyaloid artery. This vessel extends from the optic nerve to the posterior lens during embryological development of the eye. It usually regresses completely by birth. Small remnants of the hyaloid artery may persist overlying the optic nerve, producing a fibrous, elevated structure (Figure 33–3). These do not affect vision.

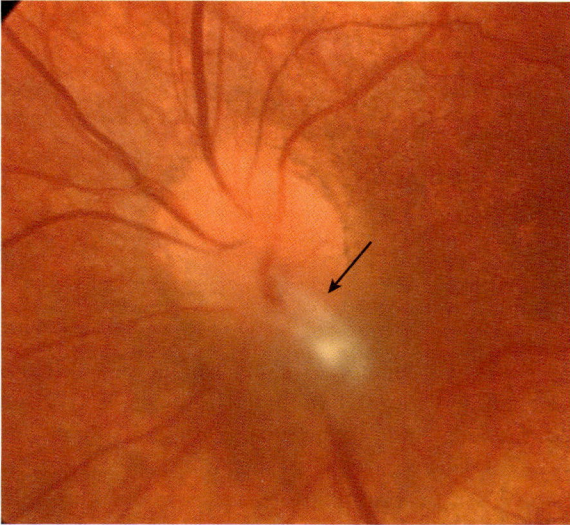

FIGURE 33–3 ■ Bergmeister's papilla (arrow). This is an elevated fibrous remnant of the hyaloid artery (which normally regresses completely by birth).

Optic nerve aplasia

True aplasia (absence) of the optic nerve is extremely rare. It usually occurs unilaterally in otherwise healthy children. It is associated with other malformations of the eye, including abnormal development of the retina. Examination reveals no visible optic nerve structures in the area where these normally should be (Figure 33–4).

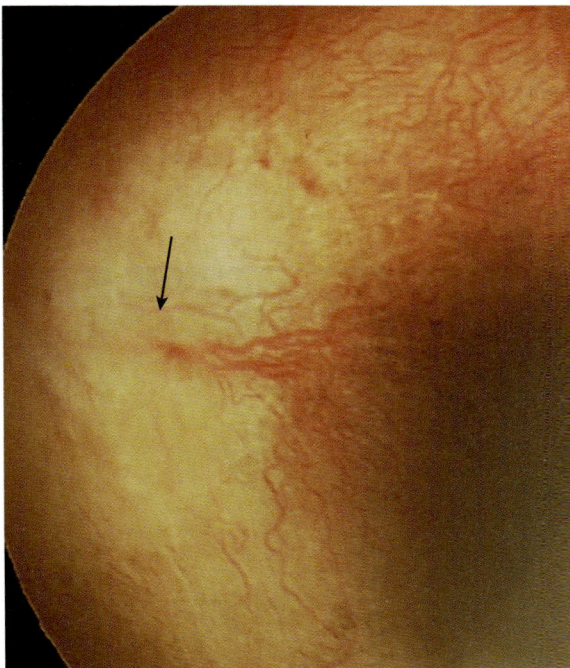

FIGURE 33–4 ■ Optic nerve aplasia. No normal optic nerve structures are visible in the area where the optic nerve normally should be (arrow).

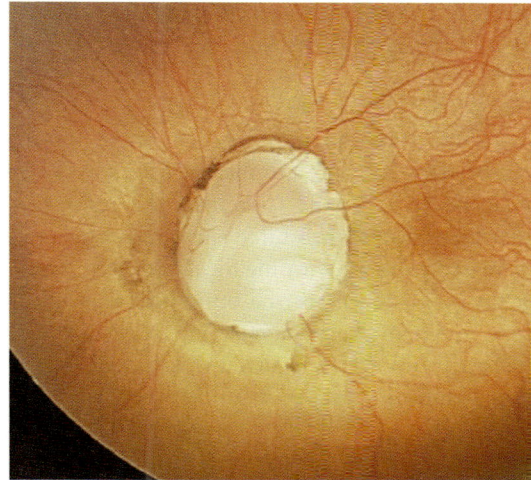

FIGURE 33–5 ■ Optic nerve coloboma

Optic nerve coloboma

Ocular colobomas occur due to incomplete folding of the embryonic fissure during ocular formation. They may include the iris, lens, retina, and optic nerve. The degree of visual impairment is primarily related to retinal involvement. Lesions that include the fovea generally cause significant loss. Surprisingly, even large optic nerve colobomas are often compatible with near normal vision if the fovea is unaffected (Figure 33–5).

Morning glory disc

This malformation is characterized by an increased number of retinal blood vessels crossing the disc in a radial pattern, with a central area of glial tissue at the site of the normal optic cup (Figure 33–5). The effects on vision

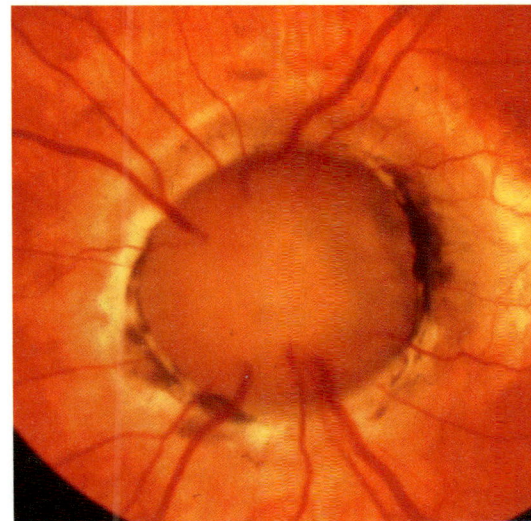

FIGURE 33–6 ■ Morning glory disc anomaly. Note the central excavation of the nerve and the radial pattern of the blood vessels as they exit the nerve.

range from minimal to marked. Systemic associations include basal encephalocele and Moyamoya disease.[1]

Optic nerve hypoplasia

ONH results from underdevelopment of the nerve during embryogenesis. The number of axons in the hypoplastic nerve is small. Therefore, the optic disc is smaller than normal. It is often surrounded by a region of decreased pigment, creating the *double-ring sign*. This ring can be mistaken for the optic disc, and the hypoplastic nerve for the optic cup (Figure 33–7A and B). Visual acuity in ONH is variably affected, but often there is significant loss.

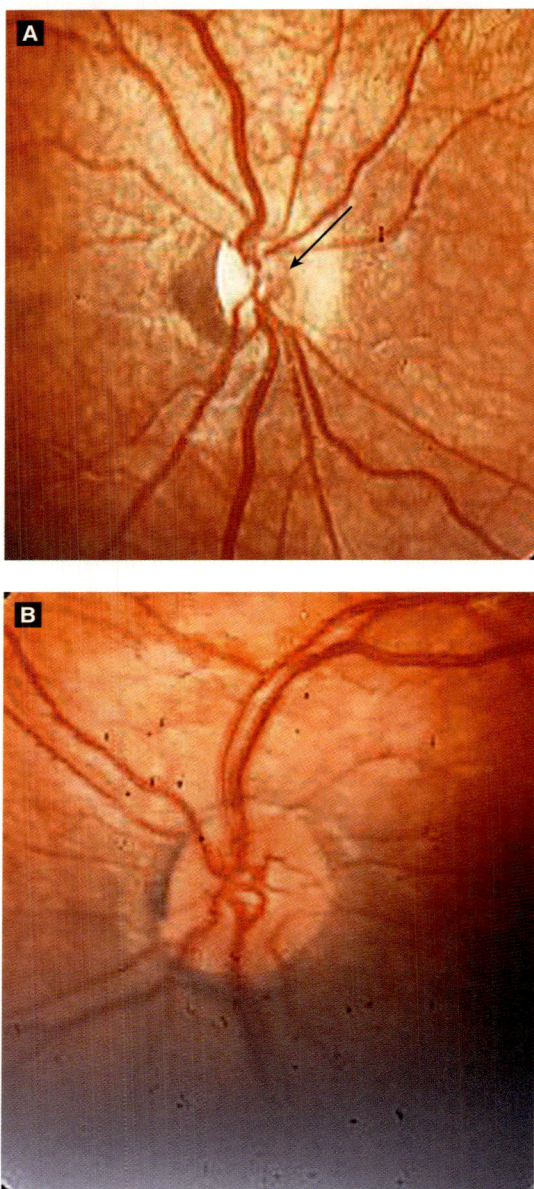

FIGURE 33–7 ■ Unilateral optic nerve hypoplasia. (A) The right optic nerve is hypoplastic with a double ring sign. The actual border of the optic nerve is marked by the arrow. (B) Normal left optic nerve.

Table 33–1.
Disorders Associated With ONH
■ Septo-optic dysplasia
■ Aniridia
■ Maternal diabetes mellitus
■ Prematurity

If ONH is bilateral, infants usually present within the first few months of life with decreased visual responsiveness and nystagmus. If it is unilateral, children frequently develop strabismus secondary to the vision loss. On examination, decreased vision and a RAPD are present.

The etiology of ONH cannot be identified in most patients, but in some cases it is associated with other abnormalities (Table 33–1). Infants whose mothers have type 1 diabetes mellitus may have *segmental ONH*. In segmental ONH the visual acuity is usually normal, but patients have visual field defects that correspond to localized areas of disc hypoplasia. Children with aniridia often have ONH as one of the associated ocular abnormalities. Children who are born prematurely and have periventricular leukomalacia may have a form of ONH characterized by a large optic cup, rather than a small disc. This results from transsynaptic degeneration of axons caused by damage to the optic nerve radiations.

The most common abnormality associated with ONH is *septo-optic dysplasia (DeMorsier syndrome)*. In this disorder, bilateral ONH is present, in addition to absence of the septum pellucidum and agenesis of the corpus callosum (Figure 33–8). Variable associations include ectopic pituitary glands (Figure 33–9A and B), schizencephaly, and cortical heterotopia (Figure 33–10).

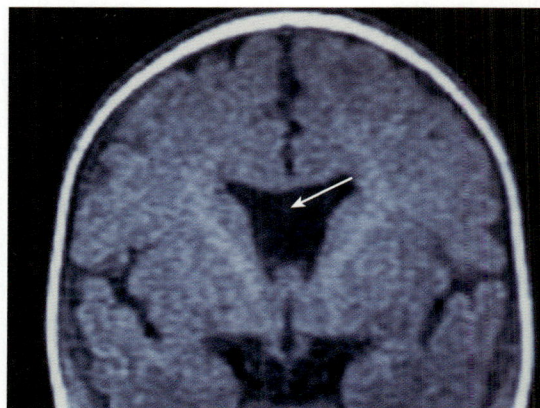

FIGURE 33–8 ■ Septo-optic dysplasia. Magnetic resonance image demonstrating absence of the septum pellucidum (the arrow points to the area where the septum pellucidum should be).

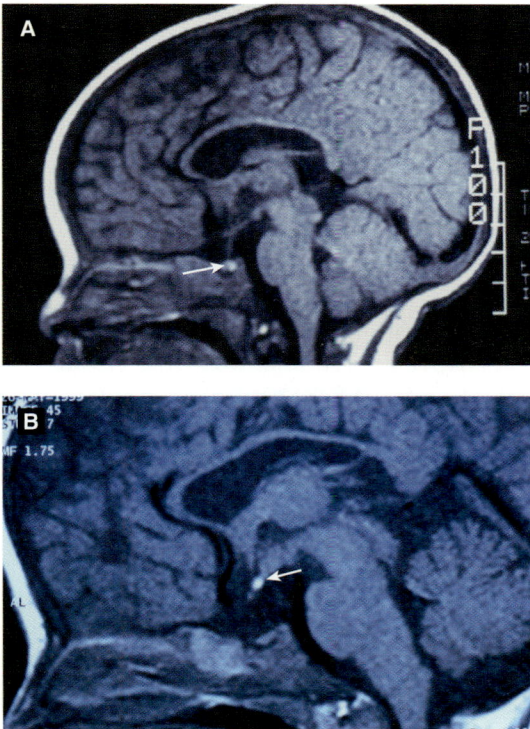

FIGURE 33–9 ■ Septo-optic dysplasia. Magnetic resonance image demonstrating ectopic pituitary gland. (A) Normal location of pituitary bright spot (arrow). (B) Ectopic location of pituitary gland (arrow) in a patient with septo-optic dysplasia.

The visual prognosis in these patients is dependent on the degree of ONH. Developmental delay and seizures may occur due to the associated CNS defects.[2] Patients with ectopic pituitary glands have endocrinological disorders, including growth hormone and adrenocortico-

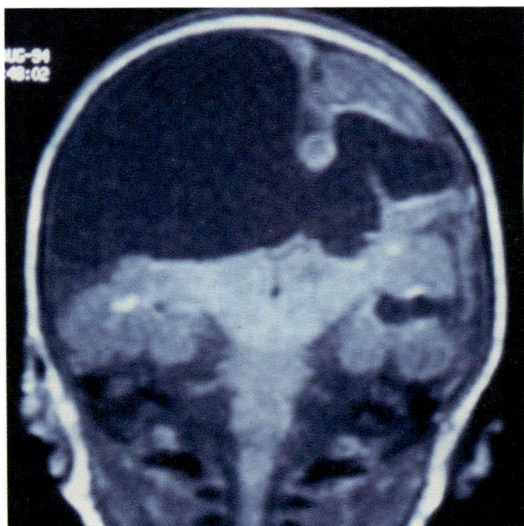

FIGURE 33–10 ■ Septo-optic dysplasia. Magnetic resonance image demonstrating marked schizencephaly and cortical heterotopia.

tropic hormone deficiency. These disorders require treatment due to the risk of developmental delay and potentially serious medical problems related to the inability to mount a normal stress response.

Optic Nerve Atrophy

The optic nerve in patients with optic nerve atrophy is of normal size, but has a pale appearance. This results from damage to the optic nerve axons. This may occur as a primary abnormality, but is usually secondary to some other problem. With acute damage, such as trauma, it typically takes several weeks before optic disc pallor becomes clinically detectable.

Dominant optic atrophy (Kjer optic atrophy)

This is an autosomal dominant disorder characterized by temporal pallor of the optic nerve (Figure 33–11A and B).

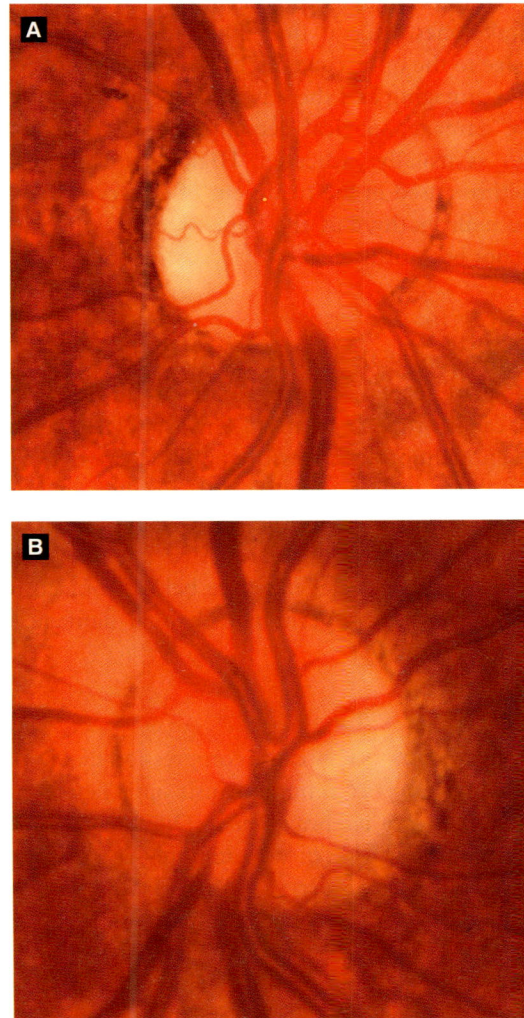

FIGURE 33–11 ■ Autosomal dominant optic atrophy (Kjer). (A) Right optic nerve, (B) Left optic nerve. Note the segmental temporal pallor of the disc in both eyes.

The onset is usually late in the first decade of life, presenting with bilateral moderately decreased vision. In addition to the characteristic appearance of the nerve, patients usually have central or pericentral visual field defects and abnormal color vision. The vision loss usually slowly progresses initially, but then stabilizes. It is usually better than 20/200. Defects in a gene on chromosome 3 (*OPA1*) have been identified in some patients with this disorder.

Compressive optic atrophy

In this condition, ganglion cell loss occurs due to compressive damage. This may result from various causes, including trauma, space-occupying lesions, optic nerve tumors, or bone disease.

Traumatic optic neuropathy

Traumatic optic neuropathy (Figure 33–12A and B) may occur due to skull fractures involving the optic canal, particularly if bone fragments impinge on the nerve. Indirect damage may occur due to trauma to the frontal bones, even if imaging studies do not show damage to the optic canal itself. If bony compression is seen on imaging and there is clinical evidence of optic nerve damage, surgical decompression and fracture repair is usually indicated. High-dose steroids are sometimes used in the treatment of indirect traumatic optic neuropathy, but the benefits of this treatment have not been proven.[3]

Space-occupying lesions

Compression of the nerve may occur due to a large number of space-occupying lesions within the orbit, optic canal, or the nerve itself. Any orbital lesion that is large enough to cause pressure on the nerve may cause this problem, including lymphangiomas, hemangiomas, enlarged extraocular muscles in thyroid eye disease, and orbital tumors. Increased ICP usually initially manifests with papilledema (see below), but chronic pressure may cause permanent axonal damage that leads to optic atrophy.

Optic nerve tumors

Optic nerve tumors may cause compression that leads to atrophy. The most common intrinsic optic nerve tumor in children is *optic pathway glioma (OPG)*. These tumors can occur primarily or, more commonly, as a manifestation of *neurofibromatosis type 1 (NF1; von Recklinghausen disease)*. NF1 is an autosomal dominant disorder caused by mutations of the neufibromin gene. There is a high rate of new mutations in NF1, such that approximately half of patients have no family history of the disease. Systemic manifestations include skin abnormalities, mild developmental delay, and bone malformations. In addition to OPGs, other ocular abnormalities associated

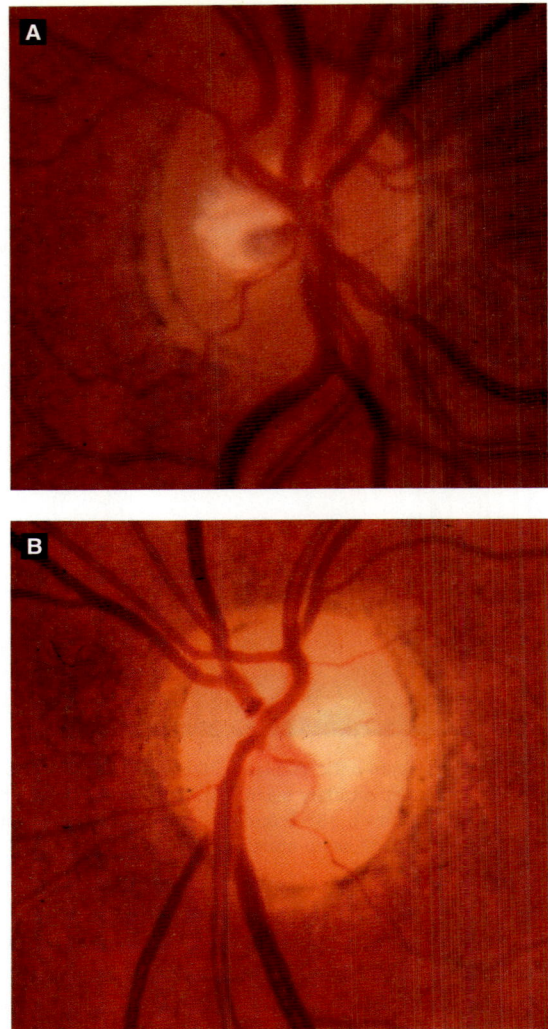

FIGURE 33–12 ■ Traumatic optic neuropathy, left eye. (A) Normal right optic nerve. (B) Left optic nerve. Note diffuse pallor and increased cup:disc ratio of left nerve compared to right.

with NF1 include iris Lisch nodules, eyelid plexiform neurofibromas, glaucoma, and hypoplasia of the sphenoid wing (Figure 33–13).

OPGs are the most serious ocular problem associated with NF1. They usually present with decreased

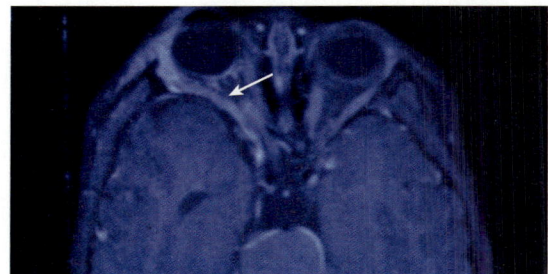

FIGURE 33–13 ■ Neurofibromatosis. Right sphenoid wing hypoplasia. Note forward displacement and distortion of lateral rectus muscle (arrow).

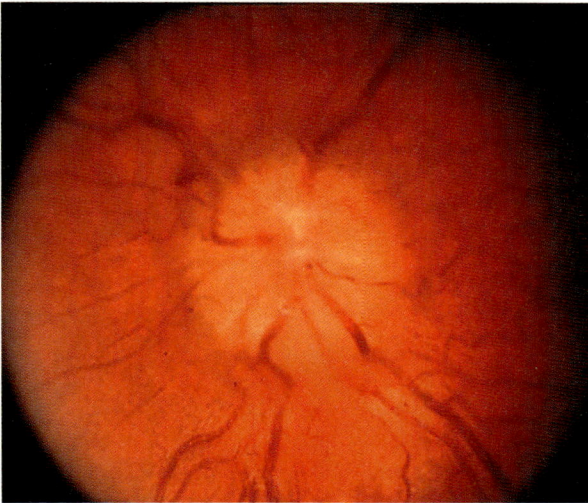

FIGURE 33–14 ■ Neurofibromatosis. Papilledema secondary to enlargement of optic nerve glioma.

vision, an RAPD, and optic nerve pallor. Papilledema sometimes is present initially, particularly if rapid enlargement of the tumor has occurred (Figure 33–14). Large tumors may cause proptosis, which may be acute. Approximately 15% of patients with NF1 have radiological evidence of OPGs, although these are often asymptomatic. Magnetic resonance imaging usually reveals diffuse enlargement of the nerve with a central core (Figure 33–15).

The natural history of primary OPGs and those associated with NF1 is different. Both types of OPG may extend intracranially, affecting the optic chiasm and hypothalamus. Primary OPGs tend to be more aggressive than those associated with NF1. In NF1, OPGs may present with an initial period of rapid growth, but they often then stabilize. They almost always appear during the first decade of life. Late spontaneous improvement may occur in NF1-associated OPGs.

The optimal treatment of OPGs, particularly those associated with NF1, is not known.[4] The natural history of these tumors is extremely variable, which makes it difficult to compare treatment regimens. Because OPGs associated with NF1 are often asymptomatic, and because there is no clear consensus on the optimal treatment, there is a difference of opinion as to whether or not patients with NF1 should be routinely screened with magnetic resonance imaging. Many centers prefer to screen patients clinically for evidence of vision problems associated with OPGs, ordering imaging studies only when vision abnormalities develop. If treatment is indicated due to vision loss or CNS extension, carboplatin-based chemotherapy is often used. Radiation therapy may be considered, but is often avoided due to associated CNS complications.

Primary optic nerve sheath meningiomas may also cause optic atrophy, but these lesions are uncommon in children. Metastatic tumors such as leukemia may involve the optic nerve.

Bone disease

Compression of the nerve within the bony optic canal may lead to optic atrophy. This may occur in craniofacial malformations, either primarily due to compression or as a result of chronic increased ICP. Primary bone disorders that may cause compression within the optic canal include *fibrous dysplasia* and *osteopetrosis*.

Osteopetrosis (Albers-Schonberg disease) is an autosomal recessive disorder in which progressive thickening of the bones occurs due to deficient osteoclastic activity. Systemic problems include deafness due to nerve compression and hematopoietic dysfunction due to displacement of the bone marrow by the abnormal bone. Children may present in early childhood with decreased vision due to optic nerve compression and atrophy. Radiographs show characteristic thickening of the bones (Figure 33–16). Bone marrow transplantation may ameliorate the disease, but the vision usually does not improve because of permanent damage to the optic nerve.

Leber's hereditary optic neuropathy (LHON): This is a mitochondrial disorder that can be diagnosed by analysis of mitochondrial DNA. It presents with central visual loss and telangiectatic vessels on the optic nerve head. It usually affects males, and often does not manifest until after age 20.

Glaucoma

Glaucomatous damage to the optic nerve is a form of optic atrophy. It results from increased intraocular pressure, which causes compression of the ganglion cells as they pass through the optic nerve head. The earliest visible sign of optic nerve damage occurs as notching of the inferior and superior temporal portions of the nerve, which correspond to arcuate visual field defects. Asymmetric cupping is present in unilateral glaucoma

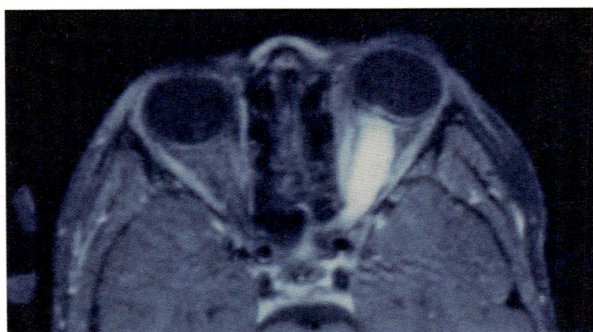

FIGURE 33–15 ■ Neurofibromatosis. Magnetic resonance image demonstrating large left optic nerve glioma (same patient as Figure 33–14).

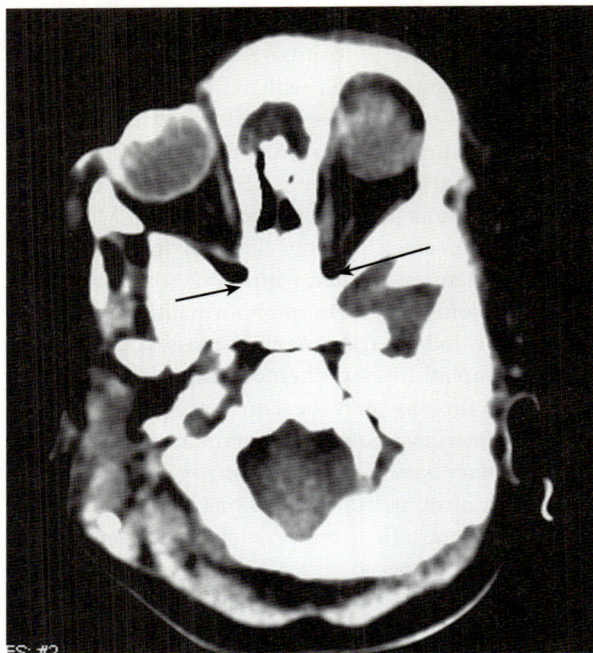

FIGURE 33–16 ■ Osteopetrosis, computed tomograph. Note diffuse marked thickening of the skull bones, including the optic canals (arrows).

(Figure 33–17A and B). Glaucoma is discussed further in Chapter 32.

Optic Neuritis

Optic neuritis results from inflammation of the optic nerve, usually due to either infection or an autoimmune reaction. It typically presents with rapid onset of marked visual loss, often to 20/200 or less. Children frequently have preceding or accompanying systemic symptoms of malaise, fever, and headache. They may report pain with eye movements. In addition to decreased vision, patients have decreased pupillary responses and central visual field defects. In children, disc swelling is usually present (Figure 33–18A and B). Magnetic resonance imaging may show signs of inflammation of the optic nerves (Figure 33–19). In some patients, leakage of fluid produces swelling of the posterior retina and lipid deposition in a star-shaped configuration around the fovea (*Leber's stellate neuroretinitis*) (Figure 33–20). Visual evoked potentials (VEPs) usually show decreased amplitudes and prolonged latencies (Figure 33–21A and B).

Unlike adults, in whom there is a strong association between optic neuritis and multiple sclerosis, children with optic neuritis usually do not develop this disease. Children may have a preceding history of viral illness or vaccinations, suggesting an autoimmune response. Stellate neuroretinitis is often associated with cat-scratch disease (*Bartonella*).

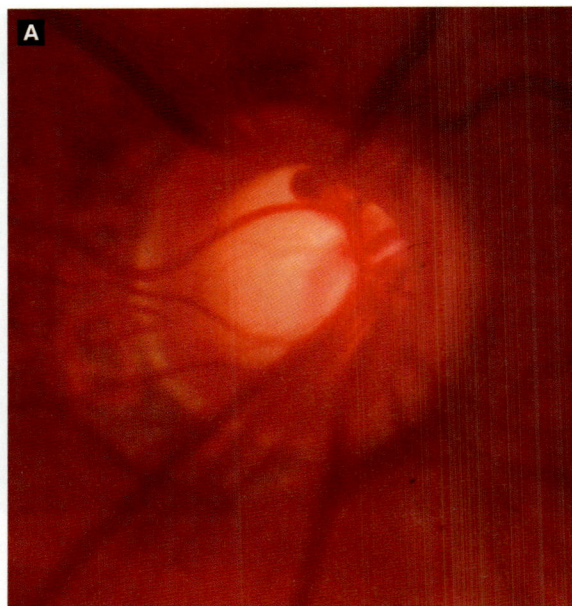

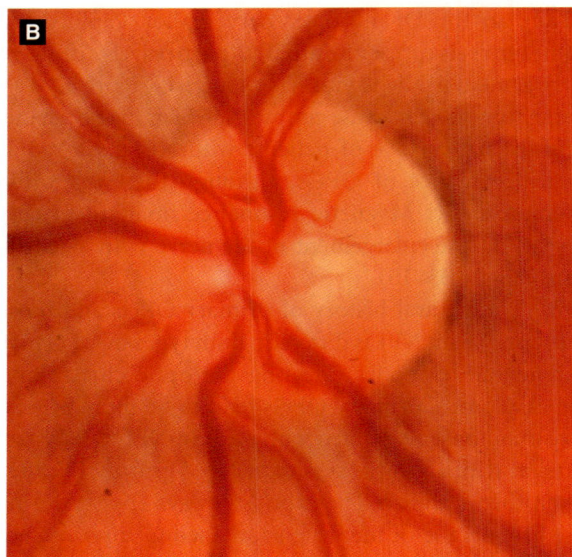

FIGURE 33–17 ■ Asymmetric optic nerve cupping in a patient with aphakic glaucoma in the right eye following infantile cataract removal. (A) Right optic nerve. (B) Normal left optic nerve.

If *Bartonella* infection is identified in a child with optic neuritis, antimicrobial therapy is indicated. The treatment of optic neuritis in other children is controversial. Many children with optic neuritis experience improvement of vision to near normal levels without any treatment (Figure 33–21). A multicentral study involving the use of corticosteroids in adults with optic neuritis (the Optic Neuritis Treatment Trial) demonstrated that intravenous corticosteroids hastened the recovery of vision and appeared to delay the onset of multiple sclerosis in some patients. The ultimate visual outcomes did not change.[5] This study did not include children, however, and therefore the benefits in pediatric patients are not known.

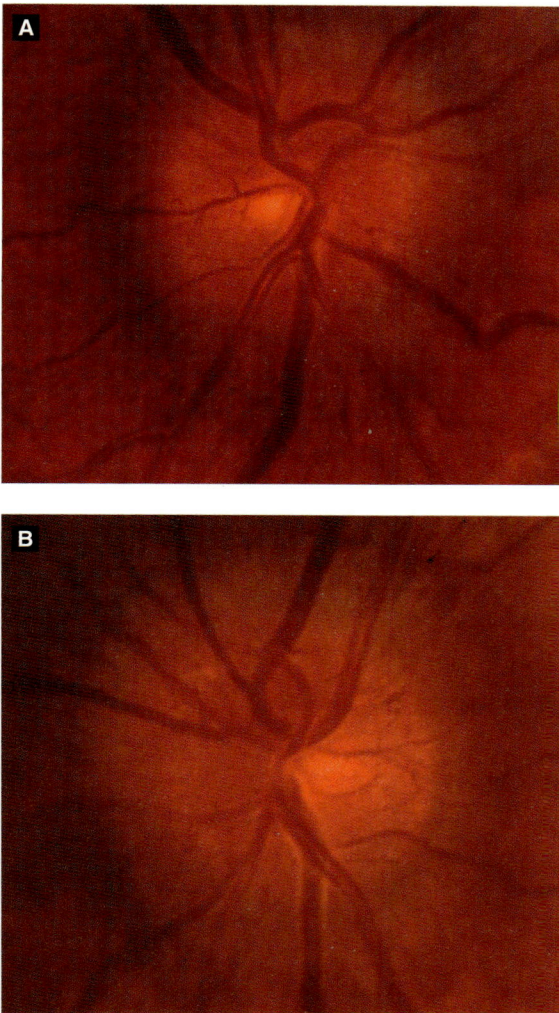

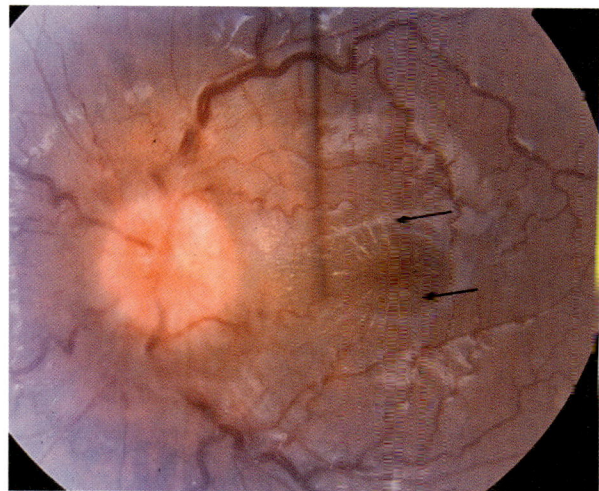

FIGURE 33–20 ■ Leber's stellate neuroretinitis in a patient with cat-scratch disease. Note swelling of optic nerve and deposition of retinal lipid in a stellate pattern (arrows) around the fovea.

FIGURE 33–18 ■ Optic neuritis. Bilateral mild swelling of optic nerves. (A) Right optic nerve. (B) Left optic nerve.

Papilledema

Papilledema is swelling of the optic nerve head that results from increased ICP. The nerve fibers become swollen, the optic cup is often not visible, the fine vessels

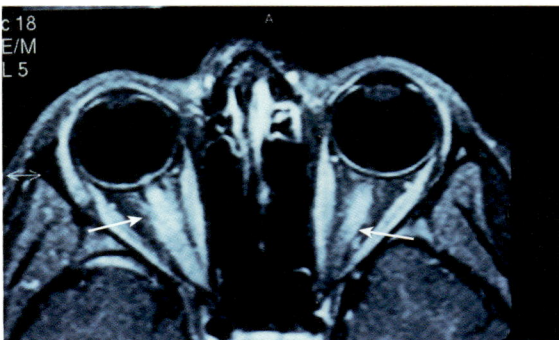

FIGURE 33–19 ■ Optic neuritis, magnetic resonance imaging with gadolinium. Bilateral enhancement of optic nerves (arrows).

overlying the optic nerve head are obscured, and there are often flame-shaped hemorrhages that follow the nerve fiber layer and cotton-wool spots surrounding the optic nerve (Figure 33–22). Associated systemic symptoms include headache, nausea, and vomiting. Transient visual obscurations (brief episodes in which the vision becomes dim) are frequently reported. Pressure on the sixth cranial nerve may cause diplopia.

The increased ICP that causes papilledema may result from a space-occupying lesion. The most common etiologies include intracranial hemorrhage and tumors. Intracranial hemorrhages usually result from trauma, but coagulopathies and bleeding from vascular malformations may also occur.

Idiopathic intracranial hypertension (pseudotumor cerebri)

In idiopathic intracranial hypertension (IIH), the increased ICP is not associated with visible structural abnormalities in the CNS. The symptoms and the ocular findings are the same as those for other patients with increased ICP, including papilledema (Figure 33–23A and B). The visual acuity is usually normal, but visual field testing may reveal an enlarged blind spot. In older patients, particularly young female adults, IIH is associated with obesity. In younger children, IIH frequently is associated with medication use. Common drugs that may cause IIH include retinoic acid, corticosteroids, tetracycline, and growth hormone.

The diagnosis of IIH is established by the characteristic historical and physical findings, normal neuroimaging, and increased ICP found on lumbar puncture. Neuroimaging is performed before lumbar

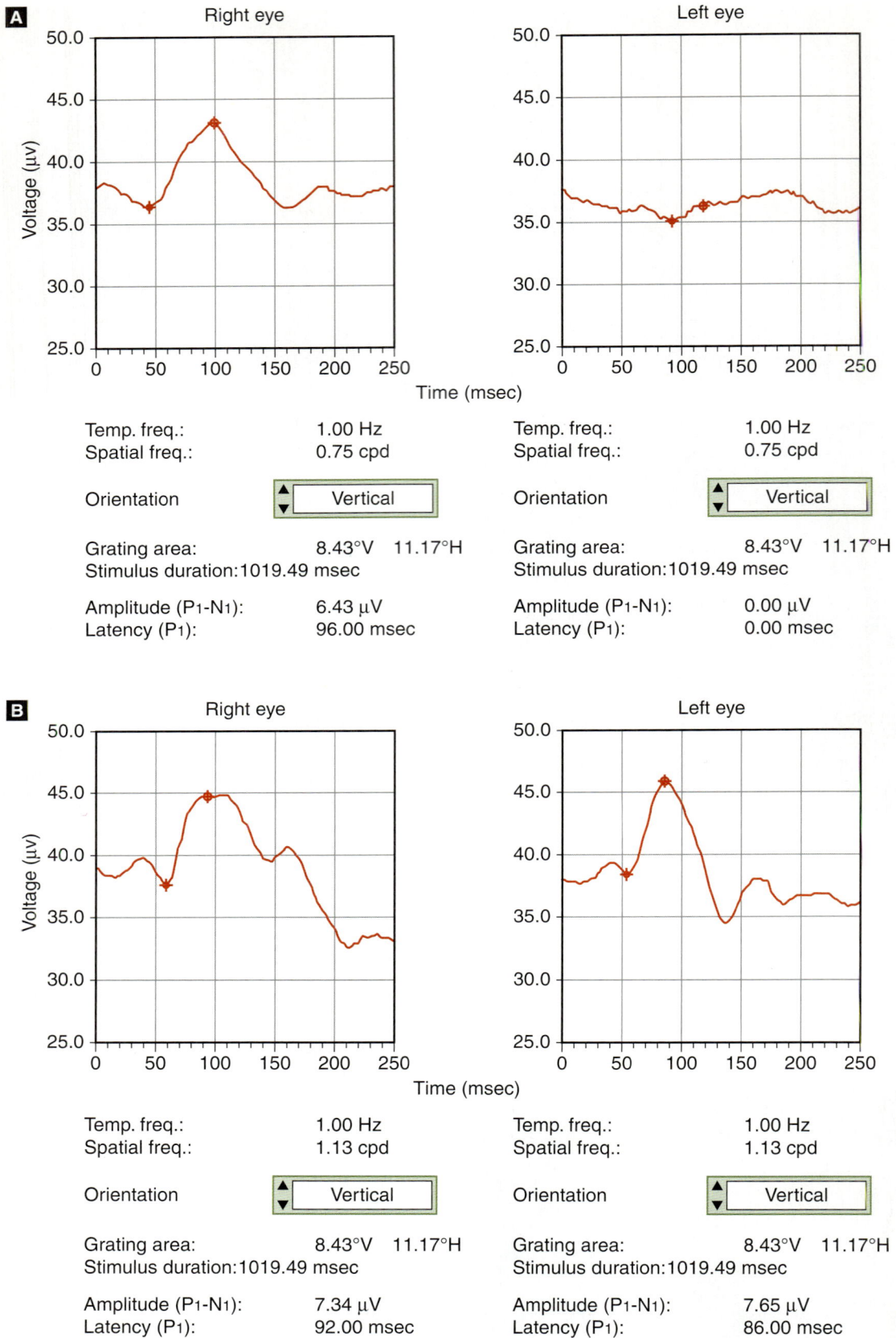

A

Right eye

Left eye

	Right eye		Left eye
Temp. freq.:	1.00 Hz	Temp. freq.:	1.00 Hz
Spatial freq.:	0.75 cpd	Spatial freq.:	0.75 cpd
Orientation	Vertical	Orientation	Vertical
Grating area:	8.43°V 11.17°H	Grating area:	8.43°V 11.17°H
Stimulus duration:	1019.49 msec	Stimulus duration:	1019.49 msec
Amplitude (P1-N1):	6.43 μV	Amplitude (P1-N1):	0.00 μV
Latency (P1):	96.00 msec	Latency (P1):	0.00 msec

B

Right eye

Left eye

	Right eye		Left eye
Temp. freq.:	1.00 Hz	Temp. freq.:	1.00 Hz
Spatial freq.:	1.13 cpd	Spatial freq.:	1.13 cpd
Orientation	Vertical	Orientation	Vertical
Grating area:	8.43°V 11.17°H	Grating area:	8.43°V 11.17°H
Stimulus duration:	1019.49 msec	Stimulus duration:	1019.49 msec
Amplitude (P1-N1):	7.34 μV	Amplitude (P1-N1):	7.65 μV
Latency (P1):	92.00 msec	Latency (P1):	86.00 msec

FIGURE 33–21 ■ Flash visual evoked potentials in a patient with left optic neuritis. (A) At presentation, the right eye is normal. The response in the left eye is barely recordable. (B) Five weeks later the VEP in the left eye has returned to normal.

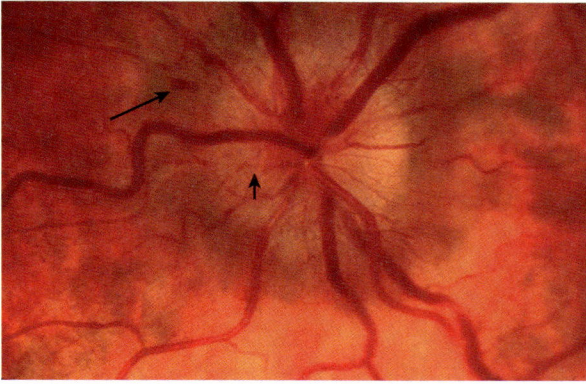

FIGURE 33–22 ■ Papilledema. Note swollen appearance of optic nerve, obscuration of small vessels as they cross the nerve (small arrow), and flame-shaped hemorrhages (long arrow).

puncture, to rule out a mass lesion, which could cause herniation if a lumbar puncture were performed. Cerebral venous sinus thrombosis may mimic the symptoms of IIH. This can be identified on imaging studies (Figure 33–24).

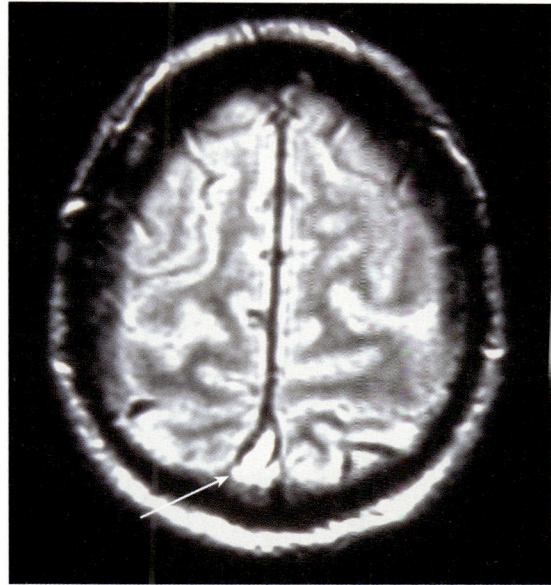

FIGURE 33–24 ■ Sagittal sinus thrombosis (arrow), magnetic resonance imaging. The presenting signs and symptoms of this disorder are the same as those in idiopathic intracranial hypertension.

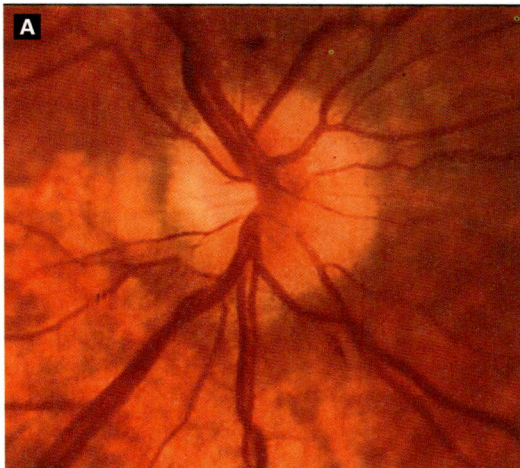

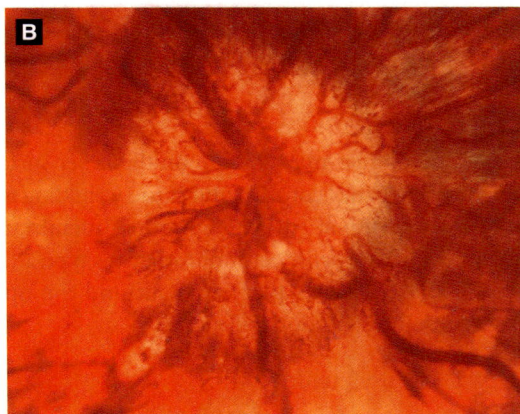

In children whose IIH is due to medication use, the disorder usually improves with discontinuation of the offending agent. If the patient has marked symptoms or visually threatening disease, other treatment may be necessary. Removal of fluid during a diagnostic lumbar puncture may provide at least temporary improvement. Serial lumbar punctures may be performed, particularly if problems persist and it is anticipated that they will improve (e.g., due to discontinuation of medication). Weight loss is usually beneficial in obese patients with IIH. Treatment with systemic acetazolamide or surgery (ventriculoperitoneal shunt, optic nerve sheath fenestration) may be indicated if a patient has persistent vision-threatening disease.

Pseudopapilledema

Pseudopapilledema describes the condition in which the optic nerve appears abnormal, with findings suggesting possible increased ICP, but the ICP is normal and the appearance is due to structural abnormalities of the nerve itself. It is important to recognize this finding, so that unnecessary tests are avoided.

Trisomy 21

One of the many ophthalmic abnormalities associated with Trisomy 21 (Down syndrome) is an anomalous appearance of the optic nerve. The nerve may appear elevated, the cup is often absent, and there are often a greater-than-normal number of vessels crossing over the disc surface (Figure 33–25). These optic nerve abnormalities cause no visual problems.

FIGURE 33–23 ■ Idiopathic intracranial hypertension. (A) Early papilledema. (B) Late papilledema.

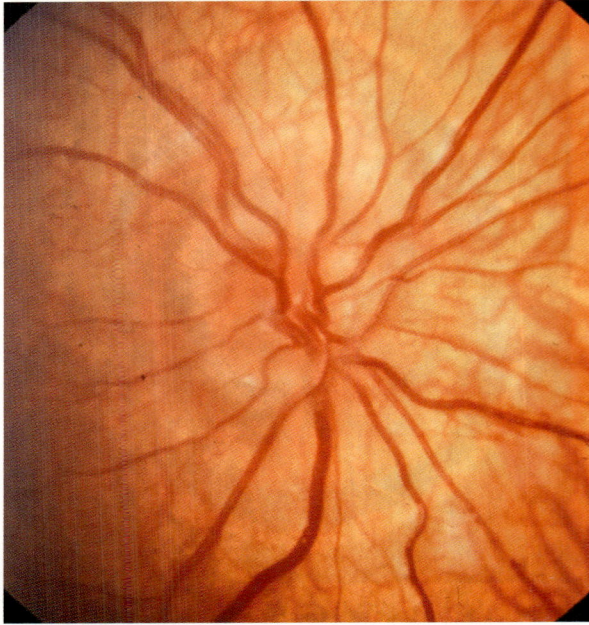

FIGURE 33–25 ■ Pseudopapilledema in a patient with Trisomy 21 (Down syndrome). Note the abnormal branching of the optic nerve blood vessels and absent cup.

Optic disc drusen

Drusen are focal areas of calcification within the substance of the optic nerve that cause an irregularly elevated, lumpy appearance of the disc (Figure 33–26). Superficial lesions may be recognized by their glistening whitish appearance (due to calcium). Buried drusen cannot be directly visualized, but may be suspected by an irregular appearance of the disc. Drusen may be

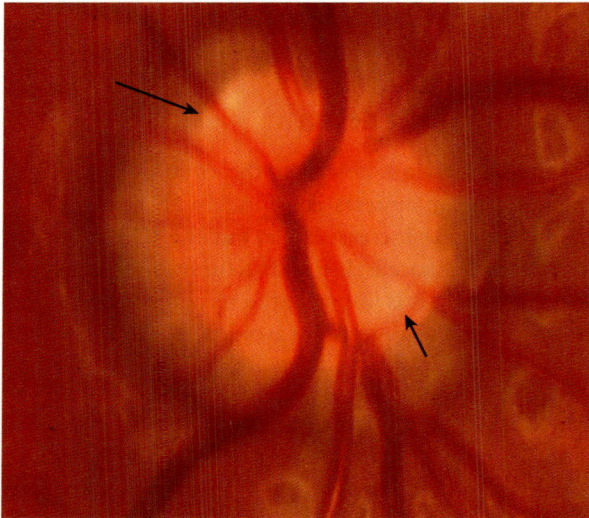

FIGURE 33–26 ■ Optic disc drusen, causing irregular elevation of optic nerve. In this patient, focal lumpy white areas are visible (arrows).

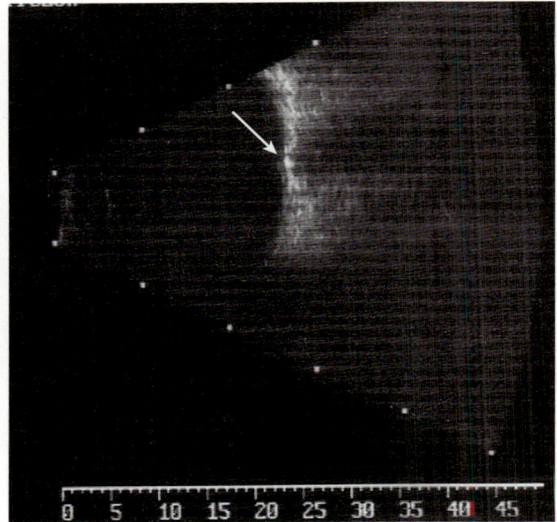

FIGURE 33–27 ■ Optic nerve drusen. B-scan ultrasonography shows a bright echo at the optic nerve head (arrow) due to calcium within the drusen. To the right of the bright spot is a shadow cast by the calcium.

inherited. The diagnosis can be established by ultrasonography, with bright echoes present within the substance of the nerve (Figure 33–27). Superficial drusen may also be diagnosed by the presence of autofluorescence when imaged with the filters used for fluorescein angiography (Figure 33–28). Drusen may cause peripheral visual field abnormalities, but these are rarely visually significant.

Myelinated nerve fibers

Myelinization of the optic nerve normally stops when the ganglion cell fibers enter the eye. In some patients, the myelin continues onto the posterior retina. The myelin is white and has an arcuate distribution that begins at the optic nerve and extends for a variable distance on the retinal surface. This is sometimes mistaken for papilledema (Figure 33–29A and B). The myelinated nerve fibers themselves do not cause visual problems, but they may be associated with amblyopia due to unequal refractive errors.

Epiretinal membrane

Epiretinal membranes may develop on the inner surface of the retina. They may contract and cause wrinkling and elevation of the retinal surface. Epiretinal membranes may occur in patients with neurofibromatosis type 2 (see Chapter 31). Membranes that occur around the optic nerve may result in pseudopapilledema.

Persistent fetal vasculature

Persistent fetal vasculature (PFV) results from incomplete regression of the hyaloid artery that is normally present during embryological development of the eye. It

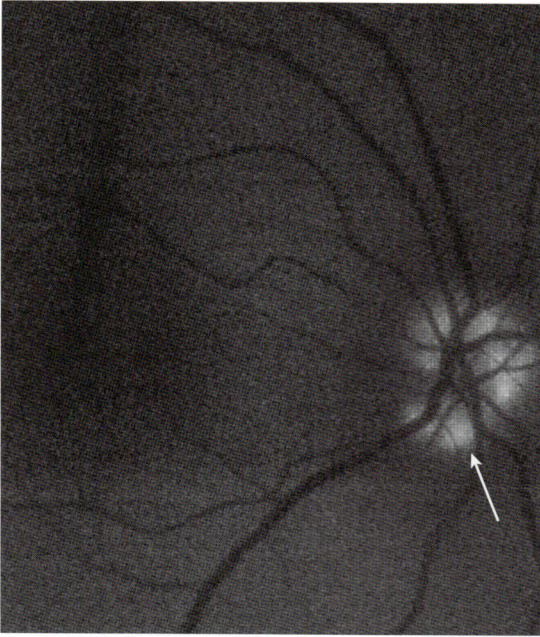

FIGURE 33–28 ■ Optic nerve drusen. Autofluorescence of optic nerve head (arrow) visible when imaged with filters used for fluorescein angiography.

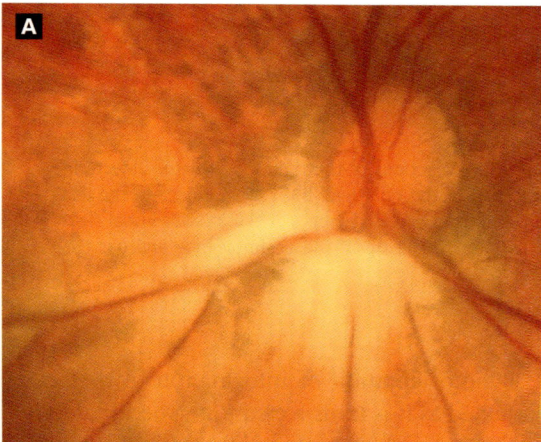

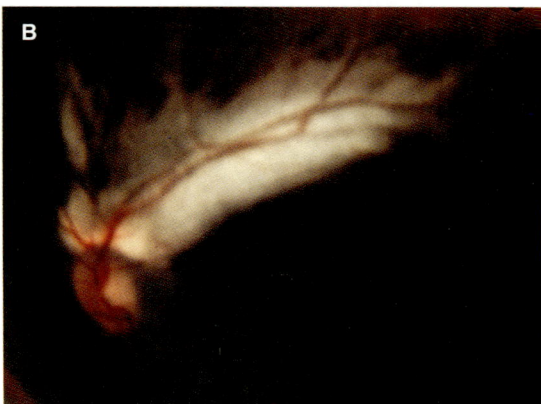

FIGURE 33–30 ■ Pseudopapilledema in a patient with persistent fetal vasculature. A stalk of tissue from the residual hyaloid artery causes traction and elevation of the tissue overlying the optic nerve.

FIGURE 33–29 ■ Myelinated nerve fibers. (A) The myelinated fibers usually are present in an arcuate pattern extending from the optic nerve head. (B) More extensive myelinated fibers in a different patient.

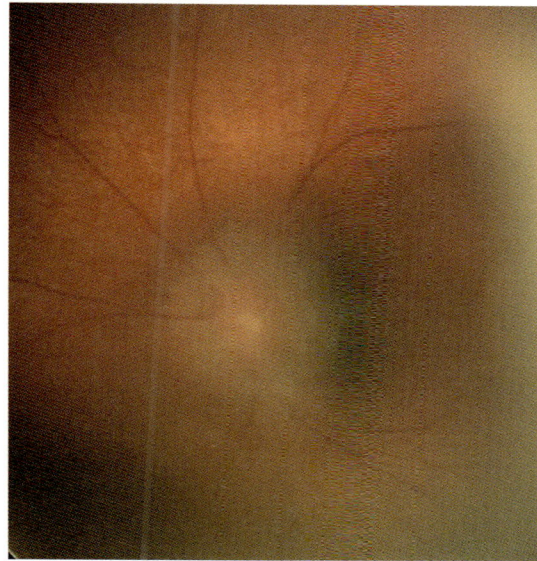

most commonly manifests as a cataract (see Chapter 30). If the stalk of tissue causes traction on the optic nerve, pseudopapilledema may occur (Figure 33–30).

DIAGNOSIS

Diagnostic Tests

In addition to the regular ocular examination, patients with suspected optic nerve problems usually require additional investigations. As noted above, careful assessment of the pupils and examination of the nerve should always be performed. If patients are old enough to be tested, color vision assessment is useful.

Visual field testing is particularly helpful in the assessment of optic nerve disorders, but formal testing requires a degree of understanding and cooperation that is often not possible in young children. If a visual field can be obtained, the type of defect may help in the differential diagnosis. Patients with compressive optic neuropathy and optic neuropathy usually have central or pericentral scotomas. Papilledema itself does not usually cause visual acuity changes, but may cause enlargement of the blind spot. Patients with optic nerve damage due to glaucoma usually have arcuate field defects.

After the optic nerve enters the brain, the pathways follow a specific pattern that can be mapped by visual field testing. At the optic chiasm, the 2 optic nerves cross. The information from the lateral half of the nerve continues to the occipital cortex on the ipsilateral side, and the information from the medial half of the nerve crosses over and travels to the contralateral occipital lobe.

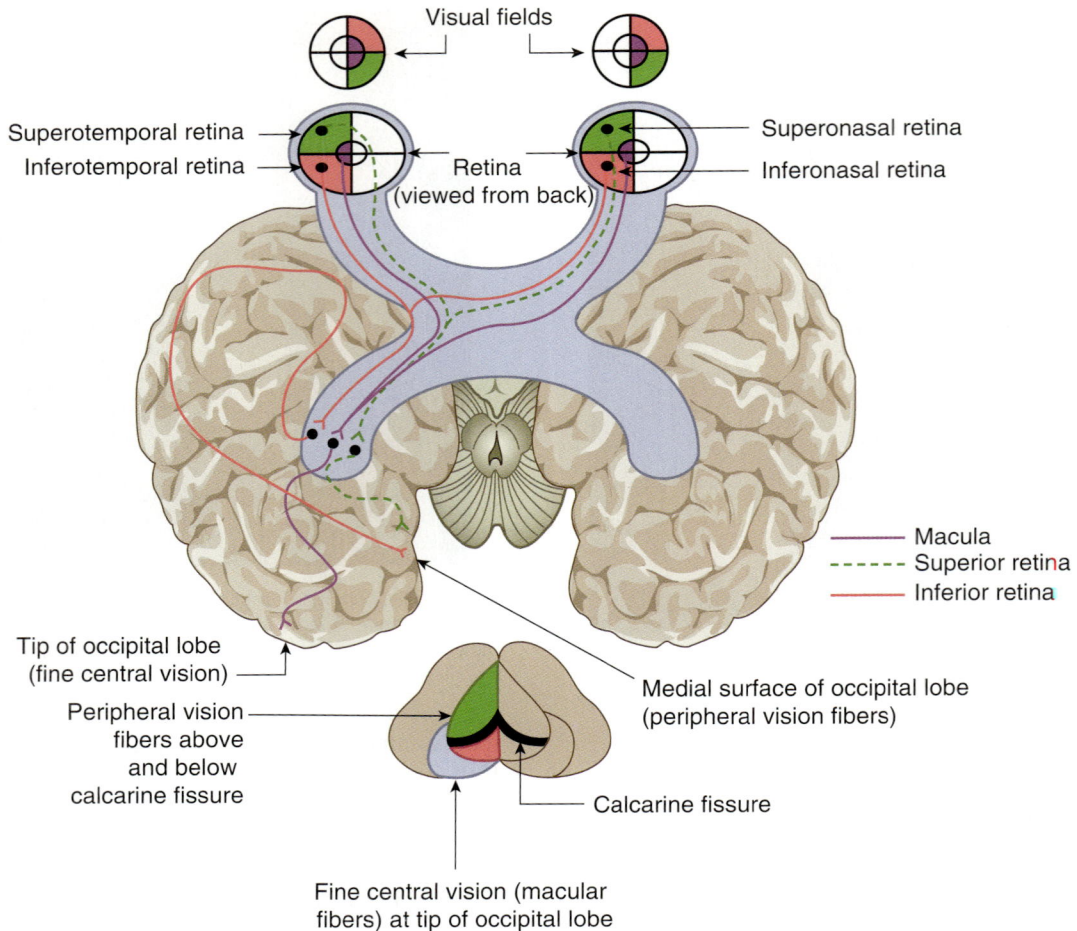

Visual fields

Superotemporal retina
Inferotemporal retina

Retina
(viewed from back)

Superonasal retina
Inferonasal retina

—— Macula
----- Superior retina
—— Inferior retina

Tip of occipital lobe
(fine central vision)

Peripheral vision
fibers above
and below
calcarine fissure

Medial surface of occipital lobe
(peripheral vision fibers)

Calcarine fissure

Fine central vision (macular
fibers) at tip of occipital lobe

FIGURE 33–31 ■ Visual field pathways. This figure demonstrates cortical projections of the right visual field. Objects in this field stimulate the temporal retina of the left eye and the nasal retina of the right eye. Both eyes project to the left occipital cortex. The superior visual field projects to the inferior portion of the occipital lobe and the inferior visual field projects to the superior occipital lobe. The macula (central vision) projects to the tip of the occipital lobe and has the largest cortical representation.

Visual information is reflected in a topographic pattern within the occipital cortex. Vertically, the upper portion receives information from the superior retina, and the inferior portion from the inferior retina. Horizontally, the right occipital lobe receives information from the temporal retina in the right eye and the nasal retina in the left eye. The opposite occurs in the left occipital lobe. The fovea and macula have a large cortical representation at the posterior portion of the occipital lobes, and the peripheral retina is represented more anteriorly (Figure 33–31).

Due to the manner in which light rays strike the eye, the location of actual objects is reversed in relation to where they are focused on the retina. Visual input from below strikes the superior retina, input from above strikes the inferior retina, input from the left strikes the right side of each retina (the nasal retina in the left eye and the temporal retina in the right eye), and vice versa for visual input from the right.

The orientation of information in the retina is maintained as it is transmitted to the occipital lobes, so that the reversal of spatial information persists. For example, information from the lower portion of the left visual field stimulates the superior occipital lobe on the right. Mapping of the visual field can therefore be used to localize CNS defects and monitor for progressive changes (Figure 33–32A–C).

Visual Evoked Potentials

Measurement of visual evoked potentials is useful in assessing the type and degree of optic nerve disease (Figure 33–31). They provide an objective measurement and can be performed even in young infants. Flash VEPs are obtained by flashing a bright light into the eyes and recording the speed and degree of response generated in the occipital lobe. Compressive lesions tend to have a greater effect on the amplitude of the response, whereas

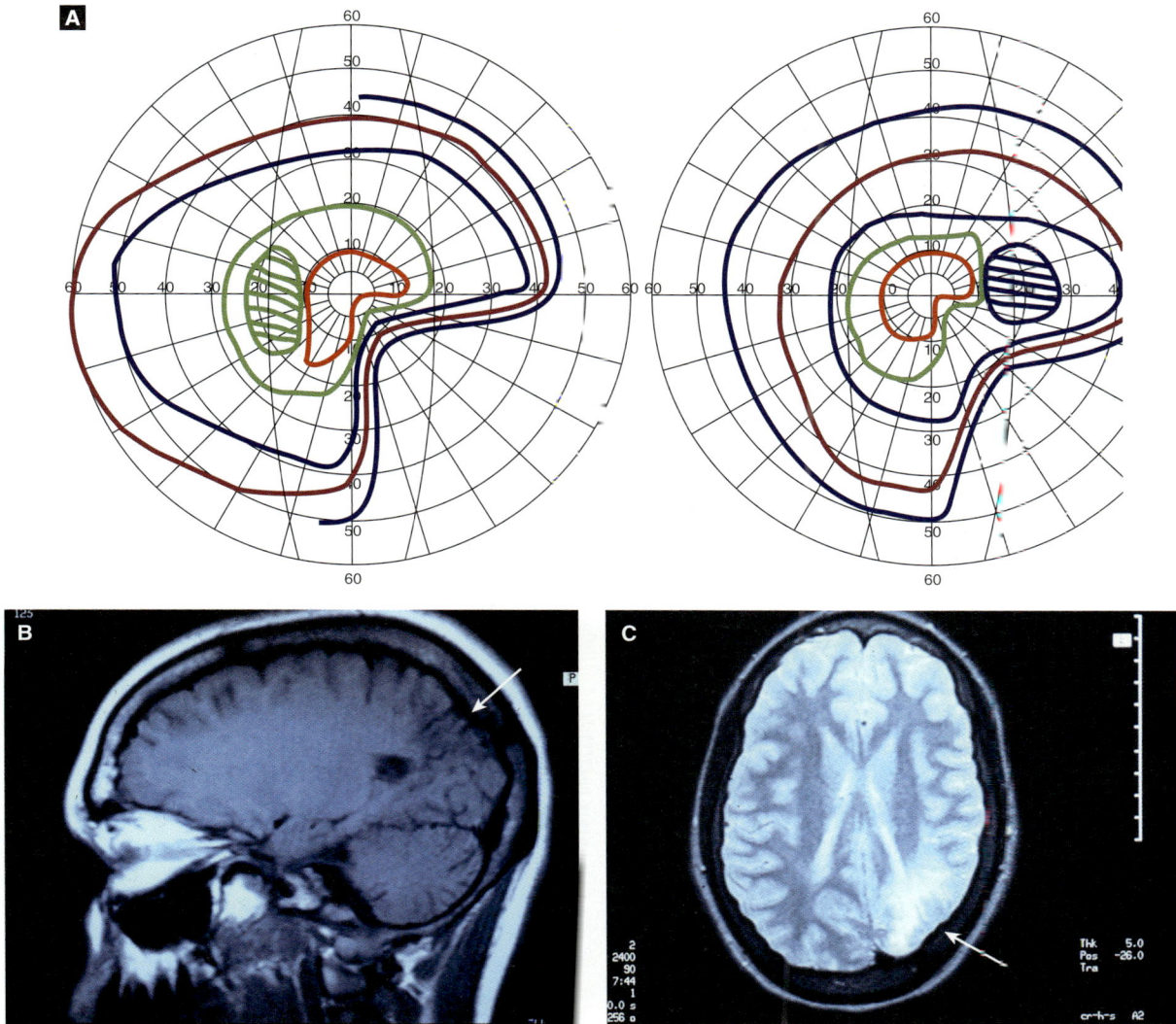

FIGURE 33–32 ■ Localization of CNS lesion based on visual field abnormalities. (A) The patient has a homonymous (symmetric) visual field defect on the lower right. This corresponds to a CNS lesion that is (B) above the calcarine fissure (arrow) and (C) in the left occipital lobe (arrow).

demyelinating processes tend to affect the latency. VEPs are discussed further in Chapter 2.

Imaging Studies

Imaging studies are often performed in patients with optic nerve disorders. Magnetic resonance imaging generally provides the most detailed images of the optic nerve and pathways. Computed tomography may be indicated in the presence of bone disease (such as fractures of the optic canal). Ultrasonography is also helpful, particularly with lesions of the optic nerve head (such as drusen).

REFERENCES

1. Bakri SJ, Siker D, Masaryk T, Luciano MG, Traboulsi EI. Ocular malformations, moyamoya disease, and midline cranial defects: a distinct syndrome. *Am J Ophthalmol.* 1999;127:356–357.
2. Brodsky MC, Glasier CM. Optic nerve hypoplasia óclinical significance of associated central nervous system abnormalities on magnetic resonance imaging. *Arch Ophthalmol.* 1993;111:66–74.
3. Levin LA, Beck RW, Joseph MP, Seiff S, Kraker R, The International Optic Nerve Trauma Study Group. The treatment of traumatic optic neuropathy. *Ophthalmology.* 1999;106:1268–1277.
4. Listernick R, Ferner RE, Liu GT, Gutmann DH. Optic pathway gliomas in neurofibromatosis 1: controversies and recommendation. *Ann Neurol.* 2007;61:189–198.
5. Beck RW, Cleary PA, Backlund JC, Group TONS. The course of visual recovery after optic neuritis: experience of the optic neuritis treatment trial. *Ophthalmology.* 1994;101:1771–1778.

CHAPTER 34

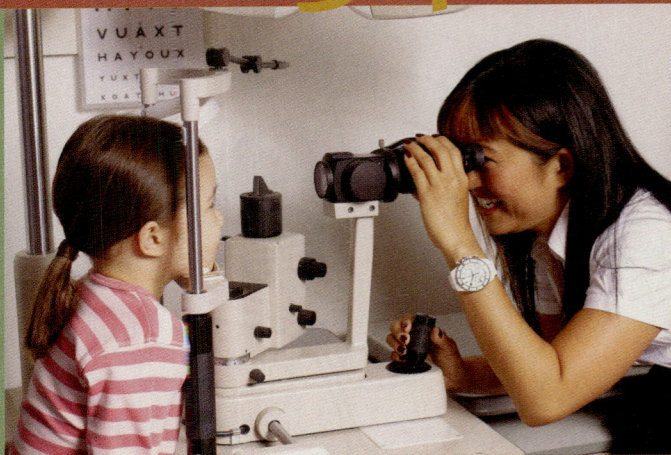

Strabismus, Amblyopia, and Nystagmus

STRABISMUS

Definitions and Epidemiology

Strabismus occurs when the visual axes of the eyes are misaligned. It is one of the most common disorders encountered in pediatric ophthalmology, estimated to affect approximately 3% to 5% of children. The type of strabismus is defined by the direction of misalignment and whether the deviation is latent, intermittent, or constant. A *phoria* describes a latent strabismus that is present when one eye is covered. The eyes return to normal alignment when the eye is uncovered and the patient views under normal binocular viewing conditions. A *tropia* describes strabismus that is present when both eyes are viewing. *Intermittent strabismus* is present when the eyes vary between being misaligned and straight.

When the eyes are horizontally misaligned, they are *esotropic* if they are turned toward each other ("cross-eyed") and *exotropic* if they are directed away from each other ("wall-eyed"). If the eyes are vertically misaligned, the type of strabismus is described by the deviating eye. If the deviating eye is lower than the straight eye, it is *hypotropic*. If it is higher than the straight eye, it is *hypertropic*. Vertical strabismus is much less common than horizontal strabismus in children.

If the eyes are aligned normally, they are *orthophoric*. A deviation is *comitant* if the amount of misalignment does not change in different positions of gaze. This is the most common situation in primary strabismus. A deviation is *incomitant* if the amount of misalignment changes as the eyes move in various directions. This occurs in patients with cranial nerve palsies or other forms of strabismus with limited extraocular movements. Horizontal eye movements are called adduction when the moves in an inward direction and abduction when it moves outward. *Pseudostrabismus* is present when the eyes appear misaligned, but they are optically straight.

Anatomy and Embryology

Eye movements result from contraction of the extraocular muscles. Horizontal movements are produced by the medial and lateral rectus muscles. Vertical movements are produced by the inferior and superior rectus muscles. The superior oblique muscle causes downward and intorsional movements. The inferior oblique muscle causes upward and extorsional movements (Figure 34–1).

Movements of the extraocular muscles are controlled by inputs from the third, fourth, and sixth cranial nerves. The third cranial nerve controls 4 of the 6 extraocular muscles (medial rectus, inferior rectus, superior rectus, and inferior oblique muscles), in addition to the sphincter muscle of the iris and the levator muscle of the eyelid. It begins in the rostral midbrain at the level of the superior colliculus, where it is composed of separate subnuclei that subserve the different muscles controlled by the nerve. The fourth cranial nerve controls the superior oblique muscle. It begins in the caudal midbrain at the level of the inferior colliculus. It has the longest intracranial course of any cranial nerve. The sixth cranial nerve controls the lateral rectus muscle. It begins in the caudal pons adjacent to the fourth ventricle.

The third, fourth, and sixth cranial nerves eventually converge in the cavernous sinus and travel through the orbital fissure to the eye. The third cranial nerve further subdivides into the superior division, which

Superior
oblique m.

Trochlea

Medial
rectus m.

Superior
rectus m.

Lateral
rectus m.

Superior
rectus

Superior
oblique

Medial
rectus

Lateral
rectus

Inferior
oblique

Inferior
rectus

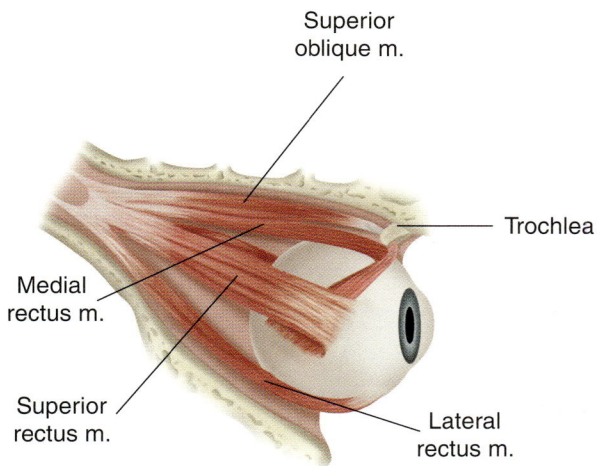

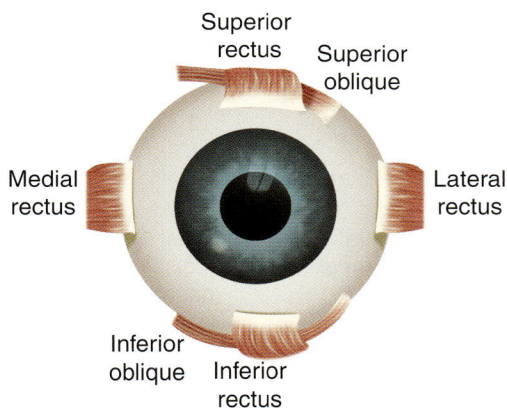

FIGURE 34–1 ■ The extraocular muscles. Top: View of right eye from above. Bottom: Frontal view of left eye.

innervates the superior rectus muscle and the levator muscle of the eyelid, and the inferior division, which innervates the sphincter muscle of the iris and the medial rectus, inferior rectus, and inferior oblique muscles.

Embryology

The extraocular muscles form from mesodermal tissue within the developing orbit. Differentiating muscle cells are present beginning at approximately the fifth week of gestation.

Pathogenesis of Strabismus

Strabismus may be caused by a number of conditions. The eyes are normally maintained in alignment by the binocular vision centers of the brain. Some patients have a latent tendency for the eyes to drift, which man-

ifests when one eye is covered (a phoria). When the eye is uncovered, the binocular vision areas of the brain recognize the misalignment and send signals to the eye muscles to realign the eyes. In the most common forms of childhood strabismus (infantile esotropia and intermittent exotropia), the extraocular muscles themselves are normal. The eyes become deviated due to abnormal signals from the binocular vision and motion processing centers of the brain. *Sensory strabismus* may develop when the vision is decreased (for any reason), and the binocular vision center has less impetus to keep the eyes aligned. In some disorders the eye muscles themselves are abnormal, creating a *restrictive strabismus*.

Cranial nerve palsies may arise from abnormalities occurring anywhere from the cranial nerve nuclei to the sites where the nerves connect to the extraocular muscles. They may be acquired or congenital. Intracranial mass lesions may directly compress a cranial nerve. Increased intracranial pressure alone may also cause dysfunction.

Proper eye alignment is necessary for normal binocular vision. Each eye sends visual information to the occipital cortex. Because the 2 eyes are slightly separate, these images are slightly different. The brain is able to compare the images and evaluate depth (*stereopsis*). If the eyes are misaligned, this binocular activity cannot function. In adults with acquired strabismus, the eye misalignment usually produces *diplopia* (double vision) because the brain is unable to reconcile the disparate images. Unlike adults, most children with strabismus *suppress* (ignore) one of the images rather than experience diplopia.

Clinical Presentation

Strabismus presents with misalignment of the eyes. This is most often first noticed by the parents. Because young children with strabismus usually do not experience diplopia, they usually have no complaints. Older children, particularly those with cranial nerve palsy and no previous history of strabismus, may report that they see 2 images of the same object. Eye deviations must reach a threshold angle to be visible to observers, usually approximately 10°. Angles between 5° and 10° may not be clinically obvious, but have the potential to interrupt binocular vision. Pediatricians may detect small angles of strabismus during well-child visits by noting asymmetry of the corneal light reflex.

Strabismus may present acutely, with the onset of a large deviation occurring over a brief period (days). Alternatively, it may begin intermittently, in which case it often gradually progresses in duration and frequency. Intermittent strabismus is most noticeable when children are fatigued, ill, or daydreaming. In young children with esotropia, the eye crossing is often most noticeable at near, whereas intermittent exotropia is usually more noticeable when the child is viewing distant objects.

The presence of associated signs and symptoms may help discriminate between primary strabismus and strabismus secondary to cranial nerve palsies or other acquired disorders. The specific findings are discussed in the individual sections below.

TYPES OF STRABISMUS

Esotropia

Physiological intermittent esotropia of the newborn

During the first 2 months of life, normal infants may have brief episodes of strabismus. This is most commonly esotropia, but intermittent exotropia may also occur. This should resolve by 3 to 4 months of age. Constant crossing is not normal, even in neonates. Any infant with constant strabismus, or intermittent strabismus that persists beyond 2-3 months of age, should be referred to an ophthalmologist.

Pseudostrabismus

This term refers to a condition in which the eyes appear to be deviated, but the visual axes of the eyes are actually aligned. The most common form is *pseudoesotropia*, in which the eyes appear to be crossed. This is common in infancy, and results from the broad, flat nasal bridge that is a normal feature of most infants' faces. Patients may have *epicanthal folds*, folds of tissue of the inner eyelid. Epicanthal folds block visualization of the normal white inner sclera, which creates an optical illusion in which the eyes appear to be crossed. The esotropia appears to be worse when the child looks to the side, because more of the white of the eye is blocked (Figure 34–2A and B). Pseudostrabismus is diagnosed by finding a symmetric corneal light reflex despite the appearance of eye crossing. Ophthalmological consultation may be indicated if the diagnosis is uncertain. The diagnosis is confirmed if no strabismus is found with cover testing and normal binocular vision responses are present.

A less common form of pseudostrabismus is *pseudoexotropia*. In one type of this condition the fovea of one eye is displaced temporally, most commonly due to retinopathy of prematurity (with dragging of the fovea toward the temporal retina). Because the fovea is displaced, the eye must rotate laterally to bring the fovea into alignment with the visual axis (Figure 34–3). The eye therefore appears exotropic, and the corneal light reflex is decentered nasally. This is known as *positive angle kappa*. The diagnosis is established by the absence of any shift of the eyes with an alternate cover test, which indicates that there is no ocular misalignment (Figure 34–4A–C).

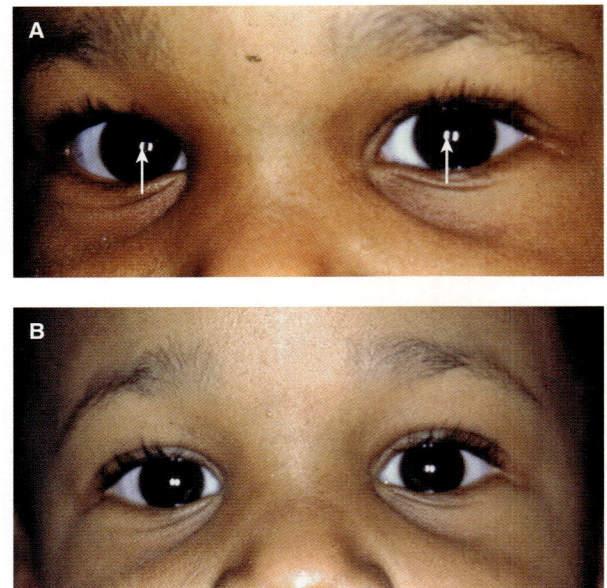

FIGURE 34–2 ■ Pseudoesotropia. (A) The right eye appears crossed when the child looks to the left. The corneal light reflexes are equal (arrows). (B) The appearance of crossing is minimal when the child looks straight ahead (the corneal light reflexes remain symmetric).

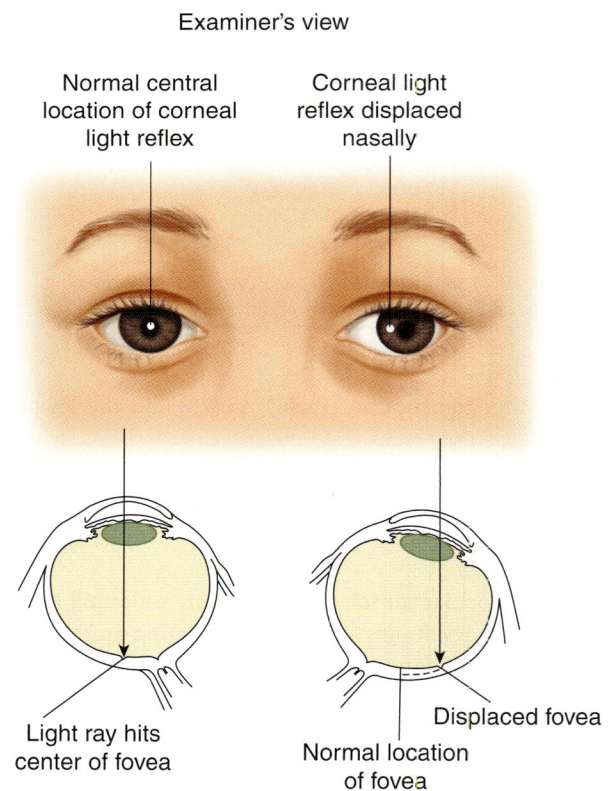

FIGURE 34–3 ■ Positive angle kappa, a form of pseudostrabismus that often results from an abnormal location of the fovea. In the left eye the fovea is displaced temporally. The eye therefore turns outward in order for light to focus on the displaced fovea, creating the appearance of exotropia.

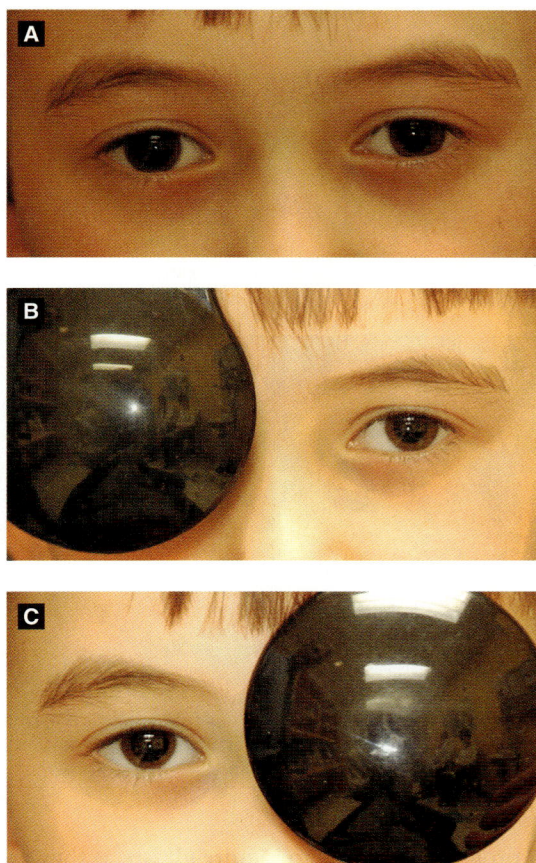

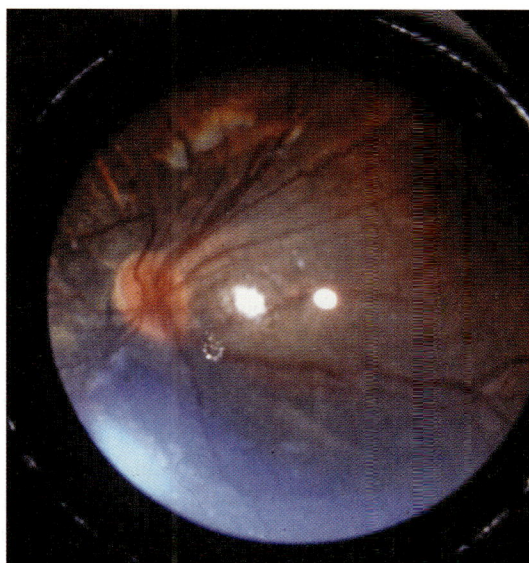

FIGURE 34–5 ■ Dragged fovea due to retinopathy of prematurity. The retinal blood vessels are pulled toward the temporal retina (to the right in this photograph), displacing the fovea temporally.

FIGURE 34–4 ■ Pseudoexotropia (positive angle kappa). (A) The left eye appears slightly exotropic, and the left corneal light reflex is nasal to the center of the cornea. There is no change in the reflex and the eyes do not move when (B) the right eye is covered or (C) the left eye is covered. This confirms the diagnosis of pseudostrabismus.

latent nystagmus (the patient develops nystagmus when one eye is covered, with the nystagmus appearing to beat toward the uncovered eye).

There is a genetic component to infantile esotropia, but it is not inherited as a classic mendelian trait. A history of infantile esotropia in other family members helps in establishing a diagnosis. Infantile esotropia also occurs more commonly in conditions such as prematurity, Trisomy 21, and other disorders associated with developmental delay.

Visible changes of the retina may be noted with ophthalmoscopy (Figure 34–5), but some children with pseudoexotropia have normal retinas.

Infantile esotropia

Infantile esotropia is not present at birth, but usually is first noted within the first 2 months of life. It may start intermittently, but rapidly progresses to constant crossing. If only one of the eyes is constantly crossed, infants develop amblyopia. This occurs in approximately half of affected patients. If the crossing spontaneously alternates, this indicates that the vision in both eyes is equal or nearly equal (Figure 34–6A and B). Some infants with large deviations have *cross-fixation*. This means that the child uses the crossed left eye to view things on their right side and the crossed right eye to view things on their left side. Other eye movement abnormalities in patients with infantile esotropia include smooth pursuit asymmetry (the eye moves more evenly when tracking objects from lateral to central gaze than vice versa) and

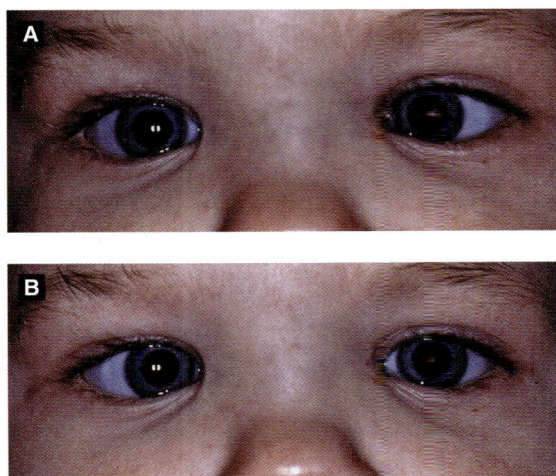

FIGURE 34–6 ■ Infantile esotropia with alternate fixation. (A) The patient is using the right eye and the left eye is crossed. (B) During the examination, the patient spontaneously shifts fixation to the left eye and the right eye becomes crossed. This indicates that the vision is equal or nearly equal between the eyes.

The goal of treatment of infantile esotropia (and, indeed, of all strabismus therapy) is to align the eyes so that binocular vision can function. The infant brain has plasticity. In general, the more promptly the eyes are realigned the better the outcome. However, even with good alignment, children with infantile esotropia almost never develop the same degree of binocular vision and depth perception that normal individuals have. Usually the best outcome is *monofixation syndrome*, in which the eyes are closely, but not perfectly, aligned and there is some degree of binocular vision.

The most common treatment for infantile esotropia is surgery, specifically weakening of the medial rectus muscles. For strabismus in general, and infantile esotropia in particular, the need for more than one surgery is common, with approximately one-third of patients requiring 2 or more procedures. Reasons a patient may need additional surgery include recurrent esotropia, *consecutive exotropia* (exotropia that develops after treatment of esotropia), or vertical misalignment (*dissociated vertical deviation* and *inferior oblique muscle overaction*—discussed below in the section on vertical strabismus).

Accommodative esotropia

Almost all children in the first few years of life are farsighted (*hyperopic*). This means that the lens of the eye must change its shape to focus (*accommodation*). This is easily accomplished in normal children with typical mild farsightedness. In addition to lens focusing, the *accommodative response* consists of inward movement of the eyes and constriction of the pupils. In normal patients the degree of inward movement corresponds appropriately to the amount of focus needed to view near objects. If the eyes are more farsighted than normal (which occurs in accommodative esotropia), the increased effort required to focus the image may be accompanied by a greater-than-normal convergence of the eyes, which produces esotropia. This can be explained to the parents as "the eyes cross because they have to focus too much."

Accommodative esotropia may develop in infancy, but usually begins after 1 year of age. It typically gradually worsens over 1 to 2 months. It is initially intermittent and most noticeable when children are viewing near objects (due to the increased focusing requirement at near). The diagnosis is established by measuring the degree of farsightedness after using dilating drops that prevent accommodation (cycloplegic refraction) and noting resolution of the esotropia when the children wear glasses to correct the farsightedness (Figure 34–7A and B).

Normal farsightedness in young children usually decreases with age. The farsightedness in children with accommodative esotropia often does not resolve, and usually changes very little as children grow older. It is important that the parents of children with accommodative esotropia understand that their child

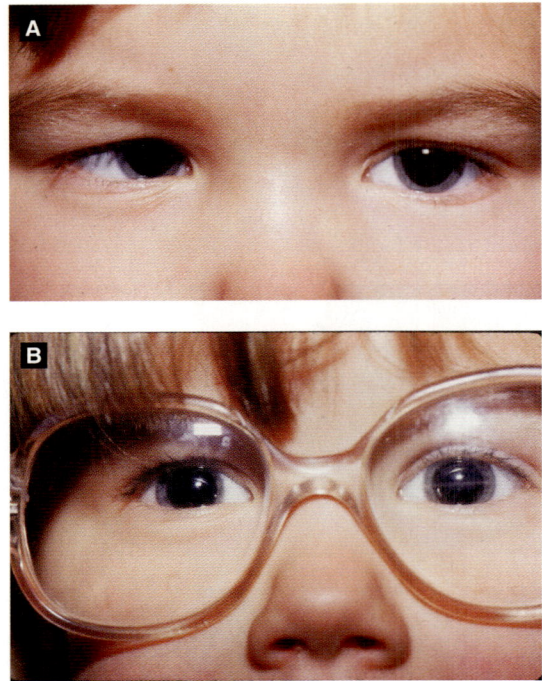

FIGURE 34–7 ■ Accommodative esotropia. The patient is hyperopic (farsighted). (A) The right eye crosses when the patient does not wear glasses. (B) The eyes are straight when glasses are worn.

will probably continue to require glasses as they grow older, and that the eyes will usually continue to cross when they are not wearing their glasses (such as while bathing or at bedtime).

Mixed mechanism esotropia

Some children have features of both infantile and accommodative esotropia. In these patients the eye crossing improves while wearing spectacles, but does not fully resolve. The treatment is surgery to correct the portion of the esotropia that persists while the glasses are worn.

Acute esotropia in older children

A less common form of esotropia develops relatively rapidly in older children (3–5 years or older). This may occur spontaneously, or after a period of occlusion of one eye (for example, when one eyelid is swollen shut after trauma or an insect bite). In most such patients the esotropia is thought to result from a previously unrecognized small-angle strabismus, which decompensates to a constant deviation. However, the possibility of an intracranial lesion or other disorder responsible for the strabismus must be considered in this situation. The absence of associated neurological symptoms and a positive family history of strabismus make this less likely. A comitant deviation (the angle of esotropia does not change in lateral gaze) also is reassuring, because this indicates that a sixth cranial nerve palsy is not present. However, acute comitant esotropia has been reported in older children with Arnold-Chiari malformation or central nervous system (CNS) tumors.[1] The presence of gaze limitation due to sixth nerve palsy (with incomitant strabismus), nystagmus, pupil defects, or optic nerve changes suggests an underlying CNS abnormality.

Imaging of the CNS (usually magnetic resonance imaging [MRI]) is sometimes performed in older children with acute esotropia due to the possibility of associated abnormalities. If no other problems are found, prompt surgical alignment of the eyes is indicated. The prognosis for improvement in binocular vision after successful surgical restoration is better than in patients with infantile esotropia.[2]

Sixth cranial nerve palsy

This is discussed below in the section on cranial nerve palsies.

Cyclic esotropia

Cyclic esotropia is a very unusual form of strabismus in which the eye alignment varies between straight and large-angle esotropia. In most children the cycles alternate daily (i.e., the eyes are straight one day and crossed the next). When the eyes are straight, the depth perception is usually normal. The patients are usually otherwise healthy. The condition responds well to surgery, with the amount of correction based on the angle of esotropia that is present on the day the eyes cross.

Exotropia

Intermittent exotropia

Intermittent exotropia is present when the eye varies between straight and outwardly deviated (Figure 34–8). It usually begins in children after 1 year of age. As the name denotes, it starts as an intermittent strabismus, but with time it may progress to a constant deviation.

There are 3 important differences between infantile esotropia and intermittent exotropia in terms of their effects on vision:

- First, amblyopia is uncommon in intermittent exotropia. Most patients have normal vision in both eyes.
- Second, when the eyes are aligned, the depth perception is usually normal (unlike infantile esotropia, in

which the binocular vision is subnormal even after successful surgical realignment).

- Third, unlike infantile esotropia, in which there is a higher incidence in patients with developmental delay, most children with intermittent exotropia are developmentally normal. An important exception to this, however, is intermittent exotropia that develops within the first year of life, which is associated with an increased incidence of developmental delay[3]

The decision regarding timing of treatment for intermittent exotropia is based on the degree and frequency of the strabismus. The visual acuity in most patients is normal. If amblyopia or a significant refractive error is found, treatment of the amblyopia and the refractive error is initiated. If this does not improve the strabismus, surgery may be considered. In general, if the family reports progressive strabismus, and the examination shows an easily elicited strabismus that the patient has difficulty controlling, surgery is recommended.

Convergence insufficiency

This is a specific type of intermittent exotropia that usually does not develop until later in childhood, often during the teenage years. In convergence insufficiency the exotropia is greater when viewing near objects, particularly with reading. Patients may report diplopia, but more commonly describe vague symptoms of eye fatigue or strain (*asthenopia*) with prolonged reading. Examination reveals good alignment when viewing distant objects and an intermittent exotropia when fixating on a near object. This type of strabismus may improve with orthoptic exercises to improve convergence.[ ] Surgery may be indicated if symptoms persist despite exercises.

Sensory strabismus

If a patient has decreased vision in one eye due to a structural abnormality of the eye, there is an increased risk of strabismus developing in that eye. Sensory strabismus can also develop if patients have an ocular disorder that affects both eyes (Figure 34–9). Any ocular

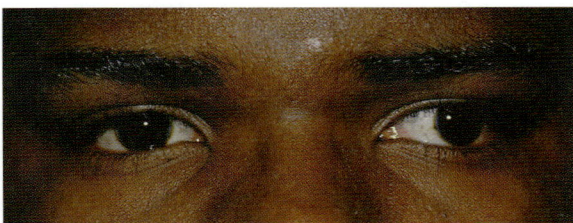

FIGURE 34–8 ■ Left exotropia.

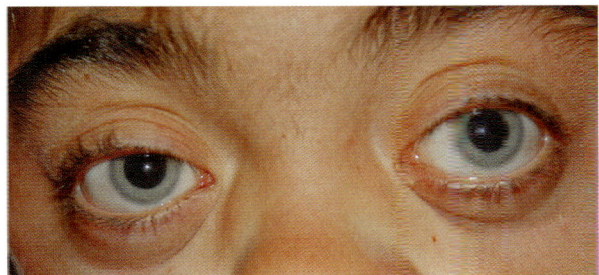

FIGURE 34–9 ■ Left exotropia in a patient with bilateral corneal clouding due to mucopolysaccharidosis.

condition that causes decreased vision may cause strabismus. In young children sensory strabismus is most commonly esotropia. In older children and adults, it is most commonly exotropia. In patients with sensory strabismus the strabismus is usually constant, the vision is decreased, and the underlying ocular defect is found on examination. Although most children with eye misalignment do not have sensory strabismus, every patient with strabismus requires a complete ophthalmic examination to rule out the presence of structural eye abnormalities.

Vertical Strabismus

Dissociated vertical deviation and inferior oblique muscle overaction

These 2 forms of vertical strabismus are usually seen in patients with infantile esotropia. They are the most common type of vertical strabismus in children. They are usually not present in early infancy (when the babies first present with infantile esotropia), but develop later during the first 1 to 2 years of life. They occur more frequently in patients whose esotropia is not corrected, but may also develop in patients whose horizontal misalignment has been successfully surgically repaired.

Dissociated vertical deviation is an intermittent slow updrifting of the eye. *Inferior oblique muscle overaction* (also termed overelevation in adduction) is an elevation of the eye when it is turned toward the nose (Figure 34–10A and B). Both forms of strabismus benefit from surgical correction. A history of infantile esotropia helps distinguish inferior oblique muscle overaction from superior oblique palsy, which has some of the same characteristics (see below).

Brown syndrome

Brown syndrome is an unusual form of vertical strabismus that results from an abnormality of the superior oblique tendon. The superior oblique muscle begins in the orbit posteriorly. Anteriorly it becomes a tendon and travels to the anterior superior portion of the orbit, where it passes through the *trochlea*. It then travels posteriorly along the superior portion of the eye to insert laterally beneath the superior rectus muscle (Figure 34–11). Contraction of the superior oblique muscle normally creates a downward movement when the eye moves toward the nose. Contraction of the inferior oblique muscle normally creates a superior movement in this direction. In order for the eye to elevate in response to inferior oblique muscle contraction, the superior oblique tendon must be able to relax and move freely through the trochlea.

In Brown syndrome, the superior oblique tendon becomes restricted, limiting elevation of the eye when it is turned in (Figure 34–12A and B). Elevation is usually better when the eye is looking up and straight ahead,

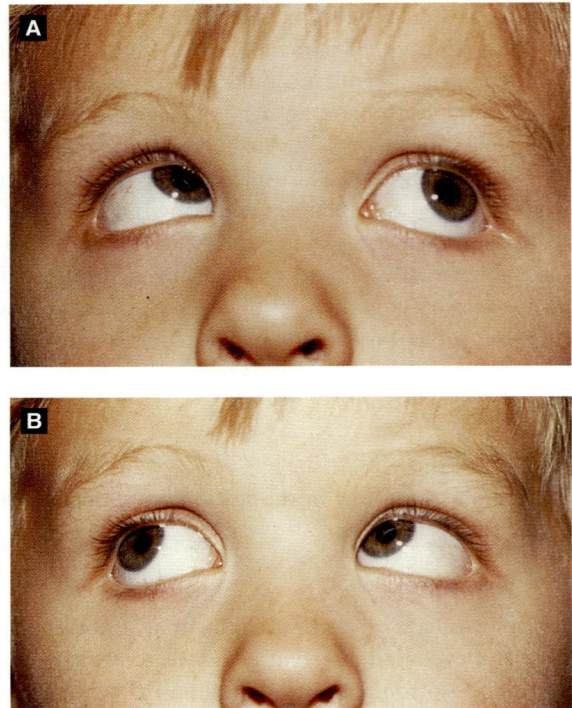

FIGURE 34–10 ■ Inferior oblique muscle overaction (seen frequently seen in patients with a history of infantile esotropia). (A) The right eye is more elevated than the left eye when the patient looks to the left. (B) The left eye is more elevated than the right eye when the patient looks to the right. Note that the corneal light reflexes are unequal (lower on the corneas of the elevated eyes).

and normal when it is looking up and out. The diagnosis of Brown syndrome is confirmed by noting restriction of the superior oblique tendon when manually rotating the eye (which is done under anesthesia at the time of surgery in children).

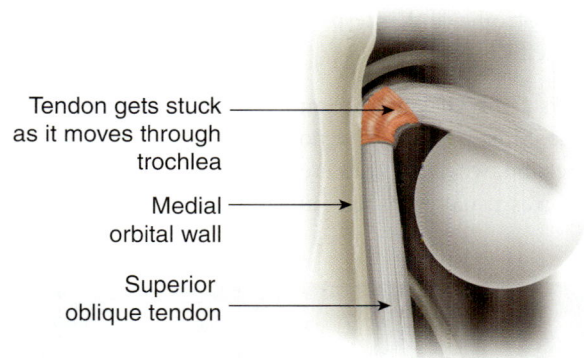

Tendon gets stuck as it moves through trochlea

Medial orbital wall

Superior oblique tendon

FIGURE 34–11 ■ Superior view of right orbit. The superior oblique tendon normally slides freely through the trochlea, like a pulley. In Brown syndrome, the tendon gets stuck when it attempts to relax and move through the trochlea, causing inability of the eye to elevate when it is turned toward the nose.

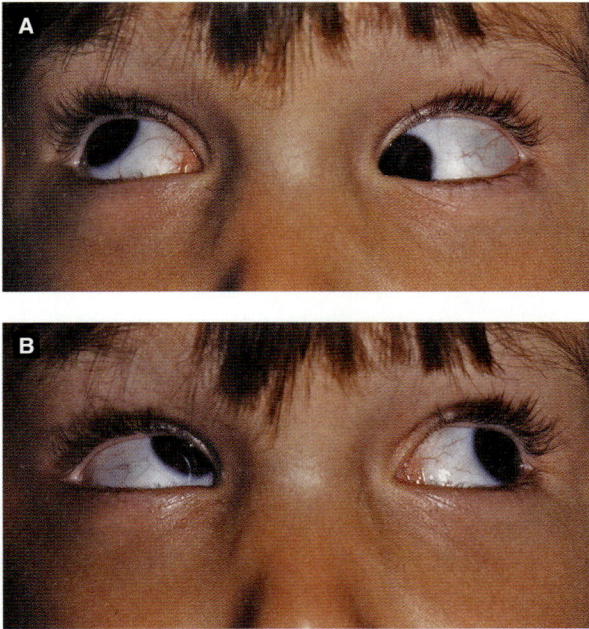

FIGURE 34–12 ■ Brown syndrome, left eye. (A) The patient is asked to look up and to the right. The right eye elevates normally and the left eye cannot elevate at all. (B) In left upgaze, the elevation of the left eye is near normal.

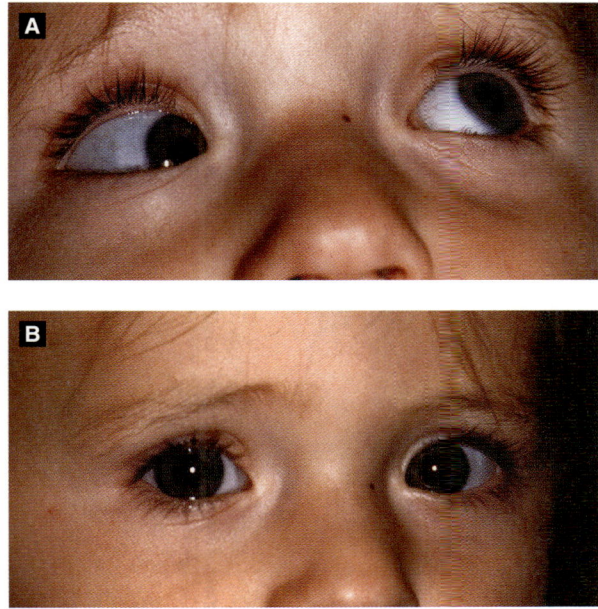

FIGURE 34–13 ■ Brown syndrome, right eye, with compensatory head turn. (A) The right eye cannot move normally when the patient looks up and to the left. (B) The patient develops a compensatory left head turn to keep the right eye outward (away from the area where its movement is restricted).

Brown syndrome is usually idiopathic, but may occur due to trauma or inflammation in the area of the trochlea. In some patients, an audible click may be heard when the patient attempts to move the eye up and in, due to movement of the restricted tendon through the trochlea. Many patients with Brown syndrome have minimal clinical problems because the misalignment only occurs when the patients look in eccentric gaze positions.

Treatment for Brown syndrome is indicated if vertical strabismus is present when the patient is looking straight ahead or if the patient adopts an abnormal head posture to avoid the gaze positions that cause problems (for instance, if the patient had a right Brown syndrome, the restriction would be most noticeable when the patient looked to the left and up; therefore, they might place their chin up to avoid upgaze, or turn their head to the left to keep their eyes to the right) (Figure 34–13A and B). In most patients who require treatment, surgical lengthening of the tendon is performed. If inflammation is present, corticosteroid injections into the area of the trochlea may improve the restriction.

Monocular elevation deficiency (double elevator palsy)

In monocular elevation deficiency (MED), the eye cannot elevate in any position (unlike Brown syndrome, in which limited elevation occurs only when the eye is turned nasally). The limited upgaze usually results from a supranuclear inability to generate normal upward movement signals. The affected eye is usually hypotropic (down), and patients may adopt a chin-up head posture to use the eyes together (Figure 34–14A and B). Ptosis is also present in many patients. In long-standing MED, the inferior rectus muscle often becomes tight, which mechanically limits upward movement of the eye. If the inferior muscle is tight, surgical correction usually requires loosening of the muscle. If it is not tight, upward transposition of the lateral and medial rectus muscles is usually performed to generate an upward force on the eye.

Orbital blow-out fracture

Patients who suffer significant ocular trauma may develop strabismus. This rarely is due to direct injury to an extraocular muscle, such as might be caused by a muscle laceration from a sharp penetrating object. More commonly, it is due to muscle restriction associated with fractures of the orbital bones, particularly the floor of the orbit. If the inferior rectus muscle becomes entrapped in the fracture, upward movement of the eye is limited, and patients experience diplopia when they attempt to look superiorly. This is sometimes accompanied by nausea and vomiting due to the oculocardiac reflex.

In the immediate posttraumatic period, extraocular muscle movements may be restricted due to hemorrhage or edema. Imaging studies are indicated to rule out a fracture. If no fracture is present, the strabismus

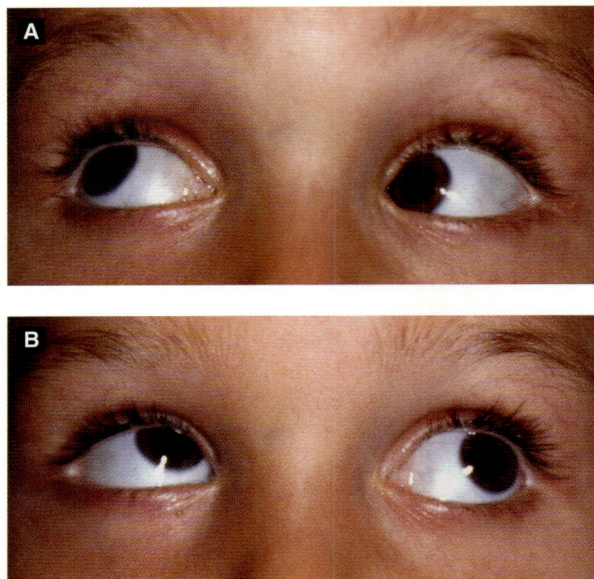

FIGURE 34–14 ■ Monocular elevation syndrome, left eye. The left eye cannot move up in either (A) right gaze or (B) left gaze.

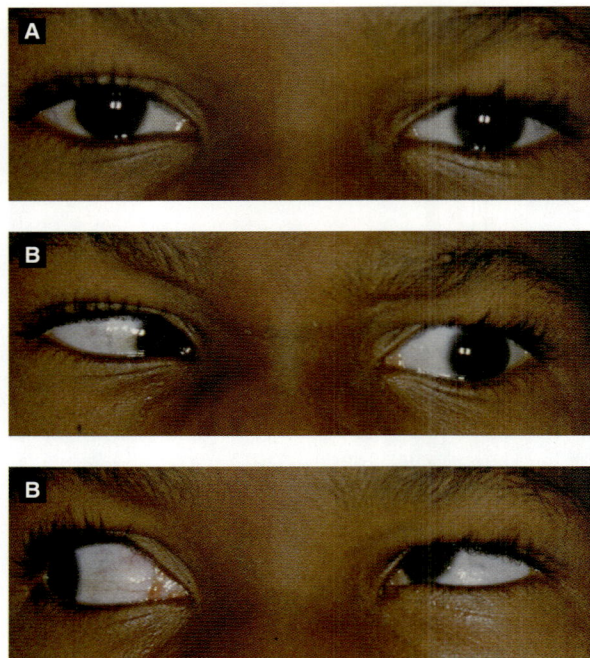

FIGURE 34–15 ■ Duane retraction syndrome, left eye. (A) The eyes are straight when the patient looks straight ahead. (B) In left gaze, there is limited outward movement of the left eye. (C) When the patient looks to the right, the space between the left eyelids (palpebral fissure) narrows due to retraction of the eye into the globe, and the left eye becomes vertically elevated (upshoot).

often resolves with time. If a fracture is present, patients are observed for 1 to 2 weeks to see whether the motility improves. Surgery may be necessary if the strabismus persists.

In children, orbital floor fractures sometimes cause acute incarceration of the muscle within the fracture. The eye in these patients usually has only mild signs of trauma. Marked restriction of elevation is present, usually accompanied by nausea and bradycardia (*white-eyed blowout fracture*). These patients require urgent surgical repair due to the risk of extraocular muscle ischemia and necrosis.

Fourth cranial nerve palsy

This is discussed below in the section on cranial nerve palsies.

Other Forms of Strabismus

Duane retraction syndrome

Duane retraction syndrome (DRS) results from miswiring of the nerves that control the extraocular muscles. It produces a strabismus characterized by limitation of eye movements. In the most common form of DRS the nucleus of the sixth cranial nerve is hypoplastic, and the lateral rectus muscle is not innervated properly. The eye does not turn out in attempted lateral gaze, which usually produces an esotropia. When the eye moves nasally, both the lateral and medial rectus muscles of the affected eye contract, which pulls the eye posteriorly into the orbit (globe retraction). This causes narrowing of the space between the eyelids (the palpebral fissure)

(Figure 34–15A–C). Vertical misalignment may also occur, most commonly an upshoot of the eye when it is turned toward the nose (Figure 34–15C). In some forms of DRS, inward movement of the eye is limited.

Most cases of DRS are sporadic and idiopathic. Familial cases may occur, and DRS is associated with intrauterine thalidomide exposure and some syndromes (Goldenhar, Wildervanck). Surgical treatment of DRS is indicated if patients have strabismus when looking straight ahead or they develop an abnormal head posture to compensate for the strabismus. The affected muscles in DRS are usually tight. Surgery consists of either loosening the tight muscles or transposing the vertical rectus muscles to generate horizontal eye movements.

Mobius syndrome

Mobius syndrome is a rare congenital abnormality in which affected children appear to have sixth and seventh cranial nerve palsies. They have a characteristic expressionless face due to the seventh nerve involvement (Figure 34–16). They usually have esotropia with limited outward movements of the eye. Clinically, the strabismus has features more suggestive of DRS than sixth nerve palsy (Figure 34–17A and B). The syndrome may be isolated or associated with limb anomalies. Surgical treatment of the strabismus requires loosening of the restricted medial rectus muscles.

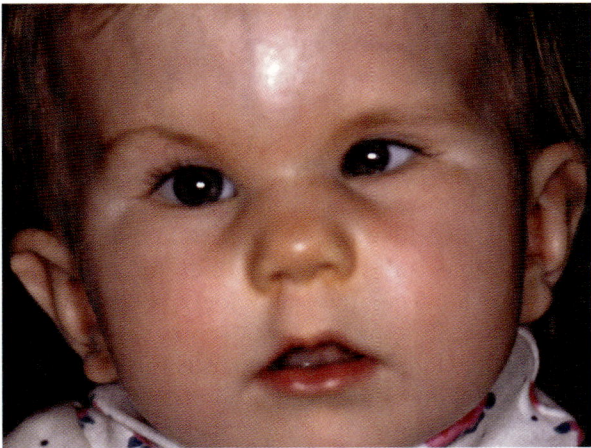

FIGURE 34–16 ■ Mobius syndrome. The patient has left esotropia and decreased contraction of the perioral muscles.

Congenital fibrosis of the extraocular muscles

This condition is characterized by early-onset, progressive restriction of the extraocular muscles, frequently in association with ptosis. Congenital fibrosis of the extraocular muscles is usually inherited as an autosomal dominant disorder. Recent studies have demonstrated that hypoplasia of the cranial nerve nuclei and dysinnervation are the likely causes of the disorder.[5] The inferior rectus muscle is most commonly affected, but

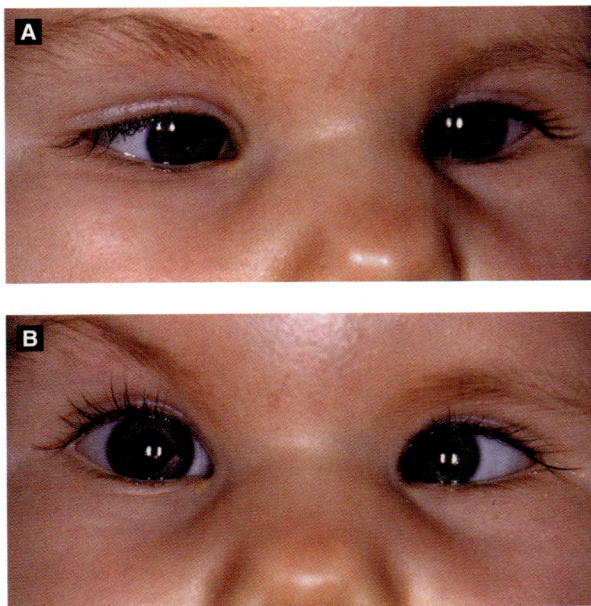

FIGURE 34–17 ■ Strabismus in Mobius syndrome. (A) In left gaze the left eye does not move fully outward, creating a right esotropia. (B) In right gaze, the right eye does not move fully outward, creating a left esotropia. Note also that the space between the eyelids (palpebral fissures) is narrower in the right eye when it looks to the left and the left eye when it looks to the right, similar to the globe retraction seen in Duane retraction syndrome.

multiple muscles may be involved. Surgical loosening of the restricted muscles is indicated if significant strabismus is present. Improvement is usually limited by the underlying muscle abnormalities.

Thyroid ophthalmopathy (Graves disease)

Thyroid ophthalmopathy is much more common in adults than in children. The ocular problems result from an autoimmune process that produces edema and inflammation of the extraocular muscles. In severe cases this may produce proptosis and compressive optic neuropathy. Strabismus results from restriction of the muscles, most commonly the inferior and medial rectus muscles. The disorder is associated with thyroid dysfunction, but the ocular abnormalities are not directly caused by abnormal thyroid hormone levels. The systemic and ocular symptoms often do not correlate. Surgical treatment of strabismus is usually delayed until the active inflammation subsides. It consists of loosening of the restricted muscles.

Myasthenia gravis

Myasthenia gravis (MG) is a disorder in which autoantibodies are directed against the acetylcholine receptors of muscles. Up to half of patients have systemic muscle involvement. Ocular effects include strabismus and ptosis (Figure 34–18). In neonates MG may occur due to transplacental transfer of antibodies, in which case spontaneous improvement should occur as the maternal antibodies are cleared.

The eye movement abnormalities associated with MG are extremely variable, and may mimic virtually any form of strabismus. Symptoms are usually worse later in the day and when the patient is fatigued. Patients with thyroid ophthalmopathy are at increased risk for developing MG, which can complicate the diagnosis.

MG is suspected when the strabismus improves after rest or an ice application. Diagnostic tests include electromyography, measurement of antiacetylcholine receptor antibodies, and improvement in the eye movements with administration of acetylcholinesterase

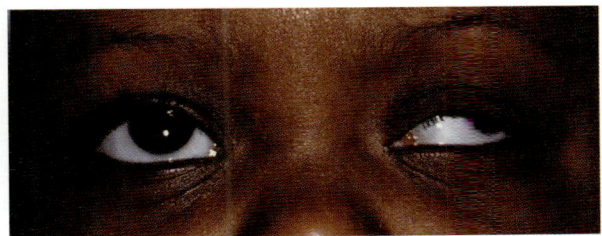

FIGURE 34–18 ■ Left exotropia and ptosis in a patient with myasthenia gravis. Note the left brow elevation the patient uses in attempt to elevate the eyelid.

inhibitors (edrophonium or neostigmine). Some patients have enlarged thymus glands, in which case thymectomy may be beneficial. Other treatment options include acetylcholinesterase inhibitors, corticosteroids, and other immunosuppressants.

Cranial Nerve Palsies

Third cranial nerve (oculomotor nerve) palsy

The third cranial nerve innervates 4 of the 6 extraocular muscles (the medial rectus, inferior rectus, inferior oblique, and superior rectus muscles), the eyelid levator muscle, and the pupil. Clinically, complete third cranial nerve palsies presents with the eye out and down (out because of preserved innervation of the lateral rectus muscle and down because of preserved innervation of the superior oblique muscle), ptosis, and a dilated pupil (Figure 34–19). If the palsy is incomplete, there may be some residual movement of the muscles. Rarely only one of the divisions of the third cranial nerve is involved, implying a lesion in the cavernous sinus or orbit. In superior division palsies, patients have ptosis and inability to elevate the eye. In inferior division palsies, the eye is exotropic and the pupil is dilated. The vertical alignment varies, depending on the amount of activity of the superior rectus, superior oblique, and inferior oblique muscles.

The most common etiology of third cranial nerve palsy in children is congenital. In these patients (and also in patients with traumatic palsies), aberrant regeneration of the nerves may occur, which produces unusual movements of the eyes in different directions (for instance, the eyelid might elevate on attempted downgaze). The pupil in many congenital cases is often small, rather than dilated. Other etiologies for third cranial nerve palsies include CNS mass lesions, trauma, postviral or postvaccination reactions, and ophthalmoplegic migraine.

Patients with acute onset of third cranial nerve palsies require an evaluation to look for underlying abnormalities. This most commonly begins with an MRI. Magnetic resonance angiography is sometimes performed to look for an aneurysm. This is an unusual problem in children compared to adults, in whom aneurysms of the posterior communicating artery are a common cause of third cranial nerve palsy.

A period of observation is usually allowed for patients with strabismus due to third cranial nerve palsies. Palsies associated with migraine or postviral phenomenon often improve over the course of several months. If the strabismus does not resolve, surgery may be indicated. Surgery for complete third cranial nerve palsies is among the most difficult problems in strabismus because only 2 of the 6 extraocular muscles function. Treatment usually includes maximal weakening of the lateral rectus muscle and medial transposition of the superior oblique tendon (to create some inward and upward pulling force). Normal eye movements can almost never be restored. The goal of surgery is to improve alignment when the eye looks straight ahead.

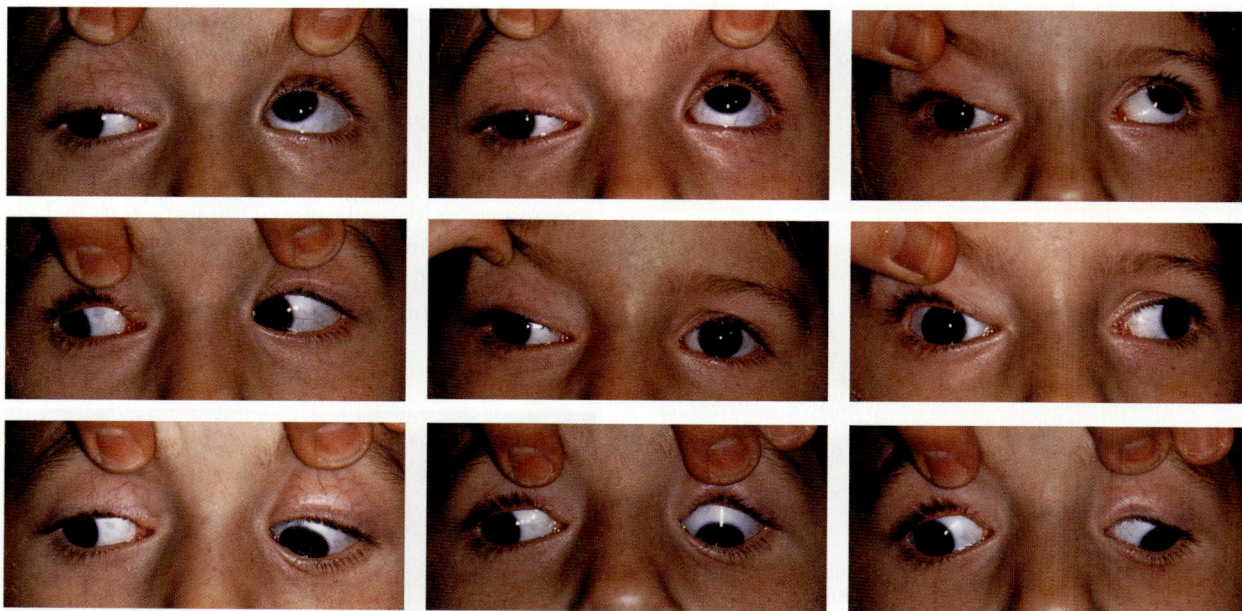

FIGURE 34–19 ■ Eye movements in a patient with a third cranial nerve palsy. The photos show the patient attempting to look in the cardinal positions of gaze. The left eye movements are normal. In the center photo the patient is looking straight ahead. The right eye can only make slight outward and downward movements (due to preserved function of the sixth and fourth cranial nerves). The patient has marked right ptosis and the eyelid is manually elevated so that the eye movements can be visualized.

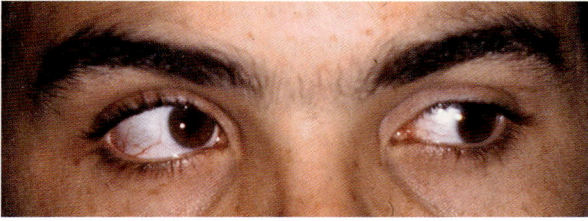

FIGURE 34–20 ■ Fourth cranial nerve palsy, right eye. The right eye cannot fully depress when the patient attempts to look down and to the left (the left eye is moving normally).

Fourth cranial nerve (superior oblique) palsy

After dissociated vertical deviation and inferior oblique muscle overaction associated with infantile esotropia, superior oblique palsy is the next most common cause of vertical strabismus in children. It results from paresis of the fourth cranial nerve, which supplies the superior oblique muscle. This produces weakness of depression of the eye when it is turned nasally (Figure 34–20). Usually overaction of the inferior oblique muscle (elevation of the eye when it is turned nasally) is more obvious than the weakness of the superior oblique muscle (decreased depression when the eye is turned nasally). The function of the superior oblique muscle is such that the vertical misalignment increases when the head is tilted toward the side of the palsy. Therefore, patients may present with a compensatory head tilt to the opposite side, which they adopt to maintain their binocular vision.

An interesting, and unexplained, feature of superior oblique palsy in children is that most patients are otherwise healthy and do not have intracranial abnormalities to account for the palsy. It is assumed that the palsy in these patients is long-standing, even congenital. The head tilt may not develop for many years, sometimes not until adulthood. Except for the strabismus, this condition is usually benign.

Although most fourth cranial nerve palsies in children are not associated with intracranial lesions, this possibility must still be considered. A long history of a head tilt is reassuring. However, in some patients the head tilt may occur so regularly that the family no longer notices it. Examination of old photographs in such instances may reveal that the tilt dates to early childhood. Another reassuring sign is the ability of the patient to control the vertical deviation. Normal individuals can only tolerate a small vertical misalignment of the eyes before diplopia develops. Patients with congenital superior oblique palsy usually have large deviations that can be elicited with cover testing, but which they control once both eyes are open and binocular vision is reestablished. Nevertheless, there is always a concern in such patients that a CNS lesion may be causing the palsy. The presence of other neurological symptoms (headache, nausea), papilledema, or associated neurological abnormalities would suggest such a lesion. If the child is otherwise well and the examination otherwise normal, then a congenital superior oblique palsy without CNS abnormalities is the likely diagnosis, and additional work-up is not necessary (Table 34–1).

Surgical treatment of the strabismus in patients with fourth cranial nerve palsies is usually required to restore normal alignment and allow the patient to function normally without a head tilt. This consists of either weakening the overacting inferior oblique muscle or strengthening the weak superior oblique tendon. In some patients who have strictly unilateral superior oblique palsy, a similar palsy will develop in the opposite eye after surgical correction of the first eye (*masked bilateral superior oblique palsy*). If a patient is found to have a CNS abnormality, surgical treatment of the strabismus is delayed until the underlying disorder is addressed.

Sixth cranial nerve (abducens) palsy

The sixth cranial nerve innervates the lateral rectus muscle. Acute sixth cranial nerve paresis presents with

Table 34–1.

Worrisome Versus Reassuring Features of Fourth Nerve Palsy

	Worrisome	Reassuring
Age of onset	Older age	Birth or infancy
Head tilt	Acute onset	Long-standing
Diplopia	Yes	No or mild/intermittent
Other neurological symptoms	Yes	No
Papilledema	Yes	No
Ability to control strabismus	No	Excellent

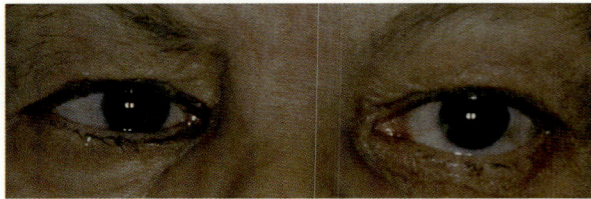

FIGURE 34–21 ■ Left sixth nerve palsy. The patient is looking to the left, and the left eye cannot move out beyond the midline. The right eye is moving normally.

a large esotropia due to inability to move the eye outward (Figure 34–21). Partial palsies present with smaller angles of strabismus and variable limitation of outward movement of the eye. The presence of increasing esotropia when the eye looks in the direction of the palsy is suggestive of a sixth cranial nerve palsy (compared with the usual comitant esotropia in childhood, in which the angle of strabismus is the same when the patient is looking straight ahead and in side gaze). Older children with acute sixth cranial nerve palsies usually complain of horizontal diplopia. Patients often turn their head toward the side of the palsy to avoid double vision (by lining the palsied eye up with the normal eye).

Sixth cranial nerve palsies may present in newborns, in which case they usually resolve spontaneously. In older children with acute sixth cranial nerve palsies, imaging studies are usually indicated to rule out an intracranial lesion. Patients with increased intracranial pressure (such as idiopathic intracranial hypertension) may have diplopia due to sixth cranial nerve palsy as part of their presentation. In approximately two-thirds of patients with sixth cranial nerve palsies no other abnormalities are found. These often develop after viral infections and are hypothesized to represent an autoimmune phenomenon.

The ocular motility abnormalities in Duane retraction syndrome (DRS) may appear similar to those due to a sixth cranial nerve palsy. In both disorders the patient is esotropic and unable to move their eye out. *Although DRS is congenital, it may not be noticed unless the eye movements are studied carefully. This occasionally occurs when a child is evaluated after a traumatic event, such as a motor vehicle accident, and DRS may be mistaken for a sixth cranial nerve palsy.* In such cases, unnecessary imaging studies may be avoided if the diagnosis of DRS is established. Features that help distinguish these 2 disorders include the degree of esotropia (very large in acute sixth cranial nerve palsies and usually small to moderate in DRS) and associated findings of DRS (eyelid retraction and vertical upshoots when the eye moves nasally) (Table 34–2).

Patients with postviral and traumatic sixth cranial nerve palsies often spontaneously improve over the course of several months. Patching may be needed during the recovery process to prevent amblyopia in young patients. If the palsy does not improve, surgery may be performed. If there is partial recovery of function, a combination of weakening the medial rectus muscle and strengthening the lateral rectus muscle is performed. If a complete paralysis persists, the inferior and superior oblique rectus muscles may be transposed laterally to generate an outward-pulling force on the eye.

STRABISMUS SURGERY

Simply put, strabismus surgery consists of either weakening or strengthening of the extraocular muscles. For the horizontal muscles (medial rectus muscle and lateral rectus muscle) and the vertical muscles (superior rectus and inferior rectus muscles), this consists of *recessions* to weaken the muscles and *resections* to strengthen the muscles (Figure 34–22). In both procedures, the

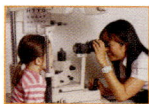

Table 34–2.

Sixth Cranial Nerve Palsy Versus Duane Retraction Syndrome

	Sixth Cranial Nerve Palsy	Duane Retraction Syndrome
Inability to move eye laterally	Yes	Yes
Age of onset	Any age	Birth (though may not be noticed in infancy)
Compensatory head turn	Yes (acute onset)	Yes (long-standing)
Angle of esotropia	Large	Small or moderate
Narrowing of eyelid fissures when affected eye turns in	No	Yes
Upshoot of affected eye when eye turns in	No	Some patients
Other neurological symptoms	Possible	No

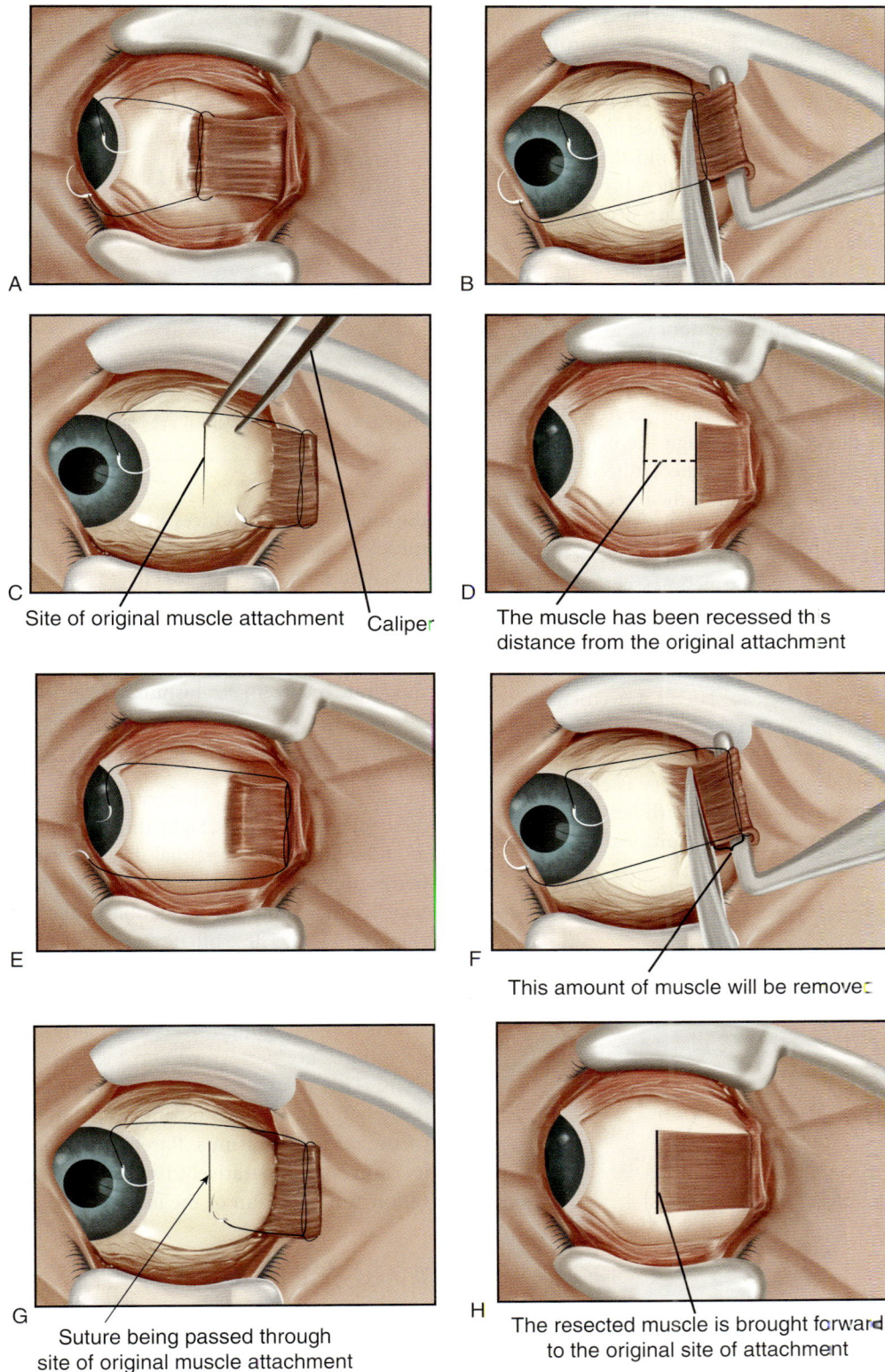

A

B

C

Site of original muscle attachment   Caliper

D

The muscle has been recessed this distance from the original attachment

E

F

This amount of muscle will be removed

G

Suture being passed through site of original muscle attachment

H

The resected muscle is brought forward to the original site of attachment

FIGURE 34–22 ■ Strabismus surgery. Recession (weakening) procedure (A-D). The muscle is weakened by moving it back from its original insertion. (A) A suture is passed through the muscle near its attachment to the eye. (B) The muscle is removed from the surface of the eye. (C) Calipers are used to measure the site of the new insertion (based on the angle of strabismus), and the sutures are passed through the sclera at this site. (D) The sutures are used to firmly attach the muscle at the new location. Resection (strengthening) procedure (E-F). The muscle is strengthened by removing a section of muscle and bringing the remaining muscle forward to the original insertion site. (E) The suture is passed through the muscle posterior to its attachment to the eye. The amount of strengthening is adjusted by how far back the sutures are placed. (F) The muscle is removed from the surface of the eye. The muscle anterior to the sutures is then removed (not shown). (G) The sutures are passed back through the site of the original attachment. (H) The muscle is brought forward and reattached to the eye.

muscle is isolated and exposed on a muscle hook. In a recession, an absorbable suture is passed through the muscle near its insertion on the sclera and secured on the borders of the muscle. The muscle is then disinserted from the eye. A new site of insertion is marked posterior to the original insertion and the sutures are passed at this site. The muscle is then brought to this new insertion site and the sutures are tied. Absorbable sutures are used, which degrade over several weeks, by which time the muscle reattaches to the sclera. Recessions weaken the effect of the muscle, causing the eye to shift in the opposite direction.

A muscle resection is similar, except that the suture is placed posterior to the insertion of the muscle. The muscle anterior to the suture is removed (resected), and the sutures are placed back through the original insertion. Because the muscle is shortened, it becomes stiffer, pulling the eye in the direction of the resected muscle.

If patients have strabismus due to cranial nerve palsies or other conditions that limit movement of the eye, *transposition* surgery is sometimes performed. In a complete sixth nerve palsy, for instance, the inferior and superior rectus muscles can be moved adjacent to the insertion of the lateral rectus muscle. This creates an outward-pulling force to increase lateral movement of the eye. Similarly, the horizontal muscles can be moved superiorly to create an upward-pulling force (Figure 34–23).

An alternative to muscle surgery is chemodenervation of the extraocular muscles with *botulinum toxin*. This is performed by direct injection of the toxin into

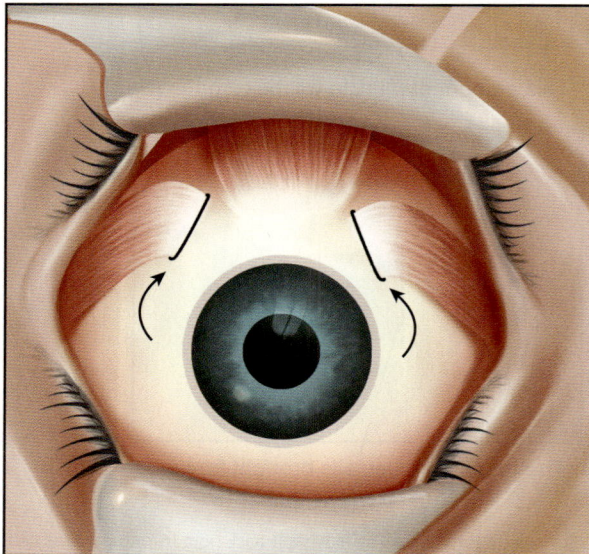

FIGURE 34–24 ■ Conjunctival pyogenic granuloma following strabismus surgery.

the muscles. This produces a chemical weakening of the muscle, causing the eye to shift in the opposite direction. Although the chemical effect wears off after several weeks, patients may experience permanent improvement in the strabismus due to a change in the muscle structure. This treatment is most useful in patients with moderate recurrent strabismus after prior surgery.

Complications of Strabismus Surgery

In general, strabismus surgery is safe, with a low incidence of complications. Sight-threatening problems, such as endophthalmitis or retinal detachment due to scleral perforation, are extremely rare. Some patients develop scarring or granuloma formation at the site of surgery (Figure 34–24). These often resolve with topical corticosteroids, but surgical excision is sometimes required.

The need for additional surgery in patients with strabismus is common, even when appropriate surgical procedures are performed and there are no complications. This is usually due to the neural mechanisms underlying the strabismus, and is an inherent part of the treatment of strabismus. Rarely, the muscle slips from its sutures postoperatively, necessitating surgical exploration and refixation of the muscle.

AMBLYOPIA ("LAZY EYE")

Definitions and Epidemiology

Amblyopia is a condition in children in which abnormal vision develops due to decreased vision input to the brain. It affects approximately 3% of children, and is the most common cause of unilateral vision loss in children. *Deprivation amblyopia* occurs when there is a structural abnormality of the eye that interferes with vision, such as a cataract or retinal defect. *Refractive*

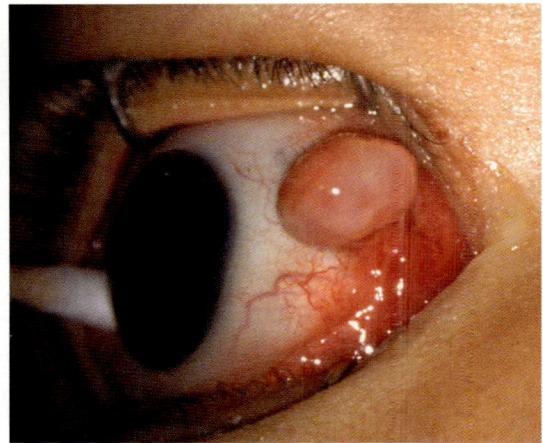

FIGURE 34–23 ■ Transposition strabismus surgery. This is done for patients who have strabismus due to minimal function of an extraocular muscle. In this case, the patient cannot elevate the eye due to monocular elevation deficiency. The lateral and medial rectus muscles are transposed (arrows) to positions adjacent to the superior rectus muscle to create an upward-pullling force.

amblyopia results from an unequal need for glasses, such as if one eye is very nearsighted and the other is not. *Strabismic amblyopia* occurs when one eye is misaligned and therefore ignored by the brain.

Pathogenesis of Amblyopia

Amblyopia is present when the visual acuity in one eye of young children is decreased because of unequal input to the visual cortex. It can develop from a variety of causes. Normal visual connections between the eye and the occipital cortex form during the first several years of life. In amblyopia, the vision from one eye is ignored. The area of the occipital cortex that represents the affected eye gradually shrinks, and the area representing the normal eye gradually enlarges. In clinical terms, this results in decreased visual acuity in the amblyopic eye. The younger the child, the more susceptible the brain is to disruptions in these connections.

Clinical Presentation

There are 3 common causes of amblyopia:

- *Strabismic amblyopia*: Children with strabismus normally do not notice the vision in the deviated eye (*suppression*). If one eye is constantly deviated in young children, this suppression causes amblyopia. It is important to understand that while amblyopia and strabismus are related, they are distinct problems requiring different treatment. The treatment for strabismus is to align the eyes (either surgically or with glasses), with the goal of improving binocular vision. The treatment for amblyopia is to make the child's brain pay more attention to the amblyopic eye, with the goal of improving visual acuity in the affected eye. Because the conditions are related, treatment of one of the conditions may cause an associated improvement in the other. For instance, if the eyes in a patient with strabismus are successfully realigned, the visual acuity may also improve because the brain no longer suppresses the eye. In many patients, however, amblyopia persists even after the eyes are aligned, and continued amblyopia treatment is needed after correction of the strabismus.
- *Refractive amblyopia*: This occurs most commonly when there is a large discrepancy in the need for glasses between the 2 eyes. This can result from any type of asymmetric refractive error, including myopia (nearsightedness), hyperopia (farsightedness), or astigmatism. The brain pays less attention to the blurred eye, with a resultant decrease in vision due to decreased occipital lobe representation of the eye. The diagnosis is made by checking the child's visual acuity after the appropriate glasses strength is identified during the examination. In normal patients with decreased vision due to refractive errors, the visual acuity measured in

the office is normal immediately after the appropriate glasses are placed on the patient. In refractive amblyopia the visual acuity remains decreased. The initial treatment for refractive amblyopia is to have the child wear their prescription glasses. Many will improve with glasses alone. If they do not, additional treatment with patching or drops is used. In some patients with developmental delay who have marked difficulty complying with glasses wear, refractive surgery may be considered.
- *Deprivation amblyopia*: Deprivation amblyopia occurs in patients who have ocular abnormalities that impair vision. Any structural defect may cause this problem, such as cataract, retinal scarring, or optic nerve lesions. These patients have decreased vision for 2 reasons. The first is the decrease caused by the underlying disorder. The second is the amblyopia superimposed on this. In these children it is often difficult to determine what portion of the vision loss is due to the structural eye problem itself, and what portion is due to amblyopia. The vision can often be improved with amblyopia treatment in such patients, but the final visual acuity is limited by the underlying problem.

Treatment of Amblyopia

The aim of amblyopia therapy is to make the brain pay more attention to the amblyopic eye. There are 2 main options for treatment. The first is occlusion of the normal eye. This is usually performed by having the child wear an adhesive patch over the good eye for a set period (usually a few hours per day) (Figure 34–25).

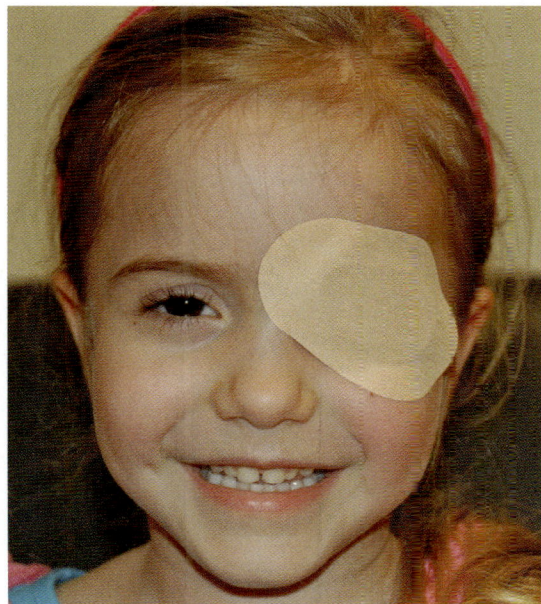

FIGURE 34–25 ■ Adhesive eye patch for treatment of amblyopia. If the patch is secured to the skin completely around the eye, peeking is not possible.

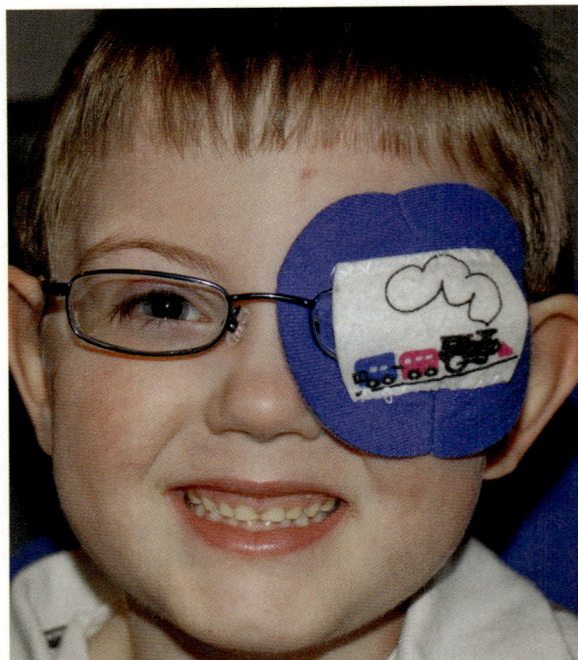

FIGURE 34–26 ■ Cloth cover over glasses, used as an alternative to an adhesive patch.

An alternative to adhesive patches is using soft material to cover one lens in children who wear glasses (Figure 34–26). The advantage of the adhesive patch is that it completely covers the eye. If soft material on the glasses is used, it is important to verify that the child does not peek around the edges (Figure 34–27).

The second option for amblyopia treatment is *optical penalization*. This is performed by instilling

cycloplegic drops (usually atropine or cyclopentolate) in the normal eye. These drops interfere with accommodation (the method by which the eye normally focuses at near), creating a blur at near. Because most young children are farsighted, the medication-induced inability to accommodate also creates a blur at distance. The blurring of the normal eye causes the brain to favor the amblyopic eye. Optical penalization is an excellent alternative to patching, particularly for children who continually pull off their patches. An important caveat is that this method does not work as well if the vision in the amblyopic eye is markedly decreased, because in this setting the vision in the normal eye that is blurred by drops will still be better than the vision in the amblyopic eye, and therefore treatment is less effective. Optical penalization is also less effective in myopic (nearsighted) patients, because they are able to focus at near even with drops in place.

In general, the earlier amblyopia treatment is initiated the more effective it is. This is believed to be due to increased plasticity of the infant visual cortex. Recent studies have also shown good visual acuity improvement in older children treated for amblyopia, particularly those who have not had prior treatment.[6]

NYSTAGMUS

Definitions

Nystagmus occurs when the eyes oscillate back and forth in a regular fashion. These movements are usually symmetric in both eyes. Nystagmus is usually either *pendular*, in which the eye movements are equal in both directions, or *jerk*, in which the eyes drift slowly in one direction, then quickly in the opposite direction. Most nystagmus occurs in the horizontal plane, but vertical and torsional forms also can occur. Nystagmus is further characterized by the frequency and amplitude of the oscillations.

Nystagmus can occur in infantile and acquired forms. The infantile form can be either primary (*infantile nystagmus syndrome; congenital motor nystagmus*) or secondary to an underlying ocular problem (*sensory defect nystagmus*). In infants, neurological problems are rarely the cause of nystagmus (unless the underlying neurological problem also causes visual loss). Many children with nystagmus discover that the nystagmus decreases in a certain position of gaze (a *null zone*). This is usually in right or left gaze, but sometimes in up- or downgaze, or with the head tilted to one side.

Clinical Presentation

The common types of childhood nystagmus are described below.

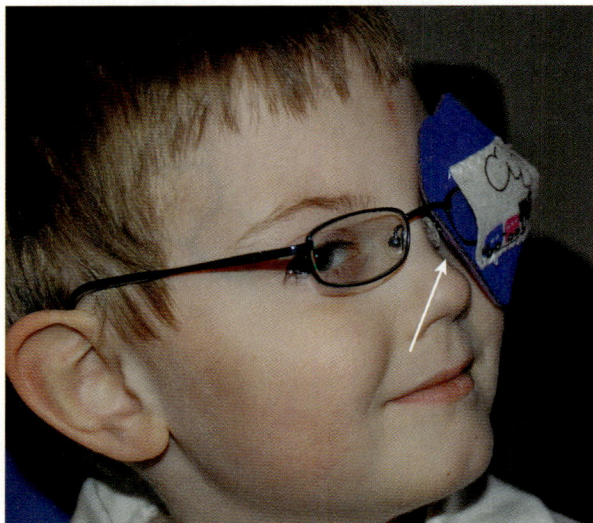

FIGURE 34–27 ■ If a cloth patch is used, the child must be monitored to be sure they are not peeking around the edges of the patch, which can be done even through a small gap (arrow).

Latent nystagmus (fusion maldevelopment nystagmus)

This is the most frequent type of nystagmus in children. It occurs almost exclusively in children with infantile esotropia, and its presence in older children with strabismus suggests that the strabismus dates to infancy. In latent nystagmus the abnormal movements are not seen when the patient has both eyes open, but is present when one is covered. The nystagmus has a slow phase in the direction of the covered eye, and a quick phase in the direction of the uncovered eye (the eye therefore appears to beat toward the uncovered eye).

An oxymoronic term is used to describe latent nystagmus that is present when both eyes are open—*manifest latent nystagmus*. This occurs when the patient has vision loss in one eye due to amblyopia or some other cause. Although the eye is not physically occluded, the decreased vision causes the child to neglect the eye, producing the same effect as if the eye were covered.

An important clinical point regarding latent nystagmus is that it may cause artificially poor results during vision screening tests. This is because most visual acuity tests are performed by occluding the eye that is not being tested. This causes increased nystagmus and therefore decreased vision in patients with latent nystagmus. The visual acuity may be 20/50 or worse when attempting to read with the opposite eye occluded, and 20/25 or better when tested with both eyes open. In the ophthalmologist's office, the visual acuity in each eye can be assessed by using blurring lenses over the opposite eye (rather than complete occlusion), which decreases the intensity of the latent nystagmus.

Infantile nystagmus syndrome (congenital motor nystagmus)

In this condition, infants have nystagmus that is not associated with strabismus or other ocular disorders. This form of nystagmus may be inherited as an autosomal dominant trait. Children usually develop nystagmus within the first 1 to 3 months of life, but are otherwise normal. The parents report that the child sees well. When children are old enough to be tested, the visual acuity may be slightly decreased, but it is usually 20/30 or better. Therefore, the infants function well visually, and the nystagmus is the only abnormality. The nystagmus in this condition is usually *uniplanar*, meaning that it remains horizontal when the patient looks up or down. Treatment is not necessary unless the patient develops a compensatory head posture due to a null zone in eccentric gaze (see below).

Sensory deprivation nystagmus

Infants who have poor vision during the first few months of life usually present because the parents note poor fixation and nystagmus. It is important that children with sensory deprivation nystagmus be differentiated from children with primary infantile nystagmus syndrome. This can usually be accomplished by an appropriate history and ophthalmological examination, but sometimes additional testing is necessary. The type of visual loss in sensory deprivation nystagmus may be severe (optic nerve hypoplasia, Leber congenital amaurosis), moderate (aniridia, ocular albinism), or mild (congenital stationary night blindness). Treatment is directed toward the underlying problem. Children with sensory nystagmus may also develop null zones, in which case surgery may be beneficial.

Other Forms of Nystagmus

Spasmus nutans

Spasmus nutans is an unusual form of nystagmus characterized by shimmering (high frequency) nystagmus, a head tilt, and head shaking. The nystagmus is bilateral, but is usually quite asymmetric (which is distinctly unusual in childhood nystagmus). Spasmus nutans normally develops within the first 2 years of life. It is usually self-limited, resolving within 2 to 3 years. Patients may have a history of premature birth. Some patients with optic pathway tumors have been reported with nystagmus that has features similar to spasmus nutans.[7] These children usually have other neurological abnormalities and their optic nerves may be pale. Imaging studies may be indicated in patients with spasmus nutans to evaluate for such lesions.

Dense amblyopia

In addition to spasmus nutans, the other disorder to be considered in the differential diagnosis of children with asymmetric nystagmus is dense amblyopia, usually to a level of 20/100 or less. The nystagmus in these children is worse in the amblyopic eye. This is a diagnosis of exclusion. Unless a clear etiology for the decreased vision is evident (a large retinal scar, for example), imaging studies may be indicated to look for other abnormalities.

Vertical nystagmus

Most nystagmus in children occurs in the horizontal plane. The presence of vertical nystagmus suggests there may be another underlying problem. This may occur in patients with inherited retinal dystrophies or CNS tumors.

Convergence-retraction nystagmus

This is one of the ocular abnormalities seen in children with *dorsal midbrain syndrome*. As the children attempt to look up, the eyes converge and retract into the orbit (see also Chapter 29).

Other causes of abnormal eye movements in children

Although these disorders are technically not nystagmus, they are included here because they also cause distinctive abnormal eye movements in children.

Opsoclonus Opsoclonus presents with random jerky eye movements that occur in any direction. It may develop as a paraneoplastic phenomenon associated with neuroblastoma. Children who present with opsoclonus need to be screened for this tumor.

Congenital ocular motor apraxia In congenital ocular motor apraxia (COMA), patients cannot generate normal saccadic eye movements (the quick eye movements that are normally used to shift gaze from straight ahead to localize objects in the peripheral visual field). In infancy, patients with COMA are sometimes thought to have poor vision because they cannot make the normal behavioral visual movements that indicate a baby is seeing. As they get older, they learn to generate eye movements by using the vestibular system in lieu of saccades. This is done by thrusting their head in the direction they wish to look, which generates eye movements via the vestibular system. They usually initially overshoot the target, then make a slow head movement back toward the object they wish to see.

COMA in general is associated with an increased risk of developmental delay. Specific disorders associated with COMA include *Joubert syndrome*, ataxia-telangiectasia, and cerebellar and other CNS lesions. CNS imaging is indicated in the evaluation of affected patients. The head thrusts used by patients with COMA are quite large and noticeable when they are young, but usually become smaller as they grow older. No treatment is available for these abnormal eye movements.

Treatment of Nystagmus

The initial treatment for nystagmus is directed at the underlying problem, if one is present. In general, patients with nystagmus are more likely to require glasses. Unfortunately, many of the disorders that cause sensory deprivation nystagmus (such as optic nerve hypoplasia) are not treatable. Early low-vision services should be offered to help affected children adapt to the best of their abilities.

Children with nystagmus who have a null zone in eccentric gaze often develop a compensatory head posture as an adaptive mechanism. This occurs because the vision is best in the area of minimal nystagmus. For example, if a patient has a null zone in right gaze, the patient may adopt a left head turn to keep their eyes to the right. If the head position is greater than 10° to 15°, patients usually benefit from surgery to shift the zone of minimal nystagmus to a straight-ahead position. This is performed by a combination of weakening and strengthening the extraocular muscles, using the same techniques described above for strabismus surgery.

REFERENCES

1. Williams AS, Hoyt CS. Acute comitant esotropia in children with brain tumors. *Arch Ophthalmol.* 1989;107:376–378.
2. Mohney BG. Acquired nonaccommodative esotropia in childhood. *JAAPOS.* 2001;5:85–89.
3. Hunter DG, Ellis FJ. Prevalence of systemic and ocular disease in infantile exotropia: comparison with infantile estropia. *Ophthalmology.* 1999;106:1951–1956.
4. Convergence Insufficiency Treatment Trial Study Group. Randomized clinical trial of treatments for symptomatic convergence insufficiency in children. *Arch Ophthalmol.* 2008;126:1336–1349.
5. Demer JL, Clark RA, Engle EC. Magnetic resonance imaging evidence for widespread orbital dysinnervation in congenital fibrosis of extraocular muscles due to mutations in KIF21A. *Invest Ophthalmol Vis Sci.* 2005;46:530–539.
6. Pediatric Eye Disease Investigator Group. Randomized trial of treatment of amblyopia in children aged 7 to 17 years. *Arch Ophthalmol.* 2005;123:437–447.
7. Albright AL, Sclabassi RJ, Slamovits TL, Bergman I. Spasmus nutans associated with optic gliomas in infants. *J Pediatr.* 1984;105:778–780.

Index

C